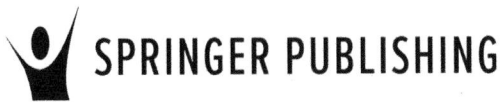

GET THE MOST FROM YOUR BOOK

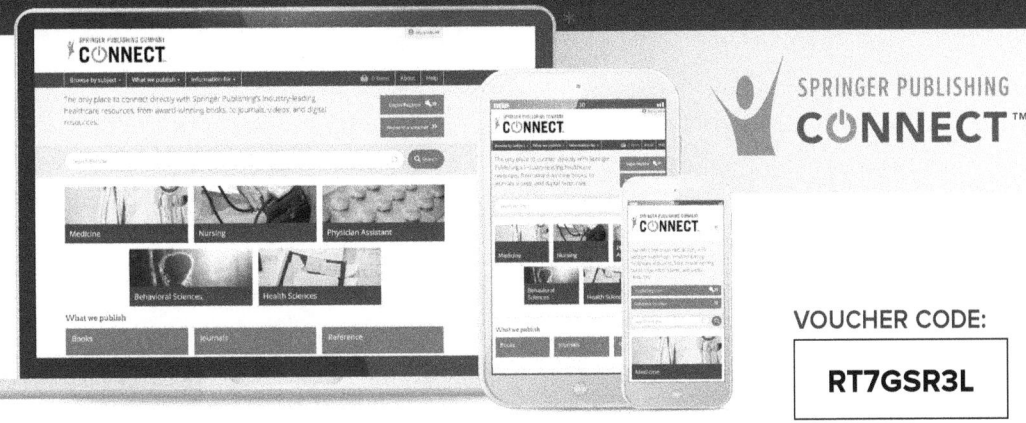

VOUCHER CODE:

RT7GSR3L

Online Access

Your print purchase of *Counseling Individuals With Co-Occurring Addictive and Mental Disorders* includes **online access via Springer Publishing Connect**™ to increase accessibility, portability, and searchability.

Insert the code at http://connect.springerpub.com/content/book/978-0-8261-5842-0 today!

Having trouble? Contact our customer service department at cs@springerpub.com

Instructor Resource Access for Adopters

Let us do some of the heavy lifting to create an engaging classroom experience with a variety of instructor resources included in most textbooks SUCH AS:

INSTRUCTOR MANUAL

POWERPOINTS

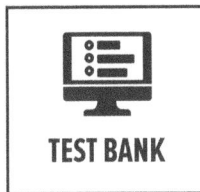

TEST BANK

Visit **https://connect.springerpub.com/** and look for the **"Show Supplementary"** button on your **book homepage** to see what is available to instructors! First time using Springer Publishing Connect?

Email **textbook@springerpub.com** to create an account and start unlocking valuable resources.

COUNSELING INDIVIDUALS WITH CO-OCCURRING ADDICTIVE AND MENTAL DISORDERS

Reginald W. Holt, PhD, is an associate professor and chair of the Department of Counselor Education and Family Therapy at Central Connecticut State University (CCSU). He completed a PhD in counseling/counselor education at the University of Missouri-St. Louis (CACREP), a MA in clinical psychology at East Tennessee State University, and a 2-year post-graduate training program in advanced psychodynamic psychotherapy at the St. Louis Psychoanalytic Institute.

He is licensed as a professional counselor in Connecticut (LPC), Illinois (LCPC), and Missouri (LPC) and credentialed as a National Certified Counselor (NCC) and Master Addictions Counselor (MAC) through the National Board of Certified Counselors (NBCC). In addition, Dr. Holt is recognized by the Connecticut Certification Board, Inc. (CCB) as an Advanced Alcohol and Drug Counselor (AADC) and by the International Certification and Reciprocity Consortium (IC&RC) as an Internationally Certified Advanced Alcohol and Drug Counselor (ICAADC).

He is an active member of several national and state professional associations, which includes working directly with the 2020–2021 President of the American Counseling Association (ACA) on the ACA Graduate Student Committee, holding elected leadership positions as the 2023–2024 Secretary of the International Association of Addictions and Offender Counseling (IAAOC) and as the 2019–2020 President of the Connecticut Association of Counselor Education and Supervision (CACES), and co-leading the development of a special interest group in addictions counseling for the Connecticut Counseling Association (CCA) that received a "Best Innovative Practice" award from ACA in 2018.

His extensive clinical career includes work conducted in behavioral healthcare hospitals, the correctional system, a top *Fortune 500* managed care organization, as well as operating his own private practice. Prior to his appointment at Central Connecticut State University, he held academic positions at the University of Missouri-St. Louis and Webster University.

In addition to his role as department chair, Dr. Holt provides graduate level instruction at CCSU with a special emphasis on implementing mindfulness-based practices into the treatment of mental and substance use disorders—which coincides with his published works and research interests. He also serves as coordinator of the department's CACREP-accredited Clinical Professional Counseling Program, administrator of The Forum for Contemplative Practices, and advisor for the Chi Alpha Mu Chapter of Chi Sigma Iota, the International Honor Society in Counseling.

Dr. Holt lives in Connecticut with his partner and their rescue dog, Jolene, who served as his muse by remaining at his deskside throughout the entire process of developing this book.

Regina R. Moro, PhD, is an associate professor of Counselor Education at St. Bonaventure University. She is licensed as a Licensed Clinical Professional Counselor in Idaho, a Licensed Clinical Addiction Specialist in North Carolina, and a Licensed Mental Health Counselor in Florida. She is also a National Certified Counselor and a board certified telemental health provider. She serves as the Practicum and Internship Coordinator for her current program, and has over 10 years of experience as a counselor educator.

Dr. Moro's clinical passion involves focusing on the full spectrum of addiction and the impact to individuals and families. She has experience working in community mental health, integrated care settings, and currently has a small telehealth private practice. As a counselor educator she is focused on educating all counseling students on the impact of addiction, regardless of which specialty area they are in. Her desire is for all counselors to be well-trained to identify and intervene when addiction is impacting their clients' lives.

Dr. Moro is an active member of the American Counseling Association, the Association of Counselor Education and Supervision, and the International Association of Addictions and Offender Counselors (IAAOC), of which she was the president for the 2017 term. She most recently completed service as a board member for the Idaho Licensing Board of Professional Counselors and Marriage and Family Therapists. Dr. Moro was recognized as the 2019 Idaho Counseling Association Counselor Educator of the Year recipient.

Dr. Moro currently lives in western Washington state where she and her partner enjoy outdoor adventures such as hiking, backpacking, and paddleboarding with their rescue dog, Barkley.

COUNSELING INDIVIDUALS WITH CO-OCCURRING ADDICTIVE AND MENTAL DISORDERS

A COMPREHENSIVE APPROACH

Reginald W. Holt, PhD

Regina R. Moro, PhD

EDITORS

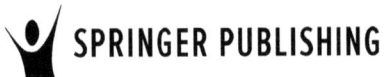

Copyright © 2024 Springer Publishing Company, LLC
All rights reserved.

No part of this publication may be reproduced, stored in a retrieval system, or transmitted in any form or by any means, electronic, mechanical, photocopying, recording, or otherwise, without the prior permission of Springer Publishing Company, LLC, or authorization through payment of the appropriate fees to the Copyright Clearance Center, Inc., 222 Rosewood Drive, Danvers, MA 01923, 978-750-8400, fax 978-646-8600, info@copyright.com or at www.copyright.com.

Springer Publishing Company, LLC
11 West 42nd Street, New York, NY 10036
www.springerpub.com
connect.springerpub.com/

Acquisitions Editor: Rhonda Dearborn
Compositor: Pajeflow

ISBN: 978-0-8261-5841-3
ebook ISBN: 978-0-8261-5842-0
DOI: 10.1891/9780826158420

SUPPLEMENTS:

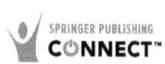 A robust set of instructor resources designed to supplement this text is located at http://connect.springerpub.com/content/book/978-0-8261-5842-0. Qualifying instructors may request access by emailing textbook@springerpub.com.

Instructor Manual: 978-0-8261-5844-4
Test Bank: 978-0-8261-5843-7
Instructor Chapter PowerPoints: 978-0-8261-5845-1

Printed by LSI

The author and the publisher of this Work have made every effort to use sources believed to be reliable to provide information that is accurate and compatible with the standards generally accepted at the time of publication. The author and publisher shall not be liable for any special, consequential, or exemplary damages resulting, in whole or in part, from the readers' use of, or reliance on, the information contained in this book. The publisher has no responsibility for the persistence or accuracy of URLs for external or third-party Internet websites referred to in this publication and does not guarantee that any content on such websites is, or will remain, accurate or appropriate.

Library of Congress Cataloging-in-Publication Data

Names: Holt, Reginald W., author. | Moro, Regina R., author.
Title: Counseling individuals with co-occurring addictive and mental
   disorders: a comprehensive approach / Reginald W. Holt, Regina R. Moro.
Description: New York, NY : Springer Publishing, [2024] | Includes
   bibliographical references and index.
Identifiers: LCCN 2022057827 (print) | LCCN 2022057828 (ebook) | ISBN
   9780826158413 (paperback) | ISBN 9780826158420 (ebook)
Subjects: MESH: Mental Disorders--therapy | Substance-Related
   Disorders--therapy | Comorbidity | Counseling
Classification: LCC RC480.5 (print) | LCC RC480.5 (ebook) | NLM WM 400 |
   DDC 616.89/1--dc23/eng/20230130
LC record available at https://lccn.loc.gov/2022057827
LC ebook record available at https://lccn.loc.gov/2022057828

Contact sales@springerpub.com to receive discount rates on bulk purchases.

***Publisher's Note*: New and used products purchased from third-party sellers are not guaranteed for quality, authenticity, or access to any included digital components.**

Printed in the United States of America.

To those individuals—including family, friends, and all others—who are impacted by co-occurring mental health and substance use disorders …

May you retain hope when challenged by despair.
May you gather courage when surrounded by fear.
May you receive compassion when facing rejection.
May you experience ease of suffering when feeling pain.
May you maintain equanimity when enduring a storm.
May you manifest resiliency when confronted by defeat.
And, above all, may you achieve sustained health of mind,
body, and spirit while traveling on the road to recovery.

To Dr. Mark Pope, I am honored you were my mentor and friend—
your sage wisdom and never-ending guidance gave me the courage
to dream big and the confidence to achieve those dreams. May
your spirit rest easy as you take your place among the stars.
To my father and mother who are no longer on this earthly plane.
Because of the loving support you provided during my early
education, your legacy lives on through this work. ~RWH

To Dr. Laura Gallo,
May all counselors embody your passion, humility,
and dedication to the helping process. ~RM

CONTENTS

Contributors   xv
Preface   xvii
Instructor Resources   xxi

SECTION I. OVERVIEW OF CO-OCCURRING DISORDERS

1. Considerations for Treating Co-Occurring Mental and Substance Use Disorders   3
Reginald W. Holt

Learning Objectives   3
Introduction   3
Prevalence, Statistics, and Demographics   4
Screening and Assessment of Co-Occurring Disorders   17
The Treatment of Co-Occurring Disorders   23
Legal and Ethical Considerations   31
Clinical Case Illustration and Discussion   34
Chapter Summary   37
Discussion Questions   37
References   38

2. Understanding Drugs of Abuse and Addiction   43
Regina R. Moro

Learning Objectives   43
Introduction   43
Drug Categories, Substance Types, and Administration Routes   45
Behavioral Addictions   57
Models of Addiction   59
General Review of the DSM-5 Classification System   61
Clinical Case Illustration and Discussion   62
Chapter Summary   65
Discussion Questions   65
References   65

3. Neuroscience of Co-Occurring Mental and Substance Use Disorders   71
Raissa Miller

Learning Objectives   71
Introduction   71
Defining the Brain and the Embodied Nervous System   72

Neuroscience of Addiction and Mental Health Disorders 78
Clinical Case Illustration and Discussion 82
Chapter Summary 84
Discussion Questions 85
References 85

SECTION II. TREATMENT APPROACHES

4. **The Comprehensive Assessment of Co-Occurring Disorders** 93
   Dilani M. Perera and Alexandra Galletti

   Learning Objectives 93
   Introduction 93
   Intake, Assessment, and the Therapeutic Relationship 94
   Biopsychosocial Evaluation 97
   Screening and Assessment Strategies and Tools 99
   Diagnosis 103
   Writing Treatment Plans and Designing Aftercare Recovery Initiatives 104
   American Society of Addiction Medicine Patient Placement Criteria 107
   Legal and Ethical Considerations 109
   Clinical Case Illustration and Discussion 111
   Chapter Summary 111
   Discussion Questions 115
   References 115

5. **Managed Care and the Use of Level of Care Guidelines for Co-Occurring Disorders** 119
   Brett Hart and Sarah A. Peipert

   Learning Objectives 119
   Introduction 119
   Historical Context of Managed Care 119
   A New Paradigm in Managed Care 120
   Insurance Plans and Population Types 122
   Insurance Benefits 123
   Levels of Care 124
   Level of Care Guidelines 127
   Utilization Management 132
   Legal and Ethical Considerations 132
   Evolving the Managed Care and Provider Relationship 133
   Managed Healthcare Innovations 134
   Clinical Case Illustration and Discussion 136
   Chapter Summary 138
   Discussion Questions 138
   References 139

6. **Treatment Engagement, Therapeutic Strategies, and Recovery Models for Co-Occurring Disorders**   *141*
   Regina R. Moro and Reginald W. Holt

   Learning Objectives   141
   Introduction   141
   Building Successful Relationships   142
   The Transtheoretical Model: Assessing the Stages of Change   142
   Motivational Interviewing/Motivational Enhancement Therapy   146
   Theoretical Approaches to Treating Co-Occurring Disorders   149
   Recognizing and Addressing Indicators of Relapse   151
   Recovery Maintenance: Consolidating Gains and Sustaining Change   152
   Legal and Ethical Considerations   153
   Clinical Case Illustration and Discussion   154
   Chapter Summary   156
   Discussion Questions   156
   References   157

7. **Psychopharmacological Interventions for Co-Occurring Disorders**   *159*
   Regina R. Moro

   Learning Objectives   159
   Introduction   159
   The Great Debate: The Question of Whether to Support an Alliance of Pharmacology Within Mental Health Treatment   159
   Principles of Psychopharmacology for the Nonprescribing Clinician   161
   Organizational Structure of the Brain   163
   Medications Utilized to Treat Co-Occurring Disorders   164
   The Psychedelic Renaissance   175
   Legal and Ethical Considerations   176
   Clinical Case Illustration and Discussion   177
   Chapter Summary   179
   Discussion Questions   179
   References   179

8. **Integrating Mindfulness-Based Practices in the Treatment of Co-Occurring Disorders**   *183*
   Reginald W. Holt and John Paulson

   Learning Objectives   183
   Introduction   183
   Historical Origins of Mindfulness   185
   Mindfulness-Based Therapies   186
   Augmenting the Treatment of Co-Occurring Mental and Substance Use Disorders With Mindfulness-Based Therapies   191

Augmenting the Counselor as a Professional and as a Person 194
Legal and Ethical Considerations 195
Clinical Case Illustration and Discussion 197
Chapter Summary 199
Discussion Questions 200
References 200

SECTION III. DIAGNOSTIC CONSIDERATIONS

9. **Co-Occurring Depressive and Substance Use Disorders** 209
   Sara W. Bailey

   Learning Objectives 209
   Introduction 209
   Depressive Disorders: DSM-5 Diagnostic Criteria and Description 209
   Substance Use Disorders: DSM-5 Diagnostic Criteria and Description 212
   Prevalence, Statistics, and Demographics 213
   Overlapping Risks, Greater Severity, and Poorer Outcomes 214
   Assessment and Diagnostic Considerations 215
   Screening and Assessment Tools 217
   Treatment Modalities 220
   Legal and Ethical Considerations 223
   Clinical Case Illustration and Discussion 224
   Chapter Summary 228
   Discussion Questions 228
   References 229

10. **Co-Occurring Bipolar and Substance Use Disorders** 233
    Nedeljko Golubovic, Lauren Flynn, Alexis Isaac, and Saundra M. Tabet

    Learning Objectives 233
    Introduction 233
    Bipolar Disorder: DSM-5 Diagnostic Criteria and Description 234
    Prevalence, Statistics, and Demographics 236
    Assessment and Diagnostic Considerations 238
    Screening and Assessment Tools 240
    Treatment Modalities 241
    Legal and Ethical Considerations 244
    Clinical Case Illustration and Discussion 245
    Chapter Summary 248
    Discussion Questions 248
    References 249

11. **Co-Occurring Anxiety and Obsessive-Compulsive Disorders and Substance Use Disorders** 253
    Geri Miller, Dominique S. Hammonds, Emily Proctor, and Miller A. Faw

    Learning Objectives 253
    Introduction 253

*Anxiety and Obsessive-Compulsive Disorders: DSM-5 Diagnostic Criteria and
    Description* 256
Prevalence, Statistics, and Demographics 258
Assessment and Diagnostic Considerations 259
Treatment Modalities 263
Legal and Ethical Considerations 265
Clinical Case Illustration and Discussion 270
Chapter Summary 271
Discussion Questions 272
References 272

12. **Co-Occurring Schizophrenia and Other Psychotic Disorders and Substance Use Disorders** 275
    Keith Morgen and Katherine Weber

    Learning Objectives 275
    Introduction 275
    Five Domains of Psychotic Disorders 276
    *Schizophrenia and Other Psychotic Disorders: DSM-5 Diagnostic Criteria and
        Description* 277
    DSM-5 Disorders and ICD-10-CM Coding 279
    Prevalence, Statistics, and Demographics 281
    Co-Occurring Schizophrenia and Substance Use Disorders 281
    Assessment and Diagnostic Considerations 283
    Screening and Assessment Tools 285
    Treatment Modalities 286
    Legal and Ethical Considerations 288
    Clinical Case Illustration and Discussion 289
    Chapter Summary 290
    Discussion Questions 290
    References 291

13. **Co-Occurring Trauma- and Stressor-Related and Substance Use Disorders** 295
    Elizabeth H. Shilling and Yasmin Gay

    Learning Objectives 295
    Introduction 295
    *Trauma- and Stressor-Related Disorders: DSM-5 Diagnostic Criteria and
        Description* 295
    Prevalence, Statistics, and Demographics 297
    Assessment and Diagnostic Considerations 300
    Screening and Assessment Tools 302
    Treatment Modalities 304
    Legal and Ethical Considerations 308
    Clinical Case Illustration and Discussion 308
    Chapter Summary 310
    Discussion Questions 310
    References 311

14. Co-Occurring Personality and Substance Use Disorders   317
    Latasha Y. Hicks Becton, Jillian Q. Van Wagenen, and Jennifer C. Barrow

    Learning Objectives   317
    Introduction   317
    Personality Disorders: DSM-5 *Diagnostic Criteria and Description   318*
    Prevalence, Statistics, and Demographics   320
    Assessment and Diagnostic Considerations   321
    Screening and Assessment Tools   323
    Treatment Modalities   326
    Legal and Ethical Considerations   330
    Clinical Case Illustration and Discussion   332
    Chapter Summary   333
    Discussion Questions   334
    References   334

SECTION IV. SPECIAL POPULATIONS

15. Lifespan Development and Co-Occurring Disorders   341
    Andrea June, Carolyn R. Fallahi, and Carissa D. Daigle

    Learning Objectives   341
    Introduction   341
    Prevalence, Statistics, and Demographics   342
    Diagnostic Considerations: Adolescents and Young Adults   344
    Diagnostic Considerations: Older Adults   346
    Treatment Considerations   350
    Multicultural Considerations   354
    Legal and Ethical Considerations   355
    Clinical Case Illustration and Discussion   357
    Chapter Summary   358
    Discussion Questions   359
    References   359

16. Gender and Co-Occurring Disorders   367
    Geneva M. Gray, Asha Dickerson, and Veronica M. Wanzer

    Learning Objectives   367
    Introduction   367
    Prevalence, Statistics, and Demographics   368
    Treatment Considerations   369
    Legal and Ethical Considerations   373
    Screening and Assessment Tools   374
    Multicultural Considerations   374
    Clinical Case Illustration and Discussion   377
    Chapter Summary   378
    Discussion Questions   379
    References   380

17. Military Population and Co-Occurring Disorders   383
Benjamin V. Noah

Learning Objectives   383
Author's Personal Statement   383
Introduction   383
Prevalence, Statistics, and Demographics   385
Screening and Assessment Tools   389
Treatment Considerations   390
Multicultural Considerations   392
Legal and Ethical Considerations   394
Clinical Case Illustration and Discussion   395
Chapter Summary   397
Discussion Questions   397
References   398

18. LGBTQ+ Communities and Co-Occurring Disorders   403
Tiffany Somerville, Breon Rose, Rattanakorn Ratanashevorn, Deb Crawford, and Susan Kashubeck-West

Learning Objectives   403
Introduction   403
Prevalence, Statistics, and Demographics   404
Multicultural Considerations   405
Legal and Ethical Considerations   408
Treatment Considerations for LGBTQ+ Individuals with Co-Occurring Disorders   411
Clinical Case Illustration and Discussion   416
Chapter Summary   417
Discussion Questions   418
References   418

Index   425

CONTRIBUTORS

Sara W. Bailey, PhD, LCMHCA (NC), NCC, Assistant Professor; College Education, Leadership Studies, and Counseling; University of Lynchburg; Lynchburg, Virginia

Jennifer C. Barrow, PhD, NCC, LCMHCS, Associate Professor, Department of Counseling and Higher Education, Counselor Education Program, North Carolina Central University, Durham, North Carolina

Deb Crawford, MEd, PhD Candidate in Counseling, Department of Education Sciences and Professional Programs, University of Missouri, St. Louis, Missouri

Carissa D. Daigle, Student, Department of Psychological Science, Central Connecticut State University, New Britain, Connecticut

Asha Dickerson, PhD, Associate Professor, Counseling Specialties, Adler Graduate School, Minnetonka, Minnesota

Carolyn R. Fallahi, PhD, Professor, Department of Psychological Science, Central Connecticut State University, New Britain, Connecticut

Miller A. Faw, MA Candidate, CMHC Track, Department of Human Development and Psychological Counseling, Appalachian State University, Boone, North Carolina

Lauren Flynn, MA, Department of Counseling and Psychological Service, College of Education and Human Development, Georgia State University, Atlanta, Georgia

Alexandra Galletti, BA, Graduate Student, Counselor Education, Fairfield University, Fairfield, Connecticut

Yasmin Gay, PhD, CCJP, LCAS, LCMHC, CRC, MAC, CCTP, CCS, Assistant Professor, Department of Surgery, Wake Forest School of Medicine, Winston-Salem, North Carolina

Nedeljko Golubovic, PhD, Counseling and Marital and Family Therapy, School of Leadership and Education Sciences, University of San Diego, San Diego, California

Geneva M. Gray, PhD, Assistant Professor, Clinical Mental Health Counseling, The Chicago School of Professional Psychology, Washington, DC

Dominique S. Hammonds, PhD, Associate Professor, Department of Human Development and Psychological Counseling, Appalachian State University, Boone, North Carolina

Brett Hart, PhD, Chief Behavioral Health Officer, Centene Corporation, St. Louis, Missouri

Latasha Y. Hicks Becton, PhD, LCMHC, LCAS, CCS, Assistant Professor, Department of Counseling and Higher Education, Counselor Education Program, North Carolina Central University, Durham, North Carolina

Reginald W. Holt, PhD, LPC, LCPC, NCC, MAC, AADC, ICAADC, Associate Professor, Department Chair, and Clinical Professional Counseling Program Coordinator, Department of Counselor Education and Family Therapy, Central Connecticut State University, New Britain, Connecticut

Alexis Isaac, BA, Counseling and Marital and Family Therapy, School of Leadership and Education Sciences, University of San Diego, San Diego, California

Andrea June, PhD, Associate Professor, Department of Psychological Science, Central Connecticut State University, New Britain, Connecticut

Susan Kashubeck-West, PhD, Professor and Chair, Department of Education Sciences and Professional Programs, University of Missouri, St. Louis, Missouri

Geri Miller, PhD, Professor, Department of Human Development and Psychological Counseling, Appalachian State University, Boone, North Carolina

Raissa Miller, PhD, Associate Professor, Department of Counselor Education, Boise State University, Boise, Idaho

Keith Morgen, PhD, LPC, ACS, Centenary University, Hackettstown, New Jersey

Regina R. Moro, PhD, LMHC, LCPC, LCAS, NCC, Associate Professor, Department of Counselor Education, St. Bonaventure University, St. Bonaventure, NY

Benjamin V. Noah, PhD, Adjunct Faculty, Clinical Mental Health Counseling, School of Social and Behavioral Sciences, Capella University, Minneapolis, Minnesota

John Paulson, ACSW, LCSW, MAC, LCAC, NCSE, CCS, HS-BCP, Associate Professor, Department of Social Work, University of Southern Indiana, Evansville, Indiana

Sarah A. Peipert, RN, BS, MBA, Vice President, Centene Corporation, St. Louis, Missouri

Dilani M. Perera, PhD, Chair and Professor, Counselor Education, Fairfield University, Fairfield, Connecticut

Emily Proctor, MA, Professor, Department of Human Development and Psychological Counseling, Appalachian State University, Boone, North Carolina

Rattanakorn Ratanashevornm, MEd, Doctoral Student in Counseling, Department of Education Sciences and Professional Programs, University of Missouri, St. Louis, Missouri

Breon Rose, MEd, Doctoral Student in Counseling, Department of Education Sciences and Professional Programs, University of Missouri, St. Louis, Missouri

Elizabeth H. Shilling, PhD, LCMCH, LCAS, CSI, Assistant Professor, Department of Surgery, Wake Forest School of Medicine, Winston-Salem, North Carolina

Tiffany Somerville, MS, Doctoral Student in Counseling, Department of Education Sciences and Professional Programs, University of Missouri, St. Louis, Missouri

Saundra M. Tabet, PhD, Counseling and Marital and Family Therapy, School of Leadership and Education Sciences, University of San Diego, San Diego, California

Jillian Q. Van Wagenen, BS, Department of Counseling and Higher Education, Counselor Education Program, North Carolina Central University, Durham, North Carolina

Veronica M. Wanzer, PhD, LCPC, Faculty, Mental Health Counseling, Minneapolis, Minnesota

Katherine Weber, MA, Centenary University, Hackettstown, New Jersey

PREFACE

This book is designed as a tool for graduate students studying to become professional counselors who will work in a variety of settings, including healthcare agencies and treatment facilities. It is highly likely that all counselors, regardless of their specialty or work environment, will encounter clients struggling with a co-occurring mental and substance use disorder. National statistics highlight this sentiment: In 2020 there were 52.9 million U.S. adults with a past-year mental illness (MI), 14.2 million with a serious mental illness (SMI), 20.9 million with a past-year substance use disorder (SUD), and an additional 17.0 million with both MI/SMI and SUD— also known as a co-occurring disorder (COD; Substance Abuse and Mental Health Services Administration [SAMHSA], 2021). While these numbers represent adults over the age of 18, adolescents also experience CODs with elements of either disorder emerging throughout adolescence and into adulthood. Professional counselors who work with clients need to be aware of the overlap between substance use disorders and mental disorders in order to identify, intervene, and provide ethical and competent treatment. This book is also a resource for established counselors who did not receive comprehensive education while in their training program yet find themselves working with clients who have CODs.

Unique to this book is the focus on the profession of counseling. Both editors and the majority of contributing authors are all professional counselors—many of whom are counselor educators and clinical supervisors—with direct care experience working with individuals diagnosed with CODs. Being grounded in the counseling profession offers a holistic, wellness perspective that is often missing from books on CODs primarily written by professionals with medical degrees or other behavioral health backgrounds.

CONTENT

This book is designed to be a straightforward, yet comprehensive text that provides counselors-in-training and counselors in clinical practice a thorough review of co-occurring mental and substance use disorders. The text is divided into four main sections:

SECTION I: CONSIDERATIONS FOR TREATING CO-OCCURRING DISORDERS

Using a step-wise fashion, the text begins by creating the groundwork by introducing the concept of CODs in Chapters 1, 2, and 3. Chapter 1 offers a general overview (including the prevalence) of CODs, describes etiological paradigms and risk factors for developing CODs, and outlines the guiding principles for working with individuals who have CODs as recommended by SAMHSA. Chapter 2 provides a brief overview of addictive disorders, both substance-related and behavioral addictions. Information includes commonly abused substance of abuse, distinct models of addiction etiology, and the *Diagnostic and Statistical Manual of Mental Disorders, Fifth Edition* (*DSM-5*) classification system. Chapter 3 provides a comprehensive introduction to the neuroscience of CODs.

SECTION II: TREATMENT APPROACHES

Section II transitions the reader to their work with future clients, including specific treatment procedures common to all counselors. This consists of chapters exploring the screening, assessment, and evaluation processes; the various levels of care in which clients may receive treatment; and useful information that clients may encounter once they enter into treatment. Chapter 4 provides an overview of screening, assessment, and evaluation of CODs. Readers will gain a general overview of treatment and recovery plan development to guide their future work with clients in the initial encounter. Chapter 5 provides details regarding the levels of care options for clients. This includes managed care admission guidelines based upon medical necessity and a discussion of the American Society of Addiction Medicine's (ASAM) six dimensions of multidimensional assessment and Patient Placement Criteria-2. In addition, this chapter explores community supports for clients with CODs. Chapter 6 introduces readers to the Transtheoretical Model of Change and explores motivational interviewing/motivational enhancement therapy. In addition, person-centered/humanistic and cognitive-behavior theories for treating CODs are discussed. Relapse mechanisms, relapse prevention, and longer-term recovery maintenance are described. Chapter 7 provides a general overview of psychopharmacology/pharmacotherapy as it relates to working with people who have CODs. This attends to both behavioral health psychotropic medications (e.g., antidepressants, anxiolytics) as well as those used in medication-assisted treatment (e.g., methadone, Suboxone). In addition, the use of pscyhedelics in the treatment of CODs is briefly explored. This section concludes with Chapter 8, which examines mindfulness as an adjunct treatment for CODs. The main mindfulness-based therapeutic programs are described, research studies supporting mindfulness are examined, and treatment integration ideas are offered.

SECTION III: DIAGNOSTIC CONSIDERATIONS

The third section focuses on diagnostic considerations for CODs. Using the *DSM-5* as a base, the following co-occurring mental and substance use disorders are explained: depressive disorders in Chapter 9; bipolar disorders in Chapter 10; anxiety and obsessive-compulsive disorders in Chapter 11; schizophrenia and other psychotic disorders in Chapter 12; trauma-related disorders, including PTSD, in Chapter 13; and personality disorders in Chapter 14. Each chapter includes information about the description of the co-occurring mental disorder, prevalence rates, specific assessment considerations, treatments unique to the disorder, and a clinical case illustration and discussion.

SECTION IV: SPECIAL POPULATIONS

The final part of the textbook emphasizes the multifaceted variables that must be considered when treating distinct groups who are diagnosed with CODs. These groups include a consideration of CODs and gender in Chapter 15; CODs across the lifespan in Chapter 16; CODs and military personnel in Chapter 17; and CODs and the LGBT+ community in Chapter 18. It is important to note that this last section attends to cultural elements of counseling practice in relation to specific groups. However, throughout the book in its entirety, chapter authors intentionally provide information that is relevant for cross-cultural competent practice by counselors.

Also infused through the book are ethical and legal implications and clinical case illustrations and discussions.

LEARNING TOOLS

Each chapter is intentionally formulated with the reader's education in mind. To begin, every chapter lists the learning objectives indicating what the reader should be able to accomplish following an indepth review of the material. Throughout the chapter content, there is a focus on helping readers understand what this means for their future work as a counselor. This is particularly prevalent in the case illustration and discussion, where readers are exposed to a clinical situation and then see how a clinical professional counselor would handle this situation. Lastly, all chapters conclude with recommended discussion questions. These questions are meant to intentionally help readers expand on the content of the chapters, use their critical thinking skills, and, if being conducted in dyads or groups, learn the art of consultation and collaboration with peers.

INSTRUCTOR RESOURCES

This textbook is accompanied with teaching tools for course instructors. PowerPoint lectures have been developed for each chapter based upon the content contained within that chapter. A test bank is provided with a combination of 10 true/false and multiple-choice questions for each chapter. In addition, each question has information related to where students can locate the correct answer. A sample syllabus is offered for how an instructor may adapt this text into a traditional 15-week semester. Finally, accreditation information specific to the *2016 Council for Accreditation of Counseling and Related Educational Programs (CACREP) Standards* is provided for each chapter.

The editors of this textbook anticipate that the publication will provide a comprehensive overview for counselors working with individuals who have CODs, which in turn will help those counselors become more competent in this much-needed area of specialization.

INSTRUCTOR RESOURCES

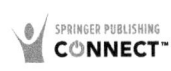 A robust set of instructor resources designed to supplement this text is located at http://connect.springerpub.com/content/book/978-0-8261-5842-0. Qualifying instructors may request access by emailing textbook@springerpub.com.

- Instructor Manual, containing a CACREP Standard Integration chart and Learning Objectives, Discussion Questions, Activities for each chapter, plus an Abbreviated Syllabus for a 15-Week Course
- Test Bank, containing Multiple-Choice and True/False questions for each chapter
- Instructor Chapter PowerPoint presentation, arranged by chapter

SECTION I

OVERVIEW OF CO-OCCURRING DISORDERS

CHAPTER 1

CONSIDERATIONS FOR TREATING CO-OCCURRING MENTAL AND SUBSTANCE USE DISORDERS

REGINALD W. HOLT

LEARNING OBJECTIVES

After reading this chapter, you will be able to:

- Recognize the prevalence of co-occurring mental and substance use disorders.
- Identify the etiological paradigms and risk factors for co-occurring mental and substance use disorders.
- Give examples of the adverse effects of co-occurring mental and substance use disorders.
- Distinguish screening procedures from the assessment process when evaluating clients for co-occurring mental and substance use disorders.
- Summarize the steps involved in the assessment process when evaluating co-occurring mental and substance use disorders.
- Discuss treatment approaches, guidelines, and levels of care for co-occurring mental and substance use disorders.
- Explain ethical and legal considerations related to counselor competencies when treating clients with co-occurring mental and substance use disorders.

INTRODUCTION

Recognizing the existence of and developing treatment models for co-occurring mental and substance use disorders have advanced over the past four decades. It was not that long ago that service providers were unaware of the extent of the problem, and, for those clients who were considered to have co-occurring mental and substance use disorders, treatment professionals lacked clear direction on how to intervene when encountering those affected by these disorders (Hendrickson et al., 2004). The profession has also evolved in the manner in which individuals with CODs are classified and discussed. For example, earlier terms such as *mentally ill substance abusers*, *substance abusing mentally ill*, and *mentally ill chemically addicted* are outdated (Substance Abuse and Mental Health Services Administration [SAMHSA], 2020). Counselors who identify their clients using language such as "having a diagnosis of co-occurring anxiety and alcohol use disorder" is a much more humanizing and person-centered approach than adopting terminology that labels others and reinforces stigma. And although the term *dual diagnosis* may be less dehumanizing than others, it is a narrow and potentially confusing conceptualization wherein it can imply the existence of no more than two disorders (e.g., one mental and one substance use; one physical and one mental; two physical). The additional constructs of *comorbidity* and *multimorbidity* are typically linked to the medical model and may indicate someone has more than one physical health illness, condition, or disease at the same time (Valderas et al., 2009). The contemporary term *co-occurring disorders* (CODs), therefore, is the one preferred for this textbook because it is best defined as no specific combination of one or more mental disorders concurrently appearing alongside one or more substance use disorders (SUDs) contained within the diagnostic classification system published by the American Psychiatric Association (APA, 2013).

PREVALENCE, STATISTICS, AND DEMOGRAPHICS

Before topics such as treatment modalities for CODs are discussed, it is important to first (a) examine the prevalence and frequency in which certain mental and substance use disorders co-occur with each other, (b) describe the primary etiological paradigms and risk factors for CODs, and (c) identity the impact that CODs have on health and level of functioning.

PREVALENCE OF CO-OCCURRING DISORDERS

Counselors-in-training who indicate they plan to only work with clients who have mental disorders (or vice versa for substance use disorders) are remiss if they believe they will not need to be cross-trained on CODs. Regardless of a counselor's preferred client population or specialization area, the informed clinician fully understands that all clients need to be screened for both mental and substance use symptomatology despite the initial chief complaint and/or self-identified presenting problem. This is evident when considering approximately 7.7 million (3.3%) adults in the United States have diagnosable co-occurring mental and substance use disorders (Han et al., 2017). It is even further made clear when reviewing the data presented by SAMHSA in its 2020 National Survey on Drug Use and Health: 17.0 million adults (6.7%) had a SUD that co-occurred with any mental illness (AMI) in the past year, and 5.7 million (2.2%) had a SUD and a serious mental illness (SMI) that significantly limited/interfered with their level of functioning (SAMHSA, 2021).

Taking into account that approximately 48% of adults with SMIs and almost 40% of those with AMIs used illicit drugs in the past year (SAMHSA, 2021), counselors should recognize that for every two clients with mental health issues who come into their office, the likelihood exists that at least one will have misused a substance recently.

Youths aged 12 to 17 are more likely to use substances if they had a major depressive episode (MDE) in the past year compared to those who did not have a MDE (28.6% vs. 10.7%).

Additionally, recognizing that 40.3 million (14.5%) people aged 12 or older in the United States had at least one SUD in 2020, counselors should remain diligent and conduct adequate substance use screenings by asking all client-types—youths and adults alike—about past and current substance use, and then provide interventions and ongoing follow-up investigations when applicable.

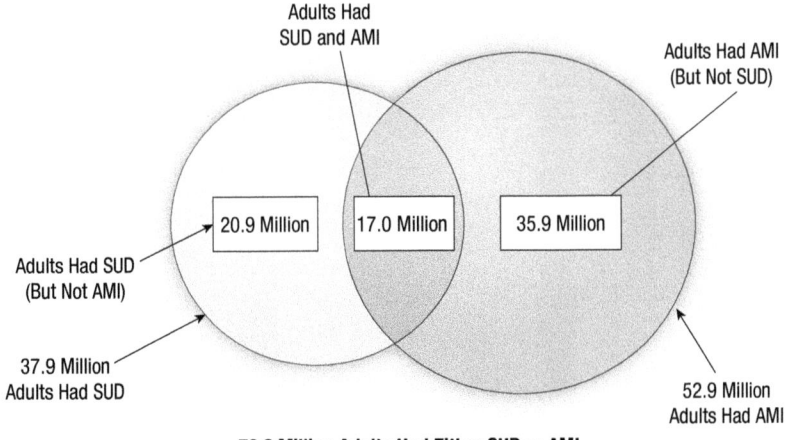

FIGURE 1.1 Past Year Substance Use Disorder (SUD) and Any Mental Illness (AMI) Among Adults Aged 18 or Older: 2020.
Source: Recreated with information from *Key Substance Use and Mental Health Indicators in the United States: Results from the 2020 National Survey on Drug Use and Health* by the Substance Abuse and Mental Health Services Administration (SAMHSA, 2021, p. 34). https://www.samhsa.gov/data/report/2020-nsduh-annual-national-report

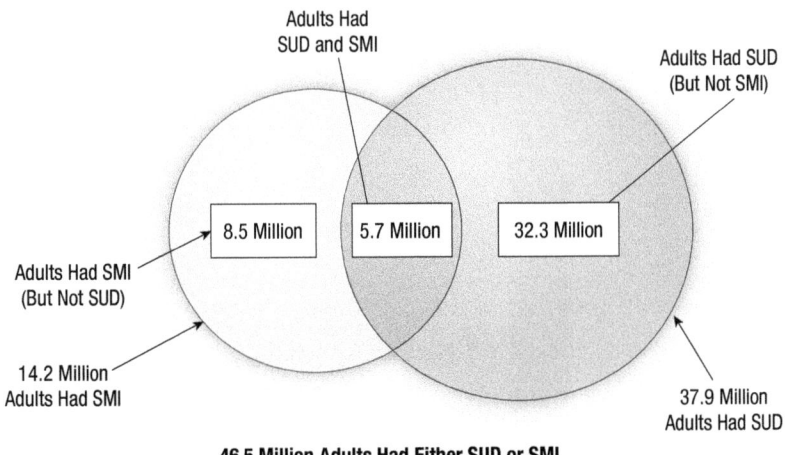

FIGURE 1.2 Past Year Substance Use Disorder (SUD) and Serious Mental Illness (SMI) Among Adults Aged 18 or Older: 2020.
Source: Recreated with information from *Key Substance Use and Mental Health Indicators in the United States: Results from the 2020 National Survey on Drug Use and Health* by the Substance Abuse and Mental Health Services Administration (SAMHSA, 2021, p. 34). https://www.samhsa.gov/data/report/2020-nsduh-annual-national-report

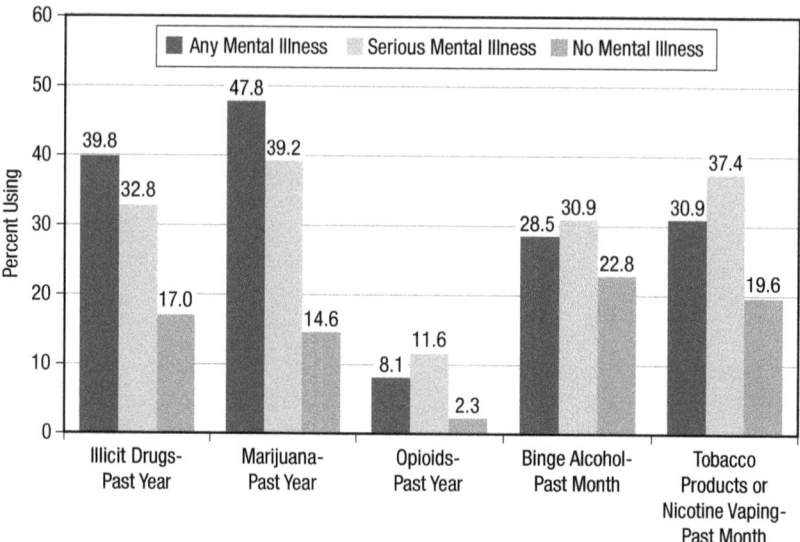

FIGURE 1.3 Substance Use Among Adults Aged 18 or Older by Mental Illness Status: 2020.
Source: Recreated with information from *Key Substance Use and Mental Health Indicators in the United States: Results from the 2020 National Survey on Drug Use and Health* by the Substance Abuse and Mental Health Services Administration (SAMHSA, 2021, p. 35). https://www.samhsa.gov/data/report/2020-nsduh-annual-national-report

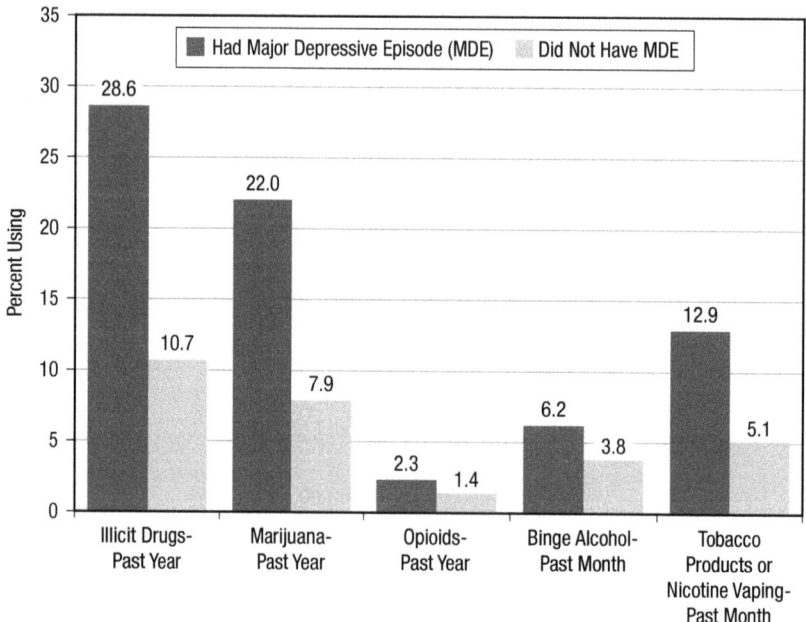

FIGURE 1.4 Substance Use Among Youths Aged 12 to 17 by Past Year Major Depressive Episode (MDE) Status: 2020.
Source: Recreated with information from *Key Substance Use and Mental Health Indicators in the United States: Results from the 2020 National Survey on Drug Use and Health* by the Substance Abuse and Mental Health Services Administration (SAMHSA, 2021, p. 33). https://www.samhsa.gov/data/report/2020-nsduh-annual-national-report

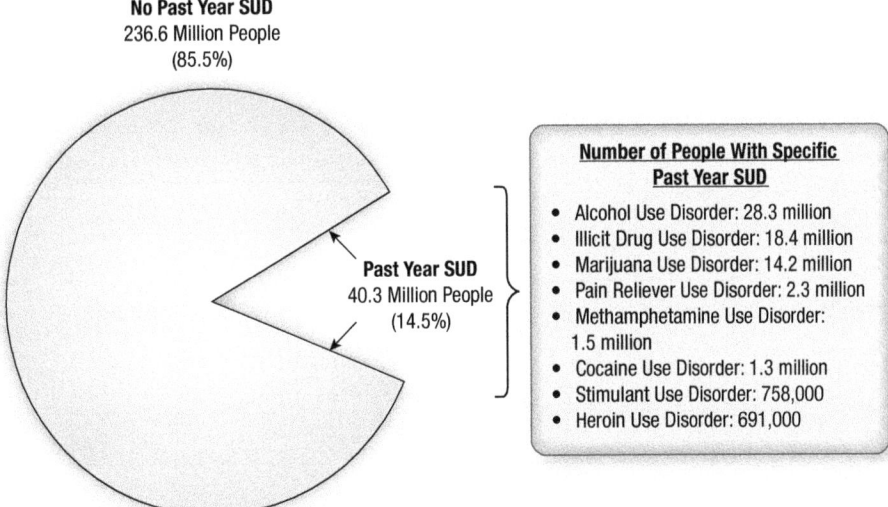

FIGURE 1.5 People Aged 12 or Older With a Past Year Substance Use Disorder (SUD): 2020.
Source: Recreated with information from *Key Substance Use and Mental Health Indicators in the United States: Results from the 2020 National Survey on Drug Use and Health* by the Substance Abuse and Mental Health Services Administration (SAMHSA, 2021, p. 29). https://www.samhsa.gov/data/report/2020-nsduh-annual-national-report

Because of the prevalence of co-occurring substance use and mental health issues in the United States, a breakdown of the data is offered to emphasize the importance of counselors being trained on the screening, assessment, and detection of CODs—and, based upon the counselor's role and credential(s), the diagnosis and treatment of *DSM* mental and substance use disorders (or, at the very least, provide brief intervention and then refer to a specialist). These responsibilities are best supported by realizing CODs are more "the rule rather than the exception" (Lai et al., 2015, p. 8) and remembering clients with SUDs have a higher probability of also having a co-occurring mental health condition. Although it is not within the capacity of this chapter to identify and thoroughly discuss every combination of mental and substance use disorder that may exist, a concise review of data presented by SAMHSA (2020) is included to highlight those disorders more commonly seen in treatment settings, as well as the substances that are primarily used based on the disorder. Counselors are encouraged to study the entire *Treatment Improvement Protocol (TIP) 42* (SAMHSA, 2020) for a more comprehensive review, including the specific research cited by SAMHSA in *TIP 42* when reporting the various data that iare graphically displayed hereinafter within the following subsections.

DEPRESSIVE DISORDERS AND SUBSTANCE USE DISORDERS

TABLE 1.1 **Prevalence of Depressive Disorders and Substance Use Disorders**

INFLUENCING DISORDER(S)	CO-OCCURRING DISORDER(S)
Lifetime major depressive disorder	SUD history (58% co-occurrence)
	AUD history (41% co-occurrence)

(continued)

TABLE 1.1 **Prevalence of Depressive Disorders and Substance Use Disorders** (*Continued*)

INFLUENCING DISORDER(S)	CO-OCCURRING DISORDER(S)
12-month or lifetime drug use disorder (SUD excluding alcohol)	Any mood disorder (1.5 to 1.9 increased odds)
	Dysthymia (1.3 to 1.5 increased odds)
	Major depressive disorder (1.2 to 1.3 increased odds)
12-month AUD	Major depressive disorder (increased risk)
	Lifetime AUD with persistent depression (increased risk)
INFLUENCING DISORDER(S)	**PRIMARY SUBSTANCE(S) USED**
Co-occurring depressive and SUDs	Variety of drugs
Depressive disorders	Cannabis (increased use is reported)

AUD, alcohol use disorder; SUDs, substance use disorders.
Source: Created with information from *Substance Use Disorder Treatment for People with Co-Occurring Disorders: Treatment Improvement Protocol (TIP) 42* by the Substance Abuse and Mental Health Services Administration (SAMHSA, 2020, pp. 75 & 76). https://store.samhsa.gov/sites/default/files/SAMHSA_Digital_Download/PEP20-02-01-004_Final_508.pdf

BIPOLAR I DISORDER AND SUBSTANCE USE DISORDERS

TABLE 1.2 **Prevalence of Bipolar I Disorder and Substance Use Disorders**

INFLUENCING DISORDER(S)	CO-OCCURRING DISORDER(S)
Bipolar I disorder	Lifetime SUD (65% co-occurrence)
	Alcohol use disorder (54% co-occurrence)
	Drug use disorder history (32% co-occurrence)
12-month or lifetime drug use disorder (SUD excluding alcohol)	Bipolar I disorder (1.4 to 1.5 increased odds)
12-month or lifetime bipolar I disorder	Lifetime SUD (2 to 5.8 times increased risk)
INFLUENCING DISORDER(S)	**PRIMARY SUBSTANCE(S) USED**
Bipolar disorder	Alcohol use disorder (30% co-occurrence)
	Cannabis use disorder (20% co-occurrence)
	Any drug use disorder (17% co-occurrence)

SUD, substance use disorder.
Source: Created with information from *Substance Use Disorder Treatment for People with Co-Occurring Disorders: Treatment Improvement Protocol (TIP) 42* by the Substance Abuse and Mental Health Services Administration (SAMHSA, 2020, p. 81). https://store.samhsa.gov/sites/default/files/SAMHSA_Digital_Download/PEP20-02-01-004_Final_508.pdf

ANXIETY DISORDERS AND SUBSTANCE USE DISORDERS

TABLE 1.3 **Prevalence of Anxiety Disorders and Substance Use Disorders**

INFLUENCING DISORDER(S)	CO-OCCURRING DISORDER(S)
12-month or lifetime drug use disorder (SUD excluding alcohol)	Any anxiety disorder (1.2 to 1.3 increased odds)
	Panic disorder (1.0 to 1.3 increased odds)
	Generalized anxiety disorder (1.2 to 1.3 increased odds)
	Social anxiety disorder (1.1 to 1.3 increased odds)
Lifetime alcohol and drug use disorders	Associated with generalized anxiety disorder
INFLUENCING DISORDER(S)	**PRIMARY SUBSTANCE(S) USED**
Generalized anxiety disorder and addiction	Higher rates of heavy alcohol use

SUD, substance use disorder.
Source: Created with information from *Substance Use Disorder Treatment for People with Co-Occurring Disorders: Treatment Improvement Protocol (TIP) 42* by the Substance Abuse and Mental Health Services Administration (SAMHSA, 2020, pp. 102 & 104). https://store.samhsa.gov/sites/default/files/SAMHSA_Digital_Download/PEP20-02-01-004_Final_508.pdf

SCHIZOPHRENIA/OTHER PSYCHOTIC DISORDERS AND SUBSTANCE USE DISORDERS

TABLE 1.4 **Prevalence of Schizophrenia/Other Psychotic Disorders and Substance Use Disorders**

INFLUENCING DISORDER(S)	CO-OCCURRING DISORDER(S)
Schizophrenia and other psychotic disorders	Lifetime SUD (55% co-occurrence)
	Alcohol abuse (17% co-occurrence)
	AUD (26% co-occurrence)
	Illicit drug abuse (13% co-occurrence)
	Illicit drug use disorder (14% co-occurrence)
INFLUENCING DISORDER(S)	**PRIMARY SUBSTANCE(S) USED**
Severe psychotic disorders	Heavy alcohol use (4 times greater risk)
	Heavy cannabis use (3.5 times greater risk)
	Recreational drug use (4.6 times greater risk)

AUD, alcohol use disorder; SUDs, substance use disorders.
Source: Created with information from *Substance Use Disorder Treatment for People with Co-Occurring Disorders: Treatment Improvement Protocol (TIP) 42* by the Substance Abuse and Mental Health Services Administration (SAMHSA, 2020, p. 107). https://store.samhsa.gov/sites/default/files/SAMHSA_Digital_Download/PEP20-02-01-004_Final_508.pdf

POSTTRAUMATIC STRESS DISORDER AND SUBSTANCE USE DISORDERS

TABLE 1.5 **Prevalence of Posttraumatic Stress Disorder and Substance Use Disorders**

INFLUENCING DISORDER(S)	CO-OCCURRING DISORDER(S)
PTSD	Lifetime SUD (36% to 52% co-occurrence)
SUDs	Lifetime PTSD (26% to 52% co-occurrence)
	Current PTSD (15% to 42% co-occurrence)
12-month or lifetime drug use disorder (SUD excluding alcohol)	PTSD (1.5 to 1.6 times increased odds)
12-month or lifetime PTSD	12-month or lifetime SUD (1.3 to 1.5 times increased odds)
INFLUENCING DISORDER(S)	**PRIMARY SUBSTANCE(S) USED**
PTSD	Cocaine
	Opioids
	Prescription medication misuse
	Cannabis
	Alcohol

PTSD, posttraumatic stress disorder; SUDs, substance use disorders.
Source: Created with information from *Substance Use Disorder Treatment for People with Co-Occurring Disorders: Treatment Improvement Protocol (TIP) 42* by the Substance Abuse and Mental Health Services Administration (SAMHSA, 2020, p. 86). https://store.samhsa.gov/sites/default/files/SAMHSA_Digital_Download/PEP20-02-01-004_Final_508.pdf

PERSONALITY DISORDERS AND SUBSTANCE USE DISORDERS

TABLE 1.6 **Prevalence of Personality Disorders and Substance Use Disorders**

INFLUENCING DISORDER(S)	CO-OCCURRING DISORDER(S)
Personality disorders	SUDs (35% to 65% co-occurrence)
	AUD detoxification (5% to 85% rate)
	AUD (up to 24% co-occurrence)
Antisocial personality disorder	SUDs (14% to 35% co-occurrence)
	AUD (more likely to co-occur in men)
	Persistent SUDs (significant association)

(continued)

TABLE 1.6 **Prevalence of Personality Disorders and Substance Use Disorders** (*Continued*)

INFLUENCING DISORDER(S)	CO-OCCURRING DISORDER(S)
Borderline personality disorder	SUDs (22% to 53% prevalence in SUD treatment settings)
	SUD-current (45% co-occurrence)
	SUD-lifetime (75% co-occurrence)
12-month or lifetime drug use disorder (SUD excluding alcohol)	Antisocial personality disorder (1.4 to 2 times increased odds)
	Borderline personality disorder (1.7 to 1.8 times increased odds)
Substance use disorders	Antisocial personality disorder (7% to 40% in men)
INFLUENCING DISORDER(S)	**PRIMARY SUBSTANCE(S) USED**
Antisocial personality disorder	Polydrug use involving: • Alcohol • Cannabis • Heroin • Cocaine • Methamphetamine
Borderline personality disorder	Opioids
	Cocaine
	Alcohol

AUD, alcohol use disorder; SUD, substance use disorder.
Source: Created with information from *Substance Use Disorder Treatment for People with Co-Occurring Disorders: Treatment Improvement Protocol (TIP) 42* by the Substance Abuse and Mental Health Services Administration (SAMHSA, 2020, pp. 92–94, & 97–98). https://store.samhsa.gov/sites/default/files/SAMHSA_Digital_Download/PEP20-02-01-004_Final_508.pdf

ETIOLOGICAL PARADIGMS AND RISK FACTORS FOR CO-OCCURRING DISORDERS

Counselors attempting to answer the age-old causality dilemma, "Which came first: the chicken or the egg?" when considering which disorder prompted the other will eventually realize a conclusive and straightforward answer cannot easily be provided. According to the National Institute on Drug Abuse (NIDA, 2018b), just because individuals who have a SUD may also have a co-occurring mental illness, it should not be always assumed that one disorder precipitated the other regardless of which emerged first. However, there are many risk factors that counselors should recognize when examining the reasons for the existence of CODs in clients. For example, *genetic factors* (e.g., DNA structure) as well as *environmental conditions* (e.g., stress, trauma, adverse childhood experiences) may change the manner in which genes are expressed from generation to generation, which subsequently alters neural networks and human behavior (NIDA, 2018b, 2020). Such epigenetic mechanisms, therefore, influence whether an individual is susceptible or predisposed to developing CODs (NIDA, 2018b, 2019).

Another possible risk factor involves the *self-medication* theory (Santucci, 2012) that postulates individuals use substances in order to manage psychiatric symptoms. An example would be a client who uses cannabis to reduce anxiety when interacting with other people in group settings. Over time, the client's frequent and ongoing use of cannabis progresses into a cannabis use disorder that now co-occurs with social anxiety disorder. However, counselors should take note that although some clients may use substances to minimize symptoms of mental illness, a cause-and-effect attribution should not be automatically assumed (SAMHSA, 2020). Furthermore, counselors are discouraged from using "self-medication" terminology (SAMHSA, 2020) because such language infers drugs of abuse (that can impair health and wellness) are on par with prescription medications (that are intended to enhance health and wellness).

Because CODs have a *bidirectional* characteristic (SAMHSA, 2020; Santucci, 2012), substance use can influence the development of a mental disorder (e.g., a client who used phencyclidine [PCP] develops PCP-induced psychotic disorder). This bidirectional influence also applies the other way around where a mental disorder that co-occurs with a medical condition advances the development of a SUD (e.g., a client with posttraumatic stress disorder [PTSD] and chronic pain regularly abuses a narcotic pain medication and eventually develops a co-occurring opioid use disorder). In addition to the bidirectional nature of CODs, research indicates that patterns of harmful substance use are correlated more highly with certain *mental disorders* such as bipolar disorder, anxiety disorder (especially social anxiety disorder), and antisocial and schizotypal personality disorders (Baigent, 2012).

In addition to those already mentioned, other variables that contribute to the existence of both mental and substance use disorders include, but are not limited to, those related to neurobiology, lifespan development, gender, and sexual orientation. It is important to highlight that even though substance use may contribute to the formation of a mental illness (and vice versa), each disorder type will more than likely impact as well as intensify the other; therefore, both require counselors to address each equally even though each disorder may not be equivalent in severity (SAMHSA, 2020).

IMPACT OF CO-OCCURRING DISORDERS

Co-occurring disorders not only impact the individual client and those around them (e.g., family members), they also negatively affect a number of other factors including treatment and recovery outcomes, employment rates, housing security status, criminal/legal system involvement, symptom severity expression, and at its worst, suicide (SAMHSA, 2020). The following information is extracted from SAMHSA (2020) to offer a representation of how CODs may cause detrimental health and socioeconomic consequences for the individual as well as the larger society. However, as previously noted, the more comprehensive *TIP 42* on CODs published by SAMHSA (2020) includes a significantly more detailed discussion of the various data while citing the large body of research selected by SAMHSA when producing the report, which should be accessed and studied by counselors working with clients who have CODs.

IMPACT OF CO-OCCURRING MENTAL DISORDERS AND SUBSTANCE USE DISORDERS

TABLE 1.7 **Impact of Co-Occurring Mental Disorders and Substance Use Disorders**

FACTOR	IMPACT
Treatment rates	42% did not complete treatment (CODs)
Unemployment rates	29% unemployed (CODs)
	50% not in the workforce (disabled, retired, student)

(continued)

TABLE 1.7 **Impact of Co-Occurring Mental Disorders and Substance Use Disorders (*Continued*)**

FACTOR	IMPACT
Homelessness rates	7.5% homelessness (ages 12 and older)
	8.3% (schizophrenia/psychotic disorders and SUD)
	7.8 (depressive disorders and SUD)
	6.9% (bipolar disorder and SUD)
Incarceration rates	48% (history of mental illness)
	26% (history of SUD)
	49% (mental illness with co-occurring SUD)
Suicide rates	46% (mental illness)
	28% (substance misuse) Of these, 1/3 (32%) had a known mental health condition

CODs, co-occurring disorders; SUDs, substance use disorders.
Source: Created with information from *Substance Use Disorder Treatment for People with Co-Occurring Disorders: Treatment Improvement Protocol (TIP) 42* by the Substance Abuse and Mental Health Services Administration (SAMHSA, 2020, p. 11). https://store.samhsa.gov/sites/default/files/SAMHSA_Digital_Download/PEP20-02-01-004_Final_508.pdf

ADVERSE EFFECTS OF DEPRESSIVE DISORDERS AND SUBSTANCE USE DISORDERS

TABLE 1.8 **Adverse Effects of Depressive Disorders and Substance Use Disorders**

CO-OCCURRING DISORDER(S)	ADVERSE EFFECTS
Depression and SUDs	More severe sleep disturbance
	Increased feelings of worthlessness
	Higher risk of suicidal ideation and suicide attempts
	Greater impairment in functioning
	Higher rates of other co-occurring mental disorders
	Increased mortality
	Less likely to receive antidepressants

SUDs, substance use disorders.
Source: Created with information from *Substance Use Disorder Treatment for People with Co-Occurring Disorders: Treatment Improvement Protocol (TIP) 42* by the Substance Abuse and Mental Health Services Administration (SAMHSA, 2020, p. 75). https://store.samhsa.gov/sites/default/files/SAMHSA_Digital_Download/PEP20-02-01-004_Final_508.pdf

ADVERSE EFFECTS OF BIPOLAR I DISORDER AND SUBSTANCE USE DISORDERS

TABLE 1.9 **Adverse Effects of Bipolar I Disorder and Substance Use Disorders**

CO-OCCURRING DISORDER(S)	ADVERSE EFFECTS
Bipolar I disorder and substance misuse	Increased symptom severity
	Poorer treatment outcomes
	Greater risk of suicide
SUD with bipolar I disorder	Lower SUD treatment adherence and retention
	Protracted mood episodes
	Poorer recovery of functional abilities
	Increased use of emergency services
	More hospitalizations
	Greater affective instability and impulsivity
	Poorer response to medications (e.g., lithium)

SUD, substance use disorder.
Source: Created with information from *Substance Use Disorder Treatment for People with Co-Occurring Disorders: Treatment Improvement Protocol (TIP) 42* by the Substance Abuse and Mental Health Services Administration (SAMHSA, 2020, p. 81). https://store.samhsa.gov/sites/default/files/SAMHSA_Digital_Download/PEP20-02-01-004_Final_508.pdf

ADVERSE EFFECTS OF ANXIETY DISORDERS AND SUBSTANCE USE DISORDERS

TABLE 1.10 **Adverse Effects of Anxiety Disorders and Substance Use Disorders**

CO-OCCURRING DISORDERS	ADVERSE EFFECTS
Anxiety and SUDs	Affect development and maintenance of co-occurring conditions
	Each disorder modifies the presentation and treatment outcomes of the other disorder
	Greater disability
	More hospitalizations and healthcare utilization
	Poorer functioning
	Greater difficulties in interpersonal relationships
	Greater symptom severity
	Worse health-related quality of life
	Poorer treatment responses

(continued)

TABLE 1.10 **Adverse Effects of Anxiety Disorders and Substance Use Disorders** (*Continued*)

CO-OCCURRING DISORDERS	ADVERSE EFFECTS
GAD and SUDs	Higher rates of alcohol use
	Higher rates of hospitalizations
	Higher rates of relapse
	Higher rates of leaving treatment against medical advice
Anxiety symptoms and anxiety disorders	Predictors of suicidal ideation and suicide attempt

GAD, generalized anxiety disorder; SUDs, substance use disorders.
Source: Created with information from *Substance Use Disorder Treatment for People with Co-Occurring Disorders: Treatment Improvement Protocol (TIP) 42* by the Substance Abuse and Mental Health Services Administration (SAMHSA, 2020, pp. 102 & 104). https://store.samhsa.gov/sites/default/files/SAMHSA_Digital_Download/PEP20-02-01-004_Final_508.pdf

ADVERSE EFFECTS OF SCHIZOPHRENIA/OTHER PSYCHOTIC DISORDERS AND SUBSTANCE USE DISORDERS

TABLE 1.11 **Adverse Effects of Schizophrenia/Other Psychotic Disorders and Substance Use Disorders**

CO-OCCURRING DISORDER(S)	ADVERSE EFFECTS
Schizophrenia/other psychotic disorders and substance misuse	Shortened mortality
	Increased likelihood of deleterious health and functional outcomes, including a higher risk for: • Self-destructive and violent behaviors • Victimization • Suicide • Housing instability • Poor physical health • Cognitive impairment • Employment problems • Legal difficulties • Unstable relationships
Substance misuse and schizophrenia	Can worsen the disease course
	May reduce adherence to antipsychotic medication

Source: Created with information from *Substance Use Disorder Treatment for People with Co-Occurring Disorders: Treatment Improvement Protocol (TIP) 42* by the Substance Abuse and Mental Health Services Administration (SAMHSA, 2020, p. 107). https://store.samhsa.gov/sites/default/files/SAMHSA_Digital_Download/PEP20-02-01-004_Final_508.pdf

ADVERSE EFFECTS OF POSTTRAUMATIC STRESS DISORDER AND SUBSTANCE USE DISORDERS

TABLE 1.12 **Adverse Effects of Posttraumatic Stress Disorder and Substance Use Disorders**

CO-OCCURRING DISORDER(S)	ADVERSE EFFECTS
PTSD and SUDs	Worse treatment outcomes
	Lower rates of remission
	Faster relapse
	Poorer treatment response
	Greater cognitive difficulties
	Worse social functioning
	Greater risk of suicide attempts
	Heightened mortality rates
PTSD and AUD	More traumatic childhoods
	More co-occurring mental disorders
	Increased suicide risk
	Greater symptom severity
	Greater disability

AUD, alcohol use disorder; PTSD, posttraumatic stress disorder; SUDs, substance use disorders.
Source: Created with information from *Substance Use Disorder Treatment for People with Co-Occurring Disorders: Treatment Improvement Protocol (TIP) 42* by the Substance Abuse and Mental Health Services Administration (SAMHSA, 2020, p. 86). https://store.samhsa.gov/sites/default/files/SAMHSA_Digital_Download/PEP20-02-01-004_Final_508.pdf

ADVERSE EFFECTS OF PERSONALITY DISORDERS AND SUBSTANCE USE DISORDERS

TABLE 1.13 **Adverse Effects of Personality Disorders and Substance Use Disorders**

CO-OCCURRING DISORDERS	ADVERSE EFFECTS
Personality and SUDs	More severe mental and substance-related symptoms
	Longer persisting substance use
	Greater likelihood of other co-occurring disorders
	Increased mortality
	Higher SUD treatment dropout

(continued)

TABLE 1.13 **Adverse Effects of Personality Disorders and Substance Use Disorders (*Continued*)**

CO-OCCURRING DISORDERS	ADVERSE EFFECTS
Antisocial personality and SUDs	Higher rates of aggression
	Higher rates of impulsivity
	Higher rates of psychopathy

SUDs, substance use disorders.
Source: Created with information from *Substance Use Disorder Treatment for People with Co-Occurring Disorders: Treatment Improvement Protocol (TIP) 42* by the Substance Abuse and Mental Health Services Administration (SAMHSA, 2020, pp. 92 & 98). https://store.samhsa.gov/sites/default/files/SAMHSA_Digital_Download/PEP20-02-01-004_Final_508.pdf

SCREENING AND ASSESSMENT OF CO-OCCURRING DISORDERS

Now that an overview of the prevalence, risk factors, and impact of CODs has been provided, the discussion now moves to the topics of screening and assessment. As stated earlier, counselors should be skilled in conducting evaluations that identify both mental and substance use problematic issues due to the widespread occurrence of CODs among clinical populations. And even if a mental health counselor is not considered to be a specialist or expert in the treatment of addiction and/or CODs (and the same for the addiction counselor who does not diagnose or treat mental disorders), all counselors should be able to effectively complete comprehensive biopsychosocial evaluations that involve screening and assessing clients who may have CODs. Every counselor whose assessment results in revealing the existence of CODs may not be expected to provide direct care services for each applicable client if it is beyond the scope of the individual counselor's education, training, and certification/licensure; however, it is expected that all counselors understand the fundamental practices involved in detecting mental and substance use conditions so that applicable clients who require specialized and integrated treatment for CODs can be identified. Problems that are not recognized cannot be addressed. This need for early detection of CODs is further evident when considering the recommendations by SAMHSA's consensus panel of experts who endorsed the following practices regarding the screening process:

1. "Substance use disorder treatment providers screen all new clients for co-occurring mental disorders" (SAMHSA, 2020, p. 41).
2. "Mental disorder treatment providers screen all new clients for any substance misuse" (SAMHSA, 2020, p. 41).

SCREENING AND ASSESSMENT: WHAT IS THE DIFFERENCE?

It has been established that screening and assessment are at the forefront of the initial (as well as ongoing) evaluation of the client. Without these essential interventions, appropriate treatment matching and effective treatment planning cannot be accomplished. Before the multilayered process of screening and assessment of CODs is outlined, counselors should be aware of the difference between the two terms. It is not unusual for the words *screening* and *assessment* to be used interchangeably during informal conversations. Although this common colloquial error may not result in the actual end of the world, it is important that counselors—especially those in training programs—understand that *screening* and *assessment* have different meanings as well as distinct procedures.

THE SCREENING PROCESS

Simply defined, *screening* is a "brief, routine process designed to identify indicators, or 'red flags,' for the presence of mental health, substance use, or other issues that reflect an individual's need for treatment" (SAMHSA, 2015, p. 19). The screening procedures designed to reveal the existence of mental and/or substance problems typically involve one or any combination of the following: (a) conducting brief, yet focused, interviews with clients; (b) using clinician-administered or client self-report screening instruments; and (c) obtaining information from collateral sources with the written consent of the client when ethically and legally applicable. The object of screening for CODs is to ask specific questions that will yield either a "yes" or "no" response in order to identify warning signs that potentially indicate the client is experiencing mental and/or substance abuse issues (SAMHSA, 2020). And for those clients whose responses yield positive results, the practitioner should either refer out or follow-up with a more comprehensive assessment to determine the severity and possible diagnoses of mental and substance use disorders. Whether or not counselors involve a variety of qualitative and quantitative methods, SAMHSA outlined the following guidelines when screening for the presence of substance misuse and mental disorders (2020, pp. 41–42):

Substance Misuse Screening

- Screen for acute safety risk related to serious intoxication or withdrawal.
- Screen for past and present substance use, substance-related problems, and substance-related disorders (i.e., SUDs and substance-induced mental disorders).

Mental Disorder Screening

- Screen for acute safety risk, including for:
  - Suicide,
  - Violence to others,
  - Inability to care for oneself,
  - Risky behaviors, and
  - Danger of physical or sexual victimization.
- Screen for past and present mental illness symptoms and disorders.
- Screen for cognitive and learning deficits.
- Regardless of setting, screen all clients for past and present victimization and trauma.

Observable Signs and Symptoms of Co-Occurring Disorders

In addition to conducting screening procedures, SAMHSA (2015) identified the following signs and symptoms associated with CODs that should be considered by counselors when observing clients during the evaluation process (p. 27):

- Unusual affect, appearance, thoughts, or speech (e.g., confusion, disorientation, rapid or slurred speech);
- Suicidal thoughts or behavior;

- Paranoid ideation;
- Impaired judgment and risk-taking behavior;
- Drug-seeking behaviors;
- Agitation or tremors;
- Impaired motor skills (e.g., unsteady gait);
- Dilated or constricted pupils;
- Elevated or diminished vital signs;
- Hyperarousal or drowsiness;
- Muscle rigidity;
- Evidence of current intoxication (e.g., alcohol on breath); and
- Needle track marks or injection sites.

THE ASSESSMENT PROCESS

Assuming the client screened positive for the presence of mental health and/or substance use issues, the counselor may still be unaware of the extent of the problem as well as the potential diagnoses that need to be considered. Because of this, a more formal assessment needs to be conducted to determine the type and severity of symptoms, understand the impact the problems have on the client's overall level of functioning, identify the variables influencing the development and perpetuation of the client's issues, and, ideally, make a provisional diagnosis of each mental and substance use disorder based upon the information revealed through the comprehensive assessment (SAMHSA, 2015). In order to accomplish these objectives, counselors need to examine all data obtained through various avenues. Sources of these data may be collected during the initial intake and screening process (completed by another treatment facility staff member or the actual counselor), obtained directly from the client via a comprehensive biopsychosocial interview (conducted by the counselor), and/or provided by third-party suppliers authorized to share historical as well as present-day information (provided by healthcare providers via records and reports and/or disclosed by collateral contacts such as family members and close friends).

Key Information: The Basics of Assessment

In order to begin seeing a fuller picture of the client's situation, basic information needs to be captured when assessing a client. This information, which may be derived in part from the intake interview, includes the following (SAMHSA, 2020, pp. 34–35):

- *Background:*
    - ☐ Family history;
    - ☐ Trauma history;
    - ☐ Domestic violence history (as either perpetrator or victim);
    - ☐ Marital status;
    - ☐ Legal involvement history;
    - ☐ Financial status;
    - ☐ Strengths and resources; and
    - ☐ Employment status.

- *Substance Use:*
    - ☐ Age of first use;
    - ☐ Primary substance(s) used, including alcohol;
    - ☐ Treatment episodes; and
    - ☐ Family history of substance use problems.
- *Mental Illness:*
    - ☐ Family history of mental illness;
    - ☐ Client history of mental illness, including diagnosis, hospitalization, and other treatment;
    - ☐ Current symptoms and mental status; and
    - ☐ Medications and medication adherence.

It is important to point out that this basic assessment information, which may be complemented by psychometric assessment instrument results, does not represent the totality of all the information needed to establish a provisional diagnosis, determine an appropriate level of care, and develop a preliminary treatment plan. A more complete assessment of the client includes, but is not limited to, chronologically documenting the history of problematic issues and applicable treatment episodes, exploring antecedents of substance use, identifying precipitating factors that contribute to the exacerbation of mental health symptoms, understanding cultural aspects, recognizing client skill deficits and limitations, and determining the stage of change for each recognized problem (SAMHSA, 2020). Furthermore, the assessment process, which should be conducted using a comprehensive biopsychosocial approach, also warrants a repeated and continued examination of the client's condition that is subject to change over time (SAMHSA, 2020).

The American Society of Addiction Medicine's Six Dimensions of Multidimensional Assessment

In order to assist in planning care and matching treatment to the client's needs, the American Society of Addiction Medicine (ASAM, n.d.) uses the six dimensions of multidimensional assessment. This strengths-based, holistic, biopsychosocial assessment considers each client's current mental/substance/medical conditions, barriers/limitations, and strengths/resources/supports in order to determine the most clinically suitable level of care across the service continuum (ASAM, n.d., para 3.). The six dimensions are:

- Dimension 1: Acute Intoxication and/or Withdrawal Potential;
- Dimension 2: Biomedical Conditions and Complications;
- Dimension 3: Emotional, Behavioral, or Cognitive Conditions and Complications;
- Dimension 4: Readiness to Change;
- Dimension 5: Relapse, Continued Use or Continued Problem Potential; and
- Dimension 6: Recovery/Living Environment.

Twelve Steps in the Assessment Process

SAMHSA (2020) identified 12 steps that should be taken when screening and assessing for the presence of co-occurring mental and substance use disorders. Each step will be succinctly listed here in order for ease of reference; however, counselors are directed to *TIP 42* (SAMHSA, 2020, pp. 39–68) for a thorough description of each of the 12 steps involved in the overall assessment process.

1. Engage the client.
2. Identify and contact collaterals (family, friends, other providers) to gather additional information.
3. Screen for and detect CODs.
4. Determine quadrant (based on severity of corresponding disorder) and locus of responsibility.
5. Determine level of care.
6. Determine diagnosis.
7. Determine disability and functional impairment.
8. Identify strengths and supports.
9. Identify cultural and linguistic needs and supports.
10. Identify problem domains.
11. Determine stage of change.
12. Plan treatment.

SCREENING TOOLS AND ASSESSMENT INSTRUMENTS

Step 3 in SAMHSA's (2020) assessment process, *screen for and detect CODs*, involves the use of various screening and assessment instruments. One resource available to assist clinicians identify tools used in screening and assessing for mental and substance use disorders is developed by the Addictions, Drug and Alcohol Institute (ADAI, 2022) at the University of Washington. The ADAI's *screening and assessment instruments database* allows users to enter keywords as they conduct their search, which then identifies the measure as well as other information such as its developer, description, and if it is in the public domain or requires access from the copyright holder. Other resources for locating information about specific instruments are the *Mental Measurements Yearbook with Tests in Print* and *APA PsycTests*, which are electronic databases available to libraries by subscription. Some of the recommended screening tools and assessment instruments offered by SAMHSA (2015, 2020) will be named here, among others, but in doing is not meant to imply it is an inclusive or exhaustive list as there are numerous tools available in the field of mental health and addiction treatment—some of which are freely available in the public domain and others require purchase and/or specialized qualifications for its use.

SCREENING TOOLS FOR MENTAL HEALTH AND SUBSTANCE USE ISSUES

- ***Client Safety Screening Tools***
  - ☐ Ask Suicide-Screening Questions (ASQ; Horowitz et al., 2012)
  - ☐ Beck Scale for Suicide Ideation (BSS; Beck & Steer, 1991)
  - ☐ Columbia-Suicide Severity Rating Scale (C-SSRS; Posner et al., 2011)

- ☐ Suicide Behaviors Questionnaire-Revised (SBQ-R; Osman et al., 2001)
- ☐ Humiliation, Afraid, Rape, and Kick (HARK; Sohal et al., 2007)

■ *Mental Disorders*
- ☐ Mental Health Screening Form-III (MHSF-III; Carroll & McGinley, 2000)
- ☐ Modified Mini Screen (MMS; Alexander et al., 2008)
- ☐ Patient Health Questionnaire-2 [for depressive disorders] (PHQ-2; Kroenke et al., 2003)
- ☐ Generalized Anxiety Disorder (GAD) 7-item (GAD-7; Spitzer et al., 2006)
- ☐ Primary Care PTSD Screen for DSM-5 (PC-PTSD-5; Prins et al., 2015)
- ☐ Brief Symptom Inventory (BSI; Derogatis & Melisaratos, 1983)
- ☐ Life Stressor Checklist-Revised (LSC-R; Wolfe & Kimerling, 1997)
- ☐ Trauma Screening Questionnaire (TSQ; Brewin, 2002)

■ *Substance Misuse*
- ☐ 10-Item Drug Abuse Screening Test (DAST-10; Skinner, 1982)
- ☐ Alcohol Use Disorders Identification Test (AUDIT; Babor et al., 2001)
- ☐ Alcohol Use Disorders Identification Test-Concise (AUDIT-C; Bush et al., 1998)
- ☐ CAGE Questionnaire Adapted to Include Drugs (CAGE-AID; Medge & Lang, 2011)
- ☐ Michigan Alcoholism Screening Test (MAST; Selzer, 1971)
- ☐ Alcohol, Smoking, and Substance Involvement Screening Test (ASSIST; Humeniuk et al., 2010)
- ☐ Simple Screening Instrument for Substance Abuse (SSI-SA; Boothroyd et al., 2015)
- ☐ The CRAFFT (Knight et al., 1999; Mitchell et al., 2014)

■ *Co-Occurring Disorders*
- ☐ Co-Occurring Disorders Screening Instrument for Mental Disorders (CODSI-MD; Sacks et al., 2007)
- ☐ The Mini International Neuropsychiatric Interview (MINI; Sheehan et al., 1998)
- ☐ Psychiatric Diagnostic Screening Questionnaire (PDSQ; Rush et al., 2013)

Assessment Instruments for Mental Health and Substance Use Issues

■ *Mental Disorders*
- ☐ *DSM-5* Cross-Cutting Symptom Measures (APA, 2013)
- ☐ Symptom Checklist 90–Revised (SCL90-R; Derogatis, 1994)
- ☐ Patient Health Questionnaire-9 [for depressive disorders] (PHQ-9; Kroenke et al., 2001)
- ☐ The PTSD Checklist for *DSM-5* (PCL-5; Weathers et al., 2013)

- **Substance Use Issues**
  - ☐ Addiction Severity Index (ASI; McLellan et al., 1992)
  - ☐ Clinical Institute Withdrawal Assessment of Alcohol Scale, Revised (CIWA-Ar; Sullivan et al., 1989)
  - ☐ Clinical Institute Narcotic Assessment Scale for Withdrawal Symptoms (CINA; Peachey, & Lei, 1988)
  - ☐ Clinical Opiate Withdrawal Scale (COWS; Wesson & Ling, 2003)
- **Co-Occurring Disorders**
  - ☐ Psychiatric Research Interview for Substance and Mental Disorders (PRISM; Hasin et al., 1996)
- **Assessing Stages of and Readiness for Change**
  - ☐ Processes of Change Questionnaire (PCQ; Prochaska et al., 1988)
    - NOTE: Alcohol, drug, and smoking versions are available (HABITS Lab, n.d.a)
  - ☐ University of Rhode Island Change Assessment Scale (URICA; DiClemente & Hughes, 1990)
    - NOTE: Psychotherapy, alcohol, and drug versions are available (HABITS Lab, n.d.b)

THE TREATMENT OF CO-OCCURRING DISORDERS

As stated earlier, it is not the intent of this chapter to provide a thorough review of CODs assessment and treatment strategies. Those interested in learning more about these topics are encouraged to read the applicable chapters provided within this textbook as well as review SAMHSA's (2020) *Substance Use Disorder Treatment for People with Co-Occurring Disorders: Treatment Improvement Protocol 42*. In the meantime, some key pieces of information regarding the treatment of CODs are included here.

Reflect on the following statistics regarding the number of individuals diagnosed with CODs who received treatment in 2020 (SAMHSA, 2021, pp. 47–48):

- Only 960,000 (5.7%) of the 17 million adults with a co-occurring SUD and AMI received *both* mental health and substance use services.
- Only 529,000 (9.3%) of the 5.7 million adults with a co-occurring SUD and a SMI received *both* mental health and substance use services.
- Only 6,000 (0.9%) of the 644,000 adolescents who experienced a SUD with a co-occurring MDE received *both* mental health and substance use services.

These data from SAMHSA are unfortunately consistent with research conducted by Han et al. (2017) who reported between 2008 and 2014 that only 9.1% of adults in the United States with CODs received both mental health and substance use treatment in the prior year. Considering there is an obvious unmet need regarding the simultaneous treatment of CODs, it is crucial for counselors to recognize the importance of clients receiving integrated services throughout the course and continuum of care.

ESTABLISHING A THERAPEUTIC RELATIONSHIP

Before evidence-based treatment strategies are implemented, the therapeutic relationship must be positively established. This is supported by research indicating a strong working alliance is correlated with positive recovery outcomes (Scanlon et al., 2022). In support of the counselor/client relationship, SAMHSA (2020, p. 142) provided a set of guidelines for treatment providers to follow when establishing a therapeutic alliance with individuals diagnosed with CODs. A detailed description of each of the 10 guidelines is available within *TIP 42* (SAMHSA, 2020); however, a concise listing is provided here:

1. Develop and use a therapeutic alliance to engage clients in treatment.
2. Maintain a recovery perspective.
3. Ensure continuity of care.
4. Address common clinical challenges (e.g., countertransference, confidentiality).
5. Monitor psychiatric symptoms (including symptoms of self-harm).
6. Use supportive and empathic counseling; adopt a multiproblem viewpoint.
7. Use culturally responsive methods.
8. Use motivational enhancement.
9. Teach relapse prevention techniques.
10. Use repetition and skill building to address deficits in functioning.

PROVIDING INTEGRATED CARE

The ASAM (as cited in SAMHSA, 2020, p. 184) identified three program types for the treatment of CODs: (a) co-occurring-capable, (b) co-occurring-enhanced, and (c) complexity-capable. Despite the program type, those offering integrated services for the treatment of co-occurring mental and substance use disorders are more effective than those who address each disorder sequentially (within the same healthcare system) or simultaneously (in separate healthcare systems; Kelly & Daley, 2013; Mangrum et al., 2006; NIDA, 2020; Otasowie, 2021; SAMHSA, 2020).

MATCHING TREATMENT TO LEVELS OF CARE

There is a large variety of levels of care across the continuum of services ranging from prevention/early intervention to medically managed intensive inpatient treatment. Clients with CODs may benefit from entering the healthcare service system at some entry point; however, every client's clinical situation will not necessitate accessing every level of care (SAMHSA, 2020). Factors that determine the most appropriate level of care for CODs include, but are not limited, to the severity of the client's symptoms, the impact CODs have on the client's level of functioning, and the client's current stage of change and readiness for change (SAMHSA, 2020). When making a level of care recommendation that matches the treatment needs of the client, SAMHSA (2020) suggests using the four quadrants of care model that considers mental illness symptom severity against SUD severity:

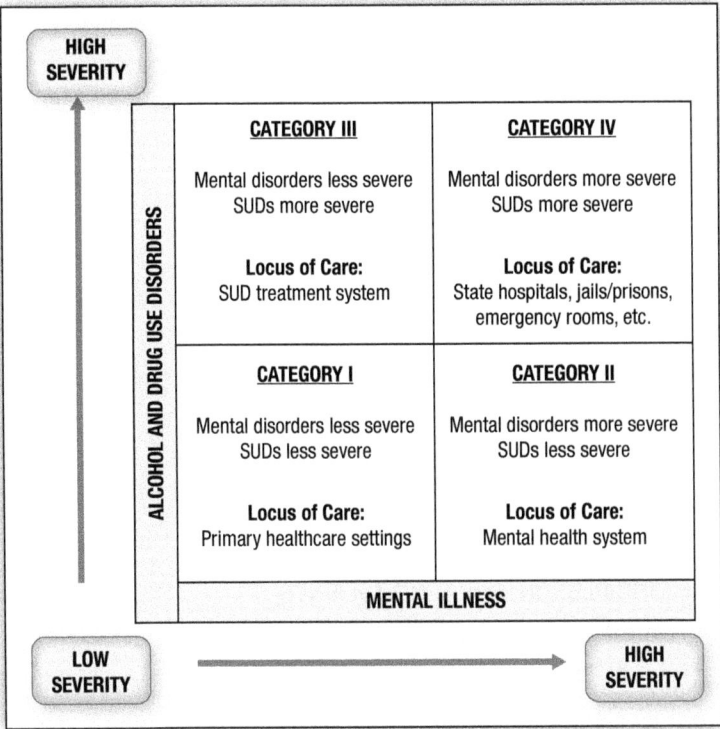

FIGURE 1.6 The Four Quadrants of Care Model.
Source: Recreated with information from *Substance Use Disorder Treatment for People with Co-Occurring Disorders: Treatment Improvement Protocol (TIP) 42* by the Substance Abuse and Mental Health Services Administration (SAMHSA, 2020, p. 185). https://store.samhsa.gov/sites/default/files/SAMHSA_Digital_Download/PEP20-02-01-004_Final_508.pdf

UNDERSTANDING TREATMENT AND BEST-PRACTICE GUIDELINES

It has been made apparent there is a prevalence of co-occurring mental and substance use disorders among client groups and within treatment settings. Because of the high rates of CODs, program administrators, service providers, healthcare professionals, and counselors alike need to recognize and implement best practice guidelines designed to identify and address client needs. And, in doing so, client health, wellness, and recovery goals may be advanced. The following sections, therefore, contain a synopsis of the various recommended best-practice guidelines for working with people who have CODs.

Providing Essential Services for People With Co-Occurring Disorders

When designing a treatment program, SAMHSA (2020, pp. 24–27) identified 10 necessary components that must be included in the provision of services if the unique needs of clients with CODs are to be addressed. These are:

1. Screening, assessment, and referral for people with CODs;
2. Physical and mental health consultation;
3. Prescribing onsite psychiatrist;
4. Psychoeducational classes;
5. Relapse prevention;
6. Case management;
7. COD-specific treatment components;
8. Continuing care services;
9. Double trouble groups (onsite); and
10. Dual recovery mutual-help groups (offsite).

Six Guiding Principles in Treating Clients With Co-Occurring Disorders

Although it may not be feasible to directly offer each of the aforementioned 10 elements in every treatment setting (such as private practices), this breakdown provides counselors an overview of the essential services needed in order to maximize client recovery outcomes. What counselors can do, regardless of the capabilities of the treatment setting in which they work, is to recognize SAMHSA's six guiding principles when considering how to best treat clients with CODs (2020, pp. 14–16):

1. Use a recovery perspective.
2. Adopt a multiproblem viewpoint.
3. Develop a phased approach to treatment.
4. Address specific real-life problems early in treatment.
5. Plan for the client's cognitive and functional impairments.
6. Use support systems to maintain and extend treatment effectiveness.

Guidelines for Counselors and Other Providers

Counselors should be aware that the six guiding principles just cited provide the foundation on which effective COD treatment may be built; however, there are six practices that counselors should adopt at the individual level (SAMHSA, 2020, pp. 16–21):

1. Providing access (using a "no wrong door" approach),
2. Completing a full assessment,
3. Providing an appropriate level of care,

4. Achieving integrated treatment,
5. Providing comprehensive services, and
6. Ensuring continuity of care.

Recognizing the Needs of Special Populations

There are certain populations who have a greater risk of developing CODs and experiencing poorer treatment outcomes. Included within these are military personnel (active duty and veterans), clients who identify as women, people experiencing homelessness, individuals involved in the criminal legal system, and those of diverse racial and ethnic backgrounds (SAMHSA, 2020). Counselors should not only be knowledgeable of the vulnerabilities associated with these groups, but they should also know how to design interventions that meet the complex needs of at-risk clients. For example, effectively offering services for CODs not only involves integrated treatment to promote recovery, it also includes collaborative care that helps identify and link clients to services based upon housing needs, medical concerns, employment issues, and legal problems (Lee et al., 2012). Therefore, counselors must understand the processes involved when collaborating/consulting with or referring to other providers, specialists, and agencies (e.g., medical/behavioral healthcare coordination). Other treatment considerations for individuals with CODs, including those who are members of special populations, are addressed within the relevant chapters contained in this textbook. However, some of the primary therapies and treatment modalities are mentioned in the following section.

DISTINGUISHING LEVELS OF CARE AND TREATMENT MODALITIES

In addition to the best-practice guidelines previously identified, research supports many levels of care and evidence-based services for treating CODs. Some services and interventions may require specialized education, training, and/or credentials that the counselor should obtain before implementing (e.g., mindfulness-based cognitive therapy) and some will be outside the scope of the professional counselor's role (e.g., prescribing medications). Nevertheless, counselors will find they have parts to play in whichever level of care they work whether they are the (a) primary party implementing the direct care intervention (e.g., counselor providing individual therapy in a private practice setting) (b) if they are a member of a multidisciplinary treatment team (e.g., lead counselor for process and relapse prevention psychoeducation groups within a partial hospitalization program); or (c) if they act as a collaborator/consultant/liaison with another healthcare professional who is the primary party implementing the direct care intervention (e.g., counselor conducts a medication inquiry at each session, recognizes potential concerns, discusses these with the client, and then coordinates a medication management session with the prescriber when necessary).

Treatment Principles and Evidence-Based Approaches: The National Institute on Drug Abuse

The NIDA identified and described 13 principles of effective treatment for drug addiction (2018a, pp. 3–6). Each of NIDA's 13 treatment principles—which should be considered by counselors working with clients who have co-occurring SUDs—are presented here:

1. Addiction is a complex but treatable disease that affects brain function and behavior.
2. No single treatment is appropriate for everyone.
3. Treatment needs to be readily available.
4. Effective treatment attends to multiple needs of the individual, not just their drug abuse.
5. Remaining in treatment for an adequate period is critical.
6. Behavioral therapies—including individual, family, or group counseling—are the most commonly used forms of drug abuse treatment.
7. Medications are an important element of treatment for many patients, especially when combined with counseling and other behavioral therapies.
8. An individual's treatment and services plan must be assessed continually and modified as necessary to ensure that it meets their changing needs.
9. Many drug-addicted individuals also have other mental disorders.
10. Medically assisted detoxification is only the first stage of addiction treatment and by itself does little to change long-term drug abuse.
11. Treatment does not need to be voluntary to be effective.
12. Drug use during treatment must be monitored continuously, as lapses during treatment do occur.
13. Treatment programs should test patients for the presence of HIV/AIDS, hepatitis B and C, tuberculosis, and other infectious diseases as well as provide targeted risk-reduction counseling, linking patients to treatment if necessary.

Treatments for Substance Use Disorders

In addition to the 13 guidelines, some of the evidence-based treatment approaches to addiction treatment identified by NIDA (2018a) are listed here. For a detailed discussion and review of these approaches, counselors should access NIDA's *Principles of Drug Addiction Treatment: A Research-Based Guide* (3rd ed.), which is freely available in the public domain.

Pharmacotherapies/Medication-Assisted Treatment

- Opioid Addiction
  - Methadone,
  - Buprenorphine,
  - Buprenorphine/naloxone (Suboxone), and
  - Naltrexone (Vivitrol, Revia).
- Alcohol Addiction
  - Naltrexone,
  - Acamprosate (Campral),
  - Disulfiram (Antabuse), and
  - Topiramate (Topamax).

- Nicotine Addiction
  - Nicotine replacement therapy (NRT),
  - Bupropion (Zyban), and
  - Varenicline (Chantix).

Behavioral Therapies

- Cognitive-Behavioral Therapy
  - Alcohol,
  - Marijuana,
  - Cocaine,
  - Methamphetamine, and
  - Nicotine.
- Contingency Management Interventions/Motivational Incentives
  - Alcohol,
  - Stimulants,
  - Opioids,
  - Marijuana, and
  - Nicotine.
- Community Reinforcement Approach (CRA) Plus Vouchers
  - Alcohol,
  - Cocaine, and
  - Opioids.
- Motivational Enhancement Therapy
  - Alcohol,
  - Marijuana,
  - Nicotine,
- The Matrix Model
  - Stimulants.
- 12-Step Facilitation Therapy
  - Alcohol,
  - Stimulants, and
  - Opiates.
- Family Behavior Therapy (FBT)

Behavioral Therapies Primarily for Adolescents

- Multisystemic Therapy (MST),
- Multidimensional Family Therapy (MDFT),
- Brief Strategic Family Therapy (BSFT),

- Functional Family Therapy (FFT), and
- Adolescent Community Reinforcement Approach (A-CRA).

Treatments for Co-Occurring Disorders

In addition to the therapies listed by NIDA for addiction treatment (2018a), NIDA also identified certain behavioral strategies that enhance the client's individual coping strategies when integrated into the treatment of CODs (NIDA, 2018b):

- Cognitive Behavioral Therapy (CBT),
- Dialectical Behavioral Therapy (DBT),
- Assertive Community Treatment (ACT),
- Therapeutic Communities (TCs), and
- Contingency Management (CM) or Motivational Incentives (MI).

These therapies, which may be used as a stand-alone service or in combination with psychopharmacological interventions prescribed for mental and/or substance use disorders, play key roles in achieving and sustaining successful treatment outcomes over time (NIDA, 2018b). Other evidence-based treatments for CODs include (a) seeking safety (Najavits, 2002) for trauma, PTSD, and substance abuse; (b) integrated group therapy (Weiss & Connery, 2001) for bipolar disorder and substance use; and (c) exposure therapy (Coffey et al., 2016) for PTSD and SUDs.

ASAM's Continuum of Care

As mentioned earlier, a wide range of treatment settings exist on the continuum of care for mental and substance use disorders. The ASAM publishes *The ASAM Criteria*, which is "the most widely used and comprehensive set of guidelines for placement, continued stay, transfer, or discharge of patients with addiction and co-occurring conditions" (n.d., para. 1). Once the multidimensional biopsychosocial assessment has been completed, the totality of the information is used to identify the most clinically appropriate level of care based upon the client's current overall needs. Although not fully comprehensive or descriptive, each available level of care (ASAM, n.d.) is shown here as a reference point.

- *Prevention/Early Intervention*
  - Early Intervention
- *Level 1: Outpatient*
  - Outpatient Services
- *Level 2: Intensive Outpatient/Partial Hospitalization*
  - Intensive Outpatient Services
  - Partial Hospitalization Services
- *Level 3: Residential/Inpatient*
  - Clinically Managed Low-Intensity Residential Services
  - Clinically Managed Population-Specific High-Intensity Residential Services
    - NOTE: This level of care only applies to adults while all others across the continuum apply to both adults and adolescents.

- Clinically Managed High-Intensity Residential Services
- Medically Monitored Intensive Inpatient Services
- *Level 4: Intensive Inpatient*
  - Medically Managed Intensive Inpatient Services

LOCATING TREATMENT FOR CO-OCCURRING DISORDERS

For counselors seeking services for clients but who may not be fully aware of all potential options in the client's area, SAMHSA developed FindTreatment.gov, a website-based database of state-licensed providers across the United States who offer treatment for mental and substance use disorders. This website provides information on searching for treatment options, reviewing the types of treatments available (as well as the cost), and understanding addiction and mental health disorders.

LEGAL AND ETHICAL CONSIDERATIONS

The American Counseling Association (ACA) is the main organization that develops the guidelines to inform the ethical practice of professional counselors, counselor supervisors, trainers, and educators, as well as counselors-in-training (2014, p. 3). Each counselor type should be familiar with the *2014 ACA Code of Ethics*, which includes detailed content related to key ethical categories. The main sections within ACA's ethical code are as follows: (a) the counseling relationship; (b) confidentiality and privacy; (c) professional responsibility; (d) relationships with other professionals; (e) evaluation, assessment, and interpretation; (f) supervision, training, and teaching; (g) research and publication; (h) distance counseling, technology, and social media; and (i) resolving ethical issues.

In addition to the ACA's code of ethics, it is an accepted fact that counselors should uphold all state and federal laws as well as adhere to the applicable ethical guidelines based upon their professional credentials (e.g., training/certification/licensure requirements). Counselors should always refer to their respective state for rules and statutes regarding scope of practice allowances and credentialing requirements; they should also review applicable certification board prerequisite and recertification requirements when seeking specialized credentials for the provision of counseling services. For the purpose of ethical and legal considerations, only a few key topics are addressed that directly relate to the content of this chapter.

PROFESSIONAL COMPETENCE

When providing services to clients with mental disorders, SUDs, or both, counselors must only practice within the boundaries of their competence; they should also only accept employment for which they are qualified and practice in specialty areas *only* after obtaining the necessary education, training, supervised experience, and applicable state/national credential(s) (ACA, 2014, p. 8). Once appropriate credentials have been obtained, continuing education is required in order to maintain competence and learn new skills, procedures, and best practices (ACA, 2014, p. 9). Beyond the many Council for Accreditation of Counseling and Related Educational Programs (CACREP)-accredited graduate-level counseling programs available across the United States, there is a variety of training and educational resources on mental health, substance use, and CODs. A few are listed here for reference; however, a more comprehensive list (including website links) may be accessed in Appendix B within *TIP 42* (SAMHSA, 2020, pp. 285–288). In addition to training resources, some credentialing organizations are also included:

Training, Specialized Credentialing, and Miscellaneous Resources

- Addiction Technology Transfer Center (ATTC) Network
- American Counseling Association (ACA)
- American Mental Health Counselors Association (AMHCA)
- International Certification & Reciprocity Consortium (IC&RC)
- NAADAC, the Association for Addiction Professionals
- National Board for Certified Counselors (NBCC)
- National Institute on Alcohol Abuse and Alcoholism (NIAAA)
- National Institute on Drug Abuse (NIDA)
- National Institute of Mental Health (NIMH)
- Substance Abuse and Mental Health Services Administration (SAMHSA)

Advanced Competencies

Beyond the education, training, supervised experience, and credentialing requirements that were just reviewed, SAMHSA (2020, p. 238) provides examples of advanced competencies that practitioners should acquire if they aspire to possess a more sophisticated and enhanced ability to offer integrated treatment to clients with CODs. These advanced competencies are:

- Understand the transtheoretical model and how client motivation and readiness to change affect behavior.
- Learn to enhance motivation via motivational interviewing and motivational enhancement therapy skills.
- Be aware of the relapse prevention model and integrating relapse prevention skills into treatments.
- Use criteria from *Diagnostic and Statistical Manual of Mental Disorders* (5th ed.; American Psychiatric Association [APA], 2013) to assess substance-related and other mental disorders.
- Understand the effects of level of functioning and degree of disability related to both substance-related and mental disorders, separately and combined.
- Apply knowledge of psychotropic medications, their actions, medical risks, side effects, and possible interactions with other substances.
- Use integrated models of assessment, intervention, and recovery for people having both substance-related and mental disorders, as opposed to sequential treatment efforts that resist integration.
- Collaboratively develop and implement an integrated treatment plan based on a thorough assessment that addresses both/all disorders and establishes sequenced goals based on urgent needs, considering the stage of recovery, stage of change, and level of engagement.

- Involve the person, family members, and other supports and service providers (including peer supports and those in the natural support system) in establishing, monitoring, and refining the current treatment plan.
- Help clients expand their social networks and systems of support.

The Use of Screening and Assessment Instruments

Whichever screening or assessment tool is utilized, the person administering it should have accessed it legally and ethically as well as fulfilled the applicable training and credentialing requirements for its use. Moreover, each chosen tool should be *valid* and *reliable*. Although healthcare providers who administer formal screening instruments do not typically require specialized credentials (SAMHSA, 2015), every counseling staff member involved in front-end intakes should be knowledgeable about the basics of COD screening (SAMHSA, 2020) and receive adequate training on conducting, scoring, and interpreting the results (SAMHSA, 2015, 2020). Furthermore, because of the clinical nature of assessing for CODs—which may involve the use of more specialized and sophisticated psychometric instruments compared to those used in the screening process—the professional conducting the assessment should not only have received supervised training and experience, but they also should have relevant graduate-level degrees with applicable certifications and/or licensure attesting to their advanced qualifications to diagnose and treat mental health disorders and substance addiction (SAMHSA, 2015). And for professional counselors and clinicians, this requirement is further emphasized by the ACA whose *2014 Code of Ethics* includes a dedicated section—*Section E. Evaluation, Assessment, and Interpretation*—that specifically identifies the expectations of counselors who perform evaluations involving the use of psychometric instruments and tests (ACA, 2014, pp. 11–12).

Pharmacotherapy

It is outside of the scope of practice for counselors to prescribe and conduct medication management sessions with their clients. Not only should counselors avoid these irresponsible practices because they violate ethical codes and medication administration laws, the untrained and unlicensed healthcare provider will jeopardize the client's safety and run the risk of causing serious (and potentially life-threatening) harm. Now, having acknowledged the limitation of the counselor's role in pharmacotherapy it not meant to imply that counselors take a hands-off approach when it comes to this topic. This point is best illustrated by SAMHSA (2020):

> *Pharmacotherapy is often a core part of COD treatment, especially for people with depression, bipolar I disorder, anxiety, schizophrenia/psychotic disorders, AUD [alcohol use disorder], or OUD [opioid use disorder]. Counselors do not prescribe medication, but they should understand what medications their clients are likely to take and the side effects clients are likely to experience so they can offer proper psychoeducation, help monitor for unsafe side effects, and refer clients to prescribers for medication management as needed. (p. xiv)*

As stated, this is not a comprehensive overview of all legal and ethical considerations counselors need to be aware of when working with clients diagnosed with CODs. There are numerous situations that will arise, and counselors need to continually monitor themselves as well as consult with other professionals/supervisors when needed.

CLINICAL CASE ILLUSTRATION AND DISCUSSION

CASE OF STEVIE

Stevie, a 32-year-old White woman who was recently divorced, arrived to attend her first counseling session in an outpatient private practice setting. When Stevie called the counselor approximately 1 week earlier, she informed the counselor that the reason she is seeking counseling is because she has been experiencing a return of depressive symptoms. Also, Stevie's primary care physician, who began prescribing duloxetine 60 mg per day 3 weeks ago, encouraged Stevie to consider talking to a mental health professional. The counselor, a licensed clinical professional counselor (LCPC) and master addiction counselor (MAC), greeted Stevie in the lobby, and then they walked to the counselor's office where a biopsychosocial assessment would be conducted.

Stevie began providing information regarding her background and history as well as present-day concerns. Stevie reported receiving brief counseling through her Employee Assistance Program (EAP) about 5 years ago after she experienced a miscarriage. She stated this was her first pregnancy, which occurred within a year of getting married to her former husband. At the time, she only attended about six sessions with the EAP counselor because she started feeling better and did not believe she needed ongoing, longer-term counseling services. Stevie recounted she based this decision on telling herself, "Hey! I'm still young and this was my first attempt at having a baby. We haven't been married that long, so there is plenty of time to have a family."

Stevie said she felt optimistic until she and her husband began having consistent difficulties in their relationship. Stevie informed a primary reason for this was because they were not able to get pregnant after trying to do so "on and off" for at least 3 years. Her husband increasingly became distant, preferring to go out with friends after work and on the weekends. Stevie became more reclusive, wanting to stay home by herself after work and on the weekends. Stevie said this pattern in their marriage eventually led them to stay in separate bedrooms. She reported her husband soon thereafter began having an affair with "Linda," a woman he met in the building where he works. About 8 months ago, her husband moved in with Linda and informed Stevie he wanted a divorce. The divorce was finalized 6 months later and since then, Stevie has consistently struggled to "feel normal." She reported having depressed mood, low energy, difficulty concentrating at work, trouble getting out of bed, and no desire to socialize with her friends. Stevie adamantly denied having any past or present thoughts of suicide: "I may be depressed, but I've never got to the point where I felt there was no way out. Besides, it would hurt my parents too much. I'm also not sure what happens after we die, so I'm not taking any chances by killing myself."

Although Stevie appeared to be open about her mental condition, she was very reluctant to answer questions related to substance use when queried by the counselor: "I'm not sure why you're focused on alcohol and drugs. I called you to talk about being depressed since my marriage fell apart!" The counselor calmly explained this was part of the overall assessment process; however, Stevie became frustrated and questioned if she made the right decision to come to counseling. The counselor, recognizing Stevie was not ready to answer all questions, offered Stevie the space to consider returning for at least one more session to talk about whatever she was willing to share. Stevie felt relieved and agreed to return for a follow-up appointment later that week.

As scheduled, Stevie returned 4 days later to meet with the counselor for the second time. Although the counselor did not press Stevie, the counselor gently reiterated the importance of gathering information in order to best help her. After the counselor spent more time with Stevie empathically listening to her story and genuinely attempting to understand her needs, barriers, and motivations, a therapeutic alliance was being formed. Stevie, now more comfortable with the counselor, admitted she fears she has a drinking problem. Stevie eventually disclosed that although she plans on only having one to two glasses of wine each evening, she usually finishes the whole bottle (which occurs at least four to five times per week for the past several months). When the counselor asked Stevie about drug use (other than alcohol), she reported never taking an illicit drug other than "a hit or two off of a joint" a few times in college. She also denied ever using or being prescribed opioid medications.

Because Stevie felt she could trust the counselor, she soon acknowledged this was not the first time in her life she experienced problems with alcohol. Because she went to the EAP 5 years ago for brief counseling, she returned about 2 years ago when she became concerned that she was drinking to cope with the problems in her marriage. Stevie, who was not drinking as much then as she is now, was recommended by the EAP counselor to engage in outpatient counseling as well as consider a 12-step facilitation group such as Alcoholics Anonymous (AA). Stevie declined counseling but agreed to check out an AA meeting. Using the AA website, she located a women's group that meets on Friday nights in the town where she lives. She said although everyone there was kind, caring, and helpful, she only attended a few meetings because she worried it would make matters worse in her marriage if her husband found out she was drinking to cope and going to AA meetings in their local area: "I didn't want to embarrass him or make him think I was weak." Over time, Stevie's use of alcohol increased in amount and frequency. She said she tried to stop on her own on a few occasions, but each time she would experience anxiety, agitation, and some shakiness in her hands. Stevie soon learned that when she returned to drinking, these issues would subside.

Because Stevie was opening up to the counselor about her situation, the counselor asked if she would allow the counselor to administer two assessment instruments designed to assess the severity of her depression and substance use, to which Stevie agreed. The two instruments were: (a) the Patient Health Questionnaire-9 (PHQ-9) for depressive symptoms and (b) the Addiction Severity Index (ASI) for substance use and addiction-related issues. Stevie's responses to the items on the PHQ-9 resulted in a score of 15 (moderately severe). Results of the ASI (which assesses medical status, employment/support status, alcohol and drug use, legal status, family history/social relationship status, and psychiatric status) yielded a composite score of 6 (considerable problem, treatment necessary) for alcohol use. The counselor discussed the results, and then made the following recommendations while involving Stevie in the decision-making process:

1. Refer Stevie to a nearby treatment facility where a wide range of levels of care are available for co-occurring mental and substance use disorders. Here, Stevie can be evaluated to determine her risk of alcohol withdrawal and assess the need for medically managed intensive inpatient treatment (i.e., detoxification services).

2. Obtain a signed release of information from Stevie so the counselor may consult/collaborate with the treatment facility to which Stevie is being referred, Stevie's primary care physician, as well as Stevie's parents.

3. Continue to engage with Stevie as she moves through the continuum of care, so Stevie can return for outpatient counseling once she no longer clinically requires a higher level of care.

Although anxious about the results, Stevie admitted she has a sense of relief knowing she is no longer hiding the extent of her problems and attempting to primarily deal with them on her own. The counselor coordinated care on behalf of Stevie, which resulted in Stevie attending an evaluation later that day at the treatment facility. After completing a comprehensive evaluation, which included using *The ASAM Criteria*, Stevie was recommended for admission for alcohol detoxification. After safety detoxing on the medically managed inpatient unit where her withdrawal symptoms were treated with a benzodiazepine and monitored using the Clinical Institute Withdrawal Assessment of Alcohol Scale-Revised (CIWA-Ar), Stevie was transitioned to the same facility's intensive outpatient program (IOP) where she received ambulatory outpatient services for both her depressive disorder and alcohol use disorder. She was also routinely seen by a psychiatrist who continued her medication regimen of duloxetine (for depressive symptoms) and initiated acamprosate (for alcohol cravings). Once she successfully completed IOP, Stevie was referred back to the counselor where she attended individual counseling sessions on a weekly basis along with medication management sessions conducted by the psychiatrist who monitored her care while at the treatment facility. Stevie's aftercare plan also included regularly attending Dual Recovery Anonymous (DRA) meetings where she would join the fellowship of other people seeking long-term recovery from CODs.

CASE DISCUSSION

Stevie arrived to counseling with a willingness to discuss and address her depression; however, it became clear to the counselor that Stevie was not willing to answer questions related to substance use. Observing this, the counselor did not pressure or argue with Stevie because the counselor recognized that resistance is a normal reaction for those clients who are ambivalent about changing their substance use behaviors. A plan was negotiated for Stevie to return for a follow-up session, which is where the counselor allowed Stevie to share her history while establishing rapport with her. Once Stevie was more engaged and trusting of the client/counselor relationship, she was able to acknowledge her alcohol problem and accept the counselor's recommendations.

Because Stevie already acknowledged having problems related to depression and alcohol, the counselor offered to conduct a more in-depth evaluation by administering the PHQ-9 and the ASI. Results of this assessment helped the counselor obtain a clearer picture of the severity of Stevie's symptoms, the impact her conditions have on her life, the potential diagnoses, and the level of care that most appropriately matches her clinical needs. This, along with other information provided by Stevie during their conversations, helped the counselor make treatment recommendations. The counselor—recognizing that Stevie only received brief counseling after the miscarriage and that her condition worsened to developing co-occurring depressive alcohol use disorders—understood that Stevie needed integrated services as well as potentially a higher level of care due to experiencing alcohol-related withdrawal symptoms when she stopped drinking on her own in the past.

Once Stevie successfully completed the higher levels of care at the treatment facility, she traveled through the continuum by returning to outpatient services where she (a) resumed individual counseling with her established counselor who used a cognitive behavioral/relapse prevention approach to address negative thought patterns and high-risk situations, (b) continued medication management sessions with Stevie's psychiatrist to treat her depressive and alcohol use disorder symptoms, and (c) began attending 12-step dual recovery group meetings to reinforce recovery and enhance support. The counselor, who also obtained consent from the client prior to the referral, acted as a consultant and collaborator to ensure all other treatment providers (i.e., integrated facility, primary care physician) as well as other collaterals (i.e., parents) were involved in the overall process. It is evident that the various actions taken by the counselor to address Stevie's needs were in alignment with the six guidelines identified by SAMHSA (2020, pp. 16–21), which serve to improve treatment outcomes:

1. Provide access (using a "no wrong door" approach).
2. Complet a full assessment.
3. Provide an appropriate level of care.
4. Achieve integrated treatment.
5. Provide comprehensive services.
6. Ensure continuity of care.

CHAPTER SUMMARY

This chapter covered a wide range of topics that should be considered by counselors working with clients in mental health and addiction treatment settings. Although individual counselors may have a preference when working with certain client populations, they will inevitably encounter clients at risk of having co-occurring mental and substance use disorders. Because of this, they should be prepared to evaluate for and detect the presence of CODs. And, in doing so, the must be knowledgeable of the best-practice guidelines that are in place for linking clients to appropriate services and/or implementing evidence-based treatments that are within the counselor's scope of practice and credentials. Various resources have been referenced herein that counselors may explore as they look to expand their knowledge of and competencies for treating clients who have co-occurring mental and substance use disorders.

DISCUSSION QUESTIONS

1. Recognizing the prevalence of co-occurring mental and substance use disorders, what additional education do you need in order to feel more competent working with this client population?
2. Among various theories regarding the etiology of co-occurring mental and substance use disorders, with which one do you most align? Explain your answer while using evidence-based research to support your stance.
3. What are the key features that distinguish screening procedures from the assessment process when evaluating clients for co-occurring mental and substance use disorders? Next, identify and describe one screening instrument designed for mental disorders, and another screening instrument designed for substance misuse.
4. After reviewing the various treatment approaches, guidelines, and levels of care for co-occurring mental and substance use disorders, which area do you believe you require the most training and supervised experience in order to work competently with clients? Describe your plan to obtain more knowledge and establish your credentials.

5. Consider the ethical and legal considerations related to counselor competencies when treating clients with co-occurring mental and substance use disorders. What steps will you take to ensure you are working within the scope of practice and boundaries of competence?

REFERENCES

Addictions, Drug & Alcohol Institute. (2022, March). *Substance use screening & assessment instruments*. University of Washington, Addictions, Drug & Alcohol Institute. http://lib.adai.uw.edu/instruments/

Alexander, M. J., Haugland, G., Lin, S. P., Bertollo, D. N., & McCorry, F. A. (2008). Mental health screening in addiction, corrections and social service settings: Validating the MMS. *International Journal of Mental Health and Addiction, 6*(1), 105–119. https://doi.org/10.1007/s11469-007-9100-x

American Counseling Association. (2014). *2014 ACA code of ethics*. https://www.counseling.org/docs/default-source/default-document-library/2014-code-of-ethics-finaladdress.pdf

American Psychiatric Association. (2013). *Diagnostic and statistical manual of mental disorders* (5th ed.). https://doi.org/10.1176/appi.books.9780890425596

American Society of Addiction Medicine. (n.d.). *About the ASAM criteria*. Retrieved July 28, 2022, from https://www.asam.org/asam-criteria/about-the-asam-criteria

Babor, T. F., Higgins-Biddle, J. C., Saunders, J. B., & Monteiro, M. G. (2001). *AUDIT: The alcohol use disorders identification test: Guidelines for use in primary care* (2nd ed.). World Health Organization.

Baigent M. (2012). Managing patients with dual diagnosis in psychiatric practice. *Current Opinion in Psychiatry, 25*(3), 201–205. https://doi.org/10.1097/YCO.0b013e3283523d3d

Beck, A. T., & Steer, R. A. (1991). *Manual for the Beck Scale for Suicide Ideation*. Psychological Corporation.

Boothroyd, R. A., Peters, R. H., Armstrong, M. I., RynearsonMoody, S., & Caudy, M. (2015). The psychometric properties of the simple screening instrument for substance abuse. *Evaluation and the Health Professions, 38*(4), 538–562. https://doi.org/10.1177/0163278713490165

Brewin, C. R., Rose, S., Andrews, B., Green, J., Tata, P., McEvedy, C., Turner, S., & Foa, E. B. (2002). Brief screening instrument for post-traumatic stress disorder. *The British Journal of Psychiatry, 181*(2), 158–162. https://doi.org/10.1017/s0007125000161896

Bush, K., Kivlahan, D. R., McDonell, M. B., Fihn, S. D., & Bradley, K. A. (1998). The AUDIT alcohol consumption questions (AUDIT-C): An effective brief screening test for problem drinking. *Archives of Internal Medicine, 158*(16), 1789–1795. https://doi.org/10.1001/archinte.158.16.1789

Carroll, J. F. X., & McGinley, J. J. (2000). *Mental health screening form-iii (MHSF-III)*. Unpublished screening instrument, Project Return Foundation, Inc.

Coffey, S. F., Schumacher, J. A., Nosen, E., Littlefield, A. K., Henslee, A. M., Lappen, A., & Stasiewicz, P. R. (2016). Trauma-focused exposure therapy for chronic posttraumatic stress disorder in alcohol and drug dependent patients: A randomized controlled trial. *Psychology of Addictive Behaviors, 30*(7), 778–790. https://doi.org/10.1037/adb0000201

Derogatis, L. R. (1994). *Symptom Checklist-90-R: Administration, scoring & procedure manual for the revised version of the SCL-90*. National Computer Systems.

Derogatis, L. R., & Melisaratos, N. (1983). The brief symptom inventory: An introductory report. *Psychological Report, 13*(3), 595–605.

DiClemente, C. C., & Hughes, J. R. (1990). Stages of change profiles in outpatient alcoholism treatment. *Journal of Substance Abuse, 2*(2), 217–235. https://doi.org/10.1016/S0899-3289(05)80057-4

HABITS Lab (n.d.a). *Processes of Change Questionnaire: Overview*. University of Maryland Baltimore County. Retrieved August 2, 2022, from https://habitslab.umbc.edu/processes-of-change-questionnaire/

HABITS Lab (n.d.b). *URICA: Overview of the URICA*. University of Maryland Baltimore County. Retrieved August 2, 2022, from https://habitslab.umbc.edu/urica/

Han, B., Compton, W. M., Blanco, C., & Colpe, L. J. (2017). Prevalence, treatment, and unmet treatment needs of US adults with mental and substance use disorders. *Health Affairs, 36*(10), 1739–1747. https://doi.org/10.1377/hlthaff.2017.0584

Hasin, D. S., Trautman, K. D., Miele, G. M., Samet, S., Smith, M., & Endicott, J. (1998). Psychiatric Research Interview for Substance and Mental Disorders (PRISM): Reliability for substance abusers. *American Journal of Psychiatry, 153*(9), 1195–1201. https://doi.org/10.1176/ajp.153.9.1195

Hendrickson, E. L., Schmal, M. S., & Ekleberry, S. C. (2004). *Treating co-occurring disorders: A handbook for mental health and substance abuse professionals*. The Haworth Press, Inc.

Horowitz, L.M., Bridge, J.A., Teach, S.J., Ballard, E., Kilma, J., Rosenstein, D. L., Wharff, E. A., Ginnis, K., Cannon, E., Joshi, P., & Peo, M. (2012). Ask Suicide-Screening Questions (ASQ): a brief instrument for the pediatric emergency department. *Archives of Pediatric and Adolescent Medicine, 166* (12), 1170–1176.

Humeniuk, R., Henry-Edwards, S., Ali, R., Poznyak, V., & Monteiro, M. (2010). *The Alcohol, Smoking and Substance Involvement Screening Test (ASSIST): Manual for use in primary care*. World Health Organization.

Kelly, T. M., & Daley, D. C. (2013). Integrated treatment of substance use and psychiatric disorders. *Social Work in Public Health, 28*(3–4). https://doi.org/10.1080/19371918.2013.774673

Knight, J., Shrier, L., Bravender, T., Farrell, M., VanderBilt, J. & Shaffer, H. (1999). A new brief screen for adolescent substance abuse. *Archives of Pediatric and Adolescent Medicine, 153*(6), 591–596. https://doi.org/10.1001/archpedi.153.6.591

Kroenke, K., Spitzer, R. L., & Williams, J. B. W. (2001). The PHQ-9: Validity of a brief depression severity measure. *Journal of General Internal Medicine, 16*(9), 606–613. https://doi.org/10.1046/j.1525-1497.2001.016009606.x

Kroenke, K., Spitzer, R. L., & Williams, J. B. W. (2003). The Patient Health Questionnaire-2: Validity of a two-item depression screener. *Medical Care, 41*(11), 1284–1292. https://doi.org/10.1097/01.MLR.0000093487.78664.3C

Lai, H. M. X., Cleary, M. Sitharthan, T., & Hunt, G. E. (2015). Prevalence of comorbid substance use, anxiety and mood disorders in epidemiological surveys, 1990–2014: A systematic review and meta-analysis. *Drug and Alcohol Dependence, 154*, 1–13. https://doi.org/10.1016/j.drugalcdep.2015.05.031

Lee, S. J., Crowther, E., Keating, C., & Kulkarni, J. (2012). What is needed to deliver collaborative care to address comorbidity more effectively with adults with severe mental illness. *Australian & New Zealand Journal of Psychiatry, 47*(4), 333–346. https://doi.org/10.1177/0004867412463975

Mangrum, L. F., Spence, R. T., & Lopez, M. (2006). Integrated versus parallel treatment of co-occurring psychiatric and substance use disorders. *Journal of Substance Abuse Treatment, 30*(1), 79–84. https://doi.org/10.1016/j.jsat.2005.10.004

McLellan, A. T., Kushner, H., Metzger, D., Peters, R. H., Smith, I., Grissom, G., & Argeriou, M. (1992). The fifth edition of the Addiction Severity Index. *Journal of Substance Abuse Treatment, 9*(3), 199–213. https://doi.org/10.1016/0740-5472(92)90062-s

Mdege, N. D., & Lang, J. (2011). Screening instruments for detecting illicit drug use/abuse that could be useful in general hospital wards: A systematic review. *Addictive Behaviors, 36*(12), 1111–1119. https://doi.org/10.1016/j.addbeh.2011.07.007

Mitchell, S. G., Kelly, S. M, Gryczynski, J., Myers, C. P., O'Grady, K. E., Kirk, A. S., & Schwartz, R. P. (2014). The CRAFFT cut-points and DSM-5 criteria for alcohol and other drugs: A re-evaluation and re-examination. *Substance Abuse, 35*(4), 376–380. https://doi.org/10.1080/08897077.2014.936992

Najavits, L. M. (2002). *Seeking safety: A treatment manual for PTSD and substance abuse*. The Guilford Press.

National Institute on Drug Abuse (2018a, January). *Principles of drug addiction treatment: A researched-based guide*. (3rd ed.). U.S. Department of Health and Human Services, National Institutes of Health. https://nida.nih.gov/sites/default/files/675-principles-of-drug-addiction-treatment-a-research-based-guide-third-edition.pdf

National Institute on Drug Abuse (2018b, August). *Comorbidity: Substance use disorders and other mental illnesses drugfacts*. U.S. Department of Health and Human Services, National Institutes of Health. https://nida.nih.gov/publications/drugfacts/comorbidity-substance-use-disorders-other-mental-illnesses

National Institute on Drug Abuse (2019, August). *Genetics and epigenetics of addiction drugfacts*. U.S. Department of Health and Human Services, National Institutes of Health. https://nida.nih.gov/publications/drugfacts/genetics-epigenetics-addiction

National Institute on Drug Abuse (2020, April). *Common comorbidities with substance use disorders research report*. Department of Health and Human Services, National Institutes of Health. https://www.ncbi.nlm.nih.gov/books/NBK571451/

Osman, A., Bagge, C. L., Gutierrez, P. M., Konick, L. C., Kopper, B. A., & Barrios, F. X. (2001). The Suicidal Behaviors Questionnaire-Revised (SBQ-R): Validation with clinical and nonclinical samples. *Assessment, 8*(4), 443–454. https://doi.org/10.1177/107319110100800409

Otasowie, J. (2021). Co-occurring mental disorder and substance use disorder in young people: Aetiology, assessment and treatment. *BJPsych Advances, 27*(4), 272–281. https://doi.org/10.1192/bja.2020.64

Peachey, J. E., & Lei, H. (1988). Assessment of opioid dependence with naloxone. *British Journal of Addiction, 83*(2), 193–201. https://doi.org/10.1111/j.1360-0443.1988.tb03981.x

Posner, K., Brown, G. K., Stanley, B., Brent, D. A., Yershova, K. V., Oquendo, M. A., Currier, G. W., Melvin, G. A., Greenhill, L., Shen, S., & Mann, J. J. (2011). The Columbia-Suicide Severity Rating Scale: Initial validity and internal consistency findings from three multisite studies with adolescents and adults. *American Journal of Psychiatry, 168*(12), 1266–1277. https://doi.org/10.1176/appi.ajp.2011.10111704

Prins, A., Bovin, M. J., Kimerling, R., Kaloupek, D. G, Marx, B. P., Pless Kaiser, A., & Schnurr, P. P. (2015). Primary Care PTSD Screen for DSM-5 (PC-PTSD-5) [Measurement instrument]. Available from https://www.ptsd.va.gov

Rush, B., Castel, S., Brands, B., Toneatto, T., & Veldhuizen, S. (2013). Validation and comparison of diagnostic accuracy of four screening tools for mental disorders in people seeking treatment for substance use disorders. *Journal of Substance Abuse Treatment, 44*(4), 375–383. https://doi.org/10.1016/j.jsat.2012.08.221

Sacks, S., Melnick, G., Coen, C., Banks, S., Friedmann, P. D., Grella, C., & Knight, K. (2007). CJDATS Co-Occurring Disorders Screening Instrument for Mental Disorders (CODSI-MD): A pilot study. *The Prison Journal, 87*(1), 86–110. https://doi.org/10.1177/0032885506299044

Santucci, K. (2012). Psychiatric disease and drug abuse. *Current Opinion in Pediatrics, 24*(2), 233–237. https://doi.org/10.1097/MOP.0b013e3283504fbf

Scanlon, F., Hirsch, S., & Morgan, R. D. (2022). The relation between the working alliance on mental illness and criminal thinking among justice-involved people with co-occurring mental illness and substance use disorders. *Journal of Consulting and Clinical Psychology, 90*(3), 282–288. https://doi.org/10.1037/ccp0000719

Selzer, M. L. (1971). The Michigan Alcoholism Screening Test: The quest for a new diagnostic instrument. *American Journal of Psychiatry, 127*(12), 1653–1658. https://doi.org/10.1176/ajp.127.12.1653

Sheehan, D. V., Lecrubier, Y., Sheehan, K. H., Amorim, P., Janavs, J., Weiller, E., Hergueta, T., Baker, R. & Dunbar, G. C. (1998). The Mini-International Neuropsychiatric Interview (M.I.N.I.): The development and validation of a structured diagnostic psychiatric interview for DSM-IV and ICD-10. *Journal of Clinical Psychiatry, 59*(Suppl. 20), 22–33.

Skinner, H. A. (1982). The Drug Abuse Screening Test. *Addictive Behaviors, 7*(4), 363–371. https://doi.org/10.1016/0306-4603(82)90005-3

Sohal, H., Eldridge, S., & Feder, G. (2007). The sensitivity and specificity of four questions (HARK) to identify intimate partner violence: A diagnostic accuracy study in general practice. *BMC Family Practice, 8*(49). https://doi.org/10.1186/1471-2296-8-49

Spitzer, R. L., Kroenke, K., Williams, J. B. W., & Lowe, B. (2006). A brief measure for assessing generalized anxiety disorder: the GAD-7. *Archives of Internal Medicine Research, 166*(10), 1092–1097. https://doi.org/10.1001/archinte.166.10.1092

Substance Abuse and Mental Health Services Administration (2015). *Screening and assessment of co-occurring disorders in the justice system*. (HHS Publication No. PEP19-SCREEN-CODJS). U.S. Department of Health and Human Services, Substance Abuse and Mental Health Services Administration. https://store.samhsa.gov/sites/default/files/d7/priv/pep19-screen-codjs.pdf

Substance Abuse and Mental Health Services Administration (2020). *Substance use disorder treatment for people with co-occurring disorders: Treatment improvement protocol (TIP) 42*. (SAMHSA Publication No. PEP20-02-01-004). U.S. Department of Health and Human Services, Substance Abuse and Mental Health Services Administration. https://store.samhsa.gov/sites/default/files/SAMHSA_Digital_Download/PEP20-02-01-004_Final_508.pdf

Substance Abuse and Mental Health Services Administration (2021). *Key substance use and mental health indicators in the United States: Results from the 2020 National Survey on Drug Use and Health* (HHS Publication No. PEP21-07-01-003, NSDUH Series H-56). Center for Behavioral Health Statistics and Quality, Substance Abuse and Mental Health Services Administration. https://www.samhsa.gov/data/report/2020-nsduh-annual-national-report

Sullivan, J. T., Sykora, K., Schneiderman, J., Naranjo, C. A., & Sellers, E. M. (1989). Assessment of alcohol withdrawal: The revised Clinical Institute Withdrawal Assessment for Alcohol scale (CIWA-Ar). *British Journal of Addiction, 84*(11), 1353–1357. https://doi.org/10.1111/j.1360-0443.1989.tb00737.x

Valderas, J. M., Starfield, B., Sibbald, B., Salisbury, C., & Roland, M. (2009) Defining comorbidity: Implications for understanding health and health services. *Annals of Family Medicine, 7*(4), 357–363. https://doi.org/10.1370/afm.983

Weathers, F.W., Litz, B.T., Keane, T.M., Palmieri, P.A., Marx, B.P., & Schnurr, P.P. (2013). *The PTSD Checklist for DSM-5 (PCL-5)*. Scale available from the National Center for PTSD at www.ptsd.va.gov.

Weiss, R. D., & Connery, H. S. (2001). *Integrated group therapy for bipolar disorder and substance abuse.* The Guilford Press.

Wesson, D. R., & Ling, W. (2003). The Clinical Opiate Withdrawal Scale (COWS). *Journal of Psychoactive Drugs, 35*(2), 253–259. https://doi.org/10.1080/02791072.2003.10400007

Wolfe, J., & Kimerling, R. (1997). Gender issues in the assessment of posttraumatic stress disorder. In J. Wilson & T. M. Keane (Eds.), *Assessing psychological trauma and PTSD* (pp. 192–238). The Guilford Press.

CHAPTER 2

UNDERSTANDING DRUGS OF ABUSE AND ADDICTION

REGINA R. MORO

LEARNING OBJECTIVES

After reading this chapter, you will be able to:

- Describe common substances of abuse, including their routes of administration and biological effects.
- Identify symptoms of addiction in clients' clinical case histories.
- Summarize the diagnostic categories and classification system of addictive disorders.
- Explain the common models of addiction including the moral model, the brain disease model, and the biopsychosocial model.

INTRODUCTION

The "Six Degrees of Kevin Bacon" game is one in which players try to connect one Hollywood actor to another, ultimately ending with the actor Kevin Bacon. The idea is that there are so many connections among those in Hollywood that it would take no more than six connections to make this happen. This game is built on the concept of *Six Degrees of Separation* where all individuals on this earth are connected via a network of no more than six people (MacMillan, 2018). When applying this concept to the world of addiction, it is highly probable that any one person is affected by addiction by at least six degrees of separation. Considering there are many individuals in the United States struggling with addiction themselves, there is an exorbitant number of family members, friends, coworkers, and other acquaintances who are touched by the addictive disease. Because of this "six degrees of addiction," counselors need to be prepared to not only serve those clients struggling with addiction using evidence-based practices, they also need to know how to support those affected indirectly via another person's addiction. The purpose of this chapter is to provide a baseline understanding of addiction to inform the work of the counseling professional.

The American Society of Addiction Medicine (ASAM, 2019) defines addiction as "a treatable, chronic medical disease involving complex interactions among brain circuits, genetics, the environment, and an individual's life experiences. People with addiction use substances or engage in behaviors that become compulsive and often continue despite harmful consequences" (para. 1). The continued use and compulsion occurs in a three-stage cycle that is repeated over and over: (a) binge/intoxication, (b) withdrawal/negative affect, and (c) preoccupation/anticipation (craving; Koob & Volkow, 2016). The ASAM continues the definition by highlighting that prevention efforts and treatment approaches are successful when compared to other chronic diseases. This definition aims to combat the stigma that surrounds addiction by positioning it as a disease that is treatable in comparison with other diseases (such as diabetes or heart disease). Stigma is pervasive in regard to addiction, resulting in individuals experiencing negative stereotyping, discrimination, and societal rejection; it affects institutional practices and policies in detrimental ways (McGinty & Barry, 2020). Considering the vast impact that addiction has on society, it is vital that counselors take all necessary steps to combat this negative image by providing competent and compassionate care for individuals affected by addiction.

Our society is drastically impacted by addiction. According to the Office of the Surgeon General of the United States (2022), the economic impact of addiction from alcohol misuse and illicit drug use is estimated to be more than $440 billion. Deaths in the United States from overdosing on drugs were recently higher than at any point in recorded history, with over 107,000 individuals dying from drug overdoses in 2021 (Ahmad et al., 2022). In 2020, over 11,600 deaths occurred in motor vehicle crashes where at least one driver was impaired by alcohol—this averages out to an alcohol-related death occurring every 45 minutes (National Center for Statistics and Analysis, 2022). Although significant attention has been poured into the opioid crisis, there is a larger epidemic occurring in this country.

The addiction epidemic is rampant with over 40.3 million people ages 12 and older meeting criteria for a diagnosis of a substance use disorder (SUD) in 2020 (Substance Abuse and Mental Health Services Administration [SAMHSA], 2021). Despite this number which represents approximately 12% of the U.S. population in 2020, it does not capture all users of substances. A review of what is involved for a diagnosis of a SUD is offered later in this chapter; however, it is important to first point out that not all who use substances go on to develop an addictive disorder. While 12% of those who used substances qualified for a SUD, 58.7% of individuals aged 12 and older (162.5 million Americans) reported using either alcohol, tobacco, or illicit drugs in the past month (SAMHSA, 2021). Additionally, the National Survey on Drug Use and Health (NSDUH; SAMHSA, 2021) provided information about the use of substances for the first time. In 2020, the number of individuals aged 12 and older began using the following substances (SAMHSA, 2021):

- 4.1 million: alcohol
- 2.8 million: marijuana
- 1.4 million: hallucinogens
- 1.2 million: prescription pain relievers
- 950,000: prescription tranquilizers
- 734,000: prescription stimulants
- 489,000: cocaine
- 153,000: methamphetamine
- 103,000: heroin

These numbers represent close to 12 million Americans who are at risk for developing future SUDs—a significant number in combination with those who have already been diagnosed with a SUD. These numbers are not presented to paint a grim picture, but to highlight the strong toll addiction has in the world, and to encourage counselors to pay attention to this issue. Addiction, or the effects of addiction, will be encountered in all settings where counselors work. It is in the client's best interest for counselors to be well informed and ready to help develop the most appropriate treatment plan possible.

DRUG CATEGORIES, SUBSTANCE TYPES, AND ADMINISTRATION ROUTES

There are many different names for the chemicals that cause mood-altering effects in the body. Psychoactive drugs, psychoactive substances, substances of abuse, and simply, drugs, are just a few. Throughout this chapter the term *substances of abuse* will primarily be used, although others may be used interchangeably. Substances of abuse are generally classified according to the effects they have on the central and peripheral nervous systems (CNS and PNS, respectively; Inaba & Cohen, 2007). The CNS, composed of the brain and the spinal cord, is "the force behind all functioning" in a human body "from reflexes to intentional movement" (Luke, 2016, p. 34). The PNS is composed of a few subsystems, notably somatic and autonomic nervous systems (Ingersoll & Rak, 2016). The focus of substances of abuse is on the CNS; however, the PNS does experience side effects (Ingersoll & Rak, 2016).

The three overarching categories on which this chapter focuses are: (a) CNS stimulants, (b) CNS depressants, and (c) psychedelics. It is important to note that most substances of abuse are derived from plants that naturally grow on Earth. The process used to derive these substances has evolved over the years, from early distilling practices that are still in use today to newer synthesizing procedures in which scientists are able to isolate and create new chemical compounds (Inaba & Cohen, 2007). Many of the psychoactive drugs used and abused today were accidentally discovered when scientists were working on other projects. This chapter does not cover all substances that are used and abused in the world today, but it will provide an overview of those substances a counselor may encounter when working with clients. To learn more about substances of abuse, readers are directed to the *Drug Wheel*, an interactive learning resource freely available on the Alcohol and Drug Foundation's website (https://adf.org.au/drug-facts/ - wheel).

CENTRAL NERVOUS SYSTEM STIMULANTS

Stimulants affect the CNS by increasing electrical and chemical activity (Inaba & Cohen, 2007). The Alcohol and Drug Foundation (2022) highlights the effect these substances can have on a person to make them feel more awake, alert, and as though they have more energy. However, at higher doses these substances can make an individual feel anxious, tense, and nauseous, as well as experience seizures and increased heart rate, blood pressure, and body temperature, among other undesirable symptoms. It is important to understand that what constitutes a high dose is dependent on factors specific to the individual user such as age, health status, weight, and tolerance level. A few of the key stimulants that are commonly abused are explored in more detail.

Amphetamines

Amphetamine was first synthesized in 1887 by a German chemist seeking to find a substitute for ephedrine, a medication used to treat asthma (Inaba & Cohen, 2007). Although this novel discovery provided relief from asthma by dilating the bronchioles, the substance also produced a feeling of euphoria for users (Kuhn & Wilson, 2008). Amphetamine use quickly became widespread, in part, due to World War II. Military personnel used amphetamine during the Second World War because it allowed them to remain alert and focused for extended periods of time (Inaba & Cohen, 2007). Amphetamine use spread after the war to civilian populations, and it was during this time that "Japan experienced the first known wave of stimulant addiction" (Kuhn & Wilson, 2008, p. 226). Amphetamines have a complicated substance profile consisting of a variety of prescription medications, as well as illegally manufactured substances (e.g., methamphetamine). Dangers associated with amphetamine abuse involve not only the risk of developing an addiction, but the possibility of overdose as well as experiencing psychotic symptoms from repeated high-dose use (Kuhn & Wilson, 2008).

Methamphetamine

Methamphetamine was synthesized from amphetamine in Japan in 1919 (Inaba & Cohen, 2007). Methamphetamine abuse is a widely known phenomenon in society, particularly following the release of the *Breaking Bad* (Gilligan, 2008–2013) television show in the mid-2000s. According to the National Institute of Drug Abuse (NIDA, 2022d), methamphetamine is available in a variety of forms (e.g., powder, crystal) as well as the manner in which it is ingested (e.g., smoking, snorting, injecting). Short-term effects of methamphetamine use include a sense of euphoria, appetite suppression, increased heart rate and breathing, more energy, and an increased body temperature. Long-term effects include anxiety, confusion, itchy skin (which can result in sores), and tooth decay (NIDA, 2022d). Common street names for methamphetamine include "meth," "crystal meth," "ice," and "speed."

Methamphetamine is considered to be highly addictive, in large part due to causing the brain to experience an intense surge of dopamine—one of the "feel-good" hormones. Another danger associated with the substance is related to its creation in illegal and clandestine laboratories. A chemical, pseudoephedrine, which is found in certain cold medicines, can be used to create illicit methamphetamine (Inaba & Cohen, 2007). Because of the wide availability of the cold medicine, many states began restricting the availability of these medications in the mid 2000s. And, in 2006, the U.S. government restricted access to these medications on a federal level (Inaba & Cohen, 2007). Methamphetamine abuse has had catastrophic consequences for users, and sadly the use continues in the United States. During 2020, over 2 million people ages 12 and older reported using methamphetamine, with the highest percentage of individuals being between 18 and 25 years old (SAMHSA, 2021).

Prescription Stimulants

Physicians may prescribe stimulants for a few medical conditions, but the focus here is on their use for the treatment of attention deficit hyperactivity disorder (ADHD). ADHD is characterized by a "persistent pattern of inattention and/or hyperactivity-impulsivity that interferes with functioning or development" (American Psychiatric Association [APA], 2013, p. 61). The prescription stimulants used to treat ADHD are methylphenidate (brand name Ritalin), dextroamphetamine sulfate (brand name Dexedrine), and amphetamine/dextroamphetamine (brand name Adderall). When prescription stimulants are used appropriately in accordance with their prescription, they can result in increased focus, attention, and alertness (NIDA, 2022g). While it may seem counterintuitive to prescribe stimulant medications to treat ADHD, it is hypothesized that prescription stimulants influence the concentration of neurotransmitters in the brain (e.g., dopamine, serotonin), which contributes to increasing focus and a sense of calmness (Inaba & Cohen, 2007).

Prescription stimulants can be abused in a few different ways. Examples include when using them in ways not recommended by the prescriber (e.g., taking more than prescribed, specifically to get high), or when taking pills that were not prescribed for the user (NIDA, 2022g). When prescription stimulants are misused, they can produce side effects such as high blood pressure, high body temperature, increased heart rate (which can lead to heart issues), disturbances in sleep, and mood disruptions (e.g., anger; NIDA, 2022g). Common street names for prescription stimulants include "addies," "vitamin R," "smarties," or "study buddies."

According to Kuhn and Wilson (2008), prescribing stimulants for treating ADHD has a controversial history that continues to this day. Some of the controversy involves concerns about medicating children in general as well as the difficulties accurately diagnosing ADHD. There is also a concern about the possibility that stimulants are being overprescribed, which is partly illuminated by the COVID-19 global pandemic and the resulting increase in telehealth utilization. While telehealth existed well before the pandemic, the lockdowns in early 2020 forced many healthcare workers to transition to remote practices, thus requiring consumers to utilize telehealth services. An online mental health company became the focus of a federal investigation in 2022, with complaints related to the prescribing of stimulants in particular (Landi, 2022). One article alleged that individual users were able to create multiple user accounts, and thus were able to obtain more prescriptions than they otherwise would have been able to as a single user (Landi, 2022). While the investigation is currently ongoing at the time of this writing, this appears to be a novel way to "doctor shop" where a consumer would go to multiple doctors to obtain more prescriptions than they would have been allowed. This specific situation highlights some of the concerns associated with prescribing practices, which may result in requiring companies to examine the safety mechanisms they have in place to mitigate the risk of addiction that could potentially result from overprescribing.

COCAINE

Cocaine is derived from the leaves of the coca bush, which is a shrub that grows naturally in the Andes Mountains of South America (Inaba & Cohen, 2007). Use of the coca leaves has occurred throughout much of history by native populations. Coca "leaves were chewed for their alerting effects and their ability to increase endurance, particularly at the high altitudes" where these individuals lived (Kuhn & Wilson, 2008, p. 224). Cocaine was isolated from the other chemicals in the coca leaf by a German graduate student in 1859 (Inaba & Cohen, 2007). Subsequently, the late 1800s and early 1900s saw widespread use of cocaine (often in liquid form) in both Europe and American (Inaba & Cohen, 2007). According to Inaba and Cohen (2007), there have been numerous waves of problematic cocaine use in society, which has continued to evolve over the years. Early cocaine use focused on beverages being infused with the substance, to switching its use to intravenous injection or snorting through the nasal passage; freebase cocaine was discovered in the mid-1970s. Although cocaine had been smoked prior to this, the freebase technique, which involves smoking a concentrated amount, preserves most of the psychoactive properties in a way the prior cigarette form was not able to do. And, because of the concentrated intensity associated with freebasing cocaine, this method is considered to be significantly more addictive.

Short-term effects of cocaine use include feeling euphoric, experiencing extreme happiness, being energized, feeling out of control, feeling annoyed, feeling paranoid or distrustful of others, increased body temperature, and experiencing hypersensitivity of senses (sight, hearing, touch). Long-term effects are associated with the mechanism used to ingest the substance and can include nasal passage disturbances (nosebleeds, loss of smell, problems swallowing) and pulmonary problems (NIDA, 2022a). Users of cocaine are also at risk for overdose, with warning signs being an irregular heart rhythm or even a heart attack, stroke, or seizure (NIDA, 2022a). The number of overdose deaths involving cocaine has risen through the years, and during 2019 approximately one in five overdose deaths in the United States involved cocaine (Centers for Disease Control and Prevention [CDC], 2021b). Common street names for cocaine often are associated with their delivery mechanism/route of administration. For example, cocaine that is snorted is referred to as "coke," "blow," "snow," or "nose candy," while freebase cocaine is known as "crack," "rock," or "base" (Inaba & Cohen, 2007, p. 96).

Tobacco/Nicotine

The use of the tobacco plant dates back thousands of years. The chemical in the tobacco plant that produces a psychoactive effect is nicotine (Inaba & Cohen, 2007). Nicotine is highly addictive, and there are many different ways users ingest tobacco (and therefore nicotine): smoking/inhaling (cigarettes, cigars, vaping devices, hookahs); chewing (chewing tobacco, dip); or sniffing (snuff; NIDA, 2022e). As a stimulant, nicotine produces effects by releasing adrenaline in a user's system, resulting in increased heart rate, blood pressure, and quickened breathing (NIDA, 2022e). Abuse of tobacco can produce significant health consequences for users including cancer, lung problems, heart disease, tooth decoloring, and serious eye conditions and ocular diseases (NIDA, 2022e).

A concerning nicotine use-related trend is the increase of adolescents and young adults who are using vaping devices. A vaping device, also called a vaporizer or vape, is a small container holding a liquid substance (flavoring and/or nicotine). The device heats up the liquid so that the user, when they inhale on the device, inhale an aerosol that contains an aerated substance such as flavoring and/or nicotine (Patrick et al., 2016). Many adults report using vaping devices to help them cut down on their cigarette use (Nicksic et al., 2019). For adolescents and younger users, there is a concerning trend of experimenting with vaping that can lead to daily use. In 2020, 1.3 million adolescents ages 12 to 17 reported use of a vape device to vape nicotine in the past month (SAMHSA, 2021). The previous year, 1.9% of 8th grade students reported they were vaping nicotine daily in comparison to 0.8% who reported smoking cigarettes daily (NIDA, 2022e). Due to the highly addictive nature of nicotine, it is not surprising that casual vape users become daily users in a short amount of time.

While there is a perception that vaping is safer than other tobacco delivery forms, this is solely a myth. Vaping can have devastating effects for users, especially adolescents by affecting the developing brain (Patrick et al., 2016). When the brain is exposed to nicotine while still developing (which lasts well into the mid-20s), brain circuit development can be interrupted, which can cause issues with attention and learning (U.S. Department of Health and Human Services [DHHS], 2016). Another problem with vaping is when a user does not know what the device contains, either because of their limited understanding of what a vape is, or because they are using someone else's device. This may result in someone thinking they are solely vaping a strawberry flavoring (which they are often led to believe via problematic marketing), and not realizing it also includes nicotine, which, according to the CDC (2022b) the majority of vapes contain. In addition, these devices are also used to vape other substances such as cannabis; when using a device that is not their own, this may result in a user inadvertently inhaling cannabis. Many vaping devices are created to be easily hidden as they mimic common items used in daily life (e.g., medical inhaler, USB flash drives, or pens). Counselors can help prevent the damage caused by vaping by providing psychoeducation to parents, adolescents, and young adults about the associated dangers.

Amphetamines, cocaine, nicotine, and prescription stimulants are some of the most commonly abused CNS stimulants; however, there are many others that were not reviewed here. These include betel nut, khat, caffeine, and pseudoephedrine. Stimulants are an interesting category with a significant number of the substances of abuse being legally available, and/or the use of them (e.g., caffeine) normalized in culture and society. Therefore, counselors need to be particularly savvy at assessing when problematic use may be occurring.

CENTRAL NERVOUS SYSTEM DEPRESSANTS

Depressants affect the CNS by decreasing electrical and chemical activity (Inaba & Cohen, 2007). In general, CNS depressants produce sedative effects such as relaxation and drowsiness, and can even induce a coma (Inaba & Cohen, 2007). CNS depressants are a highly abused category of substances that includes but is not limited to alcohol, benzodiazepines, and opioids. As a reminder, not all CNS depressants are covered here, and readers are reminded to explore more on the Drug Wheel resource mentioned at the beginning of this section.

ALCOHOL

Alcohol use has been around for thousands of years around the world. Historical reports date the first use of alcohol to approximately 10,000 to 15,000 years ago (Veach et al., 2012). It has been claimed that alcohol has the most extensive history of any psychoactive substance in the world (Heather & Stockwell, 2004). In today's society, alcohol use is quite normalized. According to SAMHSA (2021), approximately 50% of individuals ages 12 and older (138.5 million Americans) reported drinking alcohol in the past month. And although not all use is problematic, 28.6% of these individuals reported binge or heavy use. This same report indicated that 40.3 million users had an alcohol use disorder in the past year.

Alcohol comes in a variety of forms such as hard liquor, beer, wine, or malt liquors, each with their own concentration levels of alcohol. A standard drink consists of 5.0 ounces of wine, 12.0 ounces of beer, 1.5 ounces of hard liquor, and 8.0 to 10.0 ounces of malt liquor like a popular hard seltzer (National Institute of Alcohol Abuse and Alcoholism, 2016). Educating clients on standard drink sizes can provide enlightening conversations. For example, a standard pint of beer at a local bar is 16.0 ounces of beer (which is more than one standard drink). This number can also rise if the concentration of alcohol in that beer is more than a regular beer at 5.0%, which is common with craft beers. Consumers may think they are having just one drink, but the reality is quite different. Alcohol is most commonly consumed via the digestive track; however, users are continually discovering novel ways to become intoxicated such as with anal and vaginal administrations (see Stogner et al., 2014, for more information).

Alcohol affects many parts of the brain when consumed, which produce a variety of effects for the user. While there are many neurotransmitters (chemical messengers) affected by alcohol, one notable one is gamma-aminobutyric acid (GAMA), which controls inhibitory functions in the brain (Inaba & Cohen, 2007). When alcohol is consumed GAMA is activated, and this results in lowered inhibitions as well as a general slowing down of functions in the brain (Inaba & Cohen, 2007). Once alcohol is ingested, it is absorbed by the bloodstream resulting in a blood alcohol level—also known as blood alcohol concentration (BAC), which is used throughout this section. Many individuals are familiar with BACs in relation to driving privileges. A BAC of .08 or more is illegal for drivers in the United States, with some professions (truck driver, pilots) being much less (Inaba & Cohen, 2007). A BAC of .50 is high enough to result in death;

however, this author (Moro) has seen clients in a hospital setting with BACs higher than .60. Although this was out of the ordinary, these individuals were daily heavy users of alcohol and had built up a high enough tolerance to allow their BACs to get to that point. According to Inaba and Cohen (2007), any amount of alcohol in a user's system results in impairment, with lower levels impairing the body in the following ways: lowered inhibitions, loss of muscle coordination, and decreased alertness. At moderate levels, a user may experience further loss of coordination resulting in unsteady standing or walking, experiencing exaggerated emotions, and having slurred speech. At high levels, a user can experience unconsciousness, possible coma, and lung and heart failure leading to death. When alcohol is combined with other CNS depressants, the effects are increased and can be quite dangerous (Kuhn & Wilson, 2008). This is why medications (e.g., benzodiazepines, pain relievers) come with a warning to not consume alcohol while using the medication.

It is crucial that counselors are aware of the dangers associated with alcohol use, as well as with the dangers associated with alcohol withdrawal (which can be deadly). Withdrawing from alcohol, as with any substance, produces effects that are opposite to the effects experienced when actively using the substance. Therefore, withdrawing from alcohol (known as alcohol withdrawal syndrome [AWS]) mimics a stimulant and can produce the following effects in the body: headache, nausea, vomiting, tremors, sweats, tachycardia, low-grade fever, anxiety, and agitation (McKeon et al., 2007). What is significantly dangerous is when a user experiences delirium tremens, which are "dramatic symptoms [that] can include trembling over the whole body, grand mal seizures, disorientation, insomnia, and delirium, and severe auditory, visual, and tactile hallucinations" (Inaba & Cohen, 2007, p. 230). Other complications from alcohol withdrawal can ensue, although a more thorough discussion on these is beyond the scope of this chapter. Readers are directed to McKeon et al. (2007) for a more comprehensive overview of AWS. Considering the large portion of the population who use alcohol, despite many being low-risk users, it is important for counselors to be prepared to discuss alcohol use with clients as well as provide psychoeducation about its dangers when needed.

Benzodiazepines

Benzodiazepines are a classification of prescription medication used in the United States to treat anxiety disorders (Bandelow, 2020). They are also used to treat other medical conditions such as insomnia, skeletal muscular spasms, and seizures (Inaba & Cohen, 2007). Common benzodiazepines are alprazolam (brand name Xanax), lorazepam (brand name Ativan), and clonazepam (brand name Klonopin). Common street names for these substances include "benzos," "bars," or "zannies." The effects and dangers of benzodiazepine use are very similar to those associated with alcohol use. For example:

- Benzodiazepines induce similar side effects (e.g., calmness, relaxation, sedation).
- Benzodiazepines are used in the medical process of withdrawing someone off alcohol, which reduces the likelihood they will experience complications from withdrawal.
- Benzodiazepine withdrawal can be life-threatening if not medically managed.

In 2020, 1.8 million Americans over the age of 11 reported misusing benzodiazepines, with adults ages 18 to 25 the most common age group reporting misuse (SAMHSA, 2021).

Opioids

Opioids is a large classification of substances that were initially derived from the opium poppy plant (Inaba & Cohen, 2007). Two terms are used when describing these substances: opiates and opioids. The difference between the two is that *opiates* are refined from the natural poppy plant (e.g., morphine, heroin), where *opioids* (e.g., oxycodone, hydrocodone) are synthesized or created in a lab (Alcohol and Drug Policy Commission, n.d.). Both groups are narcotic drugs, and the terms are used interchangeably in the literature; however, many prefer the term *opioid* when referring to both types. Consequently, *opioid* will be used herein as an umbrella term to describe both opiates and opioids.

Heroin

There is a significant history of using opium from the poppy plant for a variety of reasons, including medical purposes and for its pleasure-inducing qualities (Inaba & Cohen, 2007). In the early 1800s morphine was isolated from the opium of the poppy plant, codeine closely followed in 1832, and heroin was isolated in 1874 (Inaba & Cohen, 2007). With the exception of codeine, all other substances refined or synthesized from the poppy plant have been considerably stronger in potency. According to NIDA (2022f), heroin can be a powder that is either white or brown, or may be a substance that is black and sticky (known as "black tar heroin"). Short-term effects of heroin include feelings of calmness, possible confusion, sedation, reduced respiratory activity (slowed breathing), and digestive issues (nausea, vomiting). Long-term effects can include lung and heart infections, constipation, decreased sexual desire, and menstrual cycle delays (Inaba & Cohen, 2007; NIDA, 2022f). Common street names for heroin include "smack," "junk," "H," "China White," and "black tar" as already mentioned.

Fentanyl

Fentanyl is an opioid that has caused significant concerns in the past few years. Fentanyl is 100 times more potent than morphine and 50 times more potent than heroin (CDC, 2022a). The side effects produced are similar to heroin; however, the risk of overdosing on fentanyl is significantly higher due to the strong potency of the substance. Fentanyl comes in different forms: pills, powder, and liquid (CDC, 2022a). One significant concern associated with fentanyl is the tendency for other substances to be laced with it. *Lacing* refers to mixing one substance with another. For example, powdered fentanyl could be sprinkled into a baggie of powdered heroin with or without the knowledge of the consumer. While the user's experience of euphoric feelings may be significantly increased, they are also at an increased risk for overdose. Another way people may be unintentionally exposed is related to the high tendency for counterfeit prescription pills, such as alprazolam or oxycodone, to contain fentanyl (Palamar et al., 2022). Although some users may understand the risks associated with taking illegal benzodiazepines, they are less likely to know when those benzodiazepines are not pure, illegally produced, and contain a number of other substances that are not remotely chemically similar to benzodiazepines (e.g., fentanyl). Fortunately, there is a harm reduction method involving strips that can be used to safety test substances for the presence of fentanyl. Local health departments are a great resource to learn about test strip availability in local areas.

Prescription Pain Medication

The management of pain is a significant concern of medical providers in the United States. Pain may be due to a recent surgical procedure, an injury, or it may be chronic. In fact, one in five U.S. adults suffers from chronic pain (Zelaya et al., 2020), such as arthritis or back pain. Prescribing opioids for chronic pain began in the late 1990s (CDC, 2017). In 2006 there was a notable increase in opioid dispensing rates with over 72 prescriptions for opioids for every 100 persons (totaling over 215 million prescriptions). This rate increased thereafter; in 2012 there were approximately 81.3 opioid prescriptions for every 100 persons, which equates to over 255 million prescriptions (CDC, 2021a). Since 2012 there has been a steady decline in opioid prescriptions, with the rate in 2020 being 43.3 prescriptions for every 100 persons, or just under 143 million prescriptions in the United States (CDC, 2021a). This decline has largely been due to educating both medical providers and the general public about the dangers of opioids—even when prescribed by a physician.

Prescription opioids are a large class of substances and include the following common medications (example brand names are included and capitalized):

- hydrocodone (Vicodin, Hycoden, Norco);
- hydromorphone (Dilaudid);
- oxycodone (Oxycontin, Percodan);
- meperidine (Demerol, Pethidine);
- methadone (Dolophine);
- fentanyl (Sublimaze);
- naloxone (Narcan);
- buprenorphine (Burpenex, Subutex, Suboxone);
- clonidine (Catapres); and
- tramadol (Ultram).

It is important to note that many of the medications listed include other active medications. For example, Vicodin is the brand name of a medication that includes hydrocodone as well as acetaminophen, or Percocet, which is the brand name for oxycodone with acetaminophen. There are also a variety of street names for prescription opioids that often reference the brand name of the intended opioid; for example, "percs/perks" for Percocet and "demmies" for Demerol. Other street names for prescription opioids include "captain cody," "pancakes and syrup," "schoolboy," "oxy," and a variety of other derivatives. Prescription medications can appear to be safe to many users, and unintentional abuse can occur when an individual begins to take the medication more than prescribed. This can happen when the medication is not achieving the desired effects. In this circumstance, clients should consult with their medical prescriber who will work collaboratively with them to develop a plan for pain management.

In 2017 the DHHS declared a public health emergency due to the national opioid crisis (DHHS, 2017). This crisis, which has also been identified as an epidemic, has been fueled, in part, by the over prescription of opioids. In recent years the epidemic has been influenced heavily by the inclusion of illegally manufactured fentanyl into other substances of abuse (e.g., pills, powders). More work will need to be done to reduce the damage that opioids of all forms are having on society, and counselors need to be prepared as the effects of this crisis will be felt for many years to come.

PSYCHEDELICS

Psychedelics, also called hallucinogens, are substances that cause disturbances to a user's perception and consciousness (Inaba & Cohen, 2007). Psychedelics have been in use for millions of years, with a long history of being taken for religious/spiritual reasons (Sexton et al., 2019). In the mid-20th century psychedelic drugs were being explored for the treatment of substance use, depressive, and personality disorders, as well as for their therapeutic potential in palliative care (Lieberman & Shalev, 2016). This research, despite many studies finding positive effects, was thwarted in 1968 when psychedelics were criminalized by the U.S. federal government (Sproul, 2021).

This criminalization was all in part due to "The War on Drugs." This campaign was sold to the American people as a combination of policy efforts that was advertised to reduce the harms of addiction in society; however, numerous problems have been associated with this "war"—not only in the United States but also globally. For example, many of the laws and policies that were either used or written to combat the so-called "war" were rooted in institutional racism (Earp et al., 2021). Significant efforts have been made to counter the harms done by the war on drugs, such as several states ending the mandatory minimum sentence associated with nonviolent drug crimes (Scully, 2021). Other jurisdictions, such as the state of Oregon and the cities of Seattle, Washington, Santa Cruz, California, and Oakland, California, have decriminalized psychedelics (Adlin, 2021). While psychedelic use continued throughout the prohibition, this resurgence of energy surrounding psychedelic use is important for counselors to pay attention to. In 2020, approximately 7.1 million Americans (ages 12 and older) reportedly used psychedelics in the past year (Substance Use and Mental Health Services Administation [SAMHSA], 2021). This resurgence is also due to numerous research efforts that are underway, exploring the therapeutic potential of psychedelics such as ketamine, MDMA (3,4-methylenedioxy-methamphetamine), psilocybin, and LSD (lysergic acid diethylamide).

Cannabis

There are many names for the cannabis plant, which is often referred to as *marijuana*. This chapter uses the term *cannabis* to reflect the scientific name of the plant and for consistency with the *Diagnostic and Statistical Manual of Mental Disorders, Fifth Edition (DSM)*. Many individuals who are familiar with cannabis are surprised to learn about its classification as a psychedelic, often believing it would like be a depressant due to the common sedating effects of the substance. Although it can have effects that are either stimulating or depressing (or both depending on the strand used), it is classified as a psychedelic due to the reality-altering properties of the substance (Inaba & Cohen, 2007).

Cannabis is a plant that contains hundreds of chemicals, notably the psychoactive chemical Δ-9-tetrahydrocannabinol (THC; Inaba & Cohen, 2007). The two popular species of the cannabis plant are *cannabis sativa* and *cannabis indica*, of which there are many different strands/strains. Short-term effects of cannabis use include relaxation, confusion, anxiety, panic, increased heart rate, increased hunger, loss of coordination, and slower reaction times. Long-term effects include problems with memory and learning activities, severe nausea and vomiting, and respiratory system distress (NIDA, 2022c). Cannabis can produce distortions of time, color, and sound, and users may experience illusions and hallucinations when consumed in high doses (Inaba & Cohen, 2007). Common street names include "pot," "weed," "ganja," "Mary Jane," "bud," "herb," "grass," and "420." Additionally, users may refer to cannabis by the strand/strain name, such as "Pineapple Express"—a strand which was made popular by the 2008 movie of the same name (Green, 2008).

A large percentage (17.9% or 49.6 million) of Americans over the age of 11 reported using cannabis in 2020. This is much larger among young adults ages 18 to 25 as evidenced by 34.5% reporting past year use (SAMHSA, 2021). Of these individuals, approximately 14.2 million had a cannabis use disorder. There are also a number of users who are prescribed cannabis for medical reasons. This may come in pill form such as dronabinol, which contains a synthetic form of THC (Inaba & Cohen, 2007). Despite numerous states legalizing cannabis for medical and recreational purposes, it is important to note that cannabis use by adolescents can severely harm brain development; therefore, most states restrict the use of recreational cannabis to users at least 21 years old (Insurance Institute for Highway Safety, n.d.).

KETAMINE

Ketamine is a substance that was developed in the mid 1960s, and has since become widely used for medical and nonmedical purposes (Morgan & Curran, 2011). Medically, ketamine is used as a dissociative anesthetic; it is also the most widely used anesthesia in veterinary medicine (Morgan & Curran, 2011). Although there are strong medical uses, ketamine has gained popularity among recreational drug users and is known by street names such as "Special K," "k," "ket," and "horse tranquilizer." Much of the strong reputation it has developed as a recreational substance is largely due to the dissociative and psychosis-like effects it can produce among users (Morgan & Curran, 2011). The side effects of ketamine are articulated by Morgan and Curran (2011):

> At low doses ketamine induces distortion of time and space, hallucinations, and mild dissociative effects…at large doses, ketamine induces a more severe dissociation commonly referred to as a "K-hole." wherein the user experiences intense detachment to the point that their perceptions appear completely divorced from their previous reality. (p. 28)

While the medical properties of ketamine are mainly for anesthesia, it is legally prescribed for "off-label" purposes such as depression, anxiety, and substance use disorders. Meta-analyses have shown positive results using ketamine for the treatment of depression (Marcantoni et al., 2020) and anxiety disorders (Whittaker et al., 2021), and a systematic review conducted by Jones et al. (2018) highlights the role ketamine treatment has in facilitating abstinence from certain drugs (i.e., alcohol, cocaine, cannabis, opioids). The use of ketamine, as well as other psychedelics for treating mental health and substance use disorders, is a growing field with significant findings frequently being published. In addition, ketamine clinics are being established across the United States in order to offer low-dose ketamine infusion therapy for the treatment of mood disorders; however, the U.S. Food and Drug Administration (FDA) has not approved ketamine for the treatment of any mental disorder (FDA, 2022). Counselors will want to stay up to date with emerging research areas and evolving treatment interventions.

LSD

Although lysergic acid diethylamide (LSD) was first extracted by Dr. Albert Hoffman in 1938, its hallucinogenic properties were not discovered until 1943 when he ingested LSD accidentally and experienced its effects while riding home on his bicycle (Inaba & Cohen, 2007). Early research into LSD was focused on the use of the chemical for treating mental illnesses and alcohol use disorder;

however, by 1966 the substance was made illegal at the federal level (Inaba & Cohen, 2007). Kuhn and Wilson (2008) offered a description of what occurs during an LSD experience (i.e., "trip"):

> *As the LSD experience begins, many people report unusual sensations, including numbness, muscle weakness, or trembling. A mild fight-or-flight response occurs: Heart rate and blood pressure increase a little, and pupils dilate. Nausea is quite common. (p. 99)*

Other common side effects of LSD include blurred vision, lack of coordination, impaired distance perception, euphoria, slowed passage of time, and, after the initial effects wear off, users can be left with a headache, feelings of lethargy, and experience a contemplative state (Kuhn & Wilson, 2008). Tolerance to the substance can occur quickly (Kuhn & Wilson, 2008); however, there is lack of consistency about the physical addictive potential of LSD (Inaba & Cohen, 2007). Similar to ketamine, there is a growing body of research examining the therapeutic potential of LSD (Liechti, 2017) that counselors will want to stay abreast of.

MDMA/Ecstasy

The chemical name of MDMA is 3,4-methylenedioxy-methamphetamine, and although it has methamphetamine in the name, the substance is classified under the psychedelics category because it has both stimulant and psychedelic properties (NIDA, 2020). Despite being discovered in the early 1900s, use of the substance did not occur until the mid-20th century (Kuhn & Wilson, 2008). Current users know the substance by the common street names of "ecstasy," "e," and "XTC." Another common street name is "Molly" referring to a pure form of MDMA. However, this is a marketing ploy by dealers because it is very rare for the substance to be pure. Up to 40% of pills tested by one research study from 2010 to 2015 did not contain any amount of MDMA (Saleemi et al., 2017), let alone being pure and, therefore, actually "Molly."

Users of MDMA experience emotional closeness, elevated mood, increased empathy, increased energy, and other biological effects such as increased heart rate and blood pressure (NIDA, 2020). In addition, users can experience other side effects such as nausea, muscle cramping, blurred vision, involuntary teeth clenching, chills, and sweats (NIDA, 2020). The effects of MDMA last about 3 to 6 hours, and some users will take a second dose to prolong the effects (NIDA, 2020). This is concerning because at high doses MDMA can cause seizures, and is particularly dangerous for individuals who have underlying cardiovascular issues as it may cause heart attacks and strokes (Kuhn & Wilson, 2008). One significant effect some users experience is the "down" which happens a few days after MDMA use. This "down" effect is represented by mood changes such as irritability, aggression, and/or depression-like symptoms (Kuhn & Wilson, 2008, p. 86). Counselors working with clients who have used MDMA will want to explore their experiences, and particularly pay attention to any risky activities in which the client may have participated while under the drug's euphoric influence.

Psilocybin

Psilocybin is the psychoactive substance found in psychedelic mushrooms, which grow in North and South America, Southeast Asia, and Europe (Inaba & Cohen, 2007). The chemical structure of psilocybin is similar to LSD (Inaba & Cohen, 2007), and this results in similar effects that are classified under the following categories with examples detailed in Table 2.1: perceptual, cognitive, emotional, and ego dissolution (Kargbo, 2020). Prior to experiencing these psychedelic effects, the user will typically experience nausea (Inaba & Cohen, 2007). The most common street names for psilocybin mushrooms are "magic mushrooms," and "shrooms," although they have also been known as "boomers," "sacred mushrooms," and "God's flesh." The potency of psilocybin in magic mushrooms is highly variable, with some mushrooms containing up to 10 times the amount when compared to others (Inaba & Cohen, 2007). There is a danger in mushroom harvesting, as there are other varieties that have no psychedelic properties but are poisonous when ingested (Inaba & Cohen, 2007). Similar to the other psychedelics reviewed here, psilocybin is being investigated for treatment of a wide range of mental health and substance use disorders. Readers interested in learning more are directed to the Johns Hopkins University's Center for Psychedelic and Consciousness Research.

TABLE 2.1 **Effects of Psilocybin**

TYPE OF EFFECT	EFFECTS EXPERIENCED BY THE USER
Perceptual	Changes in mental imagery Distorted vision Intensified perceptions Illusions Hallucinations
Cognitive	Increase in divergent thinking Sensitivity to language patterns and meaning Attribution of meaning to musical stimuli
Emotional	Intensification of feelings Expansion of range of emotions experienced Increased access to emotions Unique states of euphoria
Ego dissolution	Loss of a sense of self and/or ego loss Sense of connectivity to the universe/environment

Source: Adapted from Kargbo, R. B. (2020). Psilocybin therapeutic research: The present and future paradigm. *ACS Medicinal Chemistry Letters, 11*(4), 399–402. https://doi.org/10.1021/acsmedchemlett.0c00048

This portion of the chapter contained information about numerous substances that are abused in the world today; however, not all substances were reviewed. For example, bath salts, K2/spice (NIDA, 2022b), inhalants, and anabolic steroids are all substances that may be abused. It is important for counselors to learn about commonly abused substances in their communities, including those that are becoming more widely known such as Ayahuasca and DMT (N, N-dimethyltryptamine). For more information, please refer to Inaba and Cohen's (2007) book, *Uppers, Downers, All-Arounders*, or Kuhn and Wilson's (2008) publication, *Buzzed: The Straight Facts About the Most Used and Abused Drugs*.

ADMINISTRATION ROUTES

Administration route refers to the way a substance enters the human body (Inaba & Cohen, 2007). There are several ways this can occur including but not limited to *inhaling* a substance (involving the respiratory system) and *injecting* a substance (likely involving the circulatory system). Each administration route has a typical time it takes for a user to feel the effects. Table 2.2

TABLE 2.2. **Administration Routes and Psychoactive Effects Timeline**

	ADMINISTRATION ROUTE	PSYCHOACTIVE EFFECTS TIMELINE
Fastest	Inhalation	7 to 10 seconds
↓	Injection	15 to 30 seconds
	Mucous membrane absorption	1 to 15 minutes
	Oral ingestion	20 to 30 minutes
Slowest	Contact absorption	Up to 7 days

Sources: Created with information from Inaba, D. S., & Cohen, W. E. (2007). *Uppers, Downers, All Arounders: Physical and Mental Effects of Psychoactive Drugs.* CNS Publications; Fattinger, K, Benowitz, N. L., Jones, R. T., & Verotta, D. (2000). Nasal mucosal versus gastrointestinal absorption of nasally administered cocaine. *European Journal of Clinical Pharmacology, 56,* 305–310.

shows the most common administration routes according to the speed in which a user typically feels the effects of the substance, from fastest to slowest. Recognize that these times are all dependent on the unique characteristics of the individual user such as biological factors and history of substance use.

Inaba and Cohen (2007) outlined the major administration routes and timelines for psychoactive properties to be felt. *Inhalation* is the fastest administration route, with a user feeling the psychoactive effects of the substance within 7 to 10 seconds. Inhalation involves the respiratory system, typically smoking or vaping a substance. *Injection* is the second fastest administration route, with effects being felt in 15 to 30 seconds if administered intravenously. If the substance is injected via the muscular system (i.e., "muscling") or under the skin (i.e., "skin popping"), then the effects take longer. *Mucous membrane absorption* is the third fastest administration route, although where on the human body the mucous membrane is located will impact the absorption rate. The nasal cavity is the fastest absorption, with the oral (under the tongue or between tongue and cheek) being a bit slower at 3 to 5 minutes, and the rectal mucous membranes taking approximately 10 to 15 minutes. *Oral ingestion* involves the substance being absorbed by the digestive system, resulting in drug effects 20 to 30 minutes following ingestion. The slowest administration route is *contact absorption*, in which adhesives which have been saturated with a substance are applied to the skin. This can take up to 7 days for the effects of the substance to be experienced by the user. Most psychoactive substances can be administered in a variety of ways. For example, heroin can be smoked (inhaled), snorted (mucous membrane absorption), or injected (intravenously). It is important that counselors are talking about administration routes with clients to gain a clear picture of what their experience may be like.

BEHAVIORAL ADDICTIONS

Behavioral addictions (also referred to as process addictions in the professional literature) are those that develop as a result of a *behavior*, not due to the use of a substance. The first behavioral addiction to be recognized as a disorder was gambling in the third edition of the *DSM*; however, it was not part of the addictive disorders chapter. It was originally titled "Pathological Gambling," and classified as an impulse control disorder (Reilly & Smith, n.d.). With the *DSM-5* release in 2013, gambling disorder (GD) became the first nonsubstance addiction included in the addictive disorder chapter along with the other substance use disorders. Although there is a growing body of research comparing behavioral addictions to substance use disorders, this chapter does not provide a comprehensive overview and interested readers are directed to numerous resources to learn more.

GAMBLING ADDICTION

As mentioned, the American Psychiatric Association (APA) included gambling in the *DSM-5* among the other addictive disorders for the first time (2013). This signaled a shift in broadening the conceptualization of addiction from solely substance-related to including behavioral disorders. This was largely due to brain-imaging studies and neurochemical tests which indicated that gambling activates brain structures similar to those involved in substance addiction (Reilly & Smith, n.d.). GD is characterized by an individual "risking something of value in the hopes of obtaining something of greater value" (APA, 2013, p. 586). The *DSM-5* criteria for GD mimic those for substance use disorders, such as an individual becoming restless or irritable when attempting to cut down, or an individual being preoccupied with the activity (APA, 2013). However, these are not mirrored precisely as there are differences in the language used as well as the number of criteria describing the disorder (nine for GD, compared with 11 for SUD), and the number needed for an individual to be diagnosed (minimum of four for mild GD, compared with a minimum of two for mild SUD; APA, 2013). Prevalence of GD is variable, with estimates of 0.42% to 4.0% of the population appearing in the literature (Black & Shaw, 2019). A recommended book for counselors to learn more about gambling addiction is Custer and Milt's (1986) seminal publication, *When Luck Runs Out: Help for Compulsive Gamblers and Their Families*.

INTERNET GAMING ADDICTION

Despite GD being the only nonsubstance addictive disorder included in the *DSM-5*, internet gaming disorder (IGD) was included in the "Conditions for Further Study" chapter, which presents proposed criteria for disorders that have yet to meet the threshold for peer-reviewed research required for inclusion. However, there are indications that such disorders will be included in the future (APA, 2013). According to the APA (2013), "the essential feature of IGD is persistent and recurrent participation in computer gaming, typically group games, for many hours" (p. 796). Users typically spend a minimum of 8 to 10 hours per day in the activity, and as a result, neglect other important social, familial, vocational, or educational responsibilities (APA, 2013). The prevalence of IGD is difficult to estimate, likely because of a lack of a standard definition; however, Stevens et al. (2021) conducted a systematic review and meta-analysis and estimated the global rate of IGD to be 1.96%, which similar to some SUDs. These authors further noted there may be wide variability among certain demographic groups, with adolescents and males often accounting for higher rates. Counselors who encounter clients experiencing distress with their IGD should review the proposed criteria in the *DSM-5*, and explore the 11th edition of the *International Classification of Diseases* (*ICD*), which does include gaming disorder (Stevens et al., 2021).

SEXUAL ADDICTION

Sexual/sex addiction is not yet included in the *DSM-5* as an addictive disorder; however, there has been ongoing research exploring this (Carnes, n.d.). The American Society of Addiction Medicine (ASAM) and the *ICD* both suggest that sex can be addictive (Rosenberg et al., 2014). Despite this, there is no one agreed upon definition of sex addiction. Dr. Patrick Carnes, a notable pioneer in the sex addiction field, articulated sex addiction in the following way:

> *Within the addictive system, sexual experience becomes the reason for being- the primary relationship for the addict…the sexual experience is the source of nurturing, focus of energy, and origin of excitement. It is the remedy for pain and anxiety, the reward for success, and the means for maintaining emotional balance… addiction is truly an altered state of consciousness in which "normal" sexual behavior pales by comparison in terms of excitement and relief from troubles. (2001, pp. 26–27)*

Although there are limitations for diagnosis such as the lack of definition of sexual addiction and lack of diagnostic criteria, clients do seek counseling for self-reported sexual addiction and counselors can earn credentials specializing in this emerging field (Rosenberg et al., 2014). Rosenberg et al. (2014) detailed the treatment offered to these clients being similar to those offered for substance addiction (e.g., motivational interviewing, cognitive behavioral approaches, relapse prevention, peer recovery groups). However, it is crucial that counselors do not pathologize sexual behavior, particularly as sexuality and sexual behaviors can be uniquely connected to cultural norms (Church, 2015). This can be problematic when relying solely on the use of Carnes's original model and assessment tool (Church, 2015). Counselors are encouraged to consider embracing a sex-positive framework. Readers interested in learning more about sex addiction are referred to the following resources: Dr. Marty Klein's (n.d.) *Sexual Intelligence Blog* (found at https://www.martyklein.com/category/sexual-intelligence-blog/), *Out of the Shadows* by Dr. Patrick Carnes (2001), and *Women, Sex, and Addiction* by Dr. Charlotte S. Kasl (1990).

The inclusion of gambling, sex, and internet gaming here is not meant to be reflective of the only behavioral issues clients will present with problematic use patterns. Readers are referred to Dr. Amanda Giordano's (2022) comprehensive book, *A Clinical Guide to Treating Behavioral Addictions,* to learn more. Counselors are encouraged to review peer-reviewed research examining the specific behavioral issue that clients present with in order to form an appropriate, scientifically informed treatment plan in collaboration with the client.

MODELS OF ADDICTION

Distinct models of addiction etiology exist in order to provide insight about the causal pathway of how the disorder develops. Examples of these models are the *moral* model, the *spiritual* model, the *educational* model, the *general systems* model, the *medical* model, the *brain disease* model, and the *biopsychosocial* model. Due to their important roles in understanding addiction, three of these models are examined here: (a) the moral model, (b) the brain disease model, and (c) the biopsychosocial model.

MORAL MODEL

With advances in brain and behavior research, the moral model of addiction has become quite outdated; however, it continues to be a contributing factor in how individuals perceive addiction. And for this reason, it is explored here. According to Capuzzi et al. (2016), "the moral model explains addiction as a consequence of personal choice, and individuals who are engaging in addictive behaviors are viewed as being capable of making alternative choices" (p. 7). This model perpetuates the stigma of addiction as it places the blame on the individual struggling with addiction. Stigma toward individuals with addiction is pervasive in our society, and helping professionals are not immune from this. Conducting a review of health professions literature, van Boekel et al. (2013) found that health professionals' attitudes to be generally negative toward individuals with substance use disorders, which in turn can have inadvertent effects resulting in poorer treatment outcomes. It is important for counselors to explore their own beliefs about individuals who struggle with addiction, and then appropriately challenge those as they would any other bias. In addition, counselors can challenge the harmful narrative of the moral model by acting as advocates and speaking up about the dangers of stigma when they hear disparaging remarks about individuals with substance use disorders.

BRAIN DISEASE MODEL

The brain disease model has evolved over time; however, early language of the model was formally recognized by the American Medical Association in 1956 (Merta, 2001). This model moves away from blaming the individual struggling with the disorder as a moral failure, and instead examines how repetitive use of a substance can alter a user's brain (NIDA, 2018). Recalling the definition of addiction from earlier in this chapter, it included references to brain circuits and genetics (ASAM, 2019). According to the brain disease model, when an individual uses a substance repetitively, changes in the brain result which limit an individual's self-control and affect how they respond to urges (NIDA, 2018). This is largely due to changes in the brain reward pathway which "motivates a person to repeat behaviors needed to thrive, such as eating and spending time with loved ones" (NIDA, 2018, para. 4). The reward pathway is activated by the presence of dopamine which psychoactive substances and addictive behaviors cause to be released. This surge of dopamine signals the brain to repeat that behavior, which can lead to compulsive use of psychoactive substances or engaging in addictive behaviors (NIDA, 2018). According to Moro (2021):

> *While the initial use of a substance or behavior is typically voluntary, the changes in the brain structure after initial use or engagement result in less control for the individual; the brain has learned the route to take to "feel good" and will take that route until it learns another route. (p. 297)*

The reward pathway is not the only part of the brain affected by use/addictive behavior. Long-term use or sustained engagement in addictive behaviors affects other areas of the brain that can lead to difficulties with learning, judgment, decision-making, and memory (among other impacted functions; NIDA, 2018). The brain disease model focuses on the biological component of addiction and addictive behavior, and while it is not as comprehensive as the biopsychosocial model, which is explored next, it does offer a less stigmatizing approach to understanding addiction than the outdated moral model.

BIOPSYCHOSOCIAL MODEL

The biopsychosocial (BPS) model was presented by Engel in 1977, as an etiological framework to understanding the complexity involved with medical disease onset. According to Engel (1977), there are a variety of factors that contribute to the development and maintenance of a disease, including those factors derived from biological, psychological, and/or social domains. This model is appealing to addiction professionals as it captures the complexity of the disease.

The *biological* domain houses the brain disease model as well as honors the genetics involved in addiction. Research has identified that there can be a genetic predisposition to addiction, while at the same time there can be genetic factors that are protective against developing an addiction (Skewes & Gonzalez, 2013). Counselors want to do a thorough history to understand the genetic involvement (to the best of the client's knowledge) and consult other healthcare specialists as needed. The next domain is *psychological*. Psychological factors involve understanding the impact of adverse childhood experiences (ACES), examining operant and classical conditioning concepts and exploring the unique personality and temperament of the client, as well as other psychological concepts such as self-efficacy (Skewes & Gonzalez, 2013). The *social* domain of the biopsychosocial model involves understanding how social systems affect the development and maintenance of addiction. Social systems include families, peers, intimate partners, ethnicity, and culture (Skewes & Gonzalez, 2013). An additional domain, *spiritual* has been proposed by Sulmasy (2002) to capture the importance of spiritual elements for clients. This domain contains factors such as religiosity and spiritual/religious coping and supports. Taking into account the three (or four) domains of the biopsychosocial/spiritual model, a counselor can gain a holistic view of the client's addictive behavior in a much more comprehensive fashion than if they examined any one of the domains in isolation.

The three models presented here are not inclusive of all models to understand addiction. Counselors can conceptualize addiction solely from psychological or social theories, of which there are many. The biopsychosocial model offers a way to conceptualize a complex disease with many moving parts. In doing so, it is anticipated that this strong conceptualization will allow appropriate treatment to be planned and implemented.

GENERAL REVIEW OF THE *DSM-5* CLASSIFICATION SYSTEM

The *DSM* is a guide that mental health clinicians use to make decisions regarding a client's symptomology and resulting mental disorder. Substance use disorders have been in the *DSM* since the initial release in 1952; however, these early editions classified such disorders as being a component of other mental health issues (Robinson & Adinoff, 2016). It was not until the publication of the *DSM-III* in 1980 that substance use disorders received their own independent classification separately from mental health disorders (Robinson & Adinoff, 2016). In the third edition, and the two that followed, substance use disorders were classified as either abuse or dependence. In the 5th edition of the *DSM* (APA, 2013), a shift occurred to introduce a spectrum of SUDs as opposed to the former abuse/dependence system.

This new spectrum allows for users to be diagnosed with a mild, moderate, and severe SUD (APA, 2013). There are four main categories with 11 total criteria for counselors to assess. The main categories are *impaired control, social impairment, risky use*, and *pharmacological criteria* (APA, 2013). The impaired control category involves criteria in which an individual has limited control over their use as demonstrated in one of four ways (e.g., spending a great amount of time obtaining, using, or recovering from the substance use; APA, 2013). The second category, social impairment, involves the user experiencing negative consequences with social relationships and/or professional obligations (APA, 2013). The third category, risky use, involves use of a substance that places the individual in physical danger or will exacerbate a physical or psychological problem (APA, 2013). The last category, pharmacological, involves tolerance and withdrawal. Tolerance is

CLINICAL CASE ILLUSTRATION AND DISCUSSION

CASE OF JOANNA

Joanna is a 43-year-old divorced mother of two young children, ages 1 (Jaqueline) and 3 (John Jr.). Joanna, who has been divorced from her ex-husband for 1 year, has sole custody of the children. Her ex-husband, John, has supervised visitation every other weekend for 4 hours on Saturday morning. Joanna is currently residing with her mother, who was widowed 10 years prior. Joanna's mother, Rosa, is retired from her career as a postal worker, and she provides child care for her grandchildren during the week. Joanna is employed at the city library where she has worked for the past 16 years. When Joanna talks about her job, she lights up with a big smile and her eyes glimmer. "It is so great to help people discover new things. That is what I love most about my job—libraries are just full of adventure!" Joanna has sought out counseling services due to a recent slip she had. Joanna reports that when she dropped off her children last Saturday for their supervised visitation with their father (her ex-husband), she had a distressing interaction with him in the lobby. Later that evening, after the children were in bed, Joanna found herself pouring a glass of wine, which she drank about half of before she realized what she was doing and then quickly poured the rest down the drain. Joanna tells the counselor that she has been in recovery for 18 years. She has had a few slips and relapses throughout the years, and in order to prevent this one from spiraling, she knew it was important to get into counseling. "My old counselor retired last year, so I guess it's time to start fresh."

The counselor learns more about Joanna's history. She was raised by her mother, Rosa, and up until she was 10, also her father, Gordon. Just before Joanna's 10th birthday, her father and mother split up, which was quite distressing for Joanna. There was an infidelity in her parent's marriage, and Joanna's father subsequently moved out of the family home. Joanna was an only child, and she reports feeling quite torn during this time. "I just didn't know what was going on. I loved my mom and my dad, and it felt like I needed to choose between them." Joanna describes the next several years being difficult as her parents would often get into heated arguments when they encountered each other during custody transitions. Joanna's mother did not like when Joanna went to stay with Gordon, as he lived in an area of town that was known for violence, and she worried about Joanna's safety. Rosa's concern was valid, as on numerous occasions Joanna heard what sounded like gun shots, and it was not uncommon to fall asleep to sirens in the evening. While Joanna loved being able to see her father, she was relieved when she was able to go back home to Rosa.

Despite the difficult family dynamics, Joanna reported a healthy childhood, meeting all developmental milestones as expected, and having some close friends. However, when Joanna was 14, she and her best friend, Charlene, got into a friendship-ending argument over a boy. This caused tension in her group of friends, and Joanna reported that this distance made it hard to be around any of them. One weekend while visiting her father, Joanna met two neighborhood girls, Hannah and Laura, who were a couple years older than Joanna. The three of them became strong friends over the next year. Laura was able to drive, and she shared a car with her older brother. This meant Hannah and Laura could hang out with Joanna even when she was at her mom's house, which was more often than the times she stayed at her dad's. Joanna reports that meeting Hannah and Laura was "the best and the worst thing for me." She describes their friendship as strong and consistent, and feeling relieved to have them in her life. However, Hannah and Laura also introduced Joanna to alcohol for the first time, and Joanna states, "It was downhill from there."

Joanna describes her early alcohol use beginning around the age of 15, which consisted of drinking on the weekends. This stayed fairly consistent throughout the rest of high school, and it was after graduating that she began drinking more when she moved in with Hannah and Laura. "Maybe it's because I had so much time on my hands. I was going to community college and working part time, but it just seemed so much less structured than when I was in high school." She also describes always having access since Hannah turned 21 years old right after Joanna graduated from high school.

Joanna details a downward spiral of her relationship with alcohol. She began drinking every day, sometimes missing classes, and eventually dropping out of college altogether. She was sexually assaulted on two occasions while intoxicated, both of which she reported to the authorities yet neither resulted in charges being pressed against the perpetrators. Joanna is in tears as she describes this phase of her life, "I just don't know what happened. One day I was focused on my mom and dad, and navigating life between them, and the next I woke up at 5:00 a.m. with puke down my shirt on the stoop of our apartment. I had no clue what happened the night before, where I was, or who I was with. It was a disaster." During this time Joanna had very little contact with her mother and father, and even her relationship with Hannah and Laura became strained. Things progressed like this for the next few years with Joanna going between numerous jobs, including a cashier, barista, and server. When Joanna turned 23 years old, her parents, with the help of Hannah and Laura staged an intervention. Joanna was taken by surprise but was open to listening. After the intervention, Joanna agreed to attend an intensive outpatient treatment program (IOP). Joanna reports that during this time when her family and friends working toward intervening, her mom and dad were able to reconcile. Rosa and Gordon rekindled their relationship, attended couples counseling, and a year later, he moved back home after 13 years apart.

She reported that she graduated from the program, was active in counseling, and attended support groups consistently, which helped her maintain her sobriety for about 2 years. One night, after getting off work as a server, a group of coworkers asked her to join them for drinks next door. Joanna agreed, not intending to drink, but because she was hungry and wanted to eat. While at the restaurant Joanna's coworkers bought her a drink not knowing about her sobriety, and Joanna reported that she thought, "It's just one, I can do this." This one drink was followed by a few pitchers of beer split among the four of them, and Joanna remembers waking up the next morning just "smelling of Coors Light." She reports a few more days of partying like that before her mom stepped in and took her to a meeting. "That was 18 years ago, I've been sober since. That is, until last week."

Joanna further details her marriage difficulties, highlighting an emotionally abusive relationship with John for 7 years. In addition, John had multiple instances of infidelity. John refused to attend counseling after the second affair when Joanna requested it. Instead, he responded to Joanna that she was making it a larger issue that it was, and if only she had more self-confidence he wouldn't be lured by other women. Following the birth of her second child, her mother confronted her and offered her a place to live and child care if she would agree to leave John. It took a few months of discussions and planning. However, one evening John had become angry, hostile, and verbally aggressive toward Joanna, which prompted her to move in with her mother the next day. The following week Joanna began the process of legally separating from John, including requesting full custody to which the courts agreed during the initial process. Since then, John has been able to see the children every other Saturday for 4 hours during supervised visitation. Joanna typically does not have to see John, but this past week they encountered one another in the parking lot; he approached her and was hostile and condescending about the divorce and custody arrangement. It was following this interaction that Joanna had the slip.

CASE DISCUSSION

Joanna arrived to counseling feeling ashamed about her slip, yet hopeful about her continued recovery. Joanna's counselor spent time learning more about Joanna's addiction, as well as the biopsychosocial factors involved in the development and maintenance of her addiction. The counselor explored the biological factors, and was specifically curious about the role her parents' divorce (an ACE) had on Joanna, as well as the continued hostility between her parents. In addition, the counselor conducted a family genogram wherein relationship patterns and substance use over multiple generations of her family were explored. By completing this, the counselor learned that Joanna appeared to have a genetic predisposition to addiction, with her paternal grandfather reportedly struggling with alcohol addiction until the end of his life. In addition, she had two cousins who struggled with addiction on her paternal side of the family, and it was their parents (Gordon's sister and her spouse) who were able to recommend the interventionist that Gordon and Rosa hired to work with Joanna.

Joanna's counselor spent time examining what has worked well for her throughout these past 18 years. They examined other times she has been distressed and what she has been able to do in those situations to avoid a slip or relapse. Joanna reports that there have been other slips that have occurred, but a large differentce this time was that she did not remember purchasing the alcohol or pouring the glass. "It was like I was in a blur, and I woke up when I tasted the wine." Joanna's counselor provided psychoeducation to Joanna about the brain, and the reward pathway, highlighting that something in the interaction with her ex-husband triggered her to go back to this previous coping pattern. They worked together exploring this interaction in a way that felt safe for Joanna, and were able to connect the experience back to her adolescence. "He yelled at me, said it was my fault that he cheated on me, and if only I was not a wreck, he wouldn't have done that." Upon further conversation the counselor learned that this exchange was similar to one she overheard on multiple occasions with her parents, "But my dad wasn't so condescending." Joanna's counselor surmised this was a trigger that activated Joanna's addiction neuropathways to provide relief from her feelings of distress, which Joanna agreed with. Joanna and her counselor worked collaboratively on a treatment plan that included the following goals:

1. Refine use of previously used coping skills and develop new ones to use when experiencing high-risk situations/cravings.
2. Explore and resolve feelings of powerlessness and unmanageability which were experienced as a child and in her marriage.
3. Explore and resolve feelings of abandonment related to her parents' divorce, and the infidelity in her marriage.

Joanna and her counselor agreed to work together on a weekly basis, and then re-evaluate the treatment plan in 3 months to see what progress has been made and what Joanna's needs may be at the time.

when a user needs to take more of a substance to gain the same effects over time—something that builds with regular use (Inaba & Cohen, 2007). Withdrawal can be experienced by a person when use is discontinued after a period of prolonged and heavy use (APA, 2013). A counselor will assess a client according to the 11 criteria, and a diagnosis will be made if two or more of the criteria are met (i.e., 2–3 criteria, mild; 4–5, moderate; 6 or more, severe; APA, 2013).

CHAPTER SUMMARY

This chapter provided a general overview of substance use and addictive disorders. The definition of addiction and prevalence rates were presented to provide an overview of the scope of the problem. Substances were introduced by detailing the effects on the human body, describing the methods of ingesting substances, and identifying the street names commonly used. Models of addiction, such as the brain disease model and biopsychosocial model, were described. Clinical information was presented, such as diagnostic categorization, and a description of how addiction can present in clients' clinical histories was offered via a case study and discussion.

DISCUSSION QUESTIONS

1. Using the definition of addiction provided by ASAM (2019) and the information about the brain disease model of addiction, plan your response to a client who says, "I know it's just my fault that I can't stop drinking. I just don't have enough will power."

2. Choose one of the substances covered in this chapter that you are least familiar with. How will you assess your client to determine whether they have been using/abusing the substance?

3. As mentioned in the chapter, the moral model is outdated and does not embrace a client-centered orientation. Despite this, the moral model still appears in our everyday lives. What is an example in popular culture (e.g., TV, movies) that has perpetuated the moral model of addiction?

4. In the case of Joanna, what other factors in the biological, psychological, and social domains would a counselor need to consider when planning her treatment?

5. Considering the impact biases can have on individuals seeking addiction treatment, what personal beliefs or biases do you need to challenge about addiction? Then, identify your preliminary plans to mitigate any stereotype or bias you have about people with substance use diorders.

REFERENCES

Adlin, B. (2021, October 4). *Seattle becomes largest U.S. city to decriminalize psychedelics.* https://www.marijuanamoment.net/seattle-becomes-largest-u-s-city-to-decriminalize-psychedelics/

Ahmad, F. B., Cisewski, J. A., Roseen, L. M., & Sutton, P. (2022). *Provisional drug overdose death counts.* National Center for Health Statistics, Centers for Disease Control and Prevention. Retrieved from https://www.cdc.gov/nchs/nvss/vsrr/drug-overdose-data.htm

Alcohol and Drug Foundation. (2022). *What are stimulants?* Retrieved from https://adf.org.au/drug-facts/stimulants/

Alcohol and Drug Policy Commission. (n.d.). *Opiates or opioids- what's the difference?* Retrieved from https://www.oregon.gov/adpc/pages/opiate-opioid.aspx

American Psychiatric Association. (2013). *Diagnostic and statistical manual of mental disorders* (5th ed.). Author.

American Society of Addiction Medicine. (2019, September 15). *Definition of addiction.* Retrieved from https://www.asam.org/quality-care/definition-of-addiction

Bandelow, B. (2020). Current and novel psychopharmacological drugs for anxiety disorders. In Y.-K. Kim (Ed.) *Anxiety disorders: Rethinking and understanding recent discoveries* (pp. 347–365). Springer.

Black, D. W., & Shaw, M. (2019). The epidemiology of gambling disorder. In A. Heinz, N. Romanczuk-Seiferth, & M. Potenza (Eds.) *Gambling disorder* (pp. 29–48). Springer.

Capuzzi, D., Stauffer, M. D., & Sharpe, C. (2016). History and etiological models of addiction. In D. Capuzzi and M. D. Stauffer (Eds.), *Foundations of addiction counseling* (pp. 1–17). Pearson.

Carnes, P. (2001). *Out of the shadows: Understanding sexual addiction* (3rd ed.). Hazelden Publishing.

Carnes, S. (n.d.). *Sex addiction: Neuroscience etiology and treatment* [PowerPoint slides]. Retrieved from https://www.naadac.org/assets/2416/carnes.pdf

Centers for Disease Control and Prevention. (2017, September 26). *Opioid prescribing: Where you live matters.* Retrieved from https://www.cdc.gov/vitalsigns/opioids/index.html

Centers for Disease Control and Prevention. (2021a, November 10). *U.S. opioid dispensing rate maps.* National Center for Injury Prevention and Control. Retrieved from https://www.cdc.gov/drugoverdose/rxrate-maps/index.html#:~:text=The%20overall%20national%20opioid%20dispensing%20rate%20declined%20from%202012%20to,than%20142%20million%20opioid%20prescriptions https://www.cdc.gov/drugoverdose/rxrate-maps/index.html#:~:text=The%20overall%20national%20opioid%20dispensing%20rate%20declined%20from%202012%20to,than%20142%20million%20opioid%20prescriptions

Centers for Disease Control and Prevention. (2021b, November 18). *Other drugs.* National Center for Injury Prevention and Control. Retrieved from https://www.cdc.gov/drugoverdose/deaths/other-drugs.html

Centers for Disease Control and Prevention. (2022a, February 23). *Fentanyl facts.* Division of Drug Overdose Prevention. Retrieved from https://www.cdc.gov/stopoverdose/fentanyl/index.html

Centers for Disease Control and Prevention. (2022b, June 23). *Quick facts on the risks of e-cigarettes for kids, teens, and young adults.* Office on Smoking and Health, National Center for Chronic Disease Prevention and Health Promotion. Retrieved from https://www.cdc.gov/tobacco/basic_information/e-cigarettes/Quick-Facts-on-the-Risks-of-E-cigarettes-for-Kids-Teens-and-Young-Adults.html

Church, S. (2015, September 8). *The sex addiction model: Why an adjunct/alternative is needed.* Retrieved from https://themindembodied.com/blog/2015/8/11/the-sex-addiction-model-why-an-adjunctalternative-is-needed

Custer, R., & Milt, H. (1986). *When luck runs out: Help for compulsive gamblers and their families.* Grand Center Pub.

Earp, B., Lewis, J., & Hart, C. L. (2021). Racial justice requires ending the war on drugs. *The American Journal of Bioethics*, *21*(4), 4–19. https://doi.org/10.1080/15265161.2020.1861364

Engel, G. L. (1977). The need for a new model: A challenge for biomedicine. *Science*, *196*(4286), 129–136. https://www.science.org/doi/10.1126/science.847460

Gilligan, V. (Creator). (2008-2013). *Breaking bad* [TV series]. High Bridge Productions; Gran Via Productions; Sony Pictures Television; American Movie Classics.

Giordano, A. L. (2022). *A clinical guide to treating behavioral addictions.* Springer.

Green, D. G. (2008). *Pineapple express* [Film]. Columbia Pictures; Relativity Media; Apatow Productions.

Heather, N., & Stockwell, T. (Eds.) (2004). *The essential handbook of treatment and prevention of alcohol problems.* Wiley.

Inaba, D. S., & Cohen, W. E. (2007). *Uppers, downers, all arounders: Physical and mental effects of psychoactive drugs* (6th ed.). CNS Productions.

Ingersoll, E., & Rak, C. (2016). *Psychopharmacology for mental health professionals: An integrative approach.* (2nd ed.). Cengage.

Insurance Institute for Highway Safety. (n.d.). *Marijuana laws by state.* Retrieved from https://www.iihs.org/topics/alcohol-and-drugs/marijuana-laws-table

Jones, J. L., Mateus, C. F., Malcolm, R. J., Brady, K. T., & Black, S. E. (2018). Efficacy in ketamine in the treatment of substance use disorders: A systematic review. *Frontiers in Psychiatry, 9*, article 277, 1– https://doi.org/10.3389/fpsyt.2018.00277

Kargbo, R. B. (2020). Psilocybin therapeutic research: The present and future paradigm. *ACS Medicinal Chemistry Letters, 11*(4), 399–402. https://doi.org/10.1021/acsmedchemlett.0c00048

Kasl, C. S. (1990). *Women, sex, and addiction: A search for love and power*. HarperCollins.

Klein, M. (n.d.). *Sexual intelligence blog*. Retrieved from https://www.martyklein.com/category/sexual-intelligence-blog/

Koob, G. F., & Volkow, N. D. (2016). Neurobiology of addiction: A neurocircuitry analysis. *Lancet Psychiatry, 3*(8), 760–773. https://doi.org/10.1016/S2215-0366(16)00104-8

Kuhn, C., & Wilson, W. (2008). *Buzzed: The straight facts about the most used and abused drugs from alcohol to ecstasy* (3rd ed.). Norton.

Landi, H. (2022, May 4). *Cerebral stops prescribing Adderall for new ADHD patients as reports of DEA investigation surface*. Retrieved from https://www.fiercehealthcare.com/health-tech/truepill-cerebral-stop-prescribing-adderall-new-adhd-patients-amid-reports-mental

Lieberman, J. A., & Shalev, D. (2016). Back to the future: Research renewed on the clinical utility of psychedelic drugs. *Journal of Psychopharmacology, 30*(12), 1198–1200. https://doi.org/10.1177/0269881116675755

Liechti, M. E. (2017). Modern clinical research on LSD. *Neuropsychopharmacology, 42*, 2114–2127. https://doi.org/10.1038/npp/2017.86

Luke, C. (2016). *Neuroscience for counselors and therapists: Integrating the sciences of mind and brain*. Sage.

MacMillan, T. (2018, March 14). *The classic study that showed the world is smaller than you think*. The Cut. Retrieved from https://www.thecut.com/2018/03/the-history-of-the-six-degrees-of-separation-study.html

Marcantoni, W. S., Akoumba, B. S., Wassef, M., Mayrand, J., Lai, H., Richard-Devantoy, S., & Beauchamp, S. (2020). A systematic review and meta-analysis of the efficacy of intravenous ketamine infusion for treatment resistant depression: January 2009-January 2019. *Journal of Addictive Disorders, 277*, 831–841. https://doi.org/10.1016/j.jad.2020.09.007

Merta, R. J. (2001). Addictions counseling. *Counseling and Human Development, 33*(5), 1–24.

McGinty, E. E., & Barry, C. L. (2020). Stigma reduction to combat the addiction crisis- developing an evidence base. *New England Journal of Medicine, 382*, 1291–192. https://doi.org/10.1056/NEJMp2000227

McKeon, A., Frye, M. A., & Delanty, N. (2007). The alcohol withdrawal syndrome. *The Journal of Neurology, Neurosurgery, and Psychiatry, 79*, 854–862. https://doi.org/10.1136/jnnp.2007.128322

Morgan, C. J. A., & Curran, H. V. (2011). Ketamine use: A review. *Addiction, 107*, 27–38. https://doi.org/10.1111/j.1360-0443.2011.03576.x

Moro, R. (2021). Addiction issues in the schools. In M. A. Rausch & L. L. Gallo (Eds.), *Strengthening school counselor advocacy and practice for important populations and difficult topics* (pp. 296–314). IGI Global. https://doi.org/10.4018/978-1-7998-7319-8.ch016

National Center for Statistics and Analysis. (2022, April). *Alcohol-impaired driving: 2020 data* (Traffic Safety Facts. Report No. DOT HS 813 294). National Highway Traffic Safety Administration. Retrieved from https://crashstats.nhtsa.dot.gov/Api/Public/ViewPublication/813294

National Institute of Alcohol Abuse and Alcoholism. (2016). *Rethinking drinking: Alcohol and your health*. U.S. Department of Health and Human Services, National Institute of Health, NIH Publication No. 15-3770.

National Institute of Drug Abuse. (2018). *Understanding drug use and addiction drugfacts*. Retrieved from https://drugabuse.gov/publications/drugfacts/understanding-drug-use-addiction

National Institute of Drug Abuse. (2020, June). *MDMA (ecstasy/molly) drug facts*. National Institute of Health, Department of Health and Human Services. Retrieved from https://nida.nih.gov/publications/drugfacts/mdma-ecstasymolly

National Institute of Drug Abuse. (2022a, April). *The body's response to cocaine*. National Institute of Health, Department of Health and Human Services. Retrieved from https://nida.nih.gov/sites/default/files/NIDA_MindMatters_508_Cocaine_2022.pdf

National Institute of Drug Abuse. (2022b, April). *The body's response to K2/spice and bath salts*. National Institute of Health, Department of Health and Human Services. Retrieved from https://nida.nih.gov/sites/default/files/NIDA_MindMatters_508_K2Spice_2022.pdf

National Institute of Drug Abuse. (2022c, April). *The body's response to marijuana*. National Institute of Health, Department of Health and Human Services. Retrieved from https://nida.nih.gov/sites/default/files/NIDA_MindMatters_508_Marijuana_2022.pdf

National Institute of Drug Abuse. (2022d, April). *The body's response to methamphetamine*. National Institute of Health, Department of Health and Human Services. Retrieved from https://nida.nih.gov/sites/default/files/NIDA_MindMatters_508_Meth_2022.pdf

National Institute of Drug Abuse. (2022e, April). *The body's response to nicotine, tobacco, and vaping*. National Institute of Health, Department of Health and Human Services. Retrieved from https://nida.nih.gov/sites/default/files/NIDA_MindMatters_508_Nicotine_2022.pdf

National Institute of Drug Abuse. (2022f, April). *The body's response to opioids*. National Institute of Health, Department of Health and Human Services. Retrieved from https://nida.nih.gov/sites/default/files/NIDA_MindMatters_508_Opioids_2022.pdf

National Institute of Drug Abuse. (2022g, April). *The body's response to prescription stimulants*. National Institute of Health, Department of Health and Human Services. Retrieved from https://nida.nih.gov/sites/default/files/NIDA_MindMatters_508_RxStim_2022.pdf

Nicksic, N. E., Snell, L. M., & Barnes, A. J. (2019). *Addictive Behaviors, 93*, 93–99. https://doi.org/10.1016/j.addbeh.2019.01.037

Office of the Surgeon General. (2022, April 8). *Addiction and Substance misuse reports and publications*. Retrieved from https://www.hhs.gov/surgeongeneral/reports-and-publications/addiction-and-substance-misuse/index.html

Palamar, J. J., Ciccarone, D., Rutherford, C., Keyes, K. M., Carr, T. H., & Cottler, L. B. (2022). Trends in seizures of powders and pills containing illicit fentanyl in the United States, 2018 through 2021. *Drug and Alcohol Dependence, 234*. https://doi.org/10.1016/j.drugalcdep.2022.109398

Patrick, M. E., Miech, R. A., Carlier, C., O'Malley, P. M., Johnston, L. D., & Schulenberg, J. E. (2016). Self-reported reasons for vaping among 8th, 10th, and 12th graders in the US: Nationally-representative results. *Journal of Drug and Alcohol Dependence, 165*, 275–278. https://doi.org/10.1016/j.drugalcdep.2016.05.017

Reilly, C., & Smith, N. (n.d.). *The evolving definition of pathological gambling in the DSM-5*. National Center for Responsible Gaming. Retrieved from https://icrg.org/sites/default/files/uploads/docs/white_papers/ncrg_wpdsm5_may2013.pdf

Robinson, S. M., & Adinoff, B. (2016). The classification of substance use disorders: Historical, contextual, and conceptual considerations. *Behavioral Sciences, 6*(18), 1–23. https://doi.org/10.3390/bs6030018

Rosenberg, K. P., Carnes, P., & O'Connor, S. (2014). Evaluation and treatment of sex addiction. *Journal of Sex & Marital Therapy, 40*(2), 77–91. https://doi.org/10.1080/0092623X.2012.701268

Saleemi, S., Pennybaker, S. J., Wooldridge, M., & Johnson, M. W. (2017). Who is 'molly'? MDMA adulterants by product name and the impact of harm-reduction services at raves. *Journal of Psychopharmacology, 31*(8), 1056–1060. https://doi.org/10.1177/0269881117715596

Scully, R. (2021, October 6). *California ends mandatory minimum sentences for nonviolent drug offenses*. The Hill. Retrieved from https://thehill.com/homenews/state-watch/575517-california-ends-mandatory-minimum-sentences-for-nonviolent-drug-offenses/

Sexton, J. D., Crawford, M. S., Sweat, N. W., Varley, A., Green, E. E., & Hendricks, P. S. (2019). Prevalence and epidemiological associates of novel psychedelic use in the United States adult population. *Journal of Psychopharmacology, 33*(9), 1058–1067. https://doi.org/10.1177/0269881119827796

Skewes, M. C., & Gonzalez, V. M. (2013). The biopsychosocial model of addiction. *Principles of Addiction, 1*, 61–70. https://doi.org/10.1016/B978-0-12-398336-7.00006-1

Sproul, C. (2021). "Don't kill my buzz, man!" – Explaining the criminalization of psychedelic drugs. *Oregon Undergraduate Research Journal, 19*(1), 1–53. Retrieved from https://scholarsbank.uoregon.edu/xmlui/bitstream/handle/1794/26389/SproulDontKillMyBuzz.pdf?sequence=1&isAllowed=y#:~:text=By%201960%2C%20they%20had%20been,by%20the%20US%20federal%20government.

Stevens, M. W. R., Dorstyn, D., Delfabbro, P. H., & King, D. L. (2021). Global prevalence of gaming disorder: A systematic review and meta-analysis. *Australian & New Zealand Journal of Psychiatry, 55*(6), 553–568. https://doi.org/10.1177/0004867420962851

Stogner, J. M., Eassey, J. M., Baldwin, J. M., & Miller, B. L. (2014). Innovative alcohol use: Assessing the prevalence of alcohol without liquid and other non-oral routes of alcohol administration. *Drug and Alcohol Dependence, 142*, 74–78. https://doi.org/10.1016/j.drugalcdep.2014.05.026

Substance Abuse and Mental Health Services Administration. (2021). *Key substance use and mental health indicators in the United States: Results from the 2020 National Survey on Drug Use and Health* (HHS Publication No. PEP21-07-01-003, NSDUH Series H-56. Rockville, MD. https://www.samhsa.gov/data/sites/default/files/reports/rpt35325/NSDUHFFRPDFWHTMLFiles2020/2020NSDUHFFR1PDFW102121.pdf

Sulmasy, D. P. (2002). A biopsychosocial-spiritual model for the care of patients at the end of life. *Gerontologist, 42* (Spec. No. 3), 24–33. https://doi.org/10.1093/geront/42.suppl_3.24

U.S. Department of Health and Human Services. (2016). *E-cigarette use among youth and young adults: A report of the surgeon general.* Public Health Service, Office of the Surgeon General. Rockville, MD. Retrieved from https://www.cdc.gov/tobacco/sgr/e-cigarettes/pdfs/2016_sgr_entire_report_508.pdf

U.S. Department of Health and Human Services. (2017, October 26). *HHS acting secretary declares public health emergency to address national opioid crisis.* Retrieved from https://www.hhs.gov/about/news/2017/10/26/hhs-acting-secretary-declares-public-health-emergency-address-national-opioid-crisis.html

U.S. Food and Drug Administration. (2022, February 16). *FDA alerts health care professionals of potential risks associated with compounded ketamine nasal spray.* https://www.fda.gov/drugs/human-drug-compounding/fda-alerts-health-care-professionals-potential-risks-associated-compounded-ketamine-nasal-spray

van Boekel, L. C., Brouwers, E. P. M., van Weeghel, J., & Garretsen, H. F. L. (2013). Stigma among health professionals towards patients with substance use disorders and its consequences for healthcare delivery: Systematic review. *Drug and Alcohol Dependence, 131,* 23–35. https://doi.org/10.1016/j.drugalcdep.2013.02.018

Veach, L. J., Rogers, J. L., & Essic, E. J. (2012). Substance addictions. In D. Capuzzi & M. D. Stauffer (Eds.), *Foundations of addiction counseling* (pp. 17–40). Pearson.

Whittaker, E., Dadabayev, A. R., Joshi, S. A., & Glue, P. (2021). Systematic review and meta-analysis of randomized controlled trials of ketamine in the treatment of refractory anxiety spectrum disorders. *Therapeutic Advances in Psychopharmacology, 11,* 1–12. https://doi.org/10.1177/20451253211056743

Zelaya, C. E., Dahlhamer, J. M., Lucas, J. W., & Connor, E. M. (2020). Chronic pain and high-impact chronic pain among U.S. adults, 2019. *NCHS Data Brief,* (390), 1–8. National Center for Health Statistics, Centers for Disease Control and Prevention.

CHAPTER 3

NEUROSCIENCE OF CO-OCCURRING MENTAL AND SUBSTANCE USE DISORDERS

RAISSA MILLER

LEARNING OBJECTIVES

After reading this chapter, you will be able to:
- Identify key concepts of brain anatomy and physiology related to addiction and co-occurring mental disorders.
- Discuss the brain-based learning cycle underlying habit formation.
- Identify neural mechanisms and systems most implicated in the experience of addiction and co-occurring mental disorders.
- Apply understanding of brain and nervous system functioning in case conceptualization and treatment planning.

INTRODUCTION

Advances in technology and intentional public awareness and funding initiatives over the last three decades have resulted in significant advances in knowledge of the brain and nervous system (Erickson, 2018). Considering the evolving knowledge that is emerging from the neuroscience field, it is important for counselors to recognize how relevant this information is to the mental health professional. Bassett et al. (2020) noted that "neuroscience is—in principle—relevant to any field that seeks to understand, predict, or influence human behavior" (p. 524). Neuroscience can broaden assessment protocols, deepen case conceptualization, and inform treatment planning (Ray et al., 2020; Silvers et al., 2019). Neuroimaging studies have the potential to provide objective evidence of treatment response and specific therapeutic factors related to psychosocial interventions (Silvers et al., 2019). For example, Feldstein-Ewing et al. (2016) examined the way adolescents' brains responded to specific therapist behaviors (e.g., complex reflections vs. closed questions) and the associated behavioral outcomes (e.g., number of days drinking, number of binge drinking episodes). This type of translational research is just emerging, but it can offer promising new insight into how mental health professionals understand and treat addiction and mental health disorders.

The primary aim of this chapter is to review the basic brain and nervous system principles most relevant to addiction and co-occurring disorders so counselors can understand and apply them in practice. Areas of ongoing debate within the neuroscience and addiction fields that influence translational applications of the science are presented, and areas of ongoing research and shifting paradigms that will undoubtedly influence the next generation of mental health clinicians are identified.

DEFINING THE BRAIN AND THE EMBODIED NERVOUS SYSTEM

Neuroscience is a multidisciplinary science that is concerned with the study of the structure and function of the nervous system (Nature, n.d.). Erickson (2018) described the nervous system as "the body's control and communication network" (p. 53) with sensory and integrative functions. The nervous system monitors and interprets internal bodily cues and external inputs and, based on these interpretations, signals (via the release of hormones and other chemicals) to other bodily systems (e.g., cardiovascular, muscular, digestive). The nervous system has two parts—the central nervous system (CNS) and the peripheral nervous system (PNS). The head-located (skull) brain is part of the CNS and helps shape the flow of energy and information in the body (Siegel, 2020). Lewis (2017) defined the brain as "an open system that can develop in a multitude of directions, integrating the meaning of experience according to its own proclivities" (p. 16). The brain plays an important role in influencing mental life and behaviors. The brain, however, is part of a complex and interconnected system that can also be influenced by other factors, including the environment, relational connections, nutrition and other nonnutritional inputs (e.g., drugs, alcohol), and individual behaviors. Themes of brain complexity, integration, individual uniqueness, and bi-directional influence are noted and further expanded upon throughout this chapter.

BASIC BRAIN ANATOMY

In order to make sense of the translational neuroscience of addiction and mental health literature, it is useful to have a basic understanding of brain anatomy (e.g., brain structures, regions, general organization) and information processing principles. We can start this exploration with the most basic building blocks of the brain: glial cells and neurons (Siegel, 2020).

GLIAL CELLS

The role and value of glial cells in the brain is just beginning to be understood, but it is clear they play an essential role in maintaining brain health and responding to brain injury or pathology (Jakel & Dimou, 2017; Stellwagen et al., 2019). Glial cells constitute between 33% and 66% of the brain's mass.

NEURONS

Neurons carry signals and messages to other cells. Figure 3.1 provides a detailed picture of a neuron with labels for various parts of the cell. Extending from the cell body, there are dendrites, which carry messages toward the cell, and axons, which carry messages away from the cell. Communication between dendrites and axons happens across synapses via a process called neurotransmission. Neurotransmission relies on neurotransmitters. Scientists have identified

3: NEUROSCIENCE OF CO-OCCURRING MENTAL AND SUBSTANCE USE DISORDERS

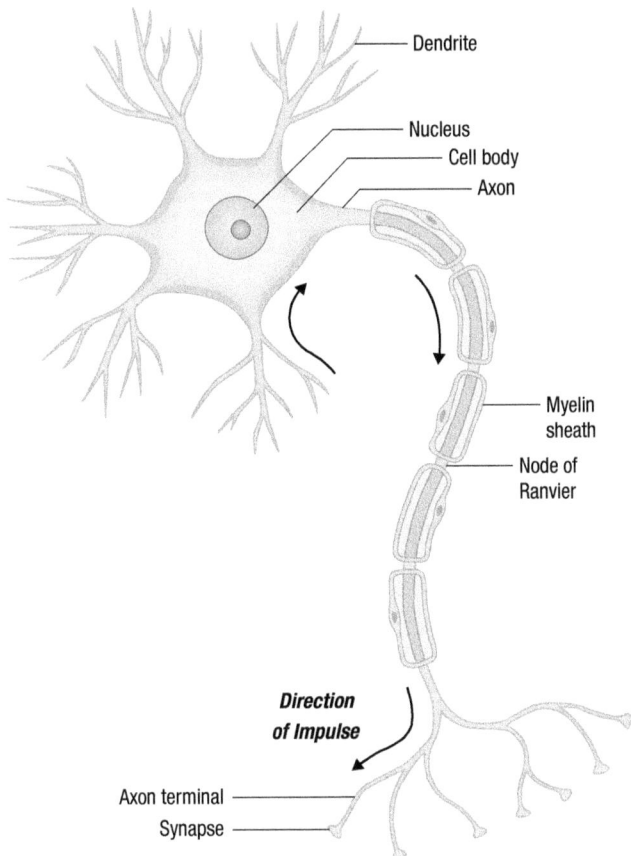

FIGURE 3.1 Detailed Picture of a Neuron.
Source: What are the parts of the nervous system? National Institutes of Health, Eunice Kennedy Shriver National Institute of Child Health and Human Development, 2018 (https://www.nichd.nih.gov/health/topics/neuro/conditioninfo/parts).

more than 60 unique neurotransmitters in the brain with various functions (Erickson, 2018). Neurotransmitters commonly implicated in addiction and the experience of mental distress include dopamine, serotonin, acetylcholine, endorphins, endocannabinoids, glutamate, and gamma aminobutyric acid (GABA).

BRAIN REGIONS AND STRUCTURES

Most broadly, the brain is divided into lower, central, and upper brain structures (Siegel, 2020) as depicted in Figure 3.2.

LOWER BRAIN

The *lower brain* includes the brainstem, thalamus, hypothalamus, and the pituitary. Structures in this part of the brain regulate basic functions essential for life, such as respiration, arousal, temperature, heart rate, and so forth. Structures in this region also play a central role in responding to perceived threat (e.g., fight, flight, freeze, faint).

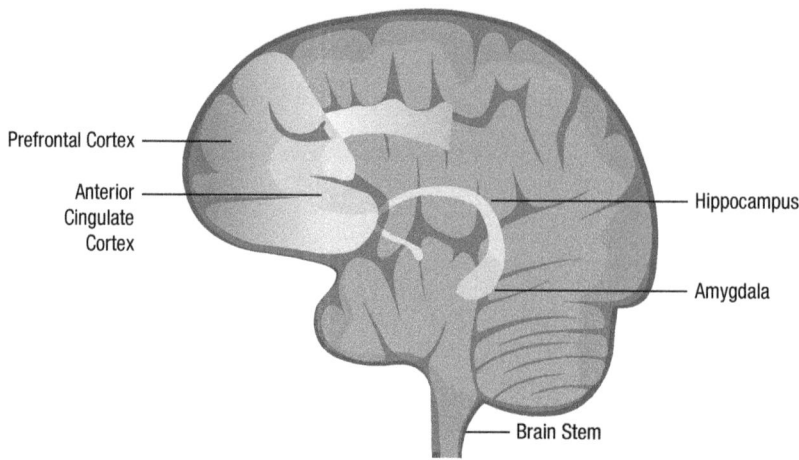

FIGURE 3.2 Brain Regions.
Source: Adapted from the National Institute of Mental Health, National Institutes of Health, Department of Health and Human Services, 2011. https://www.flickr.com/photos/nihgov/24024310606/in/album-72157662951050375/

CENTRAL BRAIN

The *central brain* area, often referred to as the limbic region, houses parts of the brain that play an important role in memory, motivation, attachment, and emotion. The hippocampus and amygdala are two specific structures in the central brain area that are often discussed in addiction and mental health literature.

UPPER BRAIN

Finally, the *upper brain* structures include the cerebral cortex, with the prefrontal cortex (PFC) receiving the most attention in translational applications. Working in connection with the subcortical regions, the PFC mediates higher-order thinking, planning, reflecting, focusing, and reasoning. These abilities are often referred to as executive functions. The PFC is further divided into lateral, ventral, and medial areas; thus, counselors may be inclined to read further about the "dorsolateral PFC" or the "orbitofrontal cortex" and the specific functions each of these localized areas is hypothesized to facilitate. Having a basic sense of these brain regions and structures is useful, but it is important to note that all of these areas are connected and, especially in healthy brains, work together in an integrated and complementary manner. Increasingly, neuroscientists are referring to the "connectome" and to brain "networks" and "systems" more so than isolated "parts."

THE CONNECTOME, NETWORKS, AND SYSTEMS

Although reducing the brain to "parts" with specific functions can be useful for simplifying explanations and understanding the impact of undifferentiated or damaged structures or regions, in reality, the brain is a complex and interconnected system (Bassett et al., 2018; Siegel, 2020).

THE CONNECTOME

Neuroscientists are increasingly emphasizing the interconnected nature of the brain and focusing on developing theories and tools that can better capture the complexity (Ekhtiari et al., 2016). For example, the term *connectome* refers to "the interconnected networks of the brain located within the head" (Siegel, 2020, p. 503) and has been the most focus of recent research efforts. Integration in the connectome has been associated with greater well-being, whereas lack of integration has been correlated with mental unhealth. Network neuroscience specifically explores how neurons connect with one another to produce specific functions and behaviors.

THREE NETWORKS

Immordino-Yang et al. (2018) outlined three networks: (a) the executive control network, (b) the default mode network, and (c) the salience network. The *executive control network*, sometimes called the frontoparietal network, is most active in goal-oriented tasks, attention and focus, and top-down regulation of thoughts, feelings, and behaviors (i.e., "cognitive control"). The *default mode network* is most active during internally directed, self-related cognitive tasks (e.g., episodic or autobiographical memory, self-reflection, interoception) and interpretative tasks (e.g., understanding thoughts and behaviors of others, imagining hypothetical or future situations; Ekhtiari et al., 2016; Zhang & Volkow, 2019). Finally, the *salience network* evaluates external and internal stimuli and facilitates mental modes and guides behavior based on the evaluation. The salience network also plays a key role in facilitating communication between the executive control network and the default mode network (Uddin, 2015).

SEVEN SYSTEMS

The Research Domain Criteria (RDoC) framework (Kozak & Cuthbert, 2016) provides an additional means to conceptualize the brain, especially as the brain relates to other levels of analysis and across diverse symptom presentation. The framework includes seven broad systems or domains: (a) the negative valence system, (b) the positive valence system, (c) cognitive systems, (d) systems that mediate social processes, (e) arousal systems, (f) regulatory systems, and (g) sensorimotor systems. Each of these systems includes specific constructs, such as threat detection and responding (*negative valence*), reward valuation and learning (*positive valence*) and attention, perception, and memory (*cognitive system*).

BRAIN AND NERVOUS SYSTEM DEVELOPMENT

Individuals are born with unique genotypes, often referred to as genetic heredity, that influence various physical features, personality traits, and vulnerability to diseases (Erickson, 2018). Despite significant funding and effort to identify genes involved in addiction and mental health concerns, the research thus far has failed to yield practically useful findings (Marsman et al., 2020). Of greater predictive validity has been the influence of experiences on development and outcome. *Experience-dependent epigenetics* is a term used to describe the role experiences play in turning off or on certain genes, leading to genetic expression and phenotype (Feinberg & Fallin, 2015). *Phenotype* is simply the state or trait we can observe.

CHILDHOOD AND ADOLESCENCE

The brain and nervous system develop most rapidly during early childhood and adolescence. Experiences that happen during these critical or sensitive periods have disproportionate and long-lasting impacts on brain structure and function (Cousijn et al., 2018; Teicher & Samson, 2016; Teicher et al., 2016). For example, children who are cared for within the context of safe, predictable, and caring relationships tend to develop brains and nervous systems that expect other people to be generally trustworthy and helpful; thus, they seek out relationships as a source of pleasure (i.e., reward) and a source of support when distressed. These children are also often able to better regulate their thoughts, feelings, and behaviors as their brains tend to function in a more integrated and connected manner. Related to their ability to better co-regulate and self-regulate, they are less vulnerable to mental health struggles or using substances to self-soothe. Conversely, experiences of relational poverty and chronic adversity can foster brain and nervous systems that are less integrated and more vulnerable to addiction and mental health struggles (Bachi et al., 2018; Strathearn et al., 2019).

Adverse Childhood Experiences

Existing literature on the impact of adverse childhood experiences (ACEs) on brain development provides some insights regarding this phenomenon. The original ACEs study was a retrospective epidemiological study that asked adults about 10 types of childhood experiences (e.g., experiences of abuse, parent with a substance use or mental health disorder, experiences of divorce) and then correlated those experiences with other physical and behavioral health outcomes (Felitti et al., 1998). The researchers found that the higher the ACE number on a scale from 1 to 10 (i.e., the more adverse circumstances the person reported), the greater likelihood for poor health outcomes. Since the original ACEs study, researchers have continued to explore this link between early adversity and later health outcomes. Neuroscientists in particular have studied the way the brain changes in response to experiences. It is largely undisputable now that chronic and/or severe adversity can result in neuroadaptations that then lead to long-term impacts on cognition, affect, and behavior (Strathearn et al., 2019). For example, neuroimaging studies examining the impact of threat exposure on the developing brain have shown alterations in the amygdala, medial prefrontal cortex (mPFC), and hippocampus resulting in heightened fear activation, problems with memory, and struggles with executive function (McLaughlin et al., 2019; Teicher et al., 2016). Experiences of deprivation (i.e., neglect) have been correlated with slightly different neurodevelopment outcomes, with a greatest impact on frontoparietal regions that play essential roles in attention, problem-solving, and working memory. Both chronic and/or severe exposure to threat and deprivation are associated with problems in cognitive control of emotions (i.e., deficits in self-regulation).

Systemic Oppression and Socioeconomic Inequality

One type of chronic adversity that has historically been overlooked by researchers is that of systemic oppression and socioeconomic inequality (Clark et al., 2018; Noble & Giebler, 2020). Although observational associations have been made between these struggles and greater vulnerability for poor physical and mental health outcomes, less was known about the mechanisms for this relationship. In an effort to address this gap in the literature, Clark et al. (2018) explored neural changes in response to experiences of discrimination and found that they were associated with higher levels of spontaneous amygdala activity and stronger connections between the amygdala and salience network nodes. This finding suggests greater threat conditioning and hyperactivity of this system, which has been associated with physical and mental health struggles over time. Another group of researchers, Tomlinson et al. (2020), found that neighborhood poverty predicted decreased activation in the *inferior frontal gyrus* (IFG). The IFG plays a critical role in response inhibition (i.e., self-control). Noble and Giebler (2020) provided a more comprehensive review of the impact of socioeconomic inequality on neurodevelopment. They highlighted mechanistic findings that offer clues to emotional and reward processing differences and executive functioning deficits in individuals with disadvantaged socioeconomic backgrounds. This line of emerging neuroscience research has great potential for increasing empathy and compassion for individuals impacted by discrimination and socioeconomic disparities and targeting interventions that will help prevent the neuroadaptations that lead to later vulnerabilities.

Social baseline theory also offers an empirical explanation for why relational poverty impacts brain development so profoundly (Beckes & Coan, 2011; Coan & Sbarra, 2015). According to this theory, being in physical and psychological contact with trusted others is what our brain expects, especially during times of stress. Being in connection when facing challenges results in less activation of the threat response system, therefore saving valuable metabolic energy. Other researchers have shown that having to chronically self-regulate (vs. co-regulate) in response to perceived threats wears down the brain and body resulting in advanced cell aging (Colich et al., 2020; Miller et al., 2015). For example, Miller et al. (2015) found that youth from low socioeconomic statuses psychologically benefited as young adults from having been exposed to psychosocial interventions aimed at fostering self-regulation during adolescence; however, they showed epigenetic aging at the cellular level. The individuals in the study could learn to competently self-regulate but all the self-regulation took a physical toll.

It is worth noting that caution should be taken in making assumptions about individuals just because of their adversity background. Many of the aforementioned studies are epidemiological in nature and not intended to be used for making any individual-level predictions. For example, researchers have strongly advocated against using the ACEs questionnaire (National Center for Injury Prevention and Control, 2021) for the purpose of qualifying individuals for services or making individual-level predictions (Anda et al., 2020). Many factors play into a single individual's experience and outcome, including the type and typing of adversity and the presence of protective factors that support resilience.

Neuroplasticity

The hopeful news is that although early experiences have an undeniable impact on brain development and functioning, individuals can change their brain and nervous system throughout the lifespan (Dahl et al., 2020). This ability is referred to as *neuroplasticity*. A robust body of literature is now emerging looking at the factors that influence positive neuroplasticity and promote optimal brain functioning. Rock et al. (2012) conceptualized these factors through *The Healthy Mind Platter* (HMP). The seven elements of the HMP include (a) sleep, (b) physical activity, (c) connection, time-in (e.g., mindfulness meditation, internal reflection), (d) focus time (e.g., engaging in a mastery or goal-oriented activity), (e) down-time (e.g., intentionally having no intention), and (f) play-time (e.g., spontaneous, novel activity). Another group of researchers with the Center for Healthy Minds identified the four core dimensions underlying plasticity of well-being: (a) awareness, (b) connection, (c) insight, and (d) purpose (Dahl et al., 2020). The common thread between these two frameworks is research demonstrating increased growth and connection in regions of the brain associated with top-down regulation of emotion, values-based decision-making, and social engagement.

With a basic understanding of neuroanatomy and neurodevelopmental processes, it is now time to turn attention to the neuroscience principles most relevant in addiction and experiences of mental distress.

NEUROSCIENCE OF ADDICTION AND MENTAL HEALTH DISORDERS

The neuroscience of addiction and mental health disorders can be most easily understood in terms of how the brain learns (Lewis, 2017). Related to the principle of plasticity, the brain is also self-organizing. Thoughts, feelings, and behaviors start out as tentative and variable in the brain, but with repeated activation, they strengthen and stabilize into expected patterns (Siegel, 2020). Prior learning influences current and future perceptions and predictions and biases experiences toward habitual expectations. This adaptive and efficient process is often referred to as *automatization*. New learning and repeated practice promote neural and synaptic *genesis* (birth of new neurons and synaptic connections), whereas lack of activation and practice results in *pruning* (the dying off of neurons and synapses). Experiences that have high motivational impact, meaning they are emotionally arousing (e.g., experiences of pleasure, threat), have the largest impact on learning. Figure 3.3 represents a brain-based learning cycle characterized by an initial emotionally arousing novel experience transitioning into a stabilized, self-perpetuating habit (Lewis, 2017). This cycle is generally representative of physiological changes related to drugs of abuse and emotional states, such as anxiety and depression.

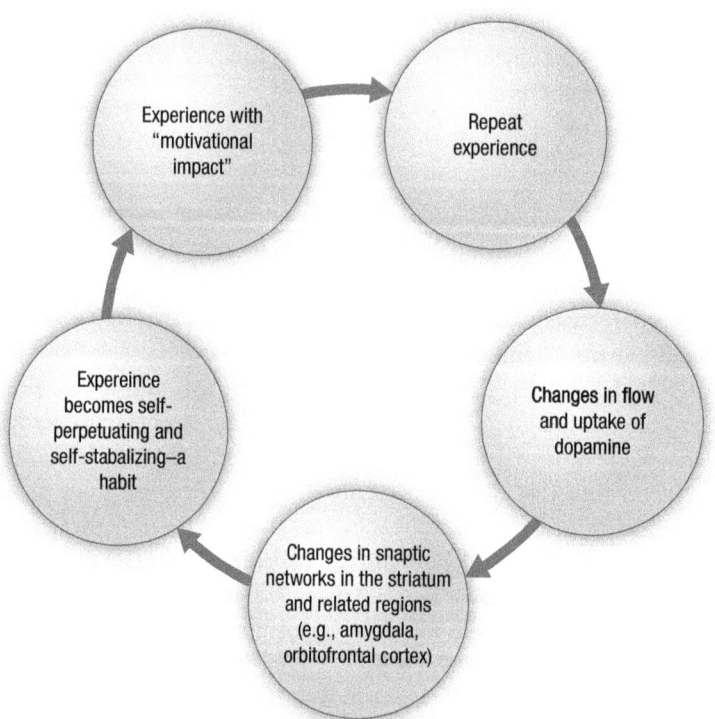

FIGURE 3.3 Brain-Based Learning Cycle.
Source: Image created from source material in Lewis, M. (2017). Addiction and the brain: Development, not disease. *Neuroethics, 10*, 7–18.

ADDICTION THROUGH THE LENS OF NEUROSCIENCE

Narrowing the lens of learning specifically to substances, the idea that certain substances are endogenously addictive has been around since at least the late 1700s. The *brain disease model of addiction* (BDMA), emerging in the mid 1900s, represents a formalization of this perspective and has become the dominant theory within the scientific and public health communities (Heather et al., 2018; Volkow et al., 2016). In 2011, the American Society of Addiction Medicine (ASAM) defined addiction as "a primary, chronic disease of brain reward, motivation, memory and related circuitry. Dysfunction in these circuits leads to characteristic biological, psychological, social and spiritual manifestations" (p. 1). The longer definition included more context (e.g., the role of culture, exposure to trauma and stressors, individual resiliency factors), but the primary focus was on malfunctioning brain circuitry. This was the message emphasized and taught within educational, public health, and treatment settings for the better part of the last decade (Volkow et al., 2016).

In 2019, ASAM revised their definition significantly, removing the notion of addiction as a primary brain disease and instead giving more equal attention to biological and ecological factors (ASAM, 2019). This organization explicitly highlighted the complexity of addition and included behaviors as potentially addictive. This change reflects advancements in neuroscience research, which paradoxically resulted in scientists acknowledging knowing *less* rather than more about the brain in relation to addiction (Heather et al., 2018). The 2019 revised short definition is, "Addiction is a treatable, chronic medical disease involving complex interactions among brain circuits, genetics, the environment, and an individual's life experiences. People with addiction use substances or engage in behaviors that become compulsive and often continue despite harmful consequences" (ASAM, 2019, p. 2). This definition shifts some of the focus, but the notion that addiction is a *disease* and that substances change the brain in ways that are nearly impossible to reverse persists (Lewis, 2017). The accuracy and value of using the term *disease* to describe the experience of addiction has received substantial attention in the literature (Hammer et al., 2013; Heather et al., 2018; Heyman, 2013; Lewis, 2017; Snoek, 2017). For the purposes of this chapter, when reviewing the science of addition literature, it will be important to keep in mind that addiction is not a one-dimensional phenomenon (e.g., solely the consequence of brain malfunction). Social and environmental factors greatly influence brain development and functioning; therefore, they play a significant role in the formation of and recovery from addition and co-occurring mental disorders.

BRAIN REGIONS AND SYSTEMS INVOLVED IN ADDICTION

The brain and nervous system do respond and adapt to substances and repeated behaviors (Lewis, 2017). Researchers have observed that drugs, and more recently, behaviors, can change the structure and function of the brain resulting in altered reward processing, impaired decision-making, and emotional dysregulation (Heather et al., 2018; Koob & Volkow, 2016). The exact nature of those changes can vary among individuals, substance or behavior, and stage of addiction, but the general idea is that chronic exposure to rewarding, pleasurable stimuli increases motivation for those rewards while at the same time decreasing behavioral control (Ersche et al., 2013; Heather et al., 2018). Researchers have identified generalized adaptations and mechanisms implicated in this experience (Hayes et al., 2020). Most of these changes have focused on neurons; however, recent research has also highlighted the critical role that glial cells (e.g., astrocytes, microglia) play in modulating neurotransmission, synaptic connectivity, and neural circuit function (Linker et al., 2018). Future research may reveal more about glial cells and specific targeting of these cells to treat addictive brain states and behaviors.

Two of the leading researchers in the neuroscience of addiction literature area are Dr. George Koob, Director of the National Institute on Alcohol Abuse and Alcoholism (NIAAA), and Dr. Nora Volkow, Director of the National Institute on Drug Abuse (NIDA). For over 30 years, Koob and Volkow have researched neuroplastic changes in brain regions and neurocircuitry adaptations underlying addiction (Koob, 2013; Koob & Volkow, 2016; Volkow et al., 2013, 2016). They have been at the forefront of advocating for the BDMA and the three-stage addiction cycle.

THREE-STAGE CYCLE

The three-stage addiction cycle offers a heuristic model of neurobiological circuit activation during the (a) *binge and intoxication*, (b) *withdrawal and negative affect*, and (c) *preoccupation and anticipation* (i.e., craving) stages of addiction (Volkow et al., 2016). Readers are invited to explore the images presented in Koob and Volkow (2016) for a comprehensive look at the brain imagery involved in this cycle. Volkow et al. (2016) proposed that individuals initially use substances voluntarily to feel good but then transition to using in order to avoid negative withdrawal symptoms and/or to subdue the agitation of craving. Hayes et al. (2020) referred to this experience as the brain seeking to achieve homeostasis and experiencing a combination of interrelated physiological and psychological symptoms (e.g., dysphoria, emotional stress, decreasing cognitive abilities) when homeostasis cannot be achieved.

A combination of genetic (e.g., tendency toward impulsivity or sensation seeking), developmental (e.g., adolescents experience greater biological drives for rewards and risk taking), and environmental/experiential (e.g., history of trauma, easy access to substances in community or friend group) influence initial use (Eme, 2017; Volkow et al., 2016). Once use has begun, individuals enter into the *binge and intoxication* stage, during which time the primary mechanism of action is dopamine and its influence on the reward and motivation system (Wise & Robble, 2020). This stage heavily involves the basal ganglia and the key subregion of the nucleus accumbens. According to Volkow et al. (2016), substance use triggers the release of dopamine and the substance and its environmental cues become associated with a high-value reward, leading to conditioned physiological processes (i.e., craving and compulsive use).

When individuals achieve tolerance to a substance and then stop using, they begin to experience *withdrawal and negative affect* mediated largely by lower levels of global dopamine in the brain (Wise & Robble, 2020) and changes to emotional processing areas of the brain (e.g., the amygdala, the basal forebrain). These changes result in less sensitivity to rewards, greater stress reactivity, and negative emotional states. The final stage of the cycle, *preoccupation and anticipation*, is characterized by alterations in the prefrontal cortical regions that further impair executive function (e.g., decision-making, emotion regulation). Specifically, there is loss of connectivity between the PFC and the striatum. Volkow et al. (2016) attributed the PFC changes to the down-regulation of dopamine signaling and changes in glutamatergic signaling.

To both elaborate on and summarize the above information, the neurocircuitry of addiction involves disruption and adaptation (i.e., substance-induced neuroplasticity) in the two interconnected systems of the mesolimbic and mesocortical regions, broadly referred to as the *mesocorticalimbic pathway*, or the brain reward system (Suckling & Nestor, 2016; Uhl et al., 2019). Specific structures implicated in these systems include the ventral tegmental area (VTA), the ventral striatum including the nucleus accumbens, the amygdala, and the medial PFC, with dopamine playing a central, albeit more convoluted, role in the development and maintenance of these changes (Hayes et al., 2020; Uhl et al., 2019). Beyond these global impacts, specific white and gray matter volume changes are often contradictory between different stages of addiction and different types of substances. Although all substances seemed to impact reward processing and inhibitory control, the exact mechanisms involved are not fully understood.

RELATIONSHIP BETWEEN SUBSTANCE USE AND MENTAL DISORDERS

Overall, there is very limited research on the neurobiology of co-occurring substance use and mental health disorders (Balhara et al., 2017; Gómez-Coronado et al., 2018). Implications from the research that does exist is limited by small and nondiverse samples. There is some research looking at specific diagnoses and specific classes of drugs (e.g., alcohol, cocaine, marijuana). For example, Gilpin and Weiner (2017) found greater structural and functional changes in the amygdala of individuals diagnosed with both posttraumatic stress disorder (PTSD) and alcohol use disorder. The researchers also identified possible hypoconnectivity in the PFC to the amygdala, hypofunction and dysregulation in the mesolimbic dopamine system, hyperarousal and heightened responsivity to stress, and hippocampal deficits impacting learning, memory, and regulation of the hypothalamic-pituitary-adrenal axis.

Eme (2017) studied individuals with an attention deficit hyperactivity disorder (ADHD) diagnosis and individuals with a substance use disorder diagnosis. The researcher found overlapping dysfunctions in the mesolimbic and neocortical dopamine systems, resulting in impaired sensitivity to reward and impaired control. Both groups of individuals became bored more easily, thus they were more motivated to seek rewards. Eme discussed how such mechanisms may help explain why ADHD increases vulnerability for addictions. Finally, Gómez-Coronado et al. (2018) examined the relationship between tobacco use and depression and found correlated dopaminergic dysfunction. The overarching theme to this emerging body of literature is that many of the same brain systems implicated in addiction are involved in mental disorders. Both addiction and mental health disorders impair optimal integration of the frontoparietal, default mode, and salience brain network systems.

IMPLICATIONS FOR TREATMENT

Fortunately, just as the brain changes in response to substance use and mental distress, so too can it change in response to new ways of thinking, feeling, and behaving (Erickson & White, 2009; Garavan et al., 2013). Lewis (2017) eloquently summarized the neuroscience of recovery stating "with the onset of addiction, plasticity is devoted to new means for acquiring pleasure or relief. With recovery, plasticity is devoted to goals with far-reaching personal value and skills necessary to attain them" (p. 14). Abstinence from substances can restore healthier brain structures and functions.

The most consistent findings in the small but growing neuroscience of recovery literature provide evidence that volume reductions in cortical and prefrontal regions common in substance use can be reversed after just a few weeks of cessation from substances (Garavan et al., 2013). This finding is perhaps not surprising given the need for activating the cortical control networks to sustain abstinence—and the more you "use" a brain structure or network (via neural firing), the stronger and better connected it becomes. For example, Ekhtiari et al. (2017) developed a neuroscience-informed psychoeducation program and noted that one of the benefits of the approach is that it intentionally engages "different neurocognitive processes, including salience/attention, memory, and self-awareness" (p. 239). Relatedly, Witkiewitz et al. (2013) provided a review of the commonly used cognitive-behavioral intervention, mindfulness-based relapse prevention (MBRP). In their review, they discussed how the neurobiology of mindfulness meditation overlaps with the neurobiology of addiction. The very systems that mindfulness meditation strengthens (e.g., connections between the prefrontal executive control systems and the ventral striatal pleasure circuitry) are the very circuits most impacted by substance use. Further evidence of this idea can be found in reviews of other cognitive, motivational, and emotional approaches to addiction treatment. Zilverstand et al. (2016) concluded that the core mechanism underlying many talk therapy interventions in the addiction field is normalizing the reward circuitry primarily by way of strengthening the brain's inhibitory control network (e.g., PFC).

Overall, the field of translating neuroscience findings into practical applications is still in its infancy. As noted in the introduction, there are very few neuroimaging studies looking at the impact of therapeutic interventions on brain structure and function (Garavan et al., 2013; Hayes et al., 2020; Morgenstern et al., 2013). An important consideration for the application of any intervention is the need to individualize treatment. Given the unique nature of brain development and functioning, inflexible manuals and protocols would not likely serve individuals with addiction and co-occurring disorders best. Along these lines, Ekhtiari el al. (2016) called for individualized treatment planning and monitoring as well as integrative approaches that incorporate cognitive, behavioral, interpersonal, and affective traditions.

In addition to these traditional talk therapy approaches, newer technology-based interventions are emerging that may provide additional support for recovery. Creed (2018) reviewed the latest findings related to neuromodulation therapies (e.g., deep brain stimulation [DBS], transcranial magnetic stimulation [TMS]), noting promising findings specifically related to protocols that target (i.e., stimulate) neural circuits in the cortico-basal ganglia network (e.g., the PFC and the nucleus accumbens). Ramlakhan et al. (2020) discussed using electroencephalography (EEG) to modulate gamma activity in individuals with addiction. Additionally, more generalized neurofeedback protocols (e.g., alpha-theta training for alcohol use disorders) have been used with success in treating addiction for many years (Marzbani et al., 2016).

CLINICAL CASE ILLUSTRATION AND DISCUSSION

CASE OF DAMION

Damion is a 41-year-old White cisgender male. He is married to a cisgender woman and has two biological teenage children; he also has a teenage step-child from his wife's first marriage. He reports feeling highly dissatisfied with his marriage and distant from all of his children. Damion has a well-paid managerial position at a large marketing firm. He commutes about 2 hours round trip to work each day. The primary symptoms he reports in his intake include anxiety (e.g., uncontrollable worry, irritability, restlessness, muscle tension) and depression with suicidal ideation (e.g., generalized depressed mood and lack of pleasure, feelings of hopelessness and worthlessness, insomnia, and recurrent thoughts of dying). Damion reports having attempted suicide 5 years prior by driving his car into a tree. He says he woke up in the emergency department and felt angry and disappointed that he was still alive. Since that time, he said he continued to think about killing himself but so far has not attempted again. Damion says he had tried taking antidepressant and antianxiety medications in the past but they did not help. Damion reports that he drinks alcohol daily to "quiet his mind." He says he keeps a bottle of vodka in his car and drinks all the way to work, during his lunch break, and all the way back home. He says he could not remember a day he had not consumed alcohol in the last 2 years. He notes that the last time he tried to stop drinking, he felt like he was "going to die." He confidently asserts that no one at his work knows he drinks alcohol and it does not impair his life—it only helps it (although he admits that the drinking has caused many arguments with his wife). When sharing about his early family history, Damion reports having a fearful relationship of his father and an emotionally detached relationship with his mother. He said he witnessed his father beating his mother frequently as a child and, on occasion, his father would turn his fist on him. Damion says his father left the family when he was 10 years old, and he has not had any contact with him for the last 30 years. Damion described his mother as "a sad, self-centered woman" who barely cared enough to make sure he ate. He says he began to drink alcohol at age 12 as an escape from his life and has only had brief periods of abstinence as an adult. Based on a thorough clinical interview, the counselor determines he meets criteria for the following *DSM-5* diagnoses:

1. **Generalized anxiety disorder**: Excessive anxiety and worry that was difficult to control. Primary symptoms included uncontrollable worry, restlessness, irritability, muscle tension, and difficulty with sleep.
2. **Major depressive disorder**: Depressed mood, loss of interest/pleasure, insomnia, feeling worthless, thoughts of suicide.
3. **Alcohol use disorder, severe**: Unsuccessful efforts to quit drinking alcohol, spending a lot of time using alcohol, craving alcohol, continuing to use even when it causes problems in relationships, development of tolerance over time, and withdrawal symptoms (e.g., shaking hands, sweating, insomnia, headache).

CASE DISCUSSION

Damion's story is unfortunately common in addiction and mental health treatment settings. He experienced significant relational poverty and abuse at a young age. His brain and nervous system learned that others could not be counted on for comfort and regulation of stress. People were a source of pain, not pleasure. Damion's mid-brain regions, including the amygdala and hypothalamic-pituitary-adrenal (HPA) system, had to remain on high alert (i.e., hypervigilant) as he was virtually on his own—it is quite dangerous to navigate the world alone, especially as a child. Anxiety was an adaptive and not unexpected outcome of having to live in a world that the brain had not evolved to thrive in (i.e., a world without the support of trusted others). Similarly, depressed mood is an expected outcome of a life void of safe and trusting relationships.

As a pre-adolescent, Damion found that alcohol was a more reliable source of reward and reprieve from distress. Although substance use may have provided perceived pleasure in the short-term, it likely inhibited further development of the frontoparietal network given the sensitive time of adolescent development on cortical/subcortical integration. And, although he began using alcohol for pleasure, over time his use was primarily driven by avoidance of withdrawal systems and the experience of negative emotions. Increasingly, his brain and body sought homeostasis and regulation through continued and progressive alcohol use. Chronic alcohol use turned into alcohol abuse and dependence, while at the same time exacerbating anxiety and interfering with close and healthy interpersonal relationships. Damion's progression from experimental use and pleasure to craving-induced abuse and dependence is consistent with the Volkow et al. (2016) three-stage addiction cycle previously discussed.

Given the vital role that sense relational connections play in an individual's sense of meaning in life and regulation of stress, it is not surprising that Damion would struggle with thoughts of killing himself. The chronic substance use and co-occurring mental disorders also likely resulted in decreased sensitivity to nonsubstance rewards via impairments to the salience network and reward pathway (e.g., food, sex, taking a walk-in nature on a beautiful day) and disruptions to the default mode network resulting in negative-based self-referential thinking and emotion. Each of these factors—early adversity, impaired neurodevelopment, impaired neural structures and functions as a result of alcohol use, ongoing relational distress—interconnected and reinforced automatic functioning that perpetuated Damion's problematic and distressing thoughts, feelings, and behaviors.

Neuroscience-informed treatment with Damion could take many directions. At its core, Damion needs to encounter affirming relational encounters in which his brain and body can begin to learn how to count on others for emotional support and connection, which, in turn, will help to mitigate his prior adverse experiences as well as challenge his beliefs. The consistency and supportive nature of the therapeutic relationship is a good place for Damion to start experiencing this type of relationship. Interventions, such as motivational interviewing and neuroscience-informed psychoeducation, that meet Damion where he is in his awareness of the problems and willingness to change could be crucial in gaining his buy-in and enhancing willingness to engage in the therapeutic process. Another priority for treatment is helping Damion cut back or abstain from alcohol use altogether so that his brain and nervous system can begin to heal. It is worth noting that Damion may need inpatient detoxification when quitting use of alcohol given his physiological dependence due to chronic use over many years. Inpatient support may also be helpful in further evaluating and addressing Damion's thoughts of suicide. Additionally, the alcohol has to be replaced with positive rewards and lifestyle behaviors that are supportive of new learning and neural growth, such as *The Healthy Mind Platter* (Rock et al., 2012) or the program from the Center for Healthy Minds described earlier in the chapter. In this sense, the reward circuitry, with dopamine activation at its core, needs to be redirected to health-promoting activities.

As Damion's brain begins to heal within the supportive therapeutic relationship and in response to lifestyle changes, traditional cognitive and behavioral interventions that help strengthen the frontoparietal network (e.g., MBRP) would be useful. These interventions could help Damion learn how to cope with cravings, reappraise negative thoughts, develop greater inhibitory control, strengthen problem-solving and decision-making abilities, and explore values and begin to set goals for living a life more in line with those values. Mindfulness-based approaches and other bottom-up interventions have also been found efficacious for treating anxiety disorder (Witkiewitz et al., 2013). Finally, adjunctive treatments, such as neurofeedback or neuromodulation therapies, may be warranted to support Damion's overall progress beyond traditional talk therapy modalities (Creed, 2018). There is no definitive time-line for healing the brain in recovery from addiction (Meyerhoff & Durazzo, 2020; Ray, 2012). Some improvements can be noted with only days or weeks of abstinence, whereas other changes take years to stabilize. The expectation should be slow, gradual changes over many months and years.

CHAPTER SUMMARY

The experience of addiction and co-occurring disorders involves a complex network of neural structures, neurotransmitters, and neuroadaptive processes. Neuroscience research is enhancing knowledge related to the mechanisms of addiction and addiction recovery, as well as co-occurring disorders, but there are still limitations to applying this research in therapeutic work. Researchers are increasingly shifting from activation and brain-mapping studies to more holistic network and connectome studies that better capture the interconnected and emergent nature of the brain (Bassett et al., 2020). There is also a growing emphasis on interindividual differences (vs. group analysis) that will allow the field to better understand interindividual variability and context. For example, are the brain differences observed in individuals with addiction the result of the substances themselves, or did the brain patterns predate the drug addiction (e.g., as a result of early adversity or exposure to toxins) and merely set the stage for vulnerability to addiction (Ersche et al., 2013)?

Furthermore, as technology becomes less invasive and more mobile, it is the hope of many researchers that they will be able to move from understanding the neurobiology of addiction through research in animal models to actual experiences of addiction and mental distress in humans, especially humans in the real-time context of their lived experiences (Hayes et al., 2020). All these areas of research progress will serve to better inform evaluation of current treatment methods and development of new effective interventions. The field of translational neuroscience is truly in its infancy and mental health counselors will no doubt need to continue updating and evolving their understanding of the neuroscience of addiction and co-occurring disorders moving into the future.

DISCUSSION QUESTIONS

1. Should neuroscience play a role in mental health professionals' understanding and treatment of co-occurring substance use and mental disorders? If so, what would this role look like?
2. How would you describe the links between early experiences, neurodevelopment, and mental health outcomes to a future client or family system?
3. How do your personal habits, positive or negative, align with Lewis's brain-based learning cycle? Share an example.
4. How does the label "brain disease" impact your view of addiction and co-occurring disorders?
5. What neuroscience information do you think is most relevant to share with clients who are diagnosed with substance use and/or co-occurring mental disorders and how do you envision integrating neuroscience principles or concepts into your counseling work?

REFERENCES

American Psychiatric Association. (2013). *Diagnostic and statistical manual of mental disorders* (5th ed.). https://doi.org/10.1176/appi.books.9780890425596

American Society of Addiction Medicine. (2011). *Public policy statement: Definition of addiction*. https://www.asam.org/docs/default-source/public-policy-statements/1definition_of_addiction_long_4-11.pdf?sfvrsn=a8f64512_4

American Society of Addiction Medicine. (2019). *Definition of addiction*. https://www.asam.org/docs/default-source/quality-science/asam's-2019-definition-of-addiction-(1).pdf?sfvrsn=b8b64fc2_2

Anda, R. F., Porter, L. E., & Brown, D. W. (2020). Inside the adverse childhood experience score: Strengths, limitations, and misapplications. *American Journal of Preventative Medicine, 59*(2), 293–295. https://doi.org/10.1016/j.amepre.2020.01.009

Bachi, K., Parvaz, M. A., Moeller, S. J., Gan, G., Zilverstand, A., Goldstein, R. Z., & Alia-Klein, N. (2018). Reduced orbitofrontal gray matter concentration as a marker of premorbid childhood trauma in cocaine use disorder. *Frontiers in Human Neuroscience, 12*(51). https://doi.org/10.3389/fnhum.2018.00051

Balhara, Y. P. S., Kuppili, P. P., & Gupta, R. (2017). Neurobiology of comorbid substance use disorders and psychiatric disorders. *International Nurses Society on Addictions, 28,* 11–26. https://doi.org/10.1097/JAN.0000000000000155

Bassett, D. S., Cullen, K. E., Eickhoff, S. B., Farah, M. J., Goda, Y., Haggard, P., Ju, H., Hurd, Y. L., Josselyn, S. A., Khakh, B. S., Knoblich, J. A., Poirazi, P., Poldrack, R. A., Prinz, M., Roelfsema, P. R., Spires-Jones, T. L., Sur, M., & Ueda, H. R. (2020). Reflections on the past two decades of neuroscience. *Nature Reviews Neuroscience, 21,* 524–534. https://doi.org/10.1038/s41583-020-0363-6

Bassett, D. S., Zurn, P., & Gold, J. I. (2018). On the nature and use of models in network neuroscience. *Nature Reviews Neuroscience, 19,* 566–578. https://doi.org/10.1038/s41583-018-0038-8

Beckes, L., & Coan, J. A. (2011). Social baseline theory: The role of social proximity in emotion and economy of action. *Social and Personality Psychology Compass, 5,* 976–988. https://doi.org/10.1111/j.1751-9004.2011.00400.x

Clark, U. S., Miller, E. R., & Hedge, R. R. (2018). Experiences of discrimination are associated with greater resting amygdala activity and functional connectivity. *Biological Psychiatry, 3,* 367–378. https://doi.org/10.1016/j.bpsc.2017.11.011

Coan, J. A., & Sbarra, D. A. (2015). Social baseline theory: The social regulation of risk and effort. *Current Opinion in Psychology, 1,* 87–91. https://doi.org/10.1016/j.copsyc.2014.12.021

Colich, N. L., Rosen, M. L., Williams, E. S., & McLaughlin, K. A. (2020). Biological aging in childhood and adolescence following experiences of threat and deprivation: A systematic review and meta-analysis. *Psychological Bulletin, 146,* 721–764. https://doi.org/10.1037/bul0000270

Cousijn, J., Luijten, M., & Feldstein Ewing, S. W. (2018). Adolescent resilience to addiction: A social plasticity hypothesis. *The Lancet Child & Adolescent Health, 2,* 69–78. https://doi.org/10.1016/S2352-4642(17)30148-7

Creed, M. (2018) Current and emerging neuromodulation therapies for addiction: Insight from pre-clinical studies. *Current Opinion in Neurobiology, 49,* 168–174. https://doi.org/10.1016/j.conb.2018.02.015

Dahl, C. J., Wilson-Mendenhall, C. D., & Davidson, R. J. (2020). The plasticity of well-being: A training-based framework for the cultivation of human flourishing. *PNAS, 117,* 32197–32206. https://doi.org/10.1073/pnas.2014859117

Ekhtiari, H., Nasseri, P., Yavari, F., Mokri, A., & Monterosso, J. (2016). Neuroscience of drug craving for addiction medicine: From circuits to therapies. *Progress in Brain Research, 223,* 115–141. https://doi.org/10.1016/bs.pbr.2015.10.002

Ekhtiari, H., Rezapour, T., Aupperle, R. L., & Paulus, M. P. (2017). Neuroscience-informed psychoeducation for addiction medicine: A neurocognitive perspective. *Progress in Brain Research, 235,* 239–264. https://doi.org/10.1016/bs.pbr.2017.08.013

Eme, R. (2017). The overlapping neurobiology of addiction and ADHD. *Mental Health and Addiction Research, 2,* 1–3. https://doi.org/10.15761/MHAR.1000129

Erickson, C. K. (2018). *The science of addiction: From neurobiology to treatment* (2nd ed). W. W. Norton & Company.

Erickson, C. K., & White, W. L. (2009). The neurobiology of addiction recovery. *Alcoholism Treatment Quarterly, 27,* 338–345. https://doi.org/10.1080/07347320903014255

Ersche, K. D., Williams, G. B., Robbins, T. W., & Bullmore, E. T. (2013). Meta-analysis of structural brain abnormalities associated with stimulant drug dependence and neuroimaging of addiction vulnerability and resilience. *Current Opinion in Neurobiology, 23,* 615–624. https://doi.org/10.1016/j.conb.2013.02.017

Feinberg, A. P., & Fallin, M. D. (2015). Epigenetics at the crossroads of genes and the environment. *JAMA, 314,* 1129–1130. https://doi.org/10.1001/jama.2015.10414

Feldstein-Ewing, S. W., Houck, J. M., Yezhuvath, U., Shokri Kojori, E., Truitt, D., & Filbey, F. M. (2016). The impact of therapists' words on the adolescent brain: In the context of addiction treatment. *Behavioural Brain Research, 297,* 359–369.

Felitti, V. J., Anda, R. F., Nordenberg, D., Williamson, D. F., Spitz, A. M., Edwards, V., Koss, M. P., & Marks, J. S. (1998). Relationship of childhood abuse and household dysfunction to many of the leading causes of death in adults: The adverse experiences (ACE) study. *American Journal of Preventative Medicine, 14*, 245–258. https://doi.org/10.1016/S0749-3797(98)00017-8

Garavan, H., Brennan, K. L., Hester, R., & Whelan, R. (2013). The neurobiology of successful abstinence. *Current Opinion in Neurobiology, 23*, 668–674. https://doi.org/10.1016/j.conb.2013.01.029

Gilpin, N. W., & Weiner, J. L. (2017). Neurobiology of comorbid post-traumatic stress disorder and alcohol-use disorder. *Genes, Brain and Behavior, 16*, 15–43. https://doi.org/10.1111/gbb.12349

Gómez-Coronado, N., Sethi, R., Bortolasci, C. C., Arancini, L., Berk, M., & Dodd, S. (2018). A review of the neurobiological underpinning of comorbid substance use and mood disorders. *Journal of Affective Disorders, 241*, 388–401. https://doi.org/10.1016/j.jad.2018.08.041

Hammer, R., Dingel, M., Ostergren, J., Partridge, B., McCormick, J., & Koenig, B. A. (2013). Addiction: Current criticism of the brain disease paradigm. *AJOB Neuroscience, 4*, 27–32. https://doi.org/10.1080/21507740.2013.796328

Hayes, A., Herlinger, K., Paterson, L., & Lingford-Hughes, A. (2020). The neurobiology of substance use and addiction: Evidence from neuroimaging and relevance to treatment. *BJPsych Advances, 26*, 367–378. https://doi.org/10.1192/bja.2020.68

Heather, N., Best, D., Kawalek, A., Field, M., Lewis, M., Rotgers, F., Wiers, R. W., & Heim, D. (2018). Challenging the brain disease model of addiction: European launch of the addiction theory network. *Addiction Research & Theory, 26*, 249–255. https://doi.org/10.1080/16066359.2017.1399659

Heyman, G. M. (2013). Addiction and choice: Theory and new data. *Frontiers in Psychiatry, 4*. https://doi.org/10.3389/fpsyt.2013.00031

Immordino-Yang, M. H., Darling-Hammond, L., & Krone, C. (2018). *The brain basics for integrated social, emotional, and academic development: How emotions and social relationships drive learning* [Research brief.]. The Aspen Institute. https://files.eric.ed.gov/fulltext/ED596337.pdf

Jakel, S., & Dimou, L. (2017). Glial cells and their function in the adult brain: A journey through the history of their ablation. *Frontiers in Cellular Neuroscience, 11*, 1–17. https://doi.org/10.3389/fncel.2017.00024

Koob, G. F. (2013). Negative reinforcement in drug addiction: The darkness within. (2013). *Current Opinion in Neurobiology, 23*, 559–563. https://doi.org/10.1016/j.conb.2013.03.011

Koob, G. F., & Volkow, N. D. (2016). Neurobiology of addiction: A neurocircuitry analysis. *Lancet Psychiatry, 3*, 760–773. https://doi.org/10.1016/S2215-0366(16)00104-8

Kozak, M. J., & Cuthbert, B. N. (2016). The NIMH research domain criteria initiative: Background, issues, and pragmatics. *Psychophysiology, 53*, 286–297. https://doi.org/10.1111/psyp.12518

Lewis, M. (2017). Addiction and the brain: Development, not disease. *Neuroethics, 10*, 7–18. https://doi.org/10.1007/s12152-016-9293-4

Linker, K. E., Cross, S. J., & Leslie, F. M. (2018). Glial mechanism underlying substance use disorders. *European Journal of Neuroscience, 50*, 2574–2589. https://doi.org/10.1111/ejn.14163

Marsman, A., Pries, L. K., ten Have, M., de Graaf, R., van Dorsselaer, S., Bak, M., Kenis, G., Lin, B. D., Luykx, J. J., Rutten, B. P. F., Guloksuz, S., & van Os, J. (2020). Do current measures of polygenic risk for mental disorders contribute to population variance in mental health? *Schizophrenia Bulletin, 46*, 1353–1362. https://doi.org/10.1093/schbul/sbaa086

Marzbani, H., Marateb, J. R., & Mansourian, M. (2016). Neurofeedback: A comprehensive review on system design, methodology, and clinical applications. *Basic and Clinical Neuroscience, 72*, 143–158. https://doi.org/10.15412/J.BCN.03070208

McLaughlin, K. A., Weissman, D., & Bitrán, D. (2019). Childhood adversity and neural development: A systematic review. *Annual Review of Developmental Psychology, 1*(1), 277–312. https://doi.org/10.1146/annurev-devpsych-121318-084950

Meyerhoff, D. J., & Durazzo, T. C. (2020). Modeling neurocognitive and neurobiological recovery in addiction. In A. Verdejo-Garcia (Ed.), *Cognition and addiction: A Researchers guide from mechanisms toward actions* (pp. 379–392). Elsevier. https://doi.org/10.1016/B978-0-12-815298-0.00028-9

Miller, G. E., Yu, T., Chen, E., & Brody, G. H. (2015). Self-control forecasts better psychosocial outcomes but faster epigenetic aging in low-SES youth. *PNAS, 112*, 10325–10330. https://doi.org/10.1073/pnas.1505063112

Morgenstern, J., Naqvi, N. H., Debellis, R., & Breiter, H. C. (2013). The contributions of cognitive neuroscience and neuroimaging to understanding mechanisms of behavior change in addiction. *Psychology of Addictive Behavior, 27,* 336–350. https://doi.org/10.1037/a0032435

National Center for Injury Prevention and Control. (2021). *Adverse childhood experiences (ACEs).* Centers for Disease Control and Prevention. Retrieved from https://www.cdc.gov/violenceprevention/aces/index.html

National Institute of Health. (2018). *What are the parts of the nervous system?* Retrieved from https://www.nichd.nih.gov/health/topics/neuro/conditioninfo/parts

Nature. (n.d.). *Neuroscience.* Retrieved from https://www.nature.com/subjects/neuroscience

Noble, K. G., & Giebler, M. A. (2020). The neuroscience of socioeconomic inequality. *Current Opinions in Behavioral Sciences, 36,* 23–28. https://doi.org/10.1016/j.cobeha.2020.05.007

Ramlakhan, J. U., Ma, M., Zomorrodi, R., Blumberger, D. M., Noda, Y., & Barr., M. S. (2020). The role of gamma oscillations in the pathophysiology of substance use disorders. *Journal of Personalized Medicine,11,* 17. https://doi.org/10.3390/jpm11010017

Ray, L. A. (2012). Clinical neuroscience of addiction: Applications to psychological science and practice. *Clinical Psychology: Science and Practice, 19,* 154–166. https://doi.org/10.1111/j.1468-2850.2012.01280.x

Ray, L. A., Grodin, E., Leggio, L., Bechtholt, A., Becker, H., Feldstein-Ewing, S., Jentsch, J. D., King, A., Mason, B., O'Malley, S., MacKillop, J., Heilig, M., & Koob, G. (2020). The future of translational research in alcohol use disorder. *Addiction Biology, 26*(2), Article e12903. https://doi.org/10.1111/adb.12903

Rock, D., Siegel, D. J., Poelmans, S. A. Y., & Payne, J. (2012). The healthy mind platter. *NeuroLeadership Journal, 4,* 1–23. https://davidrock.net/files/02_The_Healthy_Mind_Platter_US.pdf

Siegel, D. J. (2020). *The developing mind: How relationships and the brain interact to shape who we are* (3rd ed.). The Guilford Press.

Silvers, J. A., Squeglia, L. M., Rømer Thomsen, K., Hudson, K. A., & Feldstein-Ewing, S. W. (2019). Hunting for what works: Adolescents in addiction treatment. *Alcoholism: Clinical & Experimental Research, 43,* 578–592. https://doi.org/10.1111/acer.13984

Snoek, A. (2017). How to recover from a brain disease: Is addiction a disease, or is there a disease-like stage in addiction? *Neuroethics, 10,* 185–194. https://doi.org/10.1007/s12152-017-9312-0

Stellwagen, D., Kemp, G. M., Valade, S., & Chambon, J. (2019). Glial regulation of synaptic function in models of addiction. *Current Opinion in Neurobiology, 57,* 179–185. https://doi.org/10.1016/j.conb.2019.02.010

Strathearn, L., Mertens, C. E., Mayes, L., Rutherford, P. R., Xu, G., Potenza, M. N., & Kim, S. (2019). Pathways relating the neurobiology of attachment to drug addiction. *Frontiers in Psychiatry, 10,* 1–15. https://doi.org/10.3389/fpsyt.2019.00737

Suckling, J., & Nestor, L. J. (2016). The neurobiology of addiction: The perspective from magnetic resonance imaging present and future. *Addiction, 112,* 360–369. https://doi.org/10.1111/add.13474

Teicher, M. H., & Samson, J. A. (2016). Annual research review: Enduring neurobiological effects of childhood abuse and neglect. *Journal of Child Psychology and Psychiatry, 57*(3), 241–266. https://doi.org/10.1111/jcpp.12507

Teicher, M. H., Samson, J. A., Anderson, C. M., Ohashi, K. (2016). The effects of childhood maltreatment on brain structure, function, and connectivity. *Nature Reviews Neuroscience, 17,* 652–666. https://doi.org/10.1038/nrn.2016.111

Tomlinson, R. C., Burt, A., Waller, R., Jonides, J., Miller, A. L., Gearhardt, A. N., Peltier, S. J., Klump, K. L., Lumeng, J. C., & Hyde, L. W. (2020). Neighborhood poverty predicts altered neural and behavioral response inhibition. *NeuroImage, 209,* Article 116536. https://doi.org/10.1016/j.neuroimage.2020.116536

Uddin, L. Q. (2015). Salience processing and insular cortical function and dysfunction. *Nature Reviews Neuroscience, 16,* 55–61. https://doi.org/10.1038/nrn3857

Uhl, G. R., Koob, G. F., & Cable, J. (2019). The neurobiology of addiction. *Annals of the New York Academy of Sciences, 1451,* 5–28. https://doi.org/10.1111/nyas.13989

Volkow, N. D., Koob, G. F., & McLellan, A. T. (2016). Neurobiologic advances from the brain disease model of addiction. *The New England Journal of Medicine, 374*, 363–371. https://doi.org/10.1056/NEJMra1511480

Volkow, N. D., Want, G. J., Tomasi, D., & Baler, R. D. (2013). Unbalanced neuronal circuits in addiction. *Current Opinion in Neurobiology, 23*, 639–648. https://doi.org/10.1016/j.conb.2013.01.002

Wise, R. A., & Robble, M. A. (2020). Dopamine and addiction. *The Annual Review of Psychology, 71*, 79–106. https://doi.org/10.1146/annurev-psych-010418-103337

Witkiewitz, K., Lustyk, M. K. B., & Bown, S. (2013). Retraining the addicted brain: A review of hypothesized neurobiological mechanism of mindfulness-based relapse prevention. *Psychology of Addictive Behaviors, 27*(2), 351–365. https://doi.org/10.1037/a0029258

Zhang, R., & Volkow, N. D. (2019). Brain default mode network dysfunction in addiction. *NeuroImage, 15*, 313–331. https://doi.org/10.1016/j.neuroimage.2019.06.036

Zilverstand, A., Parvaz, M. A., Moeller, S. J., & Goldstein, R. Z. (2016). Cognitive interventions for addiction medicine: Understanding the underlying neurobiological mechanisms. *Progress in Brain Research, 224*, 285–304. https://doi.org/10.1016/bs.pbr.2015.07.019

SECTION II

TREATMENT APPROACHES

CHAPTER 4

THE COMPREHENSIVE ASSESSMENT OF CO-OCCURRING DISORDERS

DILANI M. PERERA AND ALEXANDRA GALLETTI

LEARNING OBJECTIVES

After reading this chapter, you will be able to:

- Explain the process of completing a thorough intake and assessment for co-occurring disorders (CODs) using a biopsychosocial model.
- Identify and evaluate screening and assessment tools and strategies for clients with CODs.
- Design treatment plans and aftercare recovery initiatives for clients with CODs.
- Apply legal and ethical knowledge to treatment for clients with CODs.

INTRODUCTION

Assessment, the process of gathering information, is an integral part of counseling. Assessment begins with the initial intake and continues until the client concludes services. The assessment process facilitates understanding of the client, the client's concerns, and the trajectory for treatment and termination. An important part of assessment is to accurately evaluate the client's level of motivation in order to develop a suitable treatment plan that culminates in a successful treatment outcome. Therefore, gathering detailed information from the client and, when possible, from family members, friends, peers, and other collateral parties, contributes to achieving a successful outcome for the client.

Co-occurring disorders (CODs), previously referred to as dual diagnosis, is the presence of both a substance use disorder and a mental disorder. Depressive, anxiety, bipolar, personality, trauma-related, and schizophrenia spectrum disorders commonly co-exist with substance use disorders (National Institute of Drug Abuse [NIDA], 2018). For example, alcohol use disorder and panic disorder, opioid use disorder and bipolar disorder, stimulant use disorder (cocaine) and major depressive disorder, and tobacco use disorder and schizophrenia are common co-occurring combinations (NIDA, 2018).

Approximately half of individuals with a mental disorder will also develop a substance use disorder at some point in their lives, and vice versa (NIDA, 2018). Risk factors for CODs include the following: history of legal issues including offender status as a minor; low educational attainment;

history of unstable housing and homelessness; suicidal intentions; history of emergency department visits; high frequency of relapse with substances; peers with antisocial traits; poor family relationships; and poor adherence to treatment (Peters et al., 2008). These common risk factors, combined with drug-induced brain changes, may contribute to the development of CODs (NIDA, 2018). It is not only necessary to conduct a comprehensive assessment to understand the various risk factors contributing to the etiology of a client's co-occurring mental and substance use condition, it is especially necessary to do so for diagnostic and case conceptualization purposes.

INTAKE, ASSESSMENT, AND THE THERAPEUTIC RELATIONSHIP

Following is a vignette of a client presenting with a possible COD that is discussed throughout this chapter:

> *Felicity is a 27-year-old, biracial (African American/Asian), heterosexual, married, cisgender female with no children, who is from the middle class. She has a bachelor's degree in education and is employed in the public school system as a high school mathematics teacher. She believes in a higher power but does not belong to any defined religion. Her support system includes her spouse and various family members. Felicity reports that she was charged with driving while intoxicated last week, and her husband threatened to leave her if she did not go to counseling. According to Felicity, "I don't know what the big fuss is because I had one small issue with the law. It was only one bad incident and drinking is not a problem." She believes her issue is due to always feeling alone; drinking simply helps her escape and be more social. Felicity indicates that she only drinks in the evenings. Upon further inquiry, she indicates that she drinks with friends and colleagues as well as drinks by herself at home. Felicity drinks five to six days of the week. She smiles and says, "There is no point wasting by leaving anything that was open"—indicating she drinks at least a bottle of wine, and sometimes two, each day. During this conversation, Felicity also shares she is not motivated to go to work on a daily basis. Although she attempts to make herself not miss work, she calls off often because she is too tired to deal with high school students all day. When inquired further, she mentions that even though she uses alcohol to help initiate sleep, she has a longstanding problem of not being able to maintain and experience a restful sleep. She has recently lost a lot of weight without intending to do so but is nonetheless pleased to have the weight loss. She stated she discussed some of these issues with her primary care physician but did not openly describe her alcohol use. She has also begun to have some hygiene issues of not showering on a regular basis, which she is very embarrassed to acknowledge. She is also questioning the value of living as evidenced by stating, "It's the same old boring life with nothing to really look forward to in the future. I don't believe anyone would really miss me if I was no longer around." It is important to note there is a family history of clinical depression with her maternal aunt committing suicide by overdose at Felicity's current age. Felicity indicates no one talks about her aunt's suicide, and most family members believe it was "just an unfortunate accident."*

INITIAL INTERVIEW (INTAKE)

Keeping Felicity in mind, refer back to the need for a thoughtful understanding of the client and the client's concerns as discussed in the chapter's introduction section. Counselors begin the assessment process with an initial interview, also known as an *intake*. Although intake forms and processes may differ slightly based on the specific work environment of the professional counselor, the process of gathering demographic information remains the same. An intake seeks to gather client's name, age, address, phone/email contact, marital status, employer/school, ethnicity, spiritual/religious preferences, sexual and gender identity, household income, method of payment, support system, referral source, and emergency contact. Other information such as presenting concerns, health history, and counseling services history (for consent to contact for continued care of services) is also collected. At the time of the initial interview, clients often are provided confidentiality, privacy, and Health Information Portability and Accountability Act (HIPAA) information as well as client financial responsibilities, and grievance procedures. The intake may be conducted by a nonlicensed office staff member and a subsequent appointment for a more comprehensive biopsychosocial assessment is later scheduled with a professional counselor.

ASSESSMENT

During the assessment, more detailed and indepth information to accurately conceptualize and appropriately plan treatment for each individual client is collected. Information may be gathered from the client and others who are knowledgeable about the client such as family, friends, peers, previous care providers, and employers with client consent. The aim is to understand the client's cultural intersectionality; motivation for treatment; biological, psychological, and social factors; and symptoms experienced.

CULTURAL CONSIDERATIONS

Culture is "the set of values and beliefs people have about how the world (both nature and society) works as well as, the norms of behavior derived from that set of values and that affects both social norms and economic behaviors" (Gorodnichenko & Roland, 2012, p. 1). Simplified, culture can be generalized into two broad categories: *individualistic* and *collectivist*. While individualism emphasizes personal freedom and achievement, collectivism emphasizes embeddedness of individuals into a larger group and conformity (Gorodnichenko & Roland, 2012). Terms such as choice, achievement, opportunity, advancement, and recognition are associated with individualistic orientation, whereas terms such as harmony, cooperation, and relations are valued in collectivist orientation.

Fifty percent of diverse clients terminate counseling after one visit (Sue & Sue, 2013). Felicity identifies as biracial; therefore, it is very important to discuss her own values and beliefs, which she has stitched together from her family's culture. Understanding a client's culture is central for a meaningful therapeutic alliance, an accurate conceptualization, a relevant treatment plan, and a beneficial treatment outcome.

THERAPEUTIC RELATIONSHIP

Because the therapeutic relationship facilitates gathering indepth information, it is necessary to begin developing this relationship starting with the initial contact for counseling and then working to strengthen and maintain this alliance until services conclude. A strong therapeutic relationship is a warm, welcoming, and accepting environment where clients feel comfortable and safe to share their concerns, values, beliefs, and take risks to facilitate change (Young, 2017). Asking too many questions, even if open-ended, may interfere with building the relationship as the client may feel they are being "interrogated." Instead, using other microskills of counseling, such as attending and encouragement, is beneficial to building and maintaining a strong therapeutic relationship (Young, 2017). Furthermore, empathy, unconditional positive regard, and genuine concern for the client are also necessary conditions for a continued therapeutic alliance (Young, 2017). The intentional development of this alliance from the start and throughout treatment is key to the return of the client for ongoing counseling, for enhancing the client's motivation to change, and for achieving a successful outcome in treatment. Additionally, intentionally using motivational interviewing (MI) techniques as clients work toward change helps to build the therapeutic relationship.

ASSESSING MOTIVATION TO CHANGE

Understanding how a client views their problem is another way to help strengthen the therapeutic relationship. For example, if a treatment plan goal for Felicity is to reduce harmful effects of drinking or eliminate drinking, it does not match her belief that she does not have a drinking problem. She is unlikely, therefore, to engage in a behavior change in an effort to meet such a goal. She may even believe that the professional counselor does not understand her situation. On the contrary, if the treatment objective focuses on tracking how much she drinks on nights she did not have restful sleep, she may be more willing to work on that goal.

The motivation for treatment may be different for each disorder when CODs are present. Motivation needs to be identified and considered for each mental and substance use disorder when developing the treatment plan. There are two frameworks that help to determine the motivational level for each disorder and assist the client to address each problem without damaging the therapeutic relationship: (a) the *stages of change model* (Prochaska & DiClemente, 1983), which helps to conceptualize the client's problem recognition and motivational level for change, and (b) *motivational interviewing* (Miller & Rollnick, 2013), which involves specific evidence-based approaches to motivate a client to resolve ambivalence and work toward actual change.

MOTIVATIONAL INTERVIEWING

MI assumes ambivalence is part of the change process and that change can be facilitated through empathic, collaborative, yet directive engagement (Miller & Rollnick, 2013). MI involves the spirit of rolling with resistance with empathy and avoiding confrontation. Grounded in principles of autonomy, collaboration, and evocation, MI offers the counselor various skills to introduce and initiate change (Miller & Rollnick, 2013).

STAGES OF CHANGE

Many clients who enter counseling do not recognize all problems and/or have motivation to change. Prochaska and DiClemente's stages of change model (also known as the transtheoretical model) is a valuable framework to use when conceptualizing and developing a treatment plan; it allows the professional counselor to know what works best when the client presents at different stages for each identified problem.

Precontemplation Stage

Clients in the *precontemplation stage* are unaware or unwilling to change. Raising awareness, rather than demanding change, is considered the best path of treatment (Krebs et al., 2018). Even though Felicity was recently charged with driving while intoxicated, she indicated that drinking is not a problem. The counselor may engage Felicity by acknowledging how alcohol may bring relief to some of her uncomfortable symptoms while offering education regarding the effects of her alcohol use (i.e., rolling with resistance). Understanding Felicity, rather than confronting her, may strengthen the therapeutic alliance and consequently aid in transitioning the client to the next stage of change.

Contemplation Stage

Clients in the *contemplation stage* are ambivalent of change, although they may see the possibility for change (Krebs et al., 2018). The hope is that Felicity may feel safe to take the risk to discuss the need to reduce her alcohol consumption as it is a temporary solution to relieve some symptoms. Still, she may be undecided on how to manage her symptoms without alcohol. Therefore, a plan to resolve ambivalence is the most appropriate intervention. Engaging Felicity in a discussion wherein she identifies other ways she may manage her symptoms without alcohol would be an appropriate course to take.

Preparation Stage

If Felicity is in the *preparation stage*, she is committed to change but may be still considering the process (Krebs et al., 2018). Helping Felicity identify and practice appropriate change strategies is useful.

Action Stage

In the *action stage*, Felicity will take steps to change although change is still unstable (Krebs et al., 2018). Felicity may demonstrate excitement and eagerness for interventions and homework.

Maintenance

Finally, if in the *maintenance stage*, Felicity has achieved her goals but can still use counseling to fine tune her life to minimize, or ideally prevent, a relapse into either disorder (Krebs et al., 2018).

Relapse

It is important to remember that *relapse* is a common part of recovery from substance use disorders. Clients may spiral backward and re-enter any of the previous stages of change (Krebs et al., 2018). Ideally, when clients relapse and return to previous behaviors, they can learn from each episode, and, in doing so, lessen the duration and impact of the relapse and subsequently enhance their future ability to sustain positive changes.

BIOPSYCHOSOCIAL EVALUATION

In order to facilitate movement through the stages of change, counselors should consider the information needed to understand the client from a holistic viewpoint. One model that helps with such conceptualization is the biopsychosocial (BPS) model (Pinel & Barnes, 2018). A BPS evaluation provides a comprehensive understanding of a client (Borrell-Carrio et al., 2004). As the name indicates, a broad base of *biological, psychological,* and *social* information is gathered to understand the client's developmental and overall level of functioning. Problems of presenting issues do not occur in a vacuum, therefore, having an overall understanding of the client and the client's environment is important. The BPS evaluation is normally an interview with the client and the family, when feasible, to obtain a holistic view of the client. Done appropriately, this assessment captures the client's culture, support systems, strengths, and challenges, which, in turn, helps develop an effective treatment plan. Such an assessment is especially beneficial with clients (like Felicity) who have co-occurring mental and substance use disorders; it aids in understanding how both disorders interact, what supports are available, and the challenges that need to be addressed in treatment.

BIOLOGY

The first component, biology, investigates the genetic and medical issues, age, developmental milestones, physical characteristics, and any variable that may negatively impact the biological self (Borrell-Carrio et al., 2004). Substance use and mental disorders both have predisposing genetic qualities, and the interview often includes a personal and family alcohol and drug use and mental health history. Similarly, substance use and mental disorders also mimic features of physical illness. Inquiring when the client last had an annual physical examination, as well as being aware of the exam results, is important. Furthermore, there is evidence that alcohol use disorder causes changes in the brain, especially in the basal ganglia, the extended amygdala, and the prefrontal cortex (Koob & Volkow, 2016). Symptoms related to these changes may mimic other mental disorders. It is easy to misdiagnose common symptoms unless an indepth inquiry is completed to identify those clients with CODs.

Some developmental stages may also mimic symptoms of mental disorders; therefore, intentionally teasing out normal development from symptoms of a disorder is very important. If maternal involvement in substance use during pregnancy is suspected, it is appropriate to seek further information, and possibly a medical evaluation, to determine if the client may have some biological consequences related to maternal substance use. Similarly, certain cultural factors also need to be carefully understood to determine if they have any biological consequence that will influence treatment. One way in which culture can affect mental illness is how clients describe their symptoms; therefore, clinicians need to consider the cultural elements that go into symptom presentation and reporting. For example, Asian clients have been found to report their somatic symptoms initially, and only after further exploration by clinicians will they then delve into emotional symptoms (Substance Abuse and Mental Health Services Administration [SAMHSA], 2001).

PSYCHOLOGY

The second component, psychology, inquires about thoughts, feelings, and behaviors (Borrell-Carrio et al., 2004). Questions will also assess for self-concept, self-esteem, and self-image. In addition, inquiries are made about physical, mental, and emotional abuse. It is vital to remember that, if allegations, suspicions, or evidence of abuse exist, professional counselors are legally and ethically bound to report this information to appropriate authorities. Conducting a mental status exam is also an important part of the assessment process. The areas to observe and explore in a mental status exam are: appearance, behavior, speech, mood, affect, thought process, thought content, cognition, and insight and judgment (Polanski & Hinkle, 2000; Trzepacz & Baker, 1993). The mental status exam can be part of the information-gathering process and does not have to be separate from the comprehensive biopsychosocial assessment.

Professional counselors also inquire about a client's past and/or present involvement in counseling services. Understanding the counseling history may highlight the need to work harder at building the relationship, or it may indicate the need to obtain permission to contact another healthcare professional for consultation, collaboration, and/or provide continuity of care.

The assessment also seeks to uncover client-identified strengths as well as limitations, barriers, and challenges. Identifying client strengths is important as they can be utilized to build hope and facilitate the treatment process. Identifying limitations and barriers will help plan ways to work around such challenges that may impede treatment. Knowledge in this case is power as it provides the professional counselor the opportunity to choose the best treatment path for the individual client.

Finally, assessing for client dangerousness, such as suicidal and homicidal ideation, is especially crucial when working with clients with CODs. The suicidal risk in those who experience CODs, especially when combined with alcohol or opioid use disorder, is high (Abroms & Sher, 2016; Rizk et al., 2021). While alcohol use increases maladaptive behaviors and reduces self-regulation, opioid use increases negative affective states (Rizk et al., 2021). For instance, in the case of Felicity, the effects of her alcohol use along with her questioning the value of life must be directly examined to determine her suicidal intent.

SOCIAL

The third component, social history, includes information on relationships with family, friends, and other social supports (such as church and community) that leads to work/life balance (Borrell-Carrio et al., 2004). Further, counselors should explore the presence and role of spirituality in the client's life. Counselors should recognize that spirituality is not necessarily affiliated with religion; therefore, an explanation may be required for the client to be able to engage in responding to this question. Spirituality brings meaning and purpose to life which is helpful in the treatment of CODs. Counselors should also inquire about the client's financial situation when conducting the social history. Finances will indicate the stress of treatment expense that the client endures. Finally, inquire about legal and military history to understand how these variables may influence treatment. All of the various components described in the social history section are useful to understand the strengths and challenges the client may experience when receiving COD treatment.

SCREENING AND ASSESSMENT STRATEGIES AND TOOLS

Outside of the BPS assessment, mental status exam, and assessing for risk of harm to self and others, there are other assessment tools available to facilitate diagnosis of and treatment planning for clients with CODs. There are many standardized documents available to complete the BPS assessment and mental status exam previously mentioned (and most healthcare agencies and organizations provide the specific assessment forms to be used by clinical counseling staff). Often, counselors gather even more information than what is listed on these forms in an effort to accurately identify the client's issues. Once sufficient information is gathered, a written report in narrative form may be required. The following information regarding screens and standardized assessments is offered to provide an understanding of how obtaining comprehensive information allows for a better recognition of a client who has both a substance use and mental disorder.

SCREENING

Screening, which is part of the evaluation process, is an efficient way of gathering information to determine if the client warrants further assessment for a possible diagnosis. The primary objectives of screening are: (a) to detect and determine current mental and/or substance use disorder symptoms and behaviors; (b) to determine if symptoms and/or behaviors warrant further assessment for a COD; (c) to examine any cognitive deficits; (d) to identify any suicidal or violent tendencies or severe medical issues that warrant immediate attention; and (e) to determine eligibility for specialized COD treatment services (Peters et al., 2008).

Screening is a set of questions that are administered and scored per the instrument's instructions, and then followed through with the affirmative or negative conclusionary steps based on the results of the screen (Co-Occurring Center for Excellence, 2007). Screens identify "red flags" of probability with answers of "*yes*" (meaning assess further), while responses of "*no*" indicate further assessment is not needed. Therefore, screening establishes the likelihood of a COD but does not determine the specific disorders. New clients can be screened for CODs using an integrated screening approach (Co-Occurring Center for Excellence, 2007). The integrated screening not only determines if CODs are present, but it also attempts to identify the related services needed (Co-Occurring Center for Excellence, 2007). Additionally, clients already diagnosed with either a substance use or mental disorder can be screened for a possible COD.

ASSESSMENT

Assessment is the next step after an affirmative conclusion is obtained after conducting a screening. Most professional counselors complete the assessment process in one or two sessions, which may be guided by policies and procedures within their place of employment. The assessment gathers further specific information to determine the presence or absence of CODs, client's strengths and challenges, level of functioning, and motivation to change (Co-Occurring Center for Excellence, 2007). The biopsychosocial and mental status exam is conducted during the assessment process, which should be concurrently performed by placing attention on cultural factors that should be considered for treatment planning purposes. This may be achieved, combined with the counselor's clinical judgment, by asking the client to complete one or more culturally appropriate standardized assessment instruments.

Information obtained from the comprehensive assessment allows for a provisional diagnosis to be made. Then, based on the diagnosis, a culturally appropriate individualized treatment plan is generated. A best-practice guideline for developing treatment plans is to involve, collaborate with, and receive input from the client. Lastly but importantly, the screening and assessment processes should continue throughout the counseling process to identify, adapt to, and address the client's changing circumstances, especially with those diagnosed with CODs.

ASSESSMENT FOR SYMPTOMS OF PSYCHOACTIVE SUBSTANCE TOXICITY, INTOXICATION, AND WITHDRAWAL

Clients who are withdrawing from substances may present symptoms of psychological or medical conditions. These symptoms may be related to a pre-existing medical or psychological condition or the direct result of substance use (SAMHSA, 2015). Withdrawal from psychoactive drugs, especially cocaine and cannabis have been demonstrated to produce sympathomimetic toxicity such as headaches, reflex bradycardia, excitability, and restless in most cases unless in combination with alcohol (Liakoni et al., 2016). When alcohol-related withdrawal symptoms occur, more severe toxicity such as impaired consciousness is present. And, for those clients experiencing severe withdrawal symptoms, death may occur unless they receive detoxification services in a medically monitored inpatient facility. Although most experience sympathomimetic toxicity, there are some fatalities (Liakoni et al., 2016). The *Diagnostic and Statistical Manual* of *Mental Disorders* (5th ed.; *DSM-5*; American Psychiatric Association, 2013) provides criteria for intoxication and withdrawal from each substance use disorder. Professional counselors should familiarize themselves with these criteria and consult addiction specialists if a substance intoxication or withdrawal, especially due to alcohol, is present. This will facilitate medically safe withdrawal for applicable clients.

PSYCHOMETRICS OF SCREENING AND ASSESSMENT TOOLS

Before diving into screening and assessment tools and strategies, it is important to discuss how to evaluate standardized screening and diagnostic assessment instruments. The instrument must be *valid* (accurate), *reliable* (repeatable), *sensitive* (can identify those with the condition accurately), and *specific* (can identify those who do not have the condition accurately). These are considered the *psychometric properties* of the assessment instrument. Reliability is provided as a coefficient on a scale from 0 to 1, with numbers closer to 1 indicating that the assessment instrument is consistent from one application to the next. Taking this into consideration, 0.9 and above is excellent; 0.8 to 0.89 is good; 0.7 to 0.79 is adequate; and below 0.7 is limited (Laux et al., 2019).

Clinicians should determine if the data provided for validity are beneficial, useful, and congruent with the purpose for which the instrument is intended (Laux et al., 2019). Validity, which is the accuracy of the instrument in measuring a defined concept (e.g., depression, anxiety), may be given in different formats. These formats include content, criterion, construct, discriminant, concurrent, and sometimes face validity. *Content validity* is the extent to which the defined construct is covered. *Criterion validity* is the extent to which a client's score is correlated with other known criteria for that disorder. *Construct validity* is the extent to which the identified construct is measured. *Concurrent validity* is achieved when criterion and construct validity are established at the same time. *Discriminant validity* is the extent to which scores are not correlated with measures of variables that are conceptually distinct. Lastly, *face validity* is the extent to which the assessment instrument appears to measure the specified concept it claims to measure (Hays, 2017).

Sensitivity is an instrument's ability to identify those with symptoms of a certain disorder, whereas *specificity* refers to the tool's ability to accurately identify those individuals without the disorder (Hays, 2017). Sensitivity and specificity, which are typically represented as percentages, have an inverse correlation: assessment instruments with higher sensitivity have lower specificity and vice versa.

Because psychometric instruments are not perfect measures, it is important to highlight the necessity of using instruments in combination with the counselor's clinical judgment. Based on the disorder for which information is gathered, some judgment will need to be executed related to what psychometrics are most valuable to benefit the client's treatment planning and well-being. And, even if the basic psychometrics (reliability, validity, specificity, and sensitivity) are adequate, the assessment instrument may not provide accurate results for a specific client due to individual client variables. Because instruments have a norming population, a "one-size-fits-all" assessment tool does not exist. Assessment instruments are only valid for the norming population for which it was designed and validated. It is important to recognize if the client is an English-language learner as well as to consider their culture, especially if the client is from an ethnic, gender, or sexual minority group. Another variable to consider is if the client is an immigrant. These groups have been underrepresented in developing and standardizing assessment instruments (i.e., not part of the norming populations). The assessment instruments may still be useful for treatment planning if used with caution and in collaboration with the client.

Counselors should choose the most appropriate assessment instrument based on the psychometrics, the norming population, and the cost and time to complete it. Consulting texts that offer reviews of assessment instruments, such as the *Mental Measurements Yearbook* or *Tests in Print*, is one way to determine appropriateness for the client. Another way to verify psychometrics is either through published peer-reviewed scholarly articles about the psychometric properties of the instrument or through the manual provided by the test's developer or publisher.

Screening and assessing for CODs is complicated by the need to explore and assess the effects of two mutually interacting disorders. Neither disorder is considered primary. While screening tools are easy to use and minimum qualifications are required, if used as the only instrument or is administered routinely, then the effectiveness may be minimized (Co-Occurring Center for Excellence, 2007). Therefore, creativity and flexibility in screening and assessing are required. There are two options to consider when screening for and assessing CODs: (a) Provide individual screens contained in a larger packet wherein some are specific to substance use while others are related to mental health conditions, or (b) adopt instruments that specifically assesses for the presence of co-occurring substance use and mental disorders.

SCREENS AND ASSESSMENT INSTRUMENTS

There are many screening tools and assessment instruments to detect the presence of either a substance use or mental disorder; therefore, counselors should be mindful of the client's individual treatment needs when considering the appropriateness of any screen or assessment tool. It is important to point out that there is a paucity of instruments that are exclusively designed to evaluate CODs; this may be a remaining historical consequence of mental health and addiction counselors working in silos. It is not the scope of this chapter to provide an exhaustive list or evaluation of each tool, but a few assessment instruments with different functions that are specifically designed for CODs are offered.

SCREENING INSTRUMENTS FOR CO-OCCURRING DISORDERS

- The Centre for Addiction and Mental Health-Concurrent Disorders Screener (CAMH-CDS; Negrete et al., 2004)
- The Co-Occurring Disorders Screening Instrument for Mental Disorders (CODSI-MD; Sacks et al., 2007)

ASSESSMENT INSTRUMENTS FOR CO-OCCURRING DISORDERS

- The MINI International Neuropsychiatric Interview (MINI; Sheehan et al., 1998)
- The Minnesota Multiphasic Personality Inventory-2 (MMPI-2; Tellegen & Ben-Porath, 2011)
- The Psychiatric Research Interview for Substance and Mental Disorders (PRISM: Hasin, 1996)

INSTRUMENTS ASSISTING IN DIAGNOSING AND TREATMENT PLANNING

- The Global Appraisal of Individual Needs (GAIN; Dennis et al., 2002)
- The Substance Use Event Survey for Severe Mental Illness (Bennett et al., 2006)
- Adult *DSM-5* Self-Rated Level 1 Cross-Cutting Symptom Measure (APA, 2013)
- Parent/Guardian-Rated Level 1 Cross-Cutting Symptom Measure for Child Age 6–17 (APA, 2013)

Instruments Assessing the Outcome of Treatment for Co-Occurring Disorders

- The Behavior and Symptom Identification Scale (BASIS-24; Mclean Hospital, 2002–2019)

DIAGNOSIS

As a reminder, a COD is the presence of both a substance use and a mental disorder(s). To arrive at a diagnosis, the client's reported and observed symptoms and behaviors, the assessment findings, and the counselor's clinical judgment should be concurrently considered. In the United States, the *DSM-5* (APA, 2013) is primarily used to diagnose mental and substance use disorders, whereas in other countries the *International Classification of Diseases and Related Health Problems-11* (ICD-11; World Health Organization [WHO], 2018) is the standard.

Once information is gathered and a diagnosis is made, a treatment plan is generated. But before moving to that step, a return to Felicity's case is needed. Gathering information from the screening tools, assessment instruments, and clinical interview, Felicity was diagnosed with the co-occurrence of major depressive disorder and alcohol use disorder. Felicity began counseling after a legal consequence of drinking and driving. Using the CAGE questionnaire to detect for alcoholism (Ewing, 1984), Felicity met criteria for further evaluation. CAGE is an acronym for four questions that focus on: attempts to Cut down on drinking, being Annoyed by the criticism of others due to the client's drinking, feeling Guilty about using alcohol, and using alcohol as an Eye opener to calm nerves or relieve a hangover.

Felicity was compelled to attend counseling because of her spouse threatening to end the marriage if she did not seek help for her alcohol use. Further, as the first counseling session progressed, Felicity was forthcoming on how she drank more to get the same affect, how her spouse had nagged her to discontinue drinking, how she had unsuccessfully tried to reduce drinking, and how she felt guilty for not being able to meet her goals. She also admitted it was difficult on certain days to get out of bed and go to work because she had a hangover. All of these symptoms are indicative of a *DSM-5* alcohol use disorder (although Felicity is certain she does not have a drinking problem).

Felicity also shared she was unable to sleep, experienced weight loss, was unable to get to work, and that her level of motivation changed (and that this was not the first time these symptoms were present). Although some of these symptoms could be as a result of her alcohol use, upon further discussion Felicity identified that some symptoms were present not only for a couple of weeks, but also for periods throughout her life—even prior to her alcohol use. This indicated a need to further evaluate Felicity for a COD, which subsequently led to a second diagnosis of major depressive disorder.

When considering the stages of change, it is not unusual for a client with CODs to be at different stages of change for each disorder. It appears Felicity was in *precontemplation* stage with her alcohol use disorder. This is evidenced by despite her willingness to share the effects of alcohol, Felicity was unable to connect and accept that she has an alcohol use problem. However, she seemed to be in the *preparation* stage with her major depressive disorder because she recognized her symptoms as problematic, was able to identify the symptoms, and had attempted to address it by discussing some of her symptoms with her primary care physician. She even tried over-the-counter supplements, such as melatonin, to help with sleep.

Further assessment of Felicity reveals her strengths as well as some challenges she is experiencing. Felicity is educated and employed; she's also concerned about her work performance. She is married, has a caring spouse, and lives in a stable home environment. Her husband is concerned about her drinking patterns. Felicity has family who are supportive of her (although most live out of state). Some of her challenges include lack of recognition and knowledge of her alcohol use disorder, husband's long work hours, limited other support system availability, family history of suicide, and her own suicidal ideation. Because of the various presenting problems, especially the severity of some symptoms, admission into an intermediate level of care, such as a partial hospitalization program (PHP), is recommended to monitor for potential alcohol withdrawal symptoms and diminish risk of client dangerousness, all while increasing her awareness of alcohol use disorder and address her major depressive disorder. Placement in PHP is also suitable due to the presence of CODs, suicidal ideation, and limited availability of familial support systems. It is important to point out that Felicity initially struggled with this placement due to being in the *precontemplative* stage for alcohol use disorder. Once her suicidal ideation was no longer an immediate concern, Felicity was transitioned to a lower level of care (intensive outpatient program; IOP), in which she willingly participated in developing a relapse prevention plan for both her alcohol use and major depressive disorders.

WRITING TREATMENT PLANS AND DESIGNING AFTERCARE RECOVERY INITIATIVES

Once detailed information is gathered and a diagnosis is determined, the next step is to work collaboratively with the client to develop an individualized treatment plan. The ultimate goal of treatment is to help the client return to a productive life (NIDA, 2018). A treatment plan is the roadmap for the client to obtain recovery. It provides direction and structure for treatment, similar to how a map used for a road trip provides direction and structure for the journey.

A treatment plan contains the client's diagnoses, identified problems, stage of change (for each problem), long-term goals, short-term objectives, and prescribed interventions with target dates to achieve the established goals. In addition, identification of client strengths and barriers are included. A goal is what has been identified collaboratively by the client and the professional counselor as needing adjustment, whereas the objectives are what the client needs to do in order to achieve the identified goal. Alternatively, writing specific, measurable, attainable, relevant, and time-limited goals, otherwise known as SMART goals (Doran, 1981), facilitates keeping the client motivated to complete treatment. Further, it allows for a measure of outcomes for clients. Felicity's treatment plan, which includes developing SMART goals, are discussed within the "Clinical Case Illustration and Discussion" section of this chapter. Until then, following is a step-by-step process to develop comprehensive and individualized treatment plans.

TWELVE-STEP ASSESSMENT PROCESS

Traditionally, clients with alcohol use disorders attended Alcoholics Anonymous (AA) where they engaged in the Twelve Step approach to recovery. Although this practice remains in place, following the AA's Twelve Step model of recovery is not the only treatment option. Similar to AA's Twelve Steps, following is a 12-step assessment process for developing a treatment plan for clients diagnosed with CODs (Co-Occurring Center for Excellence, 2007).

1. **Engage the client.** This is where building the therapeutic relationship is absolutely necessary.

2. **Gather additional information from collaterals (i.e., family, friends, other treatment providers).** Gathering the perspectives of different sources facilitates a more indepth understanding of the client. This step should only be conducted after obtaining written permission from the client.
3. **Screen and assess for CODs.** A thorough screening and assessment is needed to detect if and what CODs are present.
4. **Determine the severity of mental and substance use disorders.** Understanding the severity of each disorder will help secure the best outcome for the client by informing treatment planning, treatment placement, and the treatment sequencing.
5. **Determine the diagnoses.** Careful consideration for all information and concerns presented by the client and their support network will facilitate determining an accurate diagnosis for the client.
6. **Determine an appropriate care setting (e.g., outpatient, inpatient, or day treatment).** It is necessary to provide the best fit for the care needed by the client. If the client is at high risk, inpatient or day hospitalization may be clinically necessary, whereas if the client is at low to moderate risk, an outpatient level of care may be appropriate.
7. **Determine disability and functional impairments.** Understanding other factors, such as physical or learning disabilities and functional impairments, that impact the treatment process will be helpful for appropriate treatment planning and successful outcomes.
8. **Identify strengths and supports.** These supports and strengths can be utilized into the treatment plan to facilitate better outcomes for the client. Some strengths may be a strong support system, employment, flexibility of thought process, enthusiasm for treatment, and insightfulness.
9. **Identify the cultural and linguistic needs and supports.** Aligning treatment with client's cultural beliefs and values is paramount for a successful treatment outcome. For example, the treatment goals of a client from a collectivist culture is different than that from an individualistic culture (especially in how the goals are worded and phrased). Similarly, the client's linguistic needs and abilities also must be considered. To illustrate, the client's reading ability in the language of the assessment should be considered when choosing a tool or instrument.
10. **Identify any additional problem areas to address.** These may include but are not limited to housing, employment, education, social, physical health, spiritual, financial, and cognitive issues.
11. **Determine readiness for change.** This is crucial for the treatment plan to be effective. If the client's treatment plan does not correlate with their level of motivation and stage of change, then successful outcomes cannot be expected.
12. **Plan the treatment.** A plan with all of these steps considered is needed for the client to understand what action is required in order to achieve their short-term objectives and long-term goals.

CONSTRUCTING THE TREATMENT PLAN

An integrated treatment plan requires attention to both substance use and mental disorders as well as other services required for a successful outcome for the client. This plan must be carefully considered to determine not only what services are needed, but also what services are agreed to by the client. In addition, where the services will be provided, who will provide the services, and how the services will be coordinated and reimbursed are all factors that must be addressed.

It is important for treatment plans to be flexible by addressing changes that occur due to the client achieving, as well as not achieving, the established goals. As the name suggests, it is a plan, and plans must change to fit the needs of the individual client. The treatment plan is the roadmap for the client's recovery process. The client should be in the driver seat with the professional counselor serving as the vehicle's global positioning system (GPS) that helps the client get to the correct destination. If the client takes a wrong turn or wants to change the destination, then the professional counselor GPS may recalibrate the destination to provide a new map for the journey.

SAMHSA (2020) provides six guiding principles to comprehensively address the needs of a client with CODs for successful treatment outcome. These principles, along with a brief explanation, are provided in the following.

1. **Recovery perspective** recognizes that recovery is a long-term commitment and clients may go through stages of change. This requires that the treatment plan provides for a continuity of care over time and that strategies for different stages of change are considered.
2. **Multiproblem viewpoint** recognizes that clients with CODs have multiple issues to address and that the treatment plan includes goals for both short- and long-term needs.
3. **Phased approach to treatment** recognizes that clients require comprehensive and effective care, which may include engagement, stabilization, active treatment, and continuation of care. Also, there may be more phases depending on the client needs.
4. **Identification of specific real-life problems early in treatment** recognizes that the symptoms of cODs affect both the personal and social life of the client, and therefore, treatment may need to address more than just the symptoms of the disorder. Examples include real-life problems such as the client's employment status, support system availability, financial difficulties, and housing needs.
5. **Plan for the client's cognitive and functional impairments** requires professional counselors to be mindful that clients with CODs have cognitive and functional impairments that interfere with their ability to complete tasks. Careful assessment of impairments is needed. Gradual pacing, repeating, and documenting may be helpful strategies to work with these impairments.
6. **Use of support systems to maintain and extend treatment effectiveness** requires connecting clients with family, peers, and other supportive environments that clients with CODs may not have previously experienced. It may be also necessary to address stigma which may have ostracized the client from family support.

Once these six guiding principles have been considered, they need to be converted into a treatment plan with measurable outcomes, such as SMART goals, to determine treatment progress, change in care levels, and eventually, appropriateness for termination from treatment. Although there are numerous treatment plan formats available, components of the treatment plan should include the following: acute safety needs; severity of mental and substance use disorder; appropriate care setting; diagnosis; accessibility needs; strengths/skills; barriers/challenges; availability of continuity of recovery support; cultural context; problem priorities; and state of recovery/client's readiness to change behaviors relating to each problem.

Assessing the client's motivation to change (which was discussed earlier in the chapter as well as in the 11th step of the 12-step assessment process previously described) should be incorporated in planning treatment. According to the *stages of change model* (Prochaska & DiClemente, 1983), clients may enter treatment at any of the five stages. Motivation to change is not stable, and the client may encounter barriers, triggers, and setbacks; therefore, frequent evaluation and discussion with the client regarding motivation, as well as supporting the client when the client encounters unforeseeable challenges, are recommended (Hold, 2016). A treatment plan that is not aligned with the client's motivational stage is cause for the client and the professional counselor to experience frustration, and even worse, a poor outcome (although appropriate treatment matching has a high probability for a successful outcome).

When considering treatment matching and planning, the client's level of care that would produce the best outcomes should be determined. Both the American Society of Addiction Medicine (ASAM) and the APA have provided guidance on placement, which are discussed in the following. Suggestions for treatment planning for the case of Felicity are provided later in the "Clinical Case Illustration and Discussion" section.

AMERICAN SOCIETY OF ADDICTION MEDICINE PATIENT PLACEMENT CRITERIA

The ASAM Criteria is "the most widely used and comprehensive set of guidelines for placement, continued stay, transfer, or discharge of clients with addiction and co-occurring conditions" (ASAM, 2021, para. 1). Six dimensions are examined when completing a multidimensional assessment used to plan treatment throughout the continuum of care. The six dimensions are as follows:

1. **Dimension 1:** Considers the client's past and current use for **acute intoxication and/or withdrawal potential**.
2. **Dimension 2:** Explores the **biomedical and physical conditions** through a health history discussed in the biology component of the biopsychosocial evaluation.
3. **Dimension 3:** Explores the **cognitive, emotional, and behavioral conditions** that influence mental health issues discussed under psychological and social sections of the biopsychosocial evaluation.
4. **Dimension 4:** Assesses for **readiness to change** using the stages of change model discussed earlier in this chapter.
5. **Dimension 5:** Considers a client's **continued use of the substance and/or the relapse potential**.
6. **Dimension 6:** Evaluates the client's **recovery environment**, including people, places, and things that may be of support or a trigger for relapse.

Using these dimensions, a client's needs, challenges, as well as strengths and assets, are considered when placing the client in one of the following four levels within the continuum of care (ASAM, 2021):

1. **Level 1:** Outpatient
2. **Level 2:** Intensive Outpatient/Partial Hospitalization
3. **Level 3:** Residential/Inpatient
4. **Level 4:** Medically Managed Intensive Inpatient

If results of the assessment indicate the client does not clinically require admission into an outpatient level of care, then early intervention should be considered. Each of the four levels directs how many hours per week of treatment is provided to the client. On a weekly basis, outpatient requires less than 9 hours; intensive outpatient requires 9 hours; partial hospitalization requires 20 or more hours; residential requires 24 hour living support; and medically managed inpatient requires 24 hours of nursing and physician care (ASAM, 2021).

AMERICAN PSYCHIATRIC ASSOCIATION'S GLOBAL ASSSESMENT OF FUNCTIONING

The Global Assessment of Functioning (GAF) is a scoring system that assesses and categorizes an individual's overall level of functioning in decades from 0 to 100 for continuum of care based on client symptoms (APA, 2000). In this classification, the client with no symptoms falls between 91 to 100. At the opposite end, at 1 to 10, the client is in persistent danger to self-harm or harm others and/or is unable to maintain minimum personal hygiene (Moos et al., 2002). Because scoring can be subjective, training in the use of this assessment instrument is necessary without which the validity of placement value is questionable (Moos et al., 2002). Although no longer included in the most recent edition of the *DSM*, the GAF may still be adopted by some clinicians as an additional tool to examine the impact mental and substance use disorders have on a client's daily life. The fifth edition of the *DSM* (APA, 2013) replaced the GAF with the WHO's Disability Assessment Schedule 2.0 (WHODAS 2.0; WHO, 2012), which is a general instrument with cross-cultural applicability used to assess health and disability. Using either system for client placement of care may help determine treatment interventions and identify appropriate levels of care, which will change as clients either regress or progress through recovery.

AFTERCARE

The final part of providing assessment for CODs through the use of the various techniques and strategies discussed thus far is called aftercare. It is continued services after primary treatment has been completed and the client has moved to another stage of change (ideally *maintenance*). From the stages of change perspective, successful treatment involves mobility of the client from one stage to the next as well as transitioning through the continuum of care. Aftercare is part of the treatment continuum and affords the client counseling at the least restrictive and intense level (e.g., individual counseling, community support groups, medication management) to maintain goals accomplished during higher, more intensive levels of care. Because clients in aftercare move beyond addressing the issues of CODs to living with their disorders, aftercare incorporates wellness. Wellness is the balance of mind, body, and spirit. There is documented evidence that the mind, body, and spirit are interconnected; therefore, these concepts need to be intentionally incorporated into the client's treatment plan if sustainable change is to occur (Perera-Diltz & Moe, 2020). From the beginning of counseling, a wellness-based treatment plan should be developed by following these steps (Perera-Diltz & Moe, 2020):

1. Orienting clients to the concept of wellness.
2. Assessing wellness using a wellness screen or asking clients to rate their wellness on a scale of 1 to 10.
3. Planning a wellness-based lifestyle focusing on a few areas of underdeveloped strengths.
4. Evaluating total wellness and following up with necessary changes that incorporate wellness into the client's treatment is crucial in maintaining a new lifestyle.

With proper aftercare interventions and services, most clients change and sustain their behavior, which may include abstaining from substance use, improving social functioning, and enhancing personal relationships (SAMHSA, 2020).

LEGAL AND ETHICAL CONSIDERATIONS
ASSESSMENT CONSIDERATIONS

Professional conduct and responsibility, such as assessing and diagnosing, must be completed with professional integrity; therefore, all the previously mentioned assessment and treatment planning strategies need to be conducted within legal and ethical guidelines of professional counseling. Legal issues are related to legal mandates for assessment, such as who is qualified to provide what types of assessment and diagnosis. For example, the Licensed Professional Counselors Act within the Texas Occupations Code delineates assessment within the definition provided for the scope of practice established for licensed professional counselors:

> *"Assessment" means the selection, administration, scoring, and interpretation of an instrument designed to assess an individual's aptitudes, attitudes, abilities, achievements, interests, personal characteristics, disabilities, and mental, emotional, and behavioral disorders, and the use of methods and techniques for understanding human behavior that may include the evaluation, assessment, and treatment by counseling methods, techniques, and procedures for mental and emotional disorders, alcoholism and substance abuse, and conduct disorders. The term does not include the use of standardized projective techniques or permit the diagnosis of a physical condition or disorder.*
>
> (Texas Licensed Professional Counselor Act, 1999)

Ethical guidelines can be mandatory or aspirational professional behaviors to protect the client. The *2014 ACA Code of Ethics* (American Counseling Association [ACA], 2014) has an entire section devoted to "Evaluation, Assessment, and Interpretation" (pp. 11–12), of which counselors should be aware. In Section E, the following topics are thoroughly addressed for the ethical use of assessment in the counseling process:

1. Client welfare
2. Competence to use and interpret
3. Informed consent
4. Release of data
5. Diagnosis of mental disorders
6. Instrument selection
7. Conditions of assessment administration
8. Multicultural issues
9. Scoring and interpretation
10. Assessment security
11. Obsolete and outdated assessments
12. Construction of assessments
13. Forensic evaluation

These ethical guidelines are relevant to this chapter and are further discussed here. Client welfare is always central in all aspects of client care in professional counseling; therefore, professional counselors "do not misuse assessment results and interpretations" (ACA, 2014, p. 11). The process of assessment must be with informed consent clearly explaining to the client the nature and purpose of the assessment as well as the specific intentions for the use of results (ACA, 2014). Furthermore, it is important to only administer "those testing and assessment services for which they have been trained" (ACA, 2014, p. 11) and to use measures that are current. Although examples of screening tools and assessments have been provided in this chapter, it is important for counselors to learn how to properly use those screening tools and assessments prior to administering them with clients. For proper use of any assessment, it is necessary to investigate their psychometrics, norming populations, and cost, as well receive training from appropriately credentialed supervisors.

DIAGNOSTIC CONSIDERATIONS

Providing an accurate diagnosis of mental disorders (ACA, 2014) is both ethical and necessary for appropriate treatment. Accurate diagnosis is especially meaningful when working with clients who have a COD. According to the results from the 2020 National Survey on Drug Use and Health (SAMHSA, 2021, pp. 32–34), approximately 17 million adults have a substance use disorder while concurrently experiencing a mental, behavioral, or emotional disorder; therefore, it is important to thoroughly evaluate all symptoms and behaviors of the client to determine if they are a result of one disorder or co-occurring substance use and mental disorders.

CULTURAL CONSIDERATIONS

It is also necessary to consider a client's cultural background in this assessment process as culture affects how problems are conceptualized, experienced, verbalized, and defined (ACA, 2014). What may seem abnormal or disordered in one culture may be appropriate and normal in another culture; therefore, client's cultural demographics and socioeconomic status must be gathered and considered in selecting an assessment and determining a diagnosis. While an accurate assessment and diagnosis leads to related accurate treatment and positive outcomes for the client, misdiagnosis can lead to poor client outcomes. If a client is diagnosed with an area which is not within the professional counselor's expertise, then a referral is most appropriate (ACA, 2014).

When communicating results, the cultural background, client's understanding of the results, and the impact of the results must be considered (ACA, 2014). It is necessary to be very clear on who will receive the client's assessment results (ACA, 2014). Taking time to share results in a simple and meaningful way for the client is important. When necessary, the limitations of the validity, reliability, and norms of the assessments used must be discussed clearly so the client understands that the results may not be 100% accurate. A collaborative exploration of results is recommended, including checking if the results resonate with the client, discussing any possible discrepancies, and offering straightforward explanations.

Finally, it is necessary to maintain "the integrity and security of (any) test and assessments (used) consistent with legal and contractual obligations" (ACA, 2014, p. 12). It is not ethical to "appropriate, reproduce, or modify published assessments or parts of it for use without permission" (ACA, 2014, p. 12). In addition, it is necessary to securely store client materials including testing and assessment in compliance with state legal mandates. Most paper assessments are stored in a locked cabinet in a locked room while online assessments are securely stored in a computer that is password protected.

CLINICAL CASE ILLUSTRATION AND DISCUSSION

CASE OF FELICITY

An overview of the screening, assessment, and treatment planning processes and protocols have been provided. Now these concepts are illustrated by applying them to the case of Felicity using the 12-step assessment process of assessment outlined by Co-Occurring Center for Excellence (2007).

- **Step 1: Engage the client:** Start by engaging Felicity in her own treatment. A useful mnemonic is LEARN (Berlin & Fowkes, 1983), which stands for **l**isten with empathy so she believes she was heard; **e**xplain the professional counselor's comprehension of the problem; **a**cknowledge cultural identity; **r**ecommend treatment; and **n**egotiate agreement. Ask Felicity to identify her goals, strengths, and where she would like to see growth. This is her journey that she is planning in collaboration with the professional counselor. Next, obtain appropriate permission and paperwork while continuing to build the therapeutic relationship.

- **Step 2: Gather additional information from collaterals:** Inquire about Felicity's support system within her family and friends (especially her husband who she has already mentioned). Ask how she relates to her support system. And, with the client's permission via signed consent, contact individuals included in her primary support system and gather their perspective as well as additional information that will assist in understanding the client's situation. There may be cultural information that also needs to be considered before developing an initial treatment plan.

- **Step 3: Screen for and assess for CODs:** Choose a screen that assesses for alcohol use and another that screens for mental disorder, or select an instrument that collectively screens for co-occurring substance use and mental disorders. Earlier in the introduction of Felicity, the CAGE was described as a screen for alcohol use because Felicity presented to counseling as a result of a legal consequence of drinking (even though she believed she did not have an alcohol use problem). The CAGE results warranted further assessment, which then resulted in gathering adequate information for a *DSM-5* alcohol use disorder diagnosis. During this assessment process, other symptoms that need ongoing investigation led to the use of Beck Depression Inventory II (Beck et al., 1996). Further assessment concluded a COD of major depressive disorder. Details of Felicity's symptoms were presented earlier in the chapter within the "Intake, Assessment, and the Therapeutic Relationship" section.

- **Step 4: Determine the severity of mental and substance use disorders:** Felicity has experienced a legal consequence due to her drinking. Although she attempted to cut down on her drinking because of her spouse's concerns, her attempts were unsuccessful. She is using alcohol to escape her experienced reality of feeling lonely, sad, and empty. Felicity drinks five to six days of the week with either friends or colleagues (and sometimes alone). In addition to these symptoms, her appetite, sleep, and work are affected. Of utmost importance, she is losing the meaning of living (which is intensified due to Felicity having a family history of suicide and having a limited support system).

- **Step 5: Determine the diagnoses:** According to the *DSM-5* (APA, 2013), alcohol use disorder requires a problematic pattern within a 12-month period that is manifested by meeting at least two criteria (which Felicity meets). These include the following: (a) using in larger amounts than intended; (b) having unsuccessful attempts to control her use; (c) spending a significant amount of time drinking; (d) using despite recurrent interpersonal problems; (e) using interferes with occupational functioning; and (f) experiencing increased tolerance to alcohol. Because she presents with six symptoms, her alcohol use is considered to be severe. Felicity also meets the *DSM-5* criteria for major depressive disorder because she presents with at least six symptoms associated with this diagnosis (i.e., depressed mood; diminished interest in activities; significant weight loss; fatigue; insomnia; and feelings of worthlessness), which are more symptoms than needed for diagnosis of a major depressive disorder (APA, 2013).

- **Step 6: Determine an appropriate care setting:** Based on the assessments, the counselor's clinical judgment, and the American Society for Addiction Medicine's patient placement criteria (i.e., *The ASAM Criteria*), partial hospitalization is considered appropriate as she may be at risk for suicide, has a family history of suicide, has poor hygiene, is diagnosed with a COD, is unaware of the alcohol use disorder, is presently using alcohol, and has a limited support system. Being in treatment for approximately 20 or more hours a week is appropriate for her level of the CODs. She has a safe living environment with her spouse, so residential treatment is not necessary. She has not described or presented with alcohol withdrawal symptoms; therefore, detoxification in a medically managed inpatient unit may not be appropriate (but she can be monitored for withdrawal symptoms while in the early stage of receiving treatment within a partial hospitalization level of care).

- **Step 7: Determine disability and functional impairments:** Although she has not so far revealed a disability, it is necessary to investigate if one is present. Felicity has indicated her struggle with motivation to go to work daily, which is a functional impairment.

- **Step 8: Identify strengths and supports of the client:** Investigate other strengths that could help facilitate a successful outcome for Felicity. Felicity has identified her husband, so he may be an asset for her treatment. Although they do not reside where Felicity lives, she also reports having other supportive family members who are only a phone call away. Another strength of Felicity is that she is a college graduate employed as a mathematics teacher in the public school system.

- **Step 9: Identify the cultural and linguistic needs and supports:** Although there appears to be no specific linguistic needs, being biracial, she is straddling bicultural values and beliefs. It is significant to discuss with her how her bicultural identity is seen in her social group. Try to understand how she defines her identity for herself and how that fits with her sense of self.

- **Step 10: Identify any additional problem areas to address:** Although Felicity does not have housing, education, or cognitive issues, she acknowledged employment issues due to missing work.

- **Step 11: Determine readiness for change:** Felicity, as indicated elsewhere, is in the *precontemplation* stage for her alcohol use disorder but in the *preparation* stage for her major depressive disorder. Therefore, while helping her make more structured plans to reduce symptoms of depression and increase wellness, it is important to also educate her on the effects of alcohol on her physical and mental well-being.

- **Step 12: Plan the treatment:** Treatment planning needs to consider cultural variables, biopsychosocial details, motivation for treatment, and continuum of care. Planning treatment must not only include attending to a reduction of symptoms, but it must also focus on enhancing wellness as well as establishing and maintaining longer-term recovery. Felicity will take a brief leave of absence from work to begin a wellness and treatment and recovery plan to attend to her CODs.

CASE DISCUSSION
Felicity's Initial Treatment Plan

Presenting Problems

Felicity presents with the following presenting problems: driving while intoxicated; relationship issues due to her drinking; loneliness; drinking and socializing with friends and colleagues; missing work; motivation issues; loss of weight that was unplanned; hygiene issues; and lack of meaning of life (i.e., not looking forward to the future).

Wellness Needs

Using *The Indivisible Self*, which is an evidence-based model of wellness proposed by Myers and Sweeney (2004), the counselor should investigate Felicity's wellness needs. Considering the five factors identified by Myers and Sweeney (2004) that collectively comprise the *indivisible self* (i.e., creative self, coping self, social self, essential self, and physical self), Felicity's obvious wellness needs are: work and thinking in her *creative self*; self-worth and leisure in her *coping self*; self-care, and perhaps cultural identity, in her *essential self*; love in her *social self*; and nutrition and hygiene in her *physical self*. In order for Felicity's wellness needs to be addressed, the counselor should explore ways for her to feel connected to her inner self. Goals mutually negotiated and developed will not only ideally enhance her motivation to change, but they will also function as checkpoints for her recovery journey.

Long-Term Objectives

The long-term objectives are to address her CODs which are likely feeding off of each other as well as investigate how her cultural intersectionality is interwoven with her CODs. Establishing safety and improving her mood is a primary objective. Abstinence from alcohol use is ideal but may not be agreeable to Felicity because she does not even entertain that she has an alcohol use problem.

Short-Term Goals

Three possible short-term goals for Felicity, which are presented here as SMART goals, need to be negotiated with her. It is important to recognize these are not all inclusive as there are short-term goals that may be developed in collaboration with Felicity based on current conditions and as situations change over time.

1. By the end of week 1, Felicity will identify three support systems she can contact if she has thoughts of self-harm.
2. By the end of week 1, Felicity will identify how many nights she is using alcohol (including the amount used) to fall asleep over a 7-day period.
3. By the end of week 2, Felicity will identify two healthy alternatives to alcohol she can use to assist in falling asleep.
4. By the end of week 2, Felicity will develop a daily schedule that involves starting her day by getting out of bed within 10 minutes of waking and then attending to her daily hygiene.

Interventions

As interventions, the professional counselor would create a climate of acceptance and unconditional positive regard in which Felicity can safely explore her life and how the CODs are affecting her life. The professional counselor will also monitor the client for further suicidal ideation. The professional counselor will review user-friendly literature with Felicity to increase her knowledge to fulfil her goals. Depending on the orientation of the professional counselor, Felicity's thinking may be challenged, behaviors may be modified, and feelings may be identified and addressed. Further, the professional counselor may recommend phone apps that will allow for monitoring her progress.

CHAPTER SUMMARY

The assessment process involves gathering demographics, including all relevant cultural and biopsychosocial data, observing and documenting symptoms, arriving at a diagnosis, identifying strengths and challenges, evaluating the stage of motivation for change, and determining the severity of each disorder to determine the course of treatment and the level of care for the client (SAMHSA, 2020). It is important to gather client details, including cultural intersectionalities, to build a strong therapeutic relationship and appropriately assess and diagnose for treatment considerations. For the best treatment outcome, the client's cultural, biopsychosocial, and motivational aspects, as well as placement in the continuum of care, must all be considered. Screening, assessing, and planning treatment continually evolves as a client's circumstance unfolds and changes throughout the counseling experience. With these changes it is important to continue to build the therapeutic relationship while also continuously assessing for motivation to change.

Integrated screening, assessment, and treatment planning are appropriate for clients diagnosed with co-occurring mental and substance use disorders, especially when no one disorder is primary and the treatment process must be integrated to address the interwoven nature of both disorders within the client's values and belief systems. Such treatment should also include a wellness-oriented lifestyle that continues into aftercare. Benefits of an integrated plan include more engaged clients; meeting client needs for better client outcomes; reduction in symptoms; reduced treatment visits; independent living; steady employment; and happier lifestyle (SAMHSA, 2020).

Challenges exist when screening, assessing, and treatment planning with clients with CODs. At any given point, both disorders may not meet full diagnostic criteria but will be affecting the client's recovery plan. Furthermore, as both disorders are primary for a client with CODs, it can be challenging to "explore, determine and respond to the effects of two mutually interacting disorders" (Co-Occurring Center for Excellence, 2007, p. 2). Next, clients may be at different stages of change with the understanding and treatment readiness for each disorder. Finally, no two clients are alike. Considering the many variables that can potentially complicate the counseling process involving clients who have co-occurring substance use and mental disorders, the counselor should conduct the assessment and plan for treatment with great skill and care. This may be achieved, in part, by developing a therapeutic relationship and proficiently choosing and utilizing the appropriate tools and strategies that will assist in meeting the client's individual needs and goals.

DISCUSSION QUESTIONS

1. How would you go about building and maintaining a therapeutic relationship with Felicity so she will feel comfortable to take risks to make changes in her life? How and when would you assess the strength of the therapeutic relationship?
2. Considering Felicity's situation, what are some cultural implications that may complicate the diagnosis of a COD? How would you address these identified implications?
3. What areas will need intentional attention when conducting a biopsychosocial assessment with Felicity? What are your reasons for the areas you picked? How would you incorporate motivational interviewing into these identified areas?
4. What are some of the screens and assessments you would choose to use with Felicity? What are the psychometric properties of these instruments that make it appropriate to use with Felicity? What are possible ethical and legal implications of your choice?
5. What are three SMART goals that you would generate for Felicity? Discuss how you considered Felicity's motivation to change in generating these goals.

REFERENCES

Abroms, M., & Sher, L. (2016). Dual disorders and suicide. *Journal of Dual Diagnosis, 12*(2), 148–149. https://doi.org/10.1080/15504263.2016.1172898

American Counseling Association. (2014). *2014 ACA code of ethics.* https://www.counseling.org/docs/default-source/default-document-library/2014-code-of-ethics-finaladdress.pdf

American Psychiatric Association. (2000). *Diagnostic and statistical manual of mental disorders* (4th ed., Text Revision).

American Psychiatric Association. (2013). *Diagnostic and statistical manual of mental disorders* (5th ed.). https://doi.org/10.1176/appi.books.9780890425596

American Society of Addiction Medicine (2021). *About the ASAM Criteria.* Retrieved January 18, 2022, from https://www.asam.org/asam-criteria/about-the-asam-criteria

Beck, A. T., Steer, R. A., & Brown, G. K. (1996). *BDI-II: Beck depression Inventory Manual* (2nd ed.). Pearson.

Bennett, M. E., Bellack, A. S., & Gearon, J. S. (2006). Development of a comprehensive measure to assess clinical issues in dual diagnosis patients: The substance use event survey for severe mental illness. *Addictive Behaviors, 31*(12), 2249–2267. https://doi.org/10.1016/j.addbeh.2006.03.012

Berlin, E., & Fowkes, W. A. (1983). A teaching framework for cross-cultural health care. *Western Journal of Medicine, 139,* 934–938.

Borrell-Carrio, F., Suchman, A. M., & Epstein, R. L. (2004). The biopsychosocial model 25 years later: Principles, practice, and scientific inquiry. *Annals of Family Medicine, 2*(6), 576–582. https://doi.org/10.1370/afm.245

Co-Occurring Center for Excellence. (2007). *Screening, assessment, and treatment planning for persons with co-occurring disorders.* Substance Abuse and Mental Health Services Administration, and Center for Mental Health Services. https://www.addictioncounselorce.com/articles/101545/OP2-ScreeningandAssessment-8-13-07.pdf

Dennis, M., Titus, J., White, M., Unsicker, J., & Hodgkins, D. (2002). *Global Appraisal of Individual Needs (GAIN): Administration guide for the GAIN and related measures.* Chestnut Health Systems.

Doran, G. T. (1981). There's a S.M.A.R.T. way to write management's goals and objectives. Management Review, *70*(11), 35–36.

Ewing, J. A. (1984). Detecting alcoholism: The CAGE questionnaire. *JAMA, 252,* 1905–1907.

Gorodnichenko, Y., & Roland, G. (2012). Understanding the individualism-collectivism cleavage and its effects: Lessons from cultural psychology. In M. Aoki, T. Kuran, & G. Roland (Eds.), *Institutions and comparative economic development* (pp. 213–236). International Economic Association Series. Palgrave Macmillan. https://doi.org/10.1057/9781137034014_12

Hasin, D. S. (1996). Psychiatric research interview for substance and mental disorders (PRISM): Reliability for substance abusers. *American Journal of Psychiatry, 153*(9), 1195–1201. https://doi.org/10.1176/ajp.153.9.1195

Hays, D. G. (2017). *Assessment in counseling: Procedures and practices* (6th ed.). Alexandria, VA: American Counseling Association.

Hold, L. (2016). Co-occurring disorder assessment steps. *MOJ Immunology, 4*(2). Article 00124. https://doi.org/10.15406/moji.2016.04.00124

Koob, G. F., & Volkow, N. D. (2016). Neurobiology of addiction: A neurocircuitry analysis. *The Lancet Psychiatry, 3*(8), 760–773. https://doi.org/10.1016/S2215-0366(16)00104-8

Krebs, P., Norcross, J. C., Nicholson, J. M., & Prochaska, J. O. (2018). Stages of change and psychotherapy outcomes: A review and meta-analysis. *Journal of Clinical Psychology, 74*, 1964–1979. https://doi.org/10.1002/jclp.22683

Laux, J. M., Perera-Diltz, D. M., Calmes, S. A., Behl, M., Morgan, B. M., & Rio, J. (2019). Assessment and diagnosis of substance-related and addictive disorders. In D. Capuzzi & M. Stauffer (Eds.), *Foundations of addictions counseling* (4th ed., pp. 118–136). Pearson.

Liakoni, E., Dolder, P. C., Rentsch, K. M., & Liechti, M. E. (2016). Presentations due to acute toxicity of psychoactive substances in an urban emergency department in Switzerland: A case series. *BMC Pharmacology and Toxicology, 17* (25). https://doi.org/10.1186/s40360-016-0068-7

McLean Hospital. (2002-2019). BASIS-24. https://www.ebasis.org

Miller, W. R., & Rollnick, S. (2013). *Motivational interviewing: Helping people for change* (3rd ed.). Guilford.

Moos, R. H., Nichol, A. C., & Moos, B. S. (2002). Global assessment of functioning ratings and the allocation and outcomes of mental health services. *Psychiatric Services, 53*(6), 730–737. https://doi.org/10.1176/appi.ps.53.6.730

Myers, J. E., & Sweeney, T. J. (2004). The indivisible self: An evidence-based model of wellness. *Journal of Individual Psychology, 60*(3), 234–245.

National Institute of Drug Abuse. (2018). Comorbidity: Substance use disorders and other mental illnesses drug facts. https://www.drugabuse.gov/publications/drugfacts/comorbidity-substance-use-disorders-other-mental-illnesses

Negrete, J. C., Collins, J., Turner, N. E., & Skinner, W. (2004). The Centre for Addiction and Mental Health Concurrent Disorders Screener (CAMH-CDS). *Canadian Journal of Psychiatry, 49*(12), 843–850. https://doi.org/10.1177/070674370404901208

Perera-Diltz, D. M., & Moe, J. (2020). The wellness treatment plan. In W. W. IsHak (Ed.), *Handbook of wellness medicine*. Cambridge. https://doi.org/10.1017/9781108650182

Peters, R. H., Bartoi, M. G., & Sherman, P. B. (2008). *Screening and assessment of co-occurring disorders in the justice system*. CMHS National GAINS Center.

Pinel, J. P. J., & Barnes, S. J. (2018). *Biopsychology* (10th ed.). Pearson Education.

Polanski, P. J., & Hinkle, J. S. (2000). The mental status examination: Its use by professional counselors. *Journal of Counseling and Development, 78*, 357–364.

Prochaska, J. O., & DiClemente, C. C. (1983). Stages and processes of self-change of smoking: Toward an integrative model of change. *Journal of Consulting and Clinical Psychology, 51*(3), 390–395. https://doi.org/10.1037/0022-006X.51.3.390

Rizk, M. M., Herzog, S., Dugad, S., & Stanley, B. (2021). Suicide risk and addiction: The impact of alcohol and opioid use disorders. *Current Addiction Reports*, 1–14. Advance online publication. https://doi.org/10.1007/s40429-021-00361-z

Sacks, S., Melnick, G., Coen, C., Banks, S., Friedmann, P. D., Grella, C., & Knight, K. (2007). CJDATS co-occurring disorders screening instrument for mental disorders (CODSI-MD): A pilot study. *Prison Journal, 87*(1), 86–110. https://doi.org/10.1177/0032885506299044

Sheehan, D. V., Lecrubier, Y., Sheehan, K. H., Amorim, P., Janavs, J., Weiller, E., Hergueta, T., Baker, R., & Dunbar, G. C. (1998). The Mini-International Neuropsychiatric Interview (M.I.N.I.). *Journal of Clinical Psychiatry, 59*(20), 22–33.

Substance Abuse and Mental Health Services Administration. (2001). *Mental health: Culture, race, and ethnicity*. Rockville, MD. https://www.ncbi.nlm.nih.gov/books/NBK44243/

Substance Abuse and Mental Health Services Administration. (2015). *Detoxification and substance abuse treatment*. https://store.samhsa.gov/sites/default/files/d7/priv/sma15-4131.pdf

Substance Abuse and Mental Health Services Administration. (2020). *Substance use disorder treatment for people with co-occurring disorders: Treatment improvement protocol (TIP 42)*. https://store.samhsa.gov/sites/default/files/SAMHSA_Digital_Download/PEP20-02-01-004_Final_508.pdf

Substance Abuse and Mental Health Services Administration. (2021). *Key substance use and mental health indicators in the United States: Results from the 2020 National Survey on Drug Use and Health*. https://www.samhsa.gov/data/sites/default/files/reports/rpt35325/NSDUHFFRPDFWHTMLFiles2020/2020NSDUHFFR1PDFW102121.pdf

Sue, D. W., & Sue, D. (2013) *Counseling the culturally diverse: Theory and practice* (6th ed.). Wiley & Sons.

Tellegen, A., & Ben-Porath, Y. S. (2011). *Minnesota Multiphasic Personality Inventory-2 Restructured Form* (MMPI-2-RF). University of Minnesota Press.

Texas Licensed Professional Counselor Act. (1999). Health professions: Regulation of psychology and counseling. https://statutes.capitol.texas.gov/Docs/OC/htm/OC.503.htm

Trzepacz, P. T., & Baker, R. W. (1993). *The psychiatric mental status examination*. Oxford University Press.

World Health Organization. (2012). Measuring health and disability: Manual for WHO Disability Assessment Schedule WHODAS 2.0. https://www.who.int/publications/i/item/measuring-health-and-disability-manual-for-who-disability-assessment-schedule-(-whodas-2.0)

World Health Organization. (2018). *International classification of diseases for mortality and morbidity statistics* (11th Revision). https://icd.who.int/browse11/l-m/en

Young, M. E. (2017). *Learning the art of helping: Building blocks and techniques* (6th ed.). Pearson.

CHAPTER 5

MANAGED CARE AND THE USE OF LEVEL OF CARE GUIDELINES FOR CO-OCCURRING DISORDERS

BRETT HART AND SARAH A. PEIPERT

LEARNING OBJECTIVES

After reading this chapter, you will be able to:
- Summarize the history and function of managed care organizations (MCOs).
- Explain and distinguish between the concepts of insurance benefits, healthcare services, patient placement criteria, and levels of care.
- Explain the purpose of level of care guidelines/medical necessity criteria, which include a description of how the most commonly adopted sets of criteria are used.
- Describe how the utilization management process works as well as the ways in which managed care is beginning to evolve beyond the need for traditional utilization management.

INTRODUCTION

If you are reading this chapter, it is very likely that you are enrolled in a clinical training program with aspirations of engaging in some form of counseling. Although there are counselors who have firmly established themselves following years of experience and maintain "cash-only" clinical practices, most counselors will find that their revenue will, at least in part, flow from managed care organizations (MCOs). The relationship between MCOs and counselors has evolved significantly in recent years, such that greater alignment is being achieved between the two in order to best serve the needs of consumers. As a counselor, it is important to learn to navigate managed care requirements, including the application of medical necessity criteria and appropriate level of care placement. These concepts and tools are explored in greater depth in this chapter, but before doing so, a context for the presence of managed care within the healthcare delivery system is provided.

HISTORICAL CONTEXT OF MANAGED CARE

Insurance is ubiquitous in today's world. People have the option to insure everything from a cell phone to their own life. In the sphere of a person's health, insurance considerations touch many aspects of the care delivery experience. A consumer, for example, must be mindful of having insurance, selecting the most appropriate insurance plan, having an understanding of what is (and is not) covered, and what costs may be associated with using insurance, including co-payments and deductibles. To list a few examples, healthcare providers must give attention to becoming approved participating members of insurance panels, complying with insurance requirements in their practice, and understanding how to obtain reimbursement, limitations of coverage, and level of care criteria. As one who is training to become a behavioral healthcare professional, the world of insurance, or managed care, may seem intimidating and overwhelming. This chapter seeks to address those concerns by providing a clear understanding of managed care, the principles by which it operates, and how to navigate within the managed care framework for the ultimate benefit of future clients.

Any discussion involving managed care must begin with the question of, "What is managed care?" There is strong agreement between the *public sector* (entities partially or fully owned by the government) and the *private sector* (entities owned by an individual or group of individuals) on the definition of managed care. The federal government (public sector) defines managed care as "a health care delivery system organized to manage cost, utilization, and quality" (Medicaid.gov, n.d.). Healthinsurance.org, an organization that offers consumers reliable information about health insurance and reform, defines managed care as "a medical delivery system that attempts to manage the quality and cost of medical services that individuals receive" (Healthinsurance.org, 2022). A common denominator of these definitions is a desire to ensure that when an individual receives health services (including behavioral health and addiction treatment services), these are affordable and of the highest possible quality to ensure optimal consumer outcomes.

While the concept of health insurance dates as early as 1910 with The Western Clinic in Tacoma, Washington (Kongstvedt, 2013, p. 4), what is known today as "managed care" largely emerged in the 1970s and 1980s in response to significant medical cost inflation. This led to heightened tension in the healthcare delivery system between MCOs and healthcare providers based on an assumption that MCOs were solely concerned with profit, while health providers were solely concerned with the care they delivered and the relationship with the client. Although this was likely an oversimplified assessment of each entity's priorities, there is no question that what emerged was an adversarial relationship between MCOs and providers, with each sincerely believing they were acting in the best interest of the client. Fortunately, this adversarial relationship has diminished in recent years with a growing appreciation that all members of the healthcare delivery system—the consumer/client, the provider, and the insurer/MCO—make important contributions and play critical roles to ensure that the consumer receives an optimal healthcare experience. For example, the consumer has become much more informed and involved in healthcare choices; the provider has become more conscious of the role of efficiency and quality in healthcare delivery; and the insurer has become much more sensitive regarding the need to support clients and providers through resources and data.

A NEW PARADIGM IN MANAGED CARE

As mentioned, there has been a significant shift in attitudes on the part of insurers and providers over the last decade, with each more fully appreciating the contribution of the other in care delivery. This may stem from a recognition that each party brings unique assets and insights to the care delivery process. For example, the provider brings specialized training, clinical experience, and a relationship with the client or consumer of healthcare services. The insurer brings substantial longitudinal data insights regarding individual clients or whole populations, which are leveraged to quickly connect the client to additional resources to support care (e.g., social services, community recovery groups), facilitate medical/behavioral integration (i.e., treatment of the whole person through addressing both the physical and behavioral health issues that may be influencing one another), and case management capabilities (i.e., assessing client needs, implementing solutions, and monitoring their effects) to support the client outside the provider's office. This increasing appreciation of what each party brings to the table has served to strengthen two key concepts that positively impact consumer care: *aligned incentives* and *whole-person care*.

ALIGNED INCENTIVES

The concept of aligned incentives rests on the premise that a triad exists within the healthcare delivery system that consists of the following parties: (a) the client; (b) the provider; and (c) the insurer.

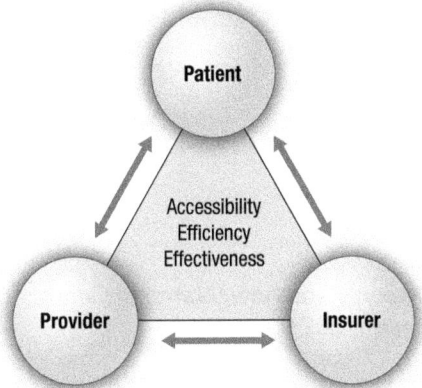

FIGURE 5.1 The Aligned Incentives Triadic Model of the Healthcare Delivery System.

It is assumed that each member of this triad desires quality healthcare services to be acknowledged, provided, and received. And, in order to accomplish this outcome, delivery systems must be:

1. **Accessible** (able to be conveniently reached and free of barriers)
2. **Efficient** (delivered in a timely, efficient manner and free of fraud, waste, or abuse)
3. **Effective** (resolves the healthcare needs to the satisfaction of the client or consumer)

If these three elements are present in all healthcare delivery scenarios, all parties achieve their desired goal: (a) *patients, clients, and consumers* are satisfied that care was obtained quickly, was affordable, and that their needs were effectively addressed; (b) *providers* are satisfied that they have a steady referral and revenue stream, are able to meet client needs in a timely manner, and can render the highest quality services; and (c) *insurers* are satisfied that their insured customers are content with sustained health and wellness at optimal cost. Thus, the incentives of each member of the triad are aligned and not at odds with one another, therefore allowing all parties to work as a team and build trust by understanding that the motives of each (i.e., getting the client timely access to efficient and effective care) are in harmony with one another.

WHOLE-PERSON CARE

The concept of whole-person care may be known by other names such as integrated care or medical/behavioral integration. As the term implies, whole-person care means viewing a client's needs not from the perspective of a specific disease state or condition; rather, it involves looking at client needs holistically and focusing on overall health and well-being (National Center for Complementary and Integrative Health, 2021).

For example, if a client were to seek care for diabetes in a traditional framework, that individual might be instructed on controlling blood sugar, maintaining appropriate diet and exercise, and administering insulin (as in the case of type 1 diabetes). A *whole-person care approach* includes an

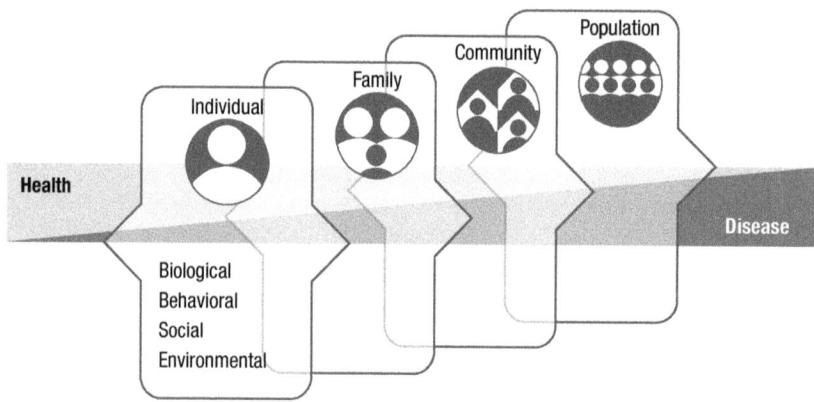

FIGURE 5.2 The Whole-Person Care View (National Center for Complementary and Integrative Health, 2021).

array of healthcare professionals working in collaboration to meet the individual's needs, which includes but is not limited to assessing and addressing behavioral health conditions, providing education, incorporating the family into care, connecting to community supports, and mitigating environmental stressors or triggers. In like manner, it is important for counselors to look at clients who present with co-occurring mental and substance use disorders from a whole-person perspective, thereby recognizing that comprehensive solutions go beyond the presenting mental health or substance misuse condition.

Now that a brief history of managed care and the ideal paradigm within which clients, providers, and insurers would operate have been discussed, attention will be placed on a more in-depth discussion of the role of the MCO with a special emphasis on managed *behavioral* healthcare.

INSURANCE PLANS AND POPULATION TYPES

Most MCOs today manage the insurance benefits for a diverse set of populations; however, MCOs typically group these populations within one of the two categories: (a) *public sector* and (b) *private insurance*.

PUBLIC SECTOR

Public sector is a category that includes individuals whose insurance coverage is through a managed, government-sponsored product such as managed Medicaid, managed Medicare, or managed marketplace/exchange (i.e., the Affordable Care Act). Each of these broad categories of coverage has a number of variations or subtypes. For example, subtypes of managed Medicaid include long-term services and supports [LTSS], Children's Health Insurance Program [CHIP], and serious mental illness [SMI]. Although other forms of public sector insurance coverage exist beyond Medicaid, Medicare, and marketplace (e.g., military health coverage, health insurance for incarcerated populations), an emphasis will be placed on the primary government-based insurance programs.

PRIVATE INSURANCE

By contrast, private insurance (sometimes referred to as "commercial" coverage) pertains to insurance coverage that individuals generally obtain either through their employer as an employment benefit or purchased independently through an insurance company. These plans are *not* government-sponsored or subsidized. As is the case with public sector plans, private insurance plans come in a number of shapes and sizes. Counselors may hear references to *health maintenance organization* (HMO), *preferred provider organization* (PPO), and *point of service* (POS) plans.

Having an *HMO* plan means an individual must obtain care from a defined group of providers in the insurance company's network, and going outside that network will generally result in no coverage. In this model, the individual's primary care physician serves as a gatekeeper for when the individual may seek a specialist or other services.

Having a *PPO* plan means that an individual can generally obtain healthcare services from any provider in or outside of the network, including specialists, without a primary care physician approval or referral. This added flexibility and freedom is generally associated with higher costs to the individual in the form of higher monthly premiums and/or deductibles in addition to co-payments.

Having a *POS* plan combines elements of both the HMO and PPO models. POS plans generally require a referral from one's chosen primary care physician to do so (as seen in the HMO model); however, it allows the insured to obtain services from providers both in and outside the network (thus offering the same flexibility as seen within a PPO plan). The result is a hybrid-type model that offers more flexibility than the HMO plan but with less cost than a PPO plan due to the retention of the primary care physician as a gatekeeper.

A further distinction within commercial health insurance plans, from the insurer's perspective, is between *fully insured* commercial plans (referring to the fact that the insurer has assumed all financial liability and risk for the expenditures of the enrolled members) and *administrative services only* (ASO) commercial plans (referring to the fact that the *employer* has assumed all financial liability and risk for the expenditures of the enrolled members). In the latter case, the insurer simply provides administrative support for the employer (e.g., providing a network of providers, authorizing care, processing claims).

INSURANCE BENEFITS

Having addressed the concept of managed care populations, based primarily on the sponsor of the plan (government versus employers) in which the individual has enrolled, the benefits associated with types of plans are now reviewed. The concept of benefits, as associated with health insurance, can be a difficult one to understand. Often, benefits are often associated within an employment context. For example, a person may accept a job that offers such benefits as paid vacation time, paid sick leave, or the option to contribute to a 401(k) with some sort of employer match. These are examples of what is often referred to as "benefits." In the context of health insurance, benefits refer to the service offerings that a government entity, employer, or individual elects to cover on behalf of their enrolled members (or oneself in the case of individually purchased insurance). For example, an employer may purchase a health insurance plan for employees that consists of coverage for free wellness visits or no-cost mammography screenings. In the context of behavioral health, benefits often include client access to outpatient mental health and substance treatment and facility-based services (e.g., outpatient care, residential treatment, inpatient hospitalization).

Increasingly, insurers are tailoring benefit options to the population needs of individuals enrolled in various types of insurance plans (e.g., commercial insurance, Medicaid, Medicare). For example, individuals insured through commercial plans who are generally considered relatively healthy and have access to basic social support may have plans that include standard health offerings such as outpatient and facility services. Individuals enrolled in a Medicaid plan, however, may lack such basic supports as shelter, food, or transportation. In these cases, insurers are increasingly making benefits available (e.g., housing allowances, food vouchers, ride share coupons) to fill these gaps to address what have become known as the *social determinants of health* (Healthy People 2030, n.d.). Likewise, individuals enrolled in a Medicare plan may have distinct needs such as nursing coverage or home health support that an individual enrolled in a commercial plan may not require. These unique or additional services, based on the population enrolled in a given type of insurance plan, may be more costly in the short-term but are generally seen as being associated with improved long-term outcomes and lower costs for individuals.

LEVELS OF CARE

Closely associated with the concept of benefits is the concept of *level of care*. While the term level of care is quite familiar to most insurance and provider community members, it may be less familiar to the general public. Level of care pertains to the type and intensity of treatment required for a physical health illness, behavioral health condition, or substance use disorder. For example, an individual experiencing mild to moderate anxiety may require an outpatient counseling or psychotherapy visit (or series of visits) to effectively address this condition. In this case, outpatient counseling would be considered a "level of care." By contrast, an individual who made a suicide attempt and remains committed to completing suicide may require treatment provided in an inpatient hospital setting to ensure safety. In this case, "inpatient" would be considered another "level of care." In the realm of behavioral healthcare, there is an array of levels of care available to meet the needs of the individual depending on one's condition and needs. Some examples, in ascending order of restrictiveness, include the following:

- **Peer Support/Community Support Groups/12-Step Programs:** Typically, a supportive environment focused on coaching, mentoring, or guidance of consumers that is led by nonclinician or fellow consumers.
- **Outpatient Counseling/Medication Management/Employee Assistance Program (EAP):** Typically, an office-based or telehealth setting in which a consumer sees a counselor or psychiatrist for 15 to 60 minutes to address nonacute mental health or substance misuse needs.
- **Intensive Outpatient Program (IOP):** Typically, a low-restriction, facility or clinic environment in which a consumer can obtain more intensive services for mental health or substance misuse (3 hours per day) than offered in traditional outpatient counseling, but less intensive than other acute care settings
- **Day Treatment/Partial Hospitalization Program (PHP):** Typically, a more acute care facility or clinic environment that serves as a substitute for inpatient care when higher, but manageable risk is present, lasting 5 to 6 hours per day, followed by the consumer

returning home for the night. This can be used for the treatment of mental health and substance misuse.

- **Residential:** Typically, an unlocked, less-monitored facility environment for longer-term treatment of mental health or substance misuse conditions that are best treated in a controlled setting away from a consumer's home due to exacerbating environmental factors that may be present.
- **Inpatient:** Typically, a locked, restricted, 24-hour monitored, acute facility environment for stabilization of life-threatening symptoms, risk, or impairment in functioning due to mental health or substance misuse. Examples of risk might include suicide plan, severe withdrawal symptoms, or severe functional impairment.

It should also be noted that within each level of care mentioned previously, many forms of service can be rendered depending on the client's condition. For example, within an outpatient level of care, services as diverse as psychological testing, counseling, medication management, detoxification, and electroconvulsive therapy (ECT) can be delivered. This is an essential illustration of the distinction that exists among benefits, services, and levels of care. A person may have an insurance plan that provides a *benefit* to cover substance detoxification, while at the same time substance detoxification can be seen as a specific *treatment service* type. However, substance detoxification can be delivered at multiple *levels of care* depending on a number of variables such as the client's current health status, interplay of co-occurring mental and substance use conditions, and existence of support systems and quality of the recovery environment.

LEVELS OF CARE CRITERIA

In order to identify which specific level of care is most appropriate for an individual client, it may be helpful to begin with a relatively simple scenario. Consider one client seeking treatment of mild anxiety; now envision another individual seeking treatment following a serious suicide attempt with a persistent desire to complete suicide. There would likely be little difficulty determining which person is more appropriate for outpatient services compared to the one who requires admission to an inpatient level of care. The decision about level of care placement, however, is not always as clear-cut as in the aforementioned example. Questions such as the following can be very challenging to answer:

- Does an individual who is experiencing severe and worsening depression but not suicidal ideation require inpatient hospitalization?
- Could this individual receive appropriate treatment in a PHP or even an intensive outpatient (IOP) level of care?
- Does the individual simply need ambulatory care/routine services from their counselor and/or a psychiatrist in an outpatient office setting?

The response to these questions may be quite subjective in nature, thus introducing the reality of bias into the level of care equation.

From a provider's perspective, the question of level of care placement may be heavily dependent on past training or the clinician's treatment orientation. For example, one provider who treats opioid dependence may adopt an *abstinence model* (i.e., complete cessation of substance use), while another may adopt a *harm reduction model* (i.e., reducing substance use and minimizing the harm done by using substances). Among physician providers and other prescribers, one may favor *medication-assisted treatment* (MAT) in a *restricted setting* for opioid dependence, while another may favor MAT in an *ambulatory setting* for the same condition (i.e., outpatient-based) setting. In the case of a hospital facility, determination of level of care placement may be influenced by what levels of care it has available to offer a client. In reality, significant variations in level of care preference having little to do with the actual consumer condition exist from region-to-region, between rural, suburban, and urban settings, and between providers representing differing treatment orientations, training backgrounds, risk tolerance, and available treatment resources.

Managed care organizations (MCOs) must also be careful to guard against a bias toward a level of care placement based on financial cost. Perhaps surprisingly, even the potential for bias by the client regarding the level of care placement must be considered. There is a strong preference for treatment in the **least restrictive** level of care possible while still receiving the **most appropriate** care for many clients. How many people would want to be hospitalized due to breaking a finger? At the other end of the continuum, there may be a bias by a client or significant other for the **most restrictive** level of care placement. For example, the parent of a minor child who has a chronic eating disorder, or the partner of an individual who has multiple substance use relapses, may press for the most restrictive level of care placement due to believing it will provide the most optimal outcome.

LEVEL OF CARE DETERMINATION

With so many variables existing that may influence level of care placement, MCOs have turned to level of care guidelines to determine the level of care the individual's insurance plan can cover. This process of using *level of care guidelines* generally begins with the provider contacting the consumer's insurance carrier to present current clinical information and make a request for a specific level of care to be covered. The insurer, or MCO, will review that clinical information against specific level of care criteria to determine whether or not coverage can be applied. It is important to emphasize that the level of care guidelines used by MCOs are in place to guide insurance coverage decisions for a requested level of care, not to dictate the final placement of a consumer or determine whether care is rendered at all. Ultimately, it is the decision of the treating provider regarding which level of care the individual will ultimately be placed for treatment. If an MCO denies coverage of a level of care, this decision can typically be appealed by the provider and/or client, which will be addressed in a later section.

Level of care guidelines are not only useful for making *initial determinations* about level of care placement at the beginning of care, but they also serve to guide decision-making regarding *continued stay* within a level of care and when it is appropriate for an individual to *discharge* and *transition* from one level of care to another. Most MCOs utilize level of care criteria that third party external organizations develop to ensure that their coverage decisions based on these criteria are not self-serving or biased. These level of care criteria are generally developed by a committee of experts (e.g., experienced practitioners, scientists, advocates) in their field who examine current scientific best practices and translate these to criteria that need to be satisfied in order to justify the placement of a consumer in a given level of care for treatment. These criteria are an attempt to establish consistent standards for level of care placement that overcome practice variations, biases, and preferences. It must be acknowledged that there is no perfect set of guidelines that can address every nuance of every treatment scenario. Most would agree, however, that level of care guidelines, at minimum, provide a useful set of scientifically derived and evidenced-based criteria that serve to resolve the majority of questions regarding level of care placement.

While most MCOs use externally derived level of care guidelines, which of these guidelines are adopted for use can depend on many factors. One factor for an MCO may be the applicability of the guidelines for the populations it serves. The cost to purchase a license for the use of the guidelines may be another consideration. Furthermore, some states mandate the use of certain level of care guidelines for individuals insured in their state. For example, many states mandate the use of the American Society of Addiction Medicine guidelines (otherwise known as *The ASAM Criteria*) for level of care placement of individuals receiving substance use treatment.

Though much of the discussion thus far has focused on the use of level of care criteria by MCOs, it would be a mistake to assume that they are the only entities to make use of level of care criteria. Most hospitals use level of care criteria to ensure that the treating provider's level of care placement recommendation aligns with objective criteria. By doing so, the hospital, facility, and/or provider can feel a greater level of confidence that when they contact an MCO to request coverage at a given level of care, there will be a high likelihood of alignment between the two entities because they will be speaking a common language to resolve any variation in interpretation.

LEVEL OF CARE GUIDELINES

While certainly not an exhaustive list of criteria, some of the more commonly utilized level of care guidelines are as follows:

- **The American Society of Addiction Medicine (ASAM) Criteria** (American Society of Addiction Medicine)
- **The Level of Care Utilization System for Psychiatric and Addiction Services** (American Association of Community Psychiatrists)
- **Child and Adolescent Level of Care Utilization System** (American Association of Community Psychiatrists)
- **Milliman Care Guidelines** (MCG Health)
- **InterQual Behavioral Health Criteria** (Change Healthcare)

In order to gain an appreciation for how such level of care criteria are utilized by MCO's and providers, ASAM's Multidimensional Assessment and ASAM Criteria Levels of Care and Continuum of Care will serve as an example. These guidelines are especially relevant for co-occurring disorders, which is the focus of this textbook.

THE ASAM CRITERIA

The American Society of Addiction Medicine's (ASAM) *ASAM Criteria* are among the most widely used sets of level of care criteria when treating members with co-occurring mental and substance use disorders (ASAM, n.d.-c.). Development of *The ASAM Criteria* began in the 1980s to create a nationally recognized set of criteria for the evidenced-based treatment of substance use disorders (ASAM, n.d.-c.). The popularity of these guidelines results from the comprehensive, multidimensional nature of the assessment and the alignment with levels of treatment "that are based on the degree of direct medical management provided, the structure, safety and security provided, and the intensity of treatment services provided" (ASAM, n.d.-c., para. 2). These criteria are uniquely designed to support the assessment of co-occurring disorders by exploring the client's needs from a "whole-person" approach to facilitate positive treatment outcomes.

THE SIX DIMENSIONS OF MULTIDIMENSIONAL ASSESSMENT

The ASAM Criteria consists of six dimensions (ASAM, n.d.-c.) that contribute to the development of a comprehensive and integrated multidimensional assessment that is used to determine care and plan treatment. The six dimensions are as follows: (a) potential for *withdrawal or acute intoxication* status; (b) the current *physical health* and potentially complicating co-occurring medical disorders; (c) *cognitive, behavioral,* or *emotional conditions* the client is experiencing and those that could complicate treatment; (d) the person's *readiness for change*; (e) *continued use* and *relapse potential*; and (f) the *recovery environment* (Mee-Lee et al., 2013).

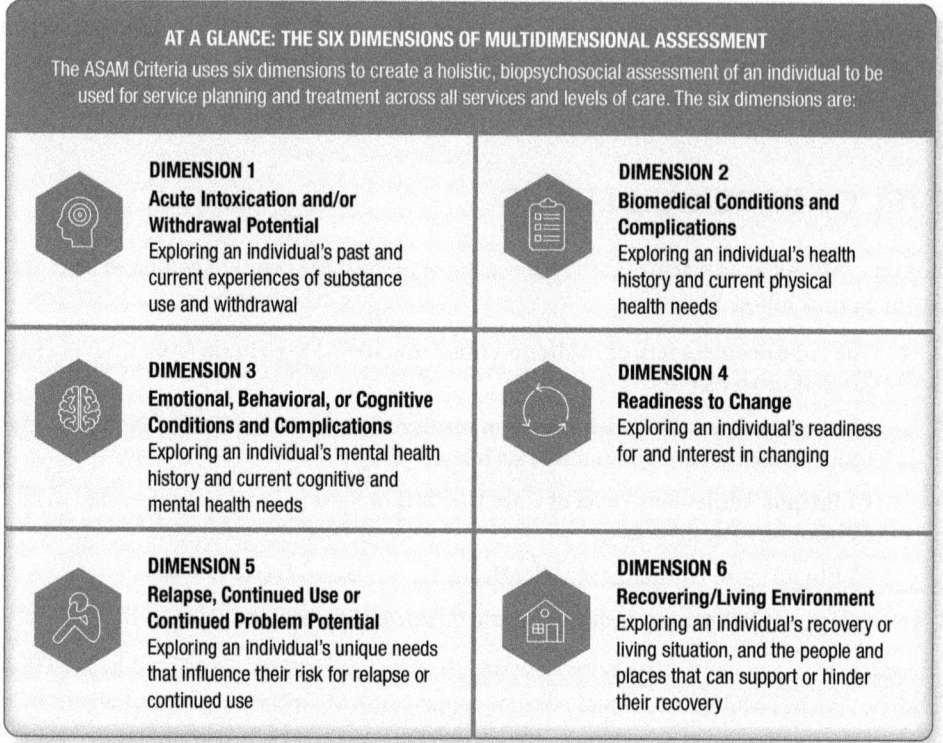

FIGURE 5.3 The Six Dimensions of Multidimensional Assessment (ASAM, n.d.-b.).
Source: *American Society of Addiction Medicine.* The Six Dimensions of Multidimensional Assessment [Infographic]. asam.org. Retrieved March 8, 2022, www.asam.org/asam-criteria/about-the-asam-criteria. *Reprinted with permission.*

These criteria assist the provider in assessing each of the six biopsychosocial categories according to a level of functioning and severity scale. The assessment and score are then utilized to build a risk rating profile that aids in the recommendation for the level of care at which treatment should occur. Risk is rated in each dimension from zero to four, with zero indicating the dimension is a non-issue or very low-risk issue. A rating of one would indicate *mild* difficulty with the problem, while a rating of two indicates some *moderate* difficulty. *Serious* issues within the dimension are rated a three, and the *highest risk* would warrant a rating of four, indicating the greatest severity or potential for imminent danger or harm (Mee-Lee et al., 2013). The severity scale rating along each of the six dimensions is then utilized to align the client's clinical presentation to the most appropriate level of care.

ASAM Continuum of Care

The ASAM Criteria defines five broad categories regarding levels of care (ASAM, n.d.-c.). It should be noted, however, this does not imply there is universal agreement that there are only five levels of care. The levels ascend in number based on the clinical severity scale along the six dimensions. The lowest score (0 to 0.5) is assigned to the least restrictive care level: early intervention. This may correspond, for example, to outpatient as the setting in which the treatment (e.g., counseling) should be delivered. The highest total score is four, which indicates a need for medically managed inpatient level of care as the setting in which treatment should be delivered (Mee-Lee et al., 2013). Once treatment for a person is initiated at a specific level of care, the provider will continually assess the member utilizing *The ASAM Criteria* to determine progress toward the individual's treatment goals that would indicate readiness for discharge from the current level of care and transition to a less restrictive level of care (the full range of levels of care is often referred to as the "continuum of care"). In some cases, application of the criteria may indicate that the client cannot meet the identified treatment goals at a given level of care or that issues have intensified, and a more intensive level of care is warranted.

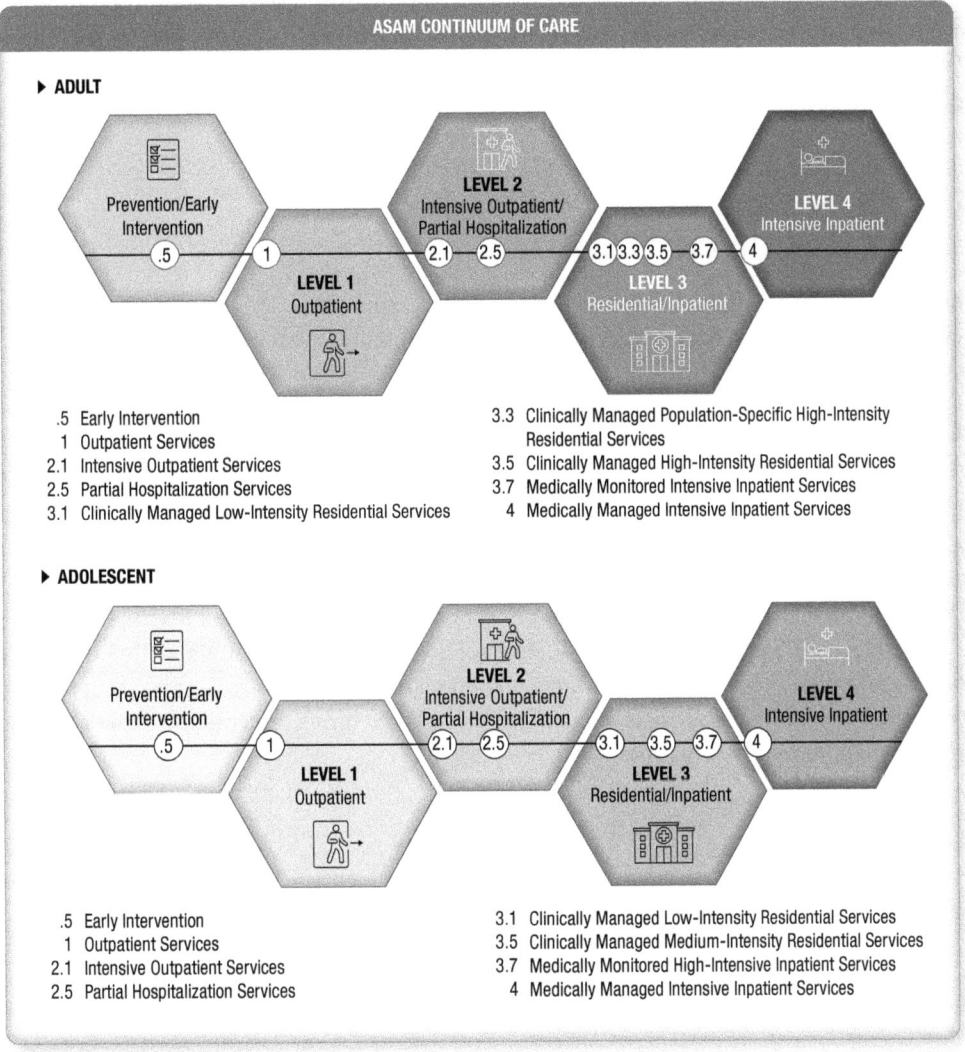

FIGURE 5.4 ASAM Levels of Care. (ASAM, n.d.-a.).
Source: *American Society of Addiction Medicine*. The Six Dimensions of Multidimensional Assessment [Infographic]. asam.org. Retrieved March 8, 2022, www.asam.org/asam-criteria/about-the-asam-criteria. Reprinted with permission.

Use of *The ASAM Criteria*, or any set of level of care criteria, is fluid. While offering a clinically sound set of guidelines to make treatment recommendations, the practitioner's expert evaluation of the client's presentation should be incorporated to create an individualized treatment plan that involves the client's participation and collaboration. The criteria are flexible to support a progression in care that is focused on positive treatment outcomes and functional change. Although *The ASAM Criteria* are popularly used among behavioral health practitioners in clinical practice settings, as well as in MCO settings, there are many other evidence-based tools in use that warrant review and discussion.

OTHER LEVEL OF CARE GUIDELINES / MEDICAL NECESSITY CRITERIA

In addition to *The ASAM Criteria*, various level of care guidelines are utilized broadly by MCOs to determine if the care level being requested by a provider meets the medical necessity criteria to receive insurance coverage for that service. These include (a) the American Association of Community Psychiatrists LOCUS and CALOCUS, (b) MCG Health's Milliman Care Guidelines, and (c) Change Healthcare's InterQual Behavioral Health Criteria.

Level of Care Utilization System for Psychiatric and Addiction Services and the Child and Adolescent Level of Care Utilization System

The Level of Care Utilization System for Psychiatric and Addiction Services (LOCUS) was developed in 1996 by the American Association of Community Psychiatrists (AACP; n.d.) to assist clinicians with assessment, placement, and continued service decisions to ensure positive treatment outcomes for adults. The Child and Adolescent Level of Care Utilization System (CALOCUS) was developed after LOCUS to support decision-making for the child and adolescent population in collaboration with the American Association of Child and Adolescent Psychiatry (AACAP). In December 2020, the AACAP and the AACP joined to create a tool that combined the CALOCUS tool and the Child and Adolescent Service Intensity Instrument (CASII) to create a simplified, standardized assessment. The new instrument for children and adolescents, called CALOCUS-CASII, is utilized for ages 6 to 18 (American Academy of Child & Adolescent Psychiatry, 2020).

Both the LOCUS and the CALOCUS-CASII are divided into three distinct sections: (a) *evaluation parameters*; (b) *level of care definitions*; and (c) *scoring methodology*. The first section, evaluation parameters, contains an assessment of the client based on six dimensions (American Association of Community Psychiatrists, 2009, p. 6–16):

1. Risk of harm;
2. Functional status;
3. Medical, addictive, and psychiatric co-morbidity
4. Recovery environment;
5. Treatment and recovery history;
6. Engagement and recovery status

Clients are scored along these six dimensions using a five-point scale, with one being the lowest acuity for each range and five the highest. Thus, total scoring could range from 6 to 30. This score then translates to one of six recommended levels of care in which treatment should occur.

This tool is quite popular and widely used among practitioners and managed care companies for initial determinations and concurrent reviews. It quickly identifies gaps in care and recovery resources needed to facilitate care transitions through all levels of care, from medically managed inpatient services to outpatient or community-based recovery and maintenance management.

MCG Care Guidelines

Formerly known as the Milliman Care Guidelines, the care guidelines from MCG Health were created to ensure that evidence-based best practices were utilized to prevent over or underutilization of services across the entire continuum of care for behavioral health and substance-related disorders (MCG Health, n.d.). The MCG care guidelines focus on diagnostic groupings using evidence-based research and treatment recommendations from practitioners and experts within the American Psychiatric Association, the American Association of Pediatrics, the ASAM, and the National Institute of Alcohol Abuse and Alcoholism, to name a few entities. More than 15 behavioral health diagnostic groups are outlined within MCG. Within those 15 groups are evidence-based summaries to determine the most appropriate level of care to treat the client. A unique feature of the MCG guidelines is detailed discharge criteria that outline specific milestones that should be achieved to warrant discharge from, and transition to a new level of care. Also included are care planning prompts that help the provider critically analyze and appropriately address social determinants of health (MCG Health, n.d.).

InterQual Behavioral Health Criteria

InterQual Behavioral Health Criteria® were created in 1978 in collaboration with a former hospital utilization review nurse, Joanne Lampry, to evaluate the appropriateness of admissions and level of service at the hospital (Mitus, 2008). Today, these criteria are used in managed care settings to evaluate the appropriate level of care placement for psychiatric conditions, substance use disorders, and dual diagnoses at the time the consumer presents for care. These are also appropriate for continued treatment determinations as well as transition of care and discharge decisions. InterQual criteria use an evidence-based approach to addressing clients' needs across their lifespans with criteria for children, adolescents, adults, geriatric individuals at all levels of care. Additionally, InterQual addresses the severity of the clinical presentation of symptoms and the client's functional status, comorbidities, and the quality of the consumer's family and community-based support systems (Change Healthcare, n.d.-a.).

The InterQual® tool (Change Healthcare, n.d.-b.) guides clinicians through the decision-making process using an evidence-based and extensive set of clinical criteria that focus on the individual's symptoms, behaviors, level of functioning, adherence to treatment, as well as the services that are available to the client. The criteria allow for decision-making across the continuum of care, meaning that if the symptoms that justified admission to a level of care have been resolved, the provider can look to the criteria as an indicator of readiness for movement to a less intensive level of care. By contrast, if the individual's symptoms are worsening, there may be a need for transition to a more intensive level of care.

COMPARING THE LEVEL OF CARE GUIDELINES

As is likely apparent, each set of criteria discussed have differing features, advantages, and limitations. However, all share two common characteristics: (a) all consist of clinical criteria used nationally to recommend appropriate level of care placement, and (b) all serve as an adjunct to the clinical expertise of both the provider requesting coverage of care and the clinician within the MCO reviewing the request for coverage. The decision regarding which guidelines are recommended or mandated varies by state and by the state departments of health and human services, though not all government entities have a position on this issue. The Center for Medicaid and Medicare Services, for example, is silent on which guidelines to use. Where there is an absence of a state policy that mandates the use of a particular criteria set, MCOs have discretion on guideline selection. They are, however, discouraged or even prohibited from using guidelines that they may develop internally that could be viewed as biased or self-serving. In the final analysis, while level of care criteria does not eliminate all disagreements between a provider and an MCO, they provide a scientifically based standard to reduce bias and encourage consistency of treatment recommendations across disciplines, geographies, and settings.

UTILIZATION MANAGEMENT

To this point, a label has not been assigned to identify the entire process by which clinical information is exchanged between a provider and an MCO, wherein the level of care criteria are applied to assist in making coverage decisions based on that clinical information. This process is referred to as *utilization management*. Utilization management often begins with obtaining relevant clinical information from the provider about the consumer's condition, including but not limited to presenting problems, current symptoms, biopsychosocial data, past and present treatment episodes, co-occurring physical, mental, and/or substance use conditions, medication regimen, etc. The MCO will generally only request enough information to allow them to apply the level of care guidelines previously described. Once applied, the MCO will generally communicate the level of care, recommended by the level of care criteria, that can be covered by the consumer's insurance benefit, and the number of sessions or days of treatment that can be covered prior to requiring a new, updated review. Ultimately, the level of care placement and extent of services is left to the provider's discretion. If the MCO does not agree with the provider's level of care request assessment, they may issue what is known as a *denial of coverage* or *adverse benefit determination* (ABD). Appeal options, such as initiating a peer-to-peer review where the treating provider may discuss utilization review concerns with the MCO's medical director/physician reviewer, are available in cases of adverse determinations based upon medical necessity.

LEGAL AND ETHICAL CONSIDERATIONS

It is important to be clear that this denial of coverage or ABD is not a prohibition of the provider rendering care to a client: a managed care organization (MCO) does not have that authority. An ABD is simply a determination that *payment* for that level of care cannot be supported by the level of care guidelines being applied. The care provider always has an ethical obligation to render or facilitate what is believed to be the appropriate care to the client regardless of the payment decision by an MCO. This would fall within the abandonment prohibition in most professional ethical standards. Specifically, even if insurance coverage is denied, a professional must provide or facilitate the acquisition of services deemed necessary by the counselor. This obligation is even more sharply defined in the case of life-threatening emergencies, where the Emergency Medical Treatment and Active Labor Act (EMTALA; CMS.gov, 2021) mandates that a consumer in need of emergency treatment be assessed and stabilized prior to transferring to other care settings regardless of payment. It should be noted that a denial of coverage determination by an MCO can almost always be appealed – often at multiple levels – and in some cases, the appeal may be reviewed by an independent reviewer unaffiliated with either the provider or MCO.

EVOLVING THE MANAGED CARE AND PROVIDER RELATIONSHIP

Historically, the process of traditional utilization management has been viewed by providers as an adversarial process. When disagreements arose over level of care guideline interpretation, providers would, at times, suspect that MCO decisions were financially driven. MCOs may have been prone to similar suspicions that a provider, due to financial considerations, might overestimate an individual's care needs or be inefficient or wasteful with healthcare dollars. While both perspectives represent errors and oversimplifications, this did not ease the tension that sometimes existed in this relationship.

Because MCOs have stewardship and fiduciary responsibilities to their customers (i.e., companies and government entities funding healthcare for their enrolled members) as well as the members themselves, it is necessary for MCO's to continue the process of conducting basic utilization management activities with treatment providers. Over the last several years, however, MCOs have begun to shift their focus toward building collaborative and supportive relationships with providers to facilitate whole-health solutions for their insured members.

ALTERNATIVE PAYMENT MODELS

One approach that has gained considerable adoption in the physical health arena and is beginning to gain traction in behavioral health is *alternative payment models*. This solution takes aim at two areas where tension can arise between providers and MCOs: (a) *reimbursement rates* and (b) *justification of payment*. Alternative payment models exist on a continuum that ranges from simple incentives to full capitation (i.e., the payment of a fixed amount to a provider for a consumer or group of consumers during a certain timeframe regardless of the number of services utilized).

INCENTIVE-BASED PAYMENT

Incentive-based payment models (sometimes called "pay for performance") generally add bonus payments to the standard, contracted reimbursement rate a provider already receives in exchange for achieving certain quality or clinical metrics with a client. For example, a provider may receive a contracted rate for the counseling service provided to a client, but if that counselor also conducts a risk screen, sees the client regularly without missed appointments, and/or prevents the need for hospitalization for a specified period, that provider may be eligible for a bonus payment. In this way, providers can reduce the time they spend participating in the utilization management process because the MCO can observe that high quality care is being delivered and positive client outcomes are being achieved through the incentives a provider is earning.

CAPITATION-BASED PAYMENT

For providers who have the highest level of confidence in their effectiveness, they may be eligible to enter into a capitated arrangement with an MCO. Generally, these providers are not required to participate in any form of utilization management because they are, essentially, managing themselves. A simplified view of capitation is that a provider is given an agreed-upon sum of money for the full course of treatment needed by a client or group of clients. The provider is disincentivized to under-deliver necessary care (or overdeliver unnecessary care) because doing so would result in poor client outcomes, which would impact the capitated rate, future referrals, and eligibility for this form of a payment model. In other words, a capitated provider is discouraged from providing unnecessary or inefficient care because doing so would prevent the provider from being profitable with the flat sum of money received.

MANAGED HEALTHCARE INNOVATIONS

There are many other payment models along the payment continuum, but what these have in common is an attempt on the part of MCOs to grant providers greater independence and remove administrative burdens, while also ensuring the best possible outcomes for consumers. By removing the financial tension that can exist between providers and MCOs, it has opened the door for both to work as partners in the evolving healthcare arena. Today, many providers work hand-in-hand with MCOs to pilot new strategies, fill the needs of specific populations, and broaden the reach of care delivery. This partnership has paved the way for significant innovation in behavioral healthcare.

CASE MANAGEMENT

One example of this evolution is the manner in which MCOs have begun to realign their own internal resources. Until the late 20th century, the majority of clinical resources held by an MCO were largely devoted to the task of utilization management described earlier. In recent years, though, these organizations have begun to shift resources away from utilization management toward case management and other client-supportive functions. Case management within an MCO often involves identifying consumers who have greater care needs or gaps in care that require closure. For example, an individual may have a co-occurring mental health and substance use disorder, or the person may have a co-occurring mental health and physical health condition (e.g., depression and diabetes). Perhaps the consumer's condition has been especially chronic and severe, or accompanied by housing or transportation barriers making it difficult to obtain care. In these and other cases, the MCO may assign a case manager to this consumer to reach out and have regular contact with the consumer to assess current functioning, identify obstacles to care, health, and well-being, and coordinate needed services between the individual and treating providers. In this way, the MCO can actually serve as a partner to the provider, assisting in coordinating care needs that the provider may not have the time or resources to address.

SOCIAL DETERMINANTS OF HEALTH

Another structural change MCOs have made includes the dedication of resources to address *social determinants of health*. Social determinants of health are the conditions in which people live their lives that can affect health and well-being (Centers for Disease Control and Prevention, 2021). These include variables such as housing availability, transportation access, disability status, social support, and safety. MCOs may work at the individual or community level to address these issues on behalf of their enrolled consumers in order to maximize health outcomes and ensure long-term stability. At the *individual level,* this may take the form of providing consumers with access to healthy food, offering free vouchers for ride-sharing options to attend a counseling appointment, or providing a free cellphone and cell service to stay connected to their case manager or treating provider. At the *community level*, examples include coordinating immunization drives or investing in the construction of safe housing alternatives.

PEER SPECIALISTS AND BEHAVIORAL HEALTH COACHES

Managed care organizations (MCOs) have also evolved in terms of making an array of care options available to consumers. The historical model of care in behavioral health consisted primarily of psychiatrists and psychotherapists or counselors seeing clients; however, MCOs have begun to support new options in care delivery to supplement traditional provider activity in light of the heightened demand for behavioral health services relative to the number of behavioral health professionals available (especially in rural and urban settings). These options include contracting with *peer specialists* and *behavioral health coaches*.

Peer specialists are individuals who are, themselves, in recovery from substance use, mental health condition, or a co-occurring disorder and serve as supports for clients involved in active care. Conversely, behavioral health coaches are generally paraprofessionals who may have some education or training in behavioral health but are generally not licensed providers. Peers and recovery coaches are often able to provide sufficient support and direction for consumers to reduce or even eliminate the need for formal treatment—this allows licensed providers to focus their efforts on those clients who are most in need of formal treatment.

POPULATION HEALTH PROGRAMS

Managed care organizations (MCOs) are also investing significantly in what is known as *population health programs,* which seek to improve behavioral health and addiction recovery outcomes. These are programs in which individuals can enroll by the hundreds, thousands, or even tens of thousands. While not a replacement for professional care, population health programs often consist of interventions that can supplement the provider's treatment efforts. For example, a population health program for substance use may provide screening, education, self-service strategies, and other resources that support an individual's overall recovery journey.

TECHNOLOGY AND TELEHEALTH

In recent years, MCOs have made considerable investments in technologies to support both providers and consumers. These technologies and their applications are vast and varied. For example, most MCOs have developed self-service portals for providers to manage common transactions in a self-service manner. Portals are also available for consumers to obtain resources and educational materials, take self-assessments, receive customer service, and obtain referrals. These organizations are also developing and partnering with technology innovators to provide individuals with digital therapies to support their treatment between sessions with counselors or other professionals.

Telehealth has emerged as a strong solution for consumers who previously found it difficult to access behavioral healthcare. Telebehavioral healthcare has exploded in popularity, helping overcome to geographic barriers to care, challenges in taking time away from work to attend appointments, or any number of other barriers to treatment. Furthermore, the types of behavioral healthcare that can be successfully delivered through the telehealth medium have expanded significantly. The COVID-19 pandemic had at least one silver lining; it sparked widespread use of tele-enabled care. While such care existed prior to COVID-19, its use skyrocketed in the midst of the pandemic and is not likely to diminish in popularity among both providers and consumers.

Today, counseling, psychiatry, substance abuse treatment (including MAT), eating disorder treatment, and school-based care can be successfully delivered through telebehavioral healthcare. MCOs are investing millions of dollars in supporting telehealth as a solution to the access challenges inherent in obtaining care in traditional brick-and-mortar office settings such as geographic distance, lack of transportation, and even stigma. Though much research is still required regarding the comparative effectiveness or office-based versus tele-enabled behavioral healthcare, this is a promising evolution in behavioral treatment.

CLINICAL CASE ILLUSTRATION AND DISCUSSION

CASE OF STEPHANIE

Stephanie, a 29-year-old female, was brought to the emergency department by the local police department. Stephanie was found in an abandoned warehouse screaming nonsensical words, was disheveled in her appearance, erratic in her behavior, and seemed to be responding to internal stimuli (i.e., hallucinations). The emergency room staff stabilized her and found that she had run away from her group home three days earlier. This was Stephanie's third runaway incident from foster care in the last year. She tested positive for the presence of methamphetamines in her system, and had been diagnosed with schizophrenia three years earlier. Stephanie was reported to be non-compliant with medications, and revealed auditory hallucinations telling her not to take her medications. The group home administrators stated they could not accept Stephanie back into the group home environment until she was fully stabilized and able to demonstrate long-term compliance with medications. The emergency room stabilized Stephanie with antipsychotic medication and held her in the emergency room's crisis unit until she was safe for transfer. She has remained stable in the crisis unit for 36 hours.

CASE DISCUSSION

The utilization reviewer at the facility contacted the MCO who manages Stephanie's benefits to request insurance coverage for acute inpatient level of care. The utilization manager at the MCO gathered all of the clinical information from the facility's utilization manager and then utilized the appropriate level of care guidelines based on level of care guidelines and medical necessity requirements. In this case, Stephanie was not at imminent risk of harming herself or someone else because she remained stable for thirty-six hours with no expressed desire or intent to harm herself or others, displayed no episodes of physical aggression, no longer appeared to be responding to internal stimuli (she also denied experiencing auditory hallucinations), was not at risk for life-threatening withdrawal from a substance, and was able to attend to self-care with the prompting of the crisis unit staff. The guidelines for acute inpatient look at symptoms in the most recent 24 hours to guide a decision about coverage for acute inpatient care. Although Stephanie had been stabilized, her social determinants of health assessment indicated that the she had a low probability of remaining stable without longer term intervention. Stephanie does not have a support system that is able to safely care for her. Although the group home management expressed a willingness to care for her, history has demonstrated that despite their best intentions, they are simply unable to ensure her stability based on a history of runaway behavior, use of illicit substances, and medication non-compliance.

After reviewing all of this clinical information, the utilization manager at the MCO stated that it appeared Stephanie did not meet the level of care criteria for acute inpatient services; however, she did appear to meet criteria for a longer-term residential treatment center (RTC) as her behaviors were chronic with a poor prognosis for safety without close monitoring by professionals. The utilization reviewer at the facility did not agree with this level of care recommendation and maintained the request for an acute inpatient level of care. Because the MCO utilization manager does not have the authority to issue a denial of insurance coverage for this level of care (only a licensed physician working for the MCO has this authority), Stephanie's case was sent to a physician for review. Before sending to the MCO physician for the review, the MCO utilization manager ensured that a residential treatment facility that could meet Stephanie's needs was available and willing to accept Stephanie for admission.

Upon receiving Stephanie's case, the MCO physician held a live conversation with the facility's attending physician who was assigned to Stephanie's care. The MCO physician shared with the facility attending physician that it did not appear Stephanie's case met level of care criteria for coverage of acute inpatient services and offered the attending physician the opportunity to provide any additional information that might alter that level of care assessment. The attending physician could offer no additional information. As a result, the MCO physician issued a denial of insurance coverage for acute inpatient treatment but reiterated that Stephanie's current clinical presentation meets criteria for residential treatment and offered to provide insurance coverage for this level of care. The facility attending physician agreed to transfer Stephanie to the residential treatment facility, which offers integrated co-occurring mental and substance use treatment. The MCO utilization manager shared this information with the facility reviewer and assisted with transfer to residential treatment after providing authorization for insurance coverage of that service.

An initial authorization for fourteen days of residential treatment was provided to allow for treatment and continued stabilization, intensive family/caregiver therapy, medication stabilization, relapse prevention, and discharge planning (which should always begin on admission). During the treatment episode, the MCO utilization manager worked with the residential treatment facility staff to coordinate outpatient follow-up care for when Stephanie is ready to discharge, assisted in coordinating with family and/or guardians in the development of a discharge plan of care, worked to fill any gaps or care coordination needs for additional mental health, substance use, and medical issues, and worked to mitigate social determinants of health that could prevent or place at risk Stephanie's ongoing stability.

A follow-up review was scheduled with the residential treatment staff after fourteen days in order to review Stephanie's condition at that time and determine if further treatment at that level of care could be covered by her insurance benefit. Stephanie continued to show improvement and ongoing stability. After two months of residential treatment level of care, the group home administrators were willing to allow her to return with the condition that Stephanie engage in weekly outpatient individual and group counseling sessions as well as regular medication management visits with a psychiatrist. Because routine outpatient services do not require prior authorization, no additional reviews were be required by the MCO utilization reviewer once Stephanie transitioned from the residential treatment setting into the outpatient level of care.

CHAPTER SUMMARY

A survey of the arena of managed behavioral healthcare has been conducted throughout this chapter. Although a special emphasis has been placed on the concept of level of care guidelines for admission and continuing stay criteria, an attempt has been made to provide this information in the more robust context of the relationship between healthcare providers and managed care entities. It is important not only to understand level of care guidelines and medical necessity criteria, but also the history and context in which they arose, limitations of their use, and the manner in which they help address bias and variation in clinical practice. Furthermore, it is important for counselors to understand how the healthcare and managed care industries are working to evolve the manner in which they partner together to address the needs of the behavioral health and addictions treatment needs of the consumer. While some people may hold on to outdated views of the relationship between MCOs and providers, the reality is that the two entities are advancing behavioral healthcare and addictions treatment outcomes by forming a collaborative partnership. Regardless of this progression, however, it is beneficial to understand the important role that level of care guidelines play. Generally developed by independent entities that have allegiances to the consumers they serve rather than to MCOs or providers, these guidelines are informed by research and professional best practices and implemented with the goal of creating effective and efficient healthcare. They serve to minimize bias in their users and reduce practice variations that can occur across disciplines, regions, and paradigms. Adopting such guidelines in a context in which all parties are working toward the best health outcomes keeps individuals who need behavioral health and addiction services in the spotlight of concern while all others remain in the appropriate role of supporting cast.

DISCUSSION QUESTIONS

1. What are some of the factors that led to the emergence of managed care? Is there still a role for managed care to play today?

2. With the emergence of tele-enabled care and digital therapies, what impacts do you anticipate for traditional levels of care (e.g., outpatient, residential, inpatient)? How do you envision behavioral healthcare delivery being impacted (positively or negatively) as a result?

3. What are the costs and benefits of relying of level of care guidelines? In what ways do you believe care delivery would be different if such guidelines did not exist?

4. As you consider the various sets of guidelines and criteria that exist, what factors do you believe should determine which should be adopted? Is there a better approach that could be used to justify level of care placement that would also reduce bias and practice variations?

5. If you were establishing a private practice today and planned to accept consumers covered by insurance, in what ways might you work with insurance companies that would differ than if you were in private practice 40 years ago?

REFERENCES

American Academy of Child & Adolescent Psychiatry. (2020, December 15). *AACAP &AACP Partner to unify CALOCUS and CASII assessment instruments.* https://www.aacap.org/AACAP/Press/Press_Releases/2020/AACAP-AACP-Partner-CALOCUS-CASII-Assessment-Instruments.aspx

American Association of Community Psychiatrists. (2009, March 20). *LOCUS Level of Care Utilization System for Psychiatric and Addiction Services*, Adult Version 2010. https://cchealth.org/mentalhealth/pdf/LOCUS.pdf

American Association of Community Psychiatry. (n.d.). *Level of care utilization system for psychiatric and addiction services.* Retrieved February 21, 2021, from https://www.communitypsychiatry.org/keystone-programs/locus

American Society of Addiction Medicine. (n.d.-a.). *ASAM Criteria.* Retrieved February 20, 2021, from https://www.asam.org/asam-criteria/about-the-asam-criteria

American Society of Addiction Medicine. (n.d.-b). *The six dimensions of multidimensional assessment.* Retrieved March 8, 2022, from https://www.asam.org/asam-criteria/about-the-asam-criteria

American Society of Addiction Medicine. (n.d.-c.). *About The ASAM Criteria.* Retrieved March 8, 2022, from https://www.asam.org/asam-criteria/about-the-asam-criteria

Centers for Disease Control and Prevention. (2021, September 30). *Social determinants of health: Know what affects health.* https://www.cdc.gov/socialdeterminants/index.htm

Change Healthcare. (n.d.-a.). *InterQual Behavioral Health Criteria.* Retrieved February 20, 2021, from https://www.changehealthcare.com/solutions/clinical-decision-support/interqual/behavioral-health-criteria

Change Healthcare. (n.d.-b.). *InterQual.* Retrieved February 13, 2022, from https://www.changehealthcare.com/clinical-decision-support/interqual

CMS.gov. (2021, December 1). *Emergency Medical Treatment & Labor Act (EMTALA).* https://www.cms.gov/Regulations-and-Guidance/Legislation/EMTALA

Healthinsurance.org (2022). *What is managed care?* https://www.healthinsurance.org/glossary/managed-care/

Healthy People 2030. (n.d.). *Social determinants of health.* Retrieved February 13, 2022, from https://health.gov/healthypeople/objectives-and-data/social-determinants-health

Kongstvedt, P. R. (2013). *Essentials of managed health care* (6th ed.). Jones & Bartlett Learning. Managed care | medicaid. (n.d.). Medicaid.gov. Retrieved March 1, 2021, from https://www.medicaid.gov/medicaid/managed-care/index.html

MCG Health. (n.d.). *Industry-leading evidence-based care guidelines.* Retrieved February 21, 2021, from https://www.mcg.com/care-guidelines/care-guidelines/

Medicaid.gov. (n.d.). *Managed care.* Retrieved February 13, 2022, from https://www.medicaid.gov/medicaid/managed-care/index.html

Mee-Lee, D., Shulman, G. D., Gastfriend, D. R., & Miller, M. M. (Eds.). (2013). *The ASAM Criteria: Treatment criteria for addictive, substance-related, and co-occurring conditions* (3rd ed.). The Change Companies.

Mitus, J. A. (2008). The birth of InterQual: Evidence-based decision support criteria that helped change healthcare. *Professional Case Management, 13*(4), 228–223. https://doi.org/10.1097/01.PCAMA.0000327413.01849.04

National Center for Complementary and Integrative Health. (2021). *Whole person health: What you need to know.* https://www.nccih.nih.gov/health/whole-person-health-what-you-need-to-know

CHAPTER 6

TREATMENT ENGAGEMENT, THERAPEUTIC STRATEGIES, AND RECOVERY MODELS FOR CO-OCCURRING DISORDERS

REGINA R. MORO AND REGINALD W. HOLT

LEARNING OBJECTIVES

After reading this chapter, you will be able to:
- Explain the transtheoretical model of change, including the individual stages of change within this model.
- Identify common counseling skills associated with motivational interviewing.
- Describe three theoretical models for the treatment of co-occurring disorders.
- Recognize signs of potential relapse among clients.
- Evaluate a client's recovery maintenance plan.

INTRODUCTION

Engaging clients in the treatment process is a necessary component for success, although it can be a complex process—especially when working with clients who have a mental disorder(s) that co-occurs with a substance use disorder(s). This chapter begins by exploring the therapeutic relationship and common ingredients for success. Then readers will be introduced to the transtheoretical model (TTM) of change, which provides a model to understand what the change process looks like for clients; it also helps counselors consider where clients may be starting at and how to engage with them there. Following the introduction of TTM, motivational interviewing (MI) is then presented to offer counselors key MI skills designed to enhance a client's motivation to change. An overview of other theoretical models will also be provided so counselors can consider how they may integrate theory into their clinical work with clients who have co-occurring disorders (CODs). The chapter also explores the concepts of relapse and recovery maintenance. The overall focus of this chapter is on engaging clients in the treatment process, and how to work with clients once they are actively involved. Legal and ethical considerations for this work are examined, specifically in relation to clients who are mandated to treatment and/or associated with the criminal legal system.

BUILDING SUCCESSFUL RELATIONSHIPS

Significant research over time has highlighted that the strength of the therapeutic relationship between the client and counselor affects how beneficial the counseling process will be (i.e., effective client outcomes; Sparks et al., 2008; Young, 2013). The stronger the relationship, the stronger the outcomes. Research has also highlighted that the client's views about the relationship strength also impact their outcomes (Sparks et al., 2008). Young (2013) outlined several unique characteristics of therapeutic relationships that distinguish these from other relationships in clients' lives:

- There is a mutual liking—or at least respect.
- The purpose of the relationship is the resolution of the client's issues.
- There is a sense of teamwork as both helper and client work toward a mutually agreed-upon goal.
- Safety and trust are established, allowing honest disclosure by the client and feedback from the helper. There is a contract specifying what will be disclosed to others outside of the relationship.
- There is an agreement about compensation for the helper.
- There is an understanding that the relationship is confined to the counseling sessions and does not overlap into the participants' personal lives.
- As a contractual relationship, the relationship can be terminated at any time. (pp. 55–56).

Fostering a strong relationship with clients is crucial for success in the therapeutic process. Dr. Carl Rogers (1957) articulated what he described as the necessary and sufficient core conditions for counseling that involve six factors associated with stimulating growth and producing beneficial outcomes for the client. Three of the six conditions are specific to the counselor, who must: (a) be congruent, (b) have unconditional positive regard for the client, and (c) have an empathic understanding of the client. In addition, the client, who is in a state of incongruence, must experience the empathy and perceive the unconditional positive regard from the counselor with whom they have made psychological contact. These three counselor factors are crucial to developing a strong relationship and helping the client. Other behaviors that foster strong relationships include: nonverbal behavior (open posture, conveying warmth); appropriate self-disclosure; limiting distractions; and reducing the hierarchy in the relationship (Young, 2013). There are many detailed skills to develop and refine the therapeutic relationship, and counselors are encouraged to consider their strengths when forming relationships with clients as well as their areas for growth regarding client relationship building.

THE TRANSTHEORETICAL MODEL: ASSESSING THE STAGES OF CHANGE

The TTM, sometimes referred to as the stages of change model, was first developed by Prochaska and DiClemente in the early 1980s as a way to understand behavior change across the many existing theoretical frameworks. The model posits that there are commonalities among theories with how the process of change occurs for clients, despite differences in the theoretical concepts and techniques/interventions used. Change occurs in six distinct stages, beginning with precontemplation and ending with termination (Prochaska & Velicer, 1997). In addition, the model highlights specific processes used by clients to enact change throughout the stages. According to the TTM, the six stages of change are: (a) precontemplation, (b) contemplation, (c) preparation, (d) action, (e) maintenance, and (f) termination (Prochaska & DiClemente, 1983; Prochaska & Velicer, 1997). The stages of changes can be seen in Figure 6.1, and example statements a counselor may hear from a client in each stage are listed in Table 6.1.

When a person is not intending to make behavioral changes in the near future, they are in the first stage known as *precontemplation*. The person's lack of having a plan for change is due to a number of reasons, unique to each individual. For example, they may be unable to see the reasons a change might be beneficial, or they might be disheartened from previous attempts at changing that were not successful. Individuals in precontemplation have traditionally been defined as "resistant or unmotivated" (Prochaska & Velicer, 1997, p. 39).

Contemplation is the second stage of change. Individuals in this stage are considering a change in the near future but are vacillating between whether or not to enact the change. Contemplation involves examining the pros of changing as well as honoring the cons of the change

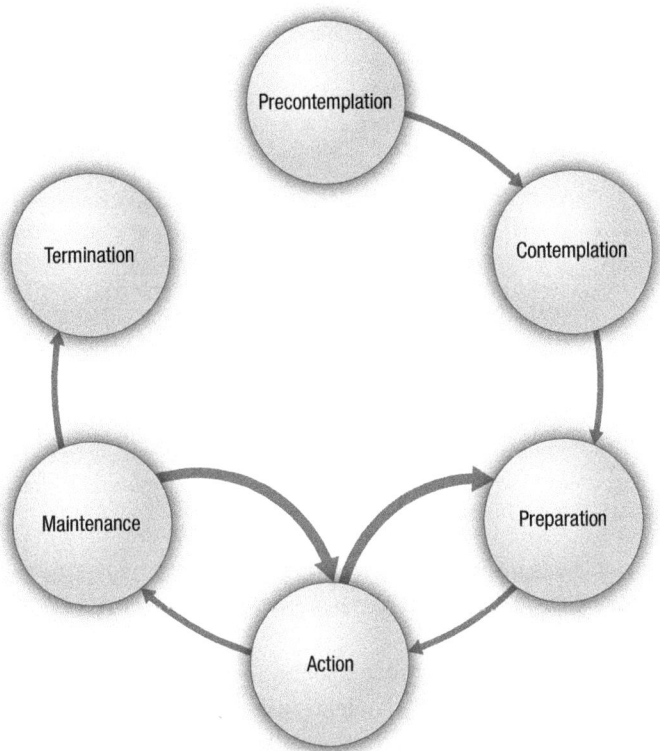

FIGURE 6.1 Stages of Change.
Note: The dark arrows inside the circle signify the possibility of relapse, which can occur in the action or maintenance stages.
Source: Adapted from Prochaska, J. O., & Velicer, W. F. (1997). The transtheoretical model of health behavior change. *American Journal of Health Promotion, 12*(1), 38–48, p. 39.

TABLE 6.1 **Example Client Statements by Corresponding Stage of Change**

STAGE OF CHANGE	EXAMPLE CLIENT QUOTE
Precontemplation	"I do not have a problem with my (insert behavior). I'm fine." "I don't experience any issues because of my (insert behavior). No one complains about it, and I'm doing great." "I tried to stop (insert behavior) before, a couple of different times. It's hopeless, I'll always be this way so it's just not worth the hassle."
Contemplation	"I'm starting to wonder if maybe I have a problem with (insert behavior). The more I think about it, I sometimes wonder if I would be better off if I stopped, but it just seems so hard." "I want to stop (insert behavior), but I just don't know how. There are so many reasons that I know it's bad for me, but I also enjoy some things about it—like being with friends. What would I do if I can't do that?!"
Preparation	"I know I want to change (insert behavior). I actually went to the bookstore and found a book describing steps I could take to stop." "I am here for counseling because I know I need to stop (insert behavior), but I just don't know how."
Action	"I have not engaged in (insert behavior) for 3 months, and I am feeling more confident every day!" "I am active in my recovery plan. I'm using my coping skills, and I have not engaged in (insert behavior) in 4 months. I am feeling like the consistency is paying off!"
Maintenance	"I have been active in my recovery from (insert behavior) for 8 months now. I am finding I do not need to think about my coping skills as much anymore; they have become integrated into who I am." "It has been 3 years since I have (insert behavior), and I am consistently working my plan. I find my urge to (insert behavior) increases in periods of stress, so I try to anticipate those beforehand in order to be prepared."
Termination	"It has been a significant amount of time since I have engaged in (insert behavior). Plus, I haven't been tempted to (insert behavior) for a very long time. I have zero desire to go back to that behavior, so it is not even an option for me now!"

Source: Created with information from Prochaska, J. O., & Velicer, W. F. (1997). The transtheoretical model of health behavior change. *American Journal of Health Promotion, 12*(1), 38–48, p. 39.

(Prochaska & Velicer, 1997), which can produce ambivalence about change. Ambivalence (which is a normal part of change) is defined as "simultaneously wanting and not wanting something, or wanting both of two incompatible things" (Miller & Rollnick, 2013, p. 6). This is characterized by feeling pulled in two directions, resulting in being immobilized or stuck.

The third stage of change is *preparation*. In this stage an individual is actively planning for a change in the immediate future. In the preparation stage, individuals have resolved the ambivalence they experienced in the contemplation stage, and have decided that the pros of changing outweigh the cons of not changing. This stage involves intentionally planning for the change, which includes analyzing what supports (e.g., people, groups, books) are needed for change to occur. Individuals in this stage of change appear motivated and are willing participants in the process.

Action is the fourth stage of change. This stage is characterized by overt changes in behavior. Prochaska and Velicer (1997) do provide context about what type of change "counts" as action steps. Small changes that are done early to help prepare an individual for a larger change would be in the preparation stage. The action stage is characterized by more large-scale behavioral changes that are in line with the overall target of change. An example would be a client who is planning to stop drinking alcohol. A behavioral change in the preparation stage may be removing all alcohol from their house, which is important, but would not meet the threshold to move someone into action. However, a behavioral change in the action stage would be the individual abstaining from alcohol in all situations for a few months. In another example, if the client was considering a reduction in the amount of alcohol they consumed (but not completely abstaining), a consistent change over a sustained period in which they drank no more than their established limit would be in the action stage. This second example is offered to highlight how important it is to recognize the individual goals of clients, and in doing so, will inform the counselor's understanding of their clients' movement through the various stages.

The fifth stage of change is *maintenance*. This stage is characterized by the individual consistently working to prevent relapsing back to the undesired behavior. Prochaska and Velicer (1997) informed this stage can last anywhere from 6 months to 5 years, which is dependent on the individual. People in this stage have built up confidence that they are able to maintain their desired behavioral change, and that confidence grows the more their change is sustained.

The final stage of change is *termination*. This stage is when "individuals have zero temptation and 100% self-efficacy" (Prochaska & Velicer, 1997, p. 39). When in the termination stage, the individual has removed the old behavior as an option for them entirely; they will not return to that behavior no matter what they experience. Prochaska (2008) highlighted that reaching termination might not be a realistic goal for all clients, so counselors may instead place the focus on the client sustaining the changes made (i.e., the maintenance stage).

The early writing of the model suggested *relapse* was a distinct stage of change. However, Prochaska and Velicer (1997) clarified that relapse is not a stage of change, but rather it is a "form of regression, which is a return to an earlier stage" (p. 39). Further clarifying this, Prochaska and Velicer pointed out that relapse may occur in either the action or maintenance stage of change.

While the stages of change are a large part of the TTM, they do not encompass the entirety of the model. A large part of the initial work of Prochaska and DiClemente (1982) was in analyzing existing models of therapy to discover similarities in how change is produced for clients. This work resulted in the identification of 10 central processes that facilitate change. The 10 processes are: (a) consciousness raising, (b) dramatic relief, (c) self-evaluation, (d) environmental re-evaluation, (e) self-liberation, (f) social liberation, (g) counterconditioning, (h) stimulus control, (i) contingency management, and (j) helping relationships (Prochaska & Velicer, 1997). Table 6.2 provides more details for each of these processes.

The early work of Prochaska and DiClemente (1982, 1983) provided a strong foundation for understanding the change process individuals go through when seeking to make a behavioral change. Research has consistently found support for the TTM as a framework for understanding behavioral change management (Hashemzadeh et al., 2019). It offers a useful framework for professional counselors, regardless of their chosen theoretical orientation, to conceptualize and work with clients on behavioral change. For counselors working with clients who have CODs, the stages of change model provides a useful blueprint when considering where their clients are in regard to their multiple disorders. Moreover, because clients with CODs may have one or more mental disorder(s) as well as one or more substance use disorder(s), it is important for counselors

TABLE 6.2 **Processes of Change From the Transtheoretical Model of Change**

PROCESS OF CHANGE	DESCRIPTION
Consciousness raising	Increasing client awareness about the precipitating events of the identified problem behavior, how the behavior has been maintained over time, and what may be needed for it to be resolved.
Dramatic relief	Processing of emotions connected to the problem behavior in order to reduce the impact of the unprocessed emotions.
Self-re-evaluation	Internal reflection of the client to examine their self-image and redefine their personal beliefs related to self.
Environmental re-evaluation	An examination of how the identified problem behavior has an impact on different systems and relationships the client is a part of (e.g., family, school, work, friendships).
Self-liberation	The personal belief that change is possible, and committing (and recommitting) to that change process.
Social liberation	Involves increasing opportunities in which systems clients are involved, and may involve advocacy efforts for clients from marginalized communities and without social support structures.
Counterconditioning	Training oneself in alternative behaviors that produce helpful effects.
Stimulus control	Involves removing temptations and inserting alternatives to help the client cope.
Contingency management	Provides consequences or rewards for certain behavioral changes.
Helping relationships	Social and professional supports who offer warmth, trust, acceptance, and validation for the client throughout the change process.

Source: From Prochaska, J. O., & Velicer, W. F. (1997). The transtheoretical model of health behavior change. *American Journal of Health Promotion, 12*(1), 38–48, p. 39.

to understand that clients may be at one stage for one disorder yet be at another stage for another problem. Due to this, each identified problem and its corresponding stage of change should be assessed and addressed accordingly. For more information and considerations, refer to the case illustration and discussion at the end of this chapter.

MOTIVATIONAL INTERVIEWING/MOTIVATIONAL ENHANCEMENT THERAPY

MI emerged in response to one of the founders, Dr. William R. Miller, engaging in a training process with clinical psychologists in Norway in 1982 (Miller & Moyers, 2017). Dr. Miller found that the questions asked by the psychologists about his own unique style of counseling highlighted his personal way of being with clients that ultimately empowered them (Miller & Moyers, 2017). This important exchange led Dr. Miller to contemplate this way of being, which resulted in a publication articulating this therapeutic approach in 1983.

MI is defined as "a person-centered counseling style for addressing the common problem of ambivalence about change" (Miller & Rollnick, 2013, p. 21). Ambivalence is feeling two opposing ways about something, which results in feeling stuck or indecisive. The work of MI is to help resolve feelings of ambivalence, and to help increase motivation for changing problematic behaviors.

Foundational to MI is the nondirective, client-centered approach of Dr. Carl Rogers, which is reflected in the underlying *spirit* of MI. The spirit of MI is a way of approaching the work of engaging clients, which distinguishes MI from being only a collection of techniques and interventions (Miller & Moyers, 2017). Miller and Rollnick (2013) articulated the four components of the spirit: (a) partnership, (b) acceptance, (c) evocation, and (d) compassion. Each component is explained in Figure 6.2. Although the spirit is considered its foundation, there are unique skills used in MI. According to Miller and Moyers (2017), a "defining difference of MI from nondirective counseling is the interviewer's intentional and strategic use of questions, reflections, affirmations, and summaries to strengthen the client's own motivations for change" (p. 758).

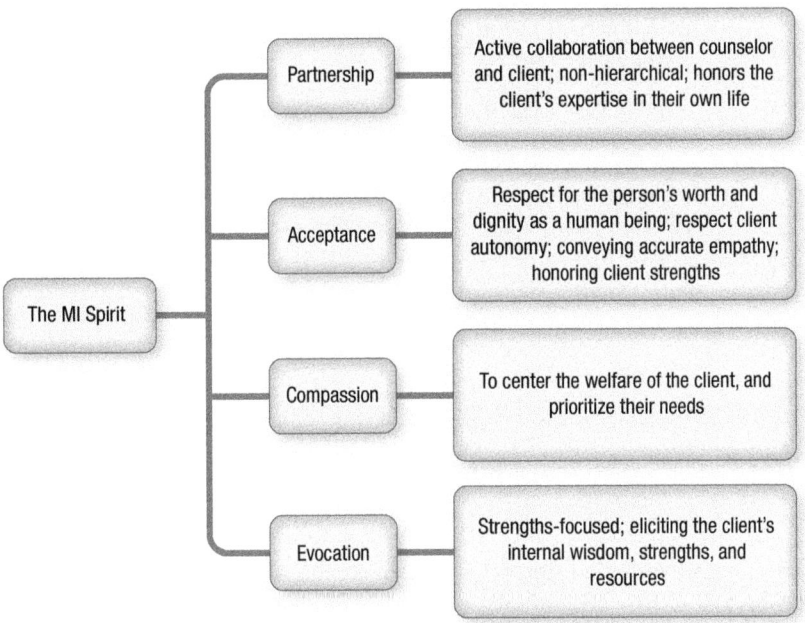

FIGURE 6.2 The Spirit of Motivational Interviewing.
Source: Created with information from Miller, W. R., & Rollnick, S. (2013). *Motivational interviewing: Helping people change.* Guilford.

Counselors who embody the spirit of MI, which is a continual and ongoing process, can intentionally use specific skills to discuss the client's behavior and ambivalence surrounding change. The fundamental counselor interaction techniques used in the MI approach are illustrated in OARS (see Table 6.3), an acronym that counselors can use to easily remember the four key skills:

TABLE 6.3 **OARS Tools**

MI SKILL	DEFINITION	EXAMPLE
Open-ended questions	A question that cannot be answered with a "yes" or "no" response. These allow more freedom on behalf of the person answering to respond however they desire.	"What brings you to counseling?" "How would you describe the problem you are experiencing?"
Affirmations	Responses that convey the counselor has noticed and acknowledged something positive about the client.	"You worked really hard on that resume and cover letter for that job application!" "You are putting in a lot of work here in counseling, and this is not easy!"
Reflections	Accurate reflections are listening to the client's storying, and then conveying your understanding and accurate empathy back to the client so they can understand it.	"You're feeling sad and depressed about this situation." "You have had a lot going on in your life these past few days."
Summaries	Provide an overall synthesis of what the client has said. Conveys understanding of multiple aspects of a client's story.	"This experience at work was frustrating for you. Not only did you get passed over for the promotion, this reminded you of the time a similar situation happened in your old job. In addition, this work stress is worsened because of the added pressure you feel with your partner going back to school in a few months. It is a lot to manage, and you are struggling to use the coping skills you have worked so hard on developing."

Source: Created with information from Miller, W. R., & Rollnick, S. (2013). *Motivational interviewing: Helping people change.* Guilford.

Researchers consistently find support for MI in comparison with other counseling interventions (Lundahl et al., 2010). For counselors working with clients who are focused on changing behaviors, there are numerous reasons an MI approach should be adopted. Some of the reasons are:

- MI can take less time to produce equal effects.
- MI is applicable to a wide range of behaviors, not only addiction.
- MI increases client's engagement in treatment.
- MI works for individuals along a spectrum of problem severity, from mild to more severe. (Lundahl et al., 2010, p. 152)

While the phrase MI has been used here, counselors interested in learning more may see MI listed as motivational enhancement therapy (MET). MET was first articulated by Miller et al. (1995) and is referred to as "MI-plus," which, in addition to embodying the spirit of MI, includes specific feedback to the client about the problem behavior they are describing (Lundahl et al., 2010). This feedback can be from any initial screenings or assessments that are done with clients that provide insight into the behavior and consequences it may have on the client's physical and/or psychological health (Miller et al., 1995). A manualized version of MET consisting of four treatment session agendas, titled *Motivational Enhancement Therapy Manual: A Clinical Research Guide for Therapists Treating Individuals with Alcohol Abuse and Dependence* (Miller et al.,1995), is reprinted and available in the public domain by the National Institute on Alcohol Abuse and Alcoholism. Readers interested in learning more about MI are also referred to the website, motivationalinterviewing.org, which offers detailed information such as training opportunities and reading resources.

The transtheoretical model of change and MI were both developed simultaneously, yet independently, by researchers. Despite this development, it has become evident how important these two models are to each other. The stages of change provide context for where a client may be, and MI provides a way of being with clients and the specific skills for counselors to use that ultimately empowers their clients to progress through the stages of change.

THEORETICAL APPROACHES TO TREATING CO-OCCURRING DISORDERS

The transtheoretical stages of change and MI models are two ways of working with clients that can be applied to other theoretical approaches. There is an abundance of theories to explain client distress and how to inform the work of counseling; however, a select few of the theoretical approaches that counselors can use to approach their work with CODs are examined here.

COGNITIVE BEHAVIORAL THEORIES

Cognitive behavioral theories are common in treating addiction and CODs. These theories are appealing to clinicians because there are specific skills and strategies associated with them, which are backed by strong research support. While cognitive behavioral therapy (CBT) is a separate and distinct treatment approach, it is also used as an umbrella term with other theories being classified as such. The focus of cognitive behavioral treatment is on challenging maladaptive cognitions that cause distress through the use of a variety of techniques (e.g., emotive, cognitive, behavioral; Corey, 2017). Cognitive therapy (CT), rational emotive behavior therapy (REBT), strengths-based CBT, dialectical behavior therapy (DBT), and acceptance and commitment therapy (ACT) are among the many approaches under the CBT umbrella.

CT was pioneered by Dr. Aaron Beck. According to Beck and Weishaar (2014), the foundation of CT is the understanding that all individuals engage in continuous information processing for survival purposes. The theory posits that people experience distress due to errors in how they process information, and in order to gain relief from the distress, they need to adjust how information is processed in their brain. Techniques involve challenging maladaptive thoughts as well as implementing behavioral techniques like assertiveness training, role playing, and exposure therapy (Beck & Weishaar, 2014).

DBT was developed by Dr. Marsha Linehan as a treatment model for individuals diagnosed with borderline personality disorder who were chronically suicidal (Corey, 2017). According to

Linehan (2015), individuals experience psychological distress due to difficulties regulating emotions and behavior. The treatment is a structured, predictable process involving skills training in four domains: (a) mindfulness, (b) interpersonal effectiveness, (c) emotional regulation, and (d) distress tolerance. Each of these domains has specific skills that are taught to clients, which they subsequently practice between sessions. The skills training of DBT may be in combination with individual/group counseling, or it may be used as a stand-alone approach.

ACT was developed by Dr. Steven Hayes in the mid 1980s. Hayes et al. (2006) describe the foundation of ACT as an understanding that distress emerges and is reinforced by the way language and thought interact in an individual's brain, which consequently creates an inflexible way of being. This inflexibility appears in a variety of ways such as an individual having weak self-knowledge, lack of values clarity, and being particularly inactive or unable to persist. The goal of ACT, therefore, is to increase psychological flexibility which is attained by the six core ACT processes: (a) acceptance, (b) cognitive defusion, (d) present moment contact, (e) self as context, (f) living a values-consistent life, and (g) committed action (Hayes et al., 2006). ACT is process-based as opposed to outcome-based, which is best illustrated by Willets (2022) who stated, "the point of ACT is not to feel better, but to better feel" (p. 7).

HUMANISTIC THEORIES

Person-centered counseling theory, Gestalt theory, and existentialism are the three main theories classified as humanistic (Fitch et al., 2001). These theoretical approaches, which are focused on the counselor/client relationship, have an underlying belief that human nature is generally positive and motivated for self-actualization (Corey, 2017). Because many counselors approach their work from an existential viewpoint, some argue it is more of a philosophy than a theory (Fitch et al., 2001); therefore, attention will be placed on person-centered and Gestalt theories.

Person-centered counseling, pioneered by Dr. Carl Rogers, was introduced earlier in this chapter due to Rogers's profound understanding of the power of the therapeutic relationship. A more detailed picture of Rogers's work is now offered. Rogers's (1957) model details the six necessary and sufficient conditions for change to occur in the therapeutic relationship:

1. Two persons are in psychological contact.
2. The first person, whom we shall term the client, is in a state of incongruence, being vulnerable or anxious.
3. The second person, whom we shall term the therapist, is congruent or integrated in the relationship.
4. The therapist experiences unconditional positive regard for the client.
5. The therapist experiences an empathic understanding of the client's internal frame of reference and endeavors to communicate this experience to the client.
6. The communication to the client of the therapist's empathic understanding and unconditional positive regard is to a minimal degree achieved. (p. 96)

The person-centered model of counseling does not have specific techniques/interventions; the sole mechanism for change rests on the six necessary and sufficient conditions (Corey, 2017). The identification of the six core conditions occurred from Rogers's dedication to the research process, transcribing and analyzing counseling sessions to discover what elements were particularly effective for client change (Corey, 2017; Miller & Moyers, 2017). In Corey's (2017) words, "He literally opened the field to research" (p. 191). It is hard to imagine the profession today without the unique contributions of Dr. Carl Rogers.

Gestalt therapy, developed by Dr. Fritz Perls, is a highly experiential process. Although it is outside the parameters of this chapter to describe it in detail, Gestalt therapy has deep philosophical beliefs rooted in field theory (Corey, 2017). In simple terms, field theory takes into account the context of an individual's environment, which is understood to influence the individual. The basic premise of Gestalt therapy is that individuals are affected by their environments, and they continuously make efforts to self-regulate their experiences—which may or may not be beneficial to them (Corey, 2017). Prior to therapy, individuals are often acting outside of their conscious awareness to manage their experiences, and the goals of Gestalt therapy include increasing awareness to help clients be more consciously engaged in their lives and take responsibility for their actions. A unique contribution of Gestalt therapy is the use of experiential techniques that are aimed at exploring the client's experiences. Common techniques include but are not limited to the empty chair, exaggeration, and making the rounds (see Corey, 2017 for more details).

This section primarily focused on cognitive behavioral therapeutic approaches and humanistic theories, which are certainly not meant to be an exhaustive list of all models of counseling and psychotherapy that are available when working with clients with CODs. These were merely offered to highlight how different theories understand human behavior and inform the therapeutic process. Counselors are encouraged to learn more about their chosen theory/approach and become experts on the process of counseling from their identified theoretical orientation.

RECOGNIZING AND ADDRESSING INDICATORS OF RELAPSE

Relapse was introduced earlier in this chapter to explain what happens when someone returns to a previous stage of change. The discussion of relapse is expanded here so counselors can consider how to help clients prevent relapse as well as plan for what happens if/when a relapse occurs. It is important for both counselors and clients to recognize that relapse is more the rule than the exception in addiction and COD treatment. This is not meant to be a pessimistic or deterministic stance suggesting that all clients will relapse, but rather more of a reality highlighting the nature of addiction being a chronically relapsing disorder.

Relapse is understood as a return to the problem behavior following a period in time in which the individual did not engage in the behavior (or did so to an extent that it was not problematic). However, what constitutes a relapse is highly variable to the unique individual. Importantly, counselors should distinguish a lapse or "slip" (momentary return to the behavior) from a relapse (prolonged, more sustained engagement in the behavior). Numerous models of relapse prevention (RP) planning exist, notably the RP model by Dr. Alan Marlatt (see Larimer et al., 1999) and the Cenaps model by Dr. Terence Gorski (2012). Donovan (2005) explained the goals of RP strategies as being twofold:

> *To prevent an initial lapse back to drinking, drug use, or other addictive behavior and to prevent initial lapse, if it does occur, from becoming more serious and prolonged by minimizing the physical, psychological, and social consequences of the return to use. (p. 5)*

Although these goals are focused on addictive behaviors, they can also be applied to mental health conditions where relapse is considered to be a return of active symptoms, problematic behaviors, and so forth.

Although proper RP planning focuses on identifying the unique individual factors that put each client at risk for returning to the behavior, there are common causes for relapse. Doweiko (2012) identified the following causes for relapse as well as the percentage of relapses that each cause accounts for:

1. Negative emotional states = 35%
2. Peer pressure = 20%
3. Interpersonal conflict = 16%
4. Craving for substance = 9%
5. Testing personal control (e.g., "I can have just one this time") = 5%
6. Negative physical states (i.e., illness, injury) = 3%

Taking into account these causes, counselors can help clients prevent relapse by asking questions about each of the six domains. For example, a counselor can discuss how their client plans to cope with negative emotional states (e.g., "What coping skills have you used in the past that helped when you started feeling angry?"). This may involve using one of the emotional regulation skills learned during DBT skills training, or it could include practicing mindfulness to cope with the emotional distress. The counselor's work here is to help prepare a client to navigate common stressors that arise without relying on the addictive behavior as a coping strategy. This will more than likely take practice for the client to integrate these skills into their everyday life; however, with time and consistency they will ideally replace harmful strategies with a more effective way of being.

RECOVERY MAINTENANCE: CONSOLIDATING GAINS AND SUSTAINING CHANGE

The dictionary defines recovery as "a return to a normal state of health, mind, or strength" (Oxford Languages, n.d.). Although this definition provides some understanding of its meaning, it is quite vague and limited when considering how to apply the concept of recovery to an individual's unique experience. A number of questions about what constitutes recovery are highlighted by White (2007):

- What are the essential, defining ingredients of the recovery process?
- Is recovery a time-limited event or a long-term process?
- Does recovery from a substance use disorder require complete and enduring abstinence?
- Does recovery require abstinence from, or a deceleration of, *all* psychoactive drug use?
- Does the use of prescribed psychoactive drugs disqualify one from the status of recovery?
- Is recovery something more than the elimination or deceleration of [alcohol or drug] problems from an otherwise unchanged life?
- Is recovery an all-or-none proposition or, as with other health conditions, something that can be achieved in degrees?
- Must recovery be conscious, voluntary, and self-managed?
- What are the temporal benchmarks of recovery? (pp. 231–235)

These questions are focused on the addictive cycle; however, these can be expanded to other disorders as well to capture how a client understands recovery in light of their COD diagnosis. Considering these questions offers a way for clients to examine their own internal understanding of recovery, which provides direction for both the client and the counselor as the treatment plan is being developed.

As clients move through their own recovery process, counselors need to proactively check in with clients about what is working and what is not working. A client may define recovery for themselves as solely maintaining abstinence from an addictive substance/behavior, and if this is their definition, the counselor should continually check in with the client regarding the effectiveness of RP strategies that were identified in previous sessions. And, if a client has a broader definition of recovery—one that means achieving recovery results in a significant change in their ability to effectively relate to family members and friends—the counselor should explore this recovery goal with the client and offer applicable services and resources as needed. Ultimately, the objective is to not only help clients sustain the changes they have made, but to also examine additional changes that may be necessary going forward. Counselors provide an important function when they offer ongoing support to clients who are traveling on the road to recovery. This road—one that is not always predictable, linear, or conclusive—is best exemplified by the saying, *"Recovery is a journey, not a destination."*

LEGAL AND ETHICAL CONSIDERATIONS

Working with all clients raises numerous legal and ethical considerations. The focus of this chapter has been on engaging clients in the therapeutic process and enacting change. The specific legal and ethical considerations to be reviewed focus on working with mandated clients, often from the criminal legal system, and how counselors can navigate the complexity of this work.

MANDATED CLIENTS

Mandated clients are those who are required to complete treatment by some external stakeholder. Although this may include clients who are issued a mandatory referral from an employer to attend an evaluation with an Employee Assistance Program (EAP) counselor due to a work-performance issue (e.g., violence in the workplace) or a work-related policy violation (e.g., positive result on a drug screening test), this section primarily focuses on those clients who are mandated to counseling by the criminal legal system. This type of mandated counseling may be as a result of a jail diversion program, part of a criminal sentence, or a condition of parole or probation. Working with mandated clients can elicit strong feelings from counselors, so it is important to be grounded in professional ethics, have awareness of and challenge all biases, strive to achieve multicultural competence, and honor the legal requirements related to working with this population.

There are certain ethical code items that are specifically relevant to working with mandated clients. In particular, the code of ethics from the American Counseling Association (ACA) states:

> *Counselors discuss the required limitations to confidentiality when working with clients who have been mandated for counseling services. Counselors also explain what type of information and with whom that information is shared prior to the beginning of counseling. The client may choose to refuse services. In this case, counselors will, to the best of their ability, discuss with the client the potential consequences of refusing counseling services. (A.2.e., 2014, p. 4)*

Central to this ethics code is that counselors must provide appropriate information about what the agreement will look like for the counselor to report to an external party. The ethical principle of autonomy, that clients have a "right to control the direction of one's life," is reflected in this item (ACA, 2014, p. 3). In addition, ACA ethics code B.2.e. requires that counselors make efforts to only disclose the minimal amount of information needed when disclosure is required. For example, if a counselor needs to report counseling involvement to a probation and parole (P&P)

officer, the counselor needs to have a clear understanding of the specific information required by the legal system so they can advise the client of these third-party expectations (including any potential consequence for not agreeing to do so) prior to disclosing information to the P&P officer. Working with court-mandated clients may not appeal to all clinicians because of the view that legal coercion negatively affects the counselor/client relationship. However, some research suggests that counselors who adopt a caring yet authoritative style that is blended with fairness is likely to achieve positive results related to the therapeutic alliance, client motivation levels, and treatment outcomes (Hatchel et al., 2019).

Legal considerations are specific to each counselor's state of practice. Best practices involve staying abreast of state laws, and if licensed and practicing in numerous states due to the power of telehealth, counselors need to be informed about all applicable state laws that may affect their work. In addition, if a counselor's credentials include numerous licenses and/or certifications, it is crucial that the practitioner understands what each of the codes of ethics says regarding the dilemma they may be experiencing. This is particularly relevant when working with CODs as the counselors may have a credential focused on mental health treatment and another one on addiction services. Counselors can consult lawyers with expertise in mental health law to ensure legal compliance.

While this section focused on mandated clients, this chapter's focus was on the entirety of the treatment process, meaning counselors need to have a solid understanding of the entire code of ethics, as each client case may challenge a counselor with ethical complexities unique to the client(s). Ultimately, professional counselors need to be prepared to handle ethical dilemmas and use an ethical decision-making model as required by ACA ethics code I.1.b.

CLINICAL CASE ILLUSTRATION AND DISCUSSION

CASE OF JASMINE

Jasmine (she/her/hers) is a 29-year-old cisgender female who is presenting to counseling for issues related to her cannabis use. Jasmine is a first-generation American, and her parents were refugees from Bosnia in the early 1990s. Jasmine currently lives with her significant other in a one-bedroom apartment in a suburb of a large metropolitan U.S. city. Jasmine reports that this is her first time in counseling. She decided to come because she was finding herself using an increased amount of cannabis, and in her words, "I get worried about my use. I mean, it's legal where I live for recreational purposes, but I just feel like I'm using more and more these days."

During the first session, Jasmine's counselor conducts a biopsychosocial assessment and specifically learns more about Jasmine's cannabis use. The counselor learns that Jasmine's early life involved strong involvement in the Bosnian community in her local town. Her parents, being refugees, had to re-establish their life in America and found having a strong Bosnian community was particularly important to them. In addition, "My dad was an engineer back in Bosnia, and he was fortunate to find a job here after taking some additional classes at the local university." Having one parent who was able to secure steady employment was a relief, especially because Jasmine was born shortly after her parents arrived in the United States. While it was a stressful transition for her parents, particularly as one was pregnant, they soon settled in to life in America. Jasmine reports having a close relationship with both of her siblings, twins that were born 2 years after her. Jasmine and one of her siblings live in a neighboring town close to where her parents and their other sibling live.

Jasmine reports a strong educational record: She graduated in the top 10% of her high school class and then completed college in only 3 years due to attending dual-enrollment classes while in high school. After earning a degree in biology, Jasmine pursued pharmacy school. Once she obtained her Doctor of Pharmacy degree (PharmD), she was hired as a pharmacist at a local hospital approximately 2 years ago. She describes the job as "rewarding but stressful," but because she is "so amped up" when she finishes her shift, she has been using cannabis to help her sleep at night.

Jasmine's counselor becomes curious about any symptoms that may be related to anxiety, and Jasmine confirms she does feel anxious quite a bit. "I am always double or triple checking my work to make sure I'm doing it right. I have this massive fear of making an error and causing someone to die." She states that she is constantly seeking reassurance from her colleagues as well as her supervisor. "I know I ask more questions than my peers, but I just get so worried." She also reports that she experiences anxiety in other situations, such as social interactions. In addition, she finds it very difficult to relax and unwind. "I try to get massages. I know I need them because my shoulders are always so tight. My massage therapist always has to say 'Relax, just relax' to remind me to unwind when I'm there. It's so frustrating!" Jasmine further reports problems with sleep. She indicates it takes her quite a long time to fall asleep, and when she eventually does, she often wakes up in the middle of the night and cannot fall back asleep. The counselor asks Jasmine to complete a standardized assessment for anxiety as part of this assessment process.

Regarding her cannabis use, Jasmine uses a vape pen. She began experimenting with cannabis while in college, but it wasn't until the end of pharmacy school that she became a more regular user ... "and by regular I just mean maybe once or twice a month. Definitely not what I'm doing now." Her use now is daily, and she reports taking about three inhalations off her vape pen each evening—sometimes even more. "It really helps me unwind and get to sleep, but I don't want to keep doing this. There has to be a better way."

Jasmine informs she has a significant other with whom she lives; however, her partner does not use cannabis nor does she approve of Jasmine's use. Because of this, they have been in numerous arguments. Jasmine says she is easily annoyed by her partner and worries about their relationship continuing. Her counselor asks about relationships with her parents and siblings. She reports strong relationships but is concerned about her irritability at times: "I've always been the one of the family that seems to be in a mood. My family even talks about it as a verb. They'll say, 'Looks like someone has a case of the Jasmines today' when someone is being cranky. They do it in a teasing way, but it's really something that has upset me for a long time."

CASE DISCUSSION

Jasmine's counselor works collaboratively to help plan out her treatment. The results of the standardized assessment instrument for anxiety show that Jasmine has clinically significant symptoms, and the counselor believes she qualifies for a diagnosis of generalized anxiety disorder based upon her symptoms (specifically muscle tension, sleep disturbances, and irritability) and the fact that she reports these symptoms being sustained for many years (although increasing in severity the past few). Jasmine's counselor also believes a diagnosis of cannabis use disorder, moderate severity, is appropriate based on her self-report. Taking all the information that was provided by the client into consideration, there is reason for the counselor to believe the two diagnoses (generalized anxiety disorder and cannabis use disorder) represent a COD.

Counseling begins with the counselor providing psychoeducation to Jasmine about CODs, including etiology, and how they are sustained. Jasmine's counselor then considers where the client is on the stages of change, and explores each of the disorders separately. Regarding her cannabis use, Jasmine says she has considered changing this behavior (contemplation stage of change). However, she also appears ambivalent about the change because of the positive effects she reports from the use (relaxation, helps sleep). The counselor explores Jasmine's sleep hygiene behaviors and her corresponding stage of change. For example, Jasmine reports sleeping with her cell phone by her bed, and says that she will frequently use her phone when she wakes up in the middle of the night to look at social media. When the counselor asks Jasmine if she perceives any problems with this pattern, she says no because this is what she has always done (precontemplation stage of change). Because Jasmine's counselor knows that there is research highlighting how using electronics before bed and while in bed can cause sleep disturbances, she asks Jasmine if this is something they can talk about, to which Jasmine agrees (shows signs of moving into the contemplation stage).

Jasmine's counselor plans to work collaboratively with her to define a treatment plan that ideally produces the desired outcomes that will benefit Jasmine. Jasmine's counselor intends to use MI strategies rooted in the spirit of MI to first discuss what changes would look like to Jasmine's cannabis use, and then explore how to enact those changes. They will repeat this strategy by targeting the cell phone behavior, and then again each time other problematic behaviors are identified. In addition, the counselor will utilize dialectical behavior skills training to help Jasmine find relief from her anxiety symptoms. The counselor and client will also examine Jasmine's potential for relapse, co-develop a plan for minimizing the risk of relapse, and explore strategies for managing relapse if/when it happens. Throughout their time together the counselor will validate the client's experience and be mindful about checking in about Jasmine's perception of the therapeutic alliance.

CHAPTER SUMMARY

This chapter began with exploring the importance of the counseling therapeutic relationship. Models of working with clients were presented, including TTM involving the stages of change, MI, and other selected counseling theoretical approaches. The chapter also explored the concepts of relapse and recovery maintenance. The overall focus of this chapter was how counselors engage clients in the treatment process, as well as how counselors may work with clients in ways that produce beneficial outcomes. Legal and ethical considerations for this work were also examined. The chapter concluded with an examination of the case of Jasmine, an individual diagnosed with generalized anxiety disorder and cannabis use disorder—a COD.

DISCUSSION QUESTIONS

1. Take time to reflect on a strong relationship you have in your life. This can be a personal relationship (e.g., significant other, friend, parent) or it can be a professional relationship (e.g., doctor, counselor, nurse). What elements of this relationship contribute to it being strong? Describe these in detail.

2. Think back to a time in your life that you made a change in your behavior. How can you see your efforts lining up with the stages of change model? Explain.
3. Working with mandated clients can elicit many different emotions for counselors. What does the idea of mandated clients bring up for you? How do you plan to resolve any feelings that would prevent you from building a therapeutic relationship with a mandated client?
4. Looking at the case of Jasmine, what other information would you want to know from the client? Who, what, or where would you get this information and how would you plan to get this information?
5. Also considering the case of Jasmine, what do you believe her risk factors for relapse are? What strategies would you suggest to help minimize the impact of these risk factors?

REFERENCES

American Counseling Association. (2014). *2014 ACA code of ethics*. Retrieved from https://www.counseling.org/docs/default-source/default-document-library/2014-code-of-ethics-finaladdress.pdf?sfvrsn=96b532c_2

Beck, A. T., & Weishaar, M. E. (2014). Cogitive therapy. In D. Wedding & R. J. Corsini (Eds.), *Current psychotherapies* (10th ed.) (pp. 231–264). Cengage.

Corey, G. (2017). *Theory and practice of counseling and psychotherapy* (10th ed.). Cengage.

Donovan, D. M. (2005). Assessment of addictive behaviors for relapse prevention. In D. M. Donovan & G. A. Marlatt (Eds.), *Assessment of addictive behaviors* (2nd ed.) (pp. 1–48). Guilford.

Doweiko, H. E. (2012). *Concepts of chemical dependency* (8th ed.). Brooks/Cole.

Fitch, T. J., Canada, R., & Marshall, J. L. (2001). The exposure of counseling practicum students to humanistic counseling theories: A survey of CACREP programs. *Journal of Humanistic Counseling, Education, and Development, 40*, 232–242.

Gorski, T. T. (2012). The Cenaps model of relapse prevention: Basic principles and procedures. *Journal of Psychoactive Drugs, 22*(2), 125–133. https://doi.org/10.1080/02791072.1990.10472538

Hashemzadeh, M., Rahimi, A., Zare-Farashbandi, F., Alavi-Naeini, A. M., & Daei, A. (2019). Transtheoretical model of health behavioral change: A systematic review. *Iranian Journal of Nursing and Midwifery Research, 24*(2), 83–90. https://doi.org/10.4103/ijnmr.IJNMR_94_17

Hatchel, H., Vogel, T., Huber, C. G. (2019). Mandated treatment and its impact on therapeutic process and outcome factors. *Frontiers in Psychiatry*, Published online 2019 Apr 12. https://doi.org/10.3389/fpsyt.2019.00219

Hayes, S. C., Luoma, J. B., Bond, F. W., Masuda, A., & Lillis, J. (2006). Acceptance and commitment therapy: Model, processes, and outcomes. *Behaviour Research and Therapy, 44*, 1–25. https://doi.org/10.1016/j.brat.2005.06.006

Larimer, M. E., Palmer, R. S., & Marlatt, G. A. (1999). Relapse prevention: An overview of Marlatt's cognitive-behavioral model. *Alcohol Research & Health, 23*(2), 151–160.

Linehan, M. M. (2015). *DBT skills training manual* (2nd ed.). Guilford Press.

Lundahl, B. W., Kunz, C., Brownell, C., Tollefson, D., & Burke, B. L. (2010). A meta-analysis of Motivational Interviewing: Twenty-five years of empirical studies. *Research on Social Work Practice, 20*(2), 137–160. https://doi.org/10.1177/1049731509347850

Miller, W. R., & Moyers, T. B. (2017). Motivational interviewing and the clinical science of Carl Rogers. *Journal of Consulting and Clinical Psychology, 85*(8), 757–766. https://doi.org/10.1037/ccp0000179

Miller, W. R., & Rollnick, S. (2013). *Motivational interviewing: Helping people change* (3rd ed.). Guilford.

Miller, W. R., Zweben, A., DiClemente, C. C., & Rychtarik, R. G. (1995). *Motivational enhancement therapy manual: A clinical research guide for therapists treating individuals with alcohol abuse and dependence*. NIH Publication No. 94-3723. U.S. Department of Health and Human Services, National Institutes of Health, National Institute on Alcohol Abuse and Alcoholism. Retrieved from https://pubs.niaaa.nih.gov/publications/projectmatch/matchintro.htm

Oxford Languages. (n.d.). *Recovery*. Retrieved from https://www.google.com/search?q=definition+of+recovery&oq=definition+of+recovery&aqs=chrome..69i57j0i512l9.2342j0j7&sourceid=chrome&ie=UTF-8

Prochaska, J. O. (2008). Decision making in the transtheoretical model of behavior change. *Medical Decision Making, 28*(6), 845–849. https://doi.org/10.1177/0272989x08327068

Prochaska, J. O., & DiClemente, C. C. (1982). Transtheoretical therapy: Toward a more integrative model of change. *Psychotherapy: Theory, Research, and Practice, 19*(3), 276–288.

Prochaska, J. O., & DiClemente, C. C. (1983). Stages and processes of self-change of smoking: Toward an integrative model of change. *Journal of Consulting and Clinical Psychology, 51*(3), 390–395.

Prochaska, J. O., & Velicer, W. F. (1997). The transtheoretical model of health behavior change. *American Journal of Health Promotion, 12*(1), 38–48.

Rogers, C. R. (1957). The necessary and sufficient conditions of therapeutic personality change. *Journal of Consulting Psychology, 21*(2), 95–104. https://doi.org/10.1037/h0045357

Sparks, J. A., Duncan, B. L., & Miller, S. D. (2008). Common factors in psychotherapy. In J. L. Lebow (Ed.) *Twenty-First Century Psychotherapies: Contemporary approaches to theory and practice* (pp. 453-497). John Wiley & Sons, Inc.

White, W. L. (2007). Addiction recovery: Its definition and conceptual boundaries. *Journal of Substance Abuse Treatment, 33*, 229–241. https://doi.org/10.1016/j.jsat.2007.04.015

Willets, A. (2022). *Advanced acceptance and commitment therapy: A guide for practitioners* [PowerPoint slides]. https://centerforchange.com/wp-content/uploads/ACT-A-Guide-for-Practitioners-PP-handout.pdf

Young, M. E. (2013). *Learning the art of helping: Building blocks and techniques* (5th ed.). Pearson.

CHAPTER 7

PSYCHOPHARMACOLOGICAL INTERVENTIONS FOR CO-OCCURRING DISORDERS

REGINA R. MORO

LEARNING OBJECTIVES

After reading this chapter, you will be able to:
- Describe common medications used to treat co-occurring disorders (CODs).
- Categorize medications according to the intended purpose.
- Explain common side effects of medications used to treat CODs.
- Compare and contrast the risks and benefits of utilizing psychopharmacological interventions.

INTRODUCTION

This chapter provides a general overview of psychopharmacology as it relates to counselors working with co-occurring disorders (CODs). Psychopharmacology is the use of medications "to treat symptoms of mental and emotional disorders" (Ingersoll & Rak, 2016, p. 4). Behavioral health medications (e.g., antidepressants, antipsychotics) as well as those used in medication-assisted treatment (MAT) are detailed in this chapter. This chapter does not provide a comprehensive education about psychopharmacology, and readers interested in learning more should utilize the resources listed throughout this chapter as a launching point.

THE GREAT DEBATE: THE QUESTION OF WHETHER TO SUPPORT AN ALLIANCE OF PHARMACOLOGY WITHIN MENTAL HEALTH TREATMENT

A significant portion of the American population uses prescription medication regularly. The National Center for Health Statistics' (NCHS; 2019) *Health, United States* reports health status data for the nation. The latest report issues data from 2015 to 2018 about the use of prescription drugs by individuals in the country:

- 48.6% of persons report using at least one prescription drug in the past 30 days,

- 24% of persons report using at least three or more prescription drugs in the past 30 days,
- 12.8% of persons report using at least five or more prescription drugs in the past 30 days (NCHS, 2019).

As these statistics highlight, a large portion of the population is using prescription medications. Although the majority of these individuals are using prescription medication as prescribed by their physician, not all of them are. In 2020, approximately 5.8% of the U.S. population 12 years of age and older reportedly misused prescription psychotherapeutic medications in the past year (Substance Abuse and Mental Health Services Administration [SAMHSA], 2021a). While this does not represent the majority of people who are prescribed a medication, it is a reason some oppose the integration of pharmacology into the mental health treatment process.

Kaut (2011) explored the rationale for integrating pharmacology into the mental health treatment process, and highlighted how there is a variety of professional attitudes surrounding this notion. "Some professionals advocate for pharmacological strategies in appropriate situations, while others might be reluctant to consider drugs as a responsible aspect of therapy" (Kaut, 2011, p. 197). Kaut embraces a strong position for the integration of psychopharmacology into the mental health landscape. One reason for this is acknowledging that many clients will already be on medication when they see a counselor for the first time. Many individuals who initially present for concerns related to mental health will do so with medical providers first, which is where they are often introduced to medication to manage their symptoms (Kaut, 2011). Hopefully these clients are also referred to a mental health provider. It is prudent for mental health providers to have this knowledge that clients may come to sessions already using medication to manage symptoms.

Kaut (2011) is an advocate for supporting integration, and one reason cited for this support is the strong advances that have been made through biomedical research that provide a foundational based in integrity. Additional support offered by Kaut involves acknowledging the benefits that some clients find from medication, which is often a key aspect of symptom reduction. Kaut also examined the critiques common among the medical/disease model. For example, it is a framework that attempts to condense symptoms down to only biological components. However, the author articulated this has been a useful position to have as a clinician, in which additional variables that are specific to the client can be attended to (e.g., demographics, educational background) to develop a robust picture of the client's life and disorder etiology (Kaut, 2011). The overall focus of Kaut's work is in support of this integration:

> *The goal of mental health care is to provide the most effective and durable treatment for clients. Depending on the etiology, intensity, and duration of symptoms, pharmacology is likely to be part of a treatment approach for many of today's clients. Given the extensive research into the underpinnings of mental disorders and into drug treatments, pharmacology should be part of modern therapies, and mental health practitioners should adapt accordingly. (p. 217)*

Offering an alternating position, Murray (2011) detailed a perspective that is highly critical of the pharmaceutical industry. Murray identified social justice implications of having medications as the first line of defense against mental health symptoms, and this is done by highlighting two investigative journalism pieces. This first article by Patricia Wen (2010), which focused on Social Security Disability Income for children, explored how the financial crisis of the early 2000s correlated to an increase among parents and families receiving financial assistance under Social Security Disability Income for their children. These children needed not only a diagnosis to qualify but often needed to be on medication for their diagnosed disorder. The second journalism article by Hunt (2011) detailed concerns of what appears to be an overprescribing of medications for children in the foster care system. Despite about 4% of the general youth population being prescribed psychiatric drugs, reports suggest a much higher prevalence rate for youth in the foster care, some even surpassing 50% (Murray, 2011). Not only are these children in foster care being prescribed much more than the general population of children, they are receiving more prescriptions—a practice called *polypharmacy* (Murray, 2011). Murray's hesitation about integrating pharmacology into mental health is further supported by highlighting problems with the pharmaceutical industry, such as the practice of *condition branding*. This practice involves creating demand for a pharmacological medication by "re-branding a condition that engenders embarrassment" (Parry [2003] as cited in Murray, 2011, p. 288). Mental health disorders and medications to treat these are key targets for this practice due to the pervasive stigma in our society. Murray (2011) confronts Kaut's confidence of the integrity in the research process of the pharmaceutical industry when he states:

> ... the industry has consistently reduced the monies spent for research and development and increased money for marketing and advertisement (Gagon & Lexchin, 2008; Witty, 2010), placing their bets on the value of branding conditions that rely on drug maintenance/sustenance models rather than actual cure and recovery. (p. 288)

Murray (2011) concluded this critical position by highlighting that the counseling process in general has been found to have strong research support, and suggested that counseling does not come with the side effects that medication may produce.

The two positions of Kaut (2011) and Murray (2011) are just that—two positions—along what might be envisioned on a spectrum. On one end are the individuals who are highly critical of the role pharmacology should play in mental health care, and on the other end are those in complete favor of medicating certain symptom profiles. It does appear both Kaut and Murray recognize there is a time and a place for medication, and both believe the importance of medication rests on understanding the unique context of the client. It is essential that counselors have awareness of their own biases regarding medication and remain inquisitive about their clients' beliefs about the use of medication for treating mental health symptoms (Kaut, 2011).

PRINCIPLES OF PSYCHOPHARMACOLOGY FOR THE NONPRESCRIBING CLINICIAN

Professional counselors do not have the legal authority to prescribe medications in the United States. This job function is typically reserved for individuals who completed medical school (e.g., psychiatrists, family medicine physicians). In some jurisdictions, clinical psychologists who have received extensive training are authorized to prescribe. Although professional counselors do not have the ability to prescribe medication, it is imperative they are competent regarding medications that are utilized to treat mental health disorders, addictive disorders, and CODs (Ingersoll & Rak, 2016). This competence is specifically necessary when working on multidisciplinary treatment teams to ensure clients are monitored appropriately (SAMHSA, 2020). Berardinelli and Mostade (2003) suggested that this competence for counselors falls in three domains: (a) assessment, (b) monitoring, and (c) advocacy (as cited in Ingersoll & Rak, 2016).

ASSESSMENT

Assessment is a "systematic approach to collecting information about a client using a variety of sources and methods" (Foster, 2015, p. 291). Counselors engage in the assessment process the moment initial contact is made and continue to do so throughout their time working with the client(s). Accurate and detailed assessment is crucial for counselors to understand the presenting problem a client brings to the counseling process. Counselors may utilize formal assessment instruments that have strong psychometric properties, and they also may engage in other assessment practices such as consulting with other providers.

To begin, counselors benefit from getting a list of all medications that clients are currently taking. Counselors will want to know the following information: (a) the name of medication (brand name or generic?); (b) the prescribed dosage (how many and/or how much?); (c) the prescribed frequency (how often?); (d) the administration form (e.g., pill, capsule, liquid); and (e) the length of time the client has been taking the medication (Ingersoll & Rak, 2016). In addition, counselors will also want to ask clients how they use the medication; it is possible that it is taken more or less than how it has been prescribed. For example, a counselor might ask a client, "I'm wondering, when it comes time for a refill for that medicine, do you typically find you are ready for the refill a few days before it can be filled or that you have plenty left over?" It is important that the client provides all medications they are currently taking (e.g., blood pressure medication, migraine medication), not only those that may be used for mental health or addictive disorders.

Counselors will also want to gain an understanding of client's history with medication use. While there may not be time initially to get the comprehensive picture of the client's entire medication history, counselors could ask about notable experiences with medicines. For example, after the client discloses all current medications, a counselor may state, "Thank you for providing that information. I'm also wondering if there is anything important for me to know about any medications you currently use or have used in the past? Perhaps something you tried that you had side effects with? Or a medication that worked great for your symptoms but you are just not taking that now?" This can help give the counselor more information about what has worked/not worked, as well as information about any current side effects the client may be experiencing.

Counselors also may want to consult (with a signed release from the client) with the prescribing physicians to learn more about the client's medication history (Ingersoll & Rak, 2016). This conversation can involve learning about the symptoms the medication is being used to treat and any pertinent information from their perspective. Consulting with other professionals provides counselors with collateral information, which can be used to supplement what they have already learned from the client. All of these actions taken by a counselor in the assessment phase will ensure they have key pieces of information relevant to medication as they move forward with clients.

MONITORING

According to Ingersoll and Rak (2016), counselors are "checking in with clients at each session about medication, updating medication information as it changes, and keeping records of medication compliance as well as the client's response to medications" (p. 62). All of these efforts are working to monitor a client's use of medication and understand how the medication may be helping or hindering the client. Counselors may also be using both their referral and consulting skills in this phase. Referrals may be used for a variety of reasons: perhaps to refer a client back to the prescriber to ask specific questions, or to make a referral to a new prescriber if the client has issues with continuing where they have been going. Counselors may also be involved in consulting with other professionals (e.g., prescribing physicians, pharmacist, supervisor) during this phase to ensure appropriate monitoring is occurring for the client. Monitoring a client's medication use is a continual process that occurs throughout the counseling relationship.

ADVOCACY

Counselor engage in advocacy work in many different ways with clients. Advocacy related to psychopharmacology is when counselors work diligently to ensure clients are getting the best service available (Ingersoll & Rak, 2016). The American Counseling Association (ACA) Advocacy Competencies (Ratts et al., 2010) provide a framework for counselors to use when deciding which advocacy domain is appropriate to specific situations. All domains are organized to either have the counselor working collaboratively *with* the client/system or on *behalf* of the client/system. According to Toporek and Daniels (2018), working collaboratively with clients/systems "facilitates greater empowerment and more helpful advocacy" in comparison to counselors working on behalf of clients/systems (para. 4). What this might look like in relation to psychopharmacology is joining a client for a doctor's appointment to discuss the client's experiences with their medication. It is imperative that a counselor is well informed prior to engaging in this advocacy work, relying on up-to-date scholarly works for information about medications.

Counselors may also engage in advocacy work by referring clients to community resources, such as case management services or medication assistance programs (Ingersoll & Rak, 2016). While engaging in this advocacy work, it is crucial that counselors do not overstep their role (Ingersoll & Rak, 2016). Counselors are not dictating medical protocols to prescribing physicians nor are they making medication recommendations to clients. What they are doing is using their counseling skills to listen, offer support for issues that arise, and work collaboratively with clients to ensure their treatment needs are being met. Readers interested in learning more to increase their competence in these domains are referred to Ingersoll and Rak's (2016) textbook titled, *Psychopharmacology for Mental Health Professionals: An Integrative Approach*.

ORGANIZATIONAL STRUCTURE OF THE BRAIN

While a comprehensive overview of the brain and neuroscience is beyond the scope of this chapter, a brief summary of the organizational structure of the brain is offered to provide context for the following discussion which highlights certain medications and how they work. The brain is a highly complex organ and is involved in all activities and functions in the human body (National Institute on Drug Abuse [NIDA], 2020). The brain is composed of billions of cells, known as neurons, which are responsible for relaying information throughout the brain and our bodies (NIDA, 2020). This information is relayed by the sending and receiving neurotransmitters (NIDA, 2020). Neurotransmitters are known as the chemical messengers in our brains. Neurotransmitters are released by neurons into what is known as the synapse, or synaptic cleft, in order to perform its function (some bind to receptor sites on other neurons and some flow in the synapse), and once it has completed the duties it is then reabsorbed by the neuron (NIDA, 2020).

All psychoactive substances (e.g., medications, drugs of abuse) work by focusing on specific neurotransmitters and/or receptor sites. Each neurotransmitter has a specific function in our body system. While over 50 neurotransmitters have been identified, there are nine that are specifically affected by psychoactive drug use, and relevant to this chapter: acetylcholine, adenosine, anandamide, dopamine, endorphins, gamma-aminobutyric acid (GABA), glutamate, norepinephrine, and serotonin (Marczinski, 2014). Table 7.1 provides information about these nine neurotransmitters and their major functions.

TABLE 7.1 **Functions of Neurotransmitters Affected by Psychoactive Substances**

NEUROTRANSMITTER	MAJOR ROLES AND FUNCTIONS
Acetylcholine	Involved in memory, attention, sensory processing, and autonomic nervous system functions (e.g., heart rate, pupil dilation/constriction, digestion)
Adenosine	Involved in suppression activities, such as decreasing arousal and promoting sleep. Also involved in regulating oxygen delivery to cells, and dilating blood vessels
Anandamide	Involved in appetite, sleep, and pain regulation
Dopamine	Involved in many functions including the regulation of pleasure, pain, movement, emotions, cognitions, and motivation
Endorphins	Associated with pain regulation and producing feelings of pleasure/euphoria
GABA	Involved in relaxation and sedation by preventing neurons from operating
Glutamate	Involved in learning and memory, associated with increasing neural activity
Norepinephrine	Involved in regulating concentration, alertness, emotional arousal, and hunger
Serotonin	Involved in regulating sleep, mood, memory, appetite, sex, body temperature, and learning activities

GABA, gamma-aminobutyric acid.
Sources: Adapted from Luke, C. (2016). *Neuroscience for counselors and therapists: Integrating the sciences of mind and brain.* Sage; Marczinski, C. A. (2014). *Drug use, misuse, and abuse: Psychopharmacology in the 21st century.* Wiley.

MEDICATIONS UTILIZED TO TREAT CO-OCCURRING DISORDERS

Proper assessment of medication usage by clients involves the need to have a basic understanding of common categories of medications. This section will provide information about medications used to treat symptoms organized by diagnostic categories. While this is organized by disorders, counselors are encouraged to focus on symptoms when discussing medication with clients, as disorders present with unique symptom presentations for each and every client (Ingersoll & Rak, 2016). In addition, clients may be prescribed a medication for symptoms despite not being diagnosed with the specific disorder.

MEDICATIONS FOR DEPRESSIVE DISORDERS AND SYMPTOMS

Depressive disorders are characterized by sadness, irritability, and/or feelings of emptiness which are in combination with physical and cognitive issues that result in functional deficits for an individual (American Psychiatric Association [APA], 2013). Medications used to treat depressive

TABLE 7.2 Example Medications Used in the Treatment of Depressive Disorders

GENERIC NAME	BRAND NAME
MONOAMINE OXIDASE INHIBITORS (MAOIs)	
Phenelzine	Nardil
Selegiline	L-Deprenyl
TRICYCLIC ANTIDEPRESSANTS (TCAs)	
Amoxapine	Asendin
Clomipramine	Anafranil
Imipramine	Tofranil
SELECTIVE SEROTONIN REUPTAKE INHIBITORS (SSRIs)	
Citalopram	Celexa
Escitalopram oxalate	Lexapro
Fluoxetine	Prozac
Sertraline	Zoloft
OTHER ANTIDEPRESSANTS	
Bupropion	Wellbutrin
Duloxetine	Cymbalta
Desvenlafaxine	Prestiq
Mirtazapine	Remeron

Note: This is not an all-inclusive list
Source: Created with information from the National Alliance on Mental Illness. (2022). *Mental health medications.* Retrieved from https://www.nami.org/About-Mental-Illness/Treatments/Mental-Health-Medications

disorders typically target serotonin, norepinephrine, and dopamine receptors. These are classified as monoamine oxidase inhibitors (MAOIs), tricyclic antidepressants (TCAs), selective serotonin reuptake inhibitors (SSRIs)/selective serotonin norepinephrine reuptake inhibitors (SNRIs), and newer third-generation antidepressants (Ingersoll & Rak, 2016) or atypical antidepressants (Hillhouse & Porter, 2015; Marczinski, 2014). Each category is explored in more detail in the following, and a brief overview can be found in Table 7.2 with common medications listed.

Monoamine Oxidase Inhibitors

MAOIs were the first classification of medication identified in the United States as a treatment for depression (Ramachandraih et al., 2011). As the name of this category suggests, MAOIs act on the enzyme monoamine oxidase (MAO). Enzymes are substances that exist within our brains (and other biological systems) that act as catalysts for chemical reactions (Blanco & Blanco, 2017). When used to treat depressive disorders, the MAO enzyme typically works to break down the neurotransmitter norepinephrine (although other neurotransmitters, such as serotonin and dopamine, are also affected), and thus, when this enzyme is inhibited, more norepinephrine is left for use (Ingersoll & Rak, 2016). Although MAOIs were the original drug category to treat depression, these have fallen out of favor with prescribers due to the possibly of experiencing serious side effects as well dangerous reactions related to certain food/drug interactions; they now are often only being prescribed when other medications have failed to produce the desired effects (Ingersoll & Rak, 2016; Ramachandraih et al., 2011).

Tricyclic Antidepressants

The discovery of TCAs occurred while chemists were focused on developing antipsychotic drugs in the mid 20th century (Hillhouse & Porter, 2015). One specific drug, imipramine (brand name Trofranil) was tested on psychiatric patients, and found no effects for psychosis; however, researchers noticed that subjects suffering from severe depression found relief (Hillhouse & Porter, 2015). Imipramine (a TCA) not only inhibits the reuptake of serotonin and norepinephrine, but it also blocks other receptor sites (adrenergic, muscarinic, and histamine; Ingersoll & Rak, 2016). It is thought that the blocking of these receptor sites contributes to the common side effects of dizziness, drowsiness, and difficulty with memory functions (Hillhouse & Porter, 2015). Prescriptions for TCAs were the second most common type of antidepressant prescribed for major depression in the mid 1990s, although these accounted for only 3.2% of prescriptions for major depression in 2015 (Luo et al., 2020). While TCAs are not the first choice by prescribers, these medications have been found to work well in combination with SSRIs when treating treatment-resistant depression (Ramachandraih, 2011).

Selective Serotonin Reuptake Inhibitors

As mentioned, MAOIs focus on norepinephrine (Ingersoll & Rak, 2016); however, serotonin and dopamine are also be affected when MAO is inhibited (Luke, 2016). Research in the mid 1900s started to examine the role that serotonin alone has in major depressive disorder (MDD) and medications targeting serotonin alone began being tested (Hillhouse & Porter, 2015). The first SSRI approved by the Food and Drug Administration (FDA) was fluoxetine (brand name Prozac) in late 1987 (Hillhouse & Porter, 2015; Ingersoll & Rak, 2016).

Serotonin is involved in many activities of the human body as highlighted in Table 7.1. SSRIs work by preventing the reuptake of the serotonin neurotransmitter by neurons (Ingersoll & Rak, 2016), thus allowing serotonin activity to be elevated (Marczinski, 2014). SSRIs are the first choice of antidepressants among prescribers often due to the limited side effects and lower potential for overdose compared with other medications (Anderson et al., 2008; Ingersoll & Rak, 2016). While these are currently the first choice, SSRIs have been the center of some controversy, specifically in relation to suicidal behaviors of adolescents. Ingersoll and Rak (2016) reported that "in 2004, the FDA issued a public warning about possible connections between adolescent suicides and SSRI medication" (p. 105), which led to the requirement for a black box warning for all SSRI antidepressants. Despite the controversy, SSRIs have accounted for the majority (ranging from 64%–74%) of antidepressant prescriptions for MDD in the United States from 1996 to 2015 (Luo et al., 2020).

Third-Generation Antidepressants

The development of antidepressants has gone through three major phases beginning with MAOIs and TCAs (Hillhouse & Porter 2015). The latest phase consists of developing a variety of chemical compounds that have shown efficacy for treating depressive disorders. One of these is bupropion (brand name Wellbutrin), which is a norepinephrine/dopamine reuptake inhibitor; however, it favors dopamine over norepinephrine (Hillhouse & Porter, 2015). A common side effect of other antidepressants (MAOIs, TCAs, SSRIs/SNRIs) is sexual dysfunction, but bupropion is not associated with this side effect (Ingersoll & Rak, 2016).

Selective SNRIs are similar to SSRIs with the addition of inhibiting norepinephrine along with serotonin. This makes SNRIs similar to TCAs; however, TCAs activate quite a few receptor sites in the brain—which is not the case with SNRIs as they have more isolated action (Hillhouse & Porter, 2015). According to Hillhouse and Porter (2015), there has been some research that found the SNRI venlafaxine (brand name Effexor) to be more effective than SSRIs in the treatment of MDD. However, despite the advantageous aspect of this SNRI, the common side effects of gastrointestinal distress and insomnia contribute to a high rate of medication discontinuation (Ingersoll & Rak, 2016). A variety of other chemical compounds exist to treat depressive disorders such as: mirtazapine (brand name Remeron) a serotonin-norepinephrine antagonist; desvenlafaxine (brand name Pristiq) a serotonin-norepinephrine reuptake inhibitor; duloxetine (brand name Cymbalta) also a serotonin-norepinephrine reuptake inhibitor; and others (Ingersoll & Rak, 2016). With over 21 million U.S. adults affected by depressive episodes in 2020 (National Institute of Mental Health, 2022), developing prescription medications will remain a top priority of pharmaceutical companies.

MEDICATIONS FOR ANXIETY DISORDERS AND SYMPTOMS

Anxiety disorders are characterized by the presence of fear and anxiety (i.e., the anticipation of a threat in the future) to a level that is not developmentally appropriate and excessive (APA, 2013). The main neurotransmitters thought to be involved in anxiety disorders are GABA, norepinephrine, and serotonin (Ingersoll & Rak, 2016). Medications used to treat anxiety and anxiety disorders are called anxiolytics (Marczinski, 2014). Barbiturates, benzodiazepines, and antihistamines are the three most common antianxiety medications; however, it is important to know that SSRIs and SNRIs are also recommended treatments for anxiety disorders (Bandelow, 2020). Since SSRIs/SNRIs have already been reviewed, the current focus is on the three other medication categories that are unique to treating anxiety disorders. These can be found in Table 7.3.

BARBITURATES

Barbiturates are not commonly prescribed today for anxiety; however, this classification of drugs has an important history in treating anxiety disorders (Ingersoll & Rak, 2016). The early 1900s saw the clinical introduction of barbiturates (López-Muñoz et al., 2005), and these were the dominant anxiolytic medications until the 1960s when concerns about dangers associated with their use were illuminated (Ingersoll & Rak, 2016). Barbiturates were used for treating insomnia, epilepsy, headaches, and migraines as well as managing tremors; they were also used in intravenous anesthesia (López-Muñoz et al., 2005). Although barbiturates are not a specific antianxiety drug, the sedating effect can bring relief for those struggling with anxiety and other symptoms, which is a reason for their common use in treating anxiety and related disorders. Common side effects include sleepiness, disrupting motor function, cognitive inhibition, and respiratory depression (among others; Ingersoll & Rak, 2016). Due to the high potential for toxicity, barbiturates have a high potential for dependence and overdose and have been involved in a number of high-profile

TABLE 7.3 **Example Medications Used in the Treatment of Anxiety Disorders**

GENERIC NAME	BRAND NAME
BARBITURATES	
Pentobarbital	Nembutal
Phenobarbital	Luminal
Secobarbital	Seconal sodium
BENZODIAZEPINES	
Alprazolam	Xanax
Clonazepam	Klonopin
Diazepam	Valium
Lorazepam	Ativan
Midazolam	Versed
ANTIHISTAMINES	
Hydroxyzine hydrochloride	Orgatrax
Hydroxyzine pamoate	Vistaril

Note: This is not an all-inclusive list
Source: Created with information from the National Alliance on Mental Illness. (2022). *Mental health medications.* Retrieved from https://www.nami.org/About-Mental-Illness/Treatments/Mental-Health-Medications

deaths by suicide (Ingersoll & Rak, 2016). Despite the dangers with barbiturates, these drugs are still utilized in medicine today (López-Muñoz et al., 2005).

Benzodiazepines

Benzodiazepines are the most common medication used to treat anxiety disorders in the United States despite the fact that most guidelines do not recommend them as a first-line treatment (Bandelow, 2020). Benzodiazepines work by focusing on the GABA neurotransmitter, facilitating binding at receptor sites (Ingersoll & Rak, 2016). These drugs have some severe side effects such as fatigue, dizziness, slowed reaction time in addition to the possibility of inducing dependence (Bandelow, 2020). Common benzodiazepines are diazepam (brand name Valium), clonazepam (brand name Klonopin), alprazolam (brand name Xanax), lorazepam (brand name Ativan) and midazolam (brand name Versed). Each of these are different compounds, varying in potency, half-life (the amount of time to clear from the body), and how long the effects are felt (Ingersoll & Rak, 2016). Most people using benzodiazepines take these medications as prescribed; however, there is still the risk of overdose due to the toxic potential (although less than barbiturates), and withdrawal from benzodiazepines can be lethal if not monitored medically (Ingersoll & Rak, 2016). Counselors need to be aware of benzodiazepine use by clients, and should be particularly concerned about any combined use of these medications with other substances that have sedating effects (e.g., alcohol, opioids; Marczinski, 2014). Although many physicians will utilize SSRIs/SNRIs for anxiety and related disorders, the long time frame for effects to be experienced (sometimes 3 to 4 weeks) may mean a benzodiazepine is prescribed in the short term as a supplement. Therefore, counselors need to inquire about the medication plan and how the medication is being consumed by the client, and then be prepared to provide psychoeducation.

ANTIHISTAMINES

Antihistamines are medications used to treat allergy reactions (e.g., itchy skin), but they have also been identified as having anxiolytic properties (Marczinski, 2014). One antihistamine, hydroxyzine (brand names Orgatrax, Vistaril) is FDA approved for treating anxiety disorders (Garakani et al., 2020). According to Garakani et al. (2020), these medications are used as alternatives to benzodiazepines in both inpatient and outpatient settings for anxiety and panic attacks as well as for sleep-related disorders. They continue highlighting that antihistamines are generally well-tolerated although there are some side effects (e.g., dry mouth, sedation, digestive issues).

With anxiety and related disorders being so prevalent in the United States, it is prudent that counselors be prepared to explore anxiety medications with clients. Specific preparation should be focused on discussing the dangers associated with withdrawing from these medications, particularly benzodiazepines, and concerns with combining their use with other substances.

MEDICATIONS FOR BIPOLAR AND RELATED DISORDERS

Bipolar and related disorders are characterized by mood disturbances, either mania or a combination of mania/depression (APA, 2013). The distinct pattern and duration of mood disturbances involving mania and depression are specific to the disorder (APA, 2013). The main medications used to treat bipolar and related disorders are known as mood stabilizers, and these focus on reducing the wide swings in mood (Marczinski, 2014). A list of common mood stabilizers can be found in Table 7.4.

TABLE 7.4 Example Medications Used in the Treatment of Bipolar and Related Disorders

GENERIC NAME	BRAND NAME
Carbamazepine	Tegretol
Lamotrigine	Lamictal
Lithium	Lithobid
Valproate	Depakote

Note: This is not an all-inclusive list
Source: Created with information from the National Alliance on Mental Illness. (2022). *Mental health medications*. Retrieved from https://www.nami.org/About-Mental-Illness/Treatments/Mental-Health-Medications

LITHIUM

Lithium, first discovered in the early 19th century, was used to treat a variety of medical issues such as kidney stones (Ingersoll & Rak, 2016). It is a complex chemical and many questions remain about its mechanism of action in the brain (Marczinski, 2014). What contributes to the confusion is that it "affects different parts of the brain differently at different times when different doses are used" (Ingersoll & Rak, 2016, p. 195). Lithium is known to affect many different neurotransmitters such as serotonin, dopamine, norepinephrine, glutamate, GABA, and has the potential to produce side effects in a variety of systems within the human body (e.g., digestive, renal, endocrine; Ingersoll & Rak, 2016). One notable concern of lithium is the toxic potential of the substance. The amount an individual has to consume to find a benefit (i.e., the therapeutic dose) is often quite high, and can be close to the dose that may be lethal, thus requiring regular monitoring of serum lithium levels in the blood (Ingersoll & Rak, 2016). While lithium was the medication of choice for several decades (Marczinski, 2014), anticonvulsants and other atypical antipsychotics have replaced it as a first choice (Ingersoll & Rak, 2016).

ANTICONVULSANTS

Anticonvulsants work by reducing the "neuronal excitability" within an individual's brain (Binder, 2021, p. 176), although the specific mechanism of action differs for each anticonvulsant. For example, carbamazepine (brand name Tegretol) decreases glutamate release and affects dopamine, norepinephrine and the neuromodulator, adenosine. Whereas a newer anticonvulsant, lamotrigine (brand name Lamictal), affects glutamate and other parts of neurons, ion channels, which help control neuron action (Ingersoll & Rak, 2016). Some anticonvulsants, such as lamotrigine, have been shown to be most useful when used in combination with lithium (Ingersoll & Rak, 2016; Shim et al., 2017). Some clients are prescribed antipsychotics for symptoms of bipolar or related disorders. Ingersoll and Rak (2016) highlight that there is debate about this practice, as questions about efficacy remain. These authors do outline the practice of using antipsychotics as an adjunct to other mood stabilizers, with at least one study (Delbello et al. [2002] as cited in Ingersoll & Rak, 2016) finding support for this practice.

It is crucial that counselors working with clients who have been diagnosed with any of the bipolar or related disorders obtain a full medication history. Often it can take many years (upward of a decade) to receive a proper diagnosis (Binder, 2021), and in the meantime, individuals may have tried many different medications for their symptoms. Also, many individuals who experience a depressive phase will also be prescribed an antidepressant (Harris et al., 2003; Shim et al., 2017). However, the support for this practice is questionable (Harris et al., 2003; Shim et al., 2017) as the research indicating the benefits is inconclusive (Shim et al., 2017). Counselors can work alongside clients to learn about their medication experiences and consider advocacy efforts when they are warranted.

MEDICATIONS FOR SCHIZOPHRENIA SPECTRUM AND OTHER PSYCHOTIC DISORDERS AND SYMPTOMS

Schizophrenia and other psychotic disorders are characterized by the presence of psychosis, which was defined by Marczinski (2014) as a "loss of contact with reality" which can occur via false beliefs (delirium) or false perceptions (hallucinations; p. 328). Before the early 1950s, when the first antipsychotic medication was discovered, there were drastic attempts made to treat psychosis (Carpenter & Davis, 2012). Perhaps the most drastic was the use of the prefrontal lobotomy—a procedure that involved disconnecting the prefrontal region of the brain from other sections in order to produce a calming effect (Carpenter & Davis, 2012; Nijensohn et al., 2012). However, this desired calming came at the expense of other vital functions, such as emotional processing (Carpenter & Davis, 2012). It was estimated that over 40,000 prefrontal lobotomies were performed worldwide during the mid 20th century, but public upheaval led to the reduction of using this procedure in the 1960s (Nijensohn et al., 2012). Fortunately, antipsychotic medications were introduced and have since been continually developed. There are three categories of medication used to treat psychotic symptoms: (a) traditional antipsychotics, (b) second-generation (atypical) antipsychotics, and (c) third-generation antipsychotics (Marczinski, 2014). Table 7.5 provides an overview of these medications.

TABLE 7.5 **Medications Used in the Treatment of Schizophrenia and Other Psychotic Disorders**

GENERIC NAME	BRAND NAME
TRADITIONAL ANTIPSYCHOTICS	
Chlorpromazine	Thorazine
Haloperidol	Haldol
Pimozide	Orap
Promazine	Prazine
SECOND-GENERATION ANTIPSYCHOTICS	
Clozapine	Clozaril
Quetiapine	Seroquel
Risperidone	Risperdal
THIRD-GENERATION ANTIPSYCHOTIC	
Aripiprazole	Abilify

Note: This is not an all-inclusive list
Source: Created with information from the National Alliance on Mental Illness. (2022). *Mental health medications.* Retrieved from https://www.nami.org/About-Mental-Illness/Treatments/Mental-Health-Medications

Traditional Antipsychotics

The use of chlorpromazine (brand name Thorazine) was revolutionary in the treatment of psychotic symptoms. This drug was initially discovered and reported on by physicians in France in 1952, and the use quickly spread worldwide (Carpenter & Davis, 2012). Until the widespread use of this medication, many individuals were placed in hospitals for the remainder of their lives. Because this medication was so successful at reducing psychotic symptoms and other undesirable symptoms (violence), many hospitals were downsized or closed (Carpenter & Davis, 2012).

Chlorpromazine and other early neuroleptics (another term for traditional antipsychotics) are dopamine antagonists (Ingersoll & Rak, 2016). This means that these substances decrease dopamine activity (Marczinski, 2014). Despite the early successes of chlorpromazine and other neuroleptics, such as haloperidol (brand name Haldol), promazine (brand name Prazine), and pimozide (brand name Orap), significant negative side effects made these substances less desirable (Marczinski, 2014). For example, over 7% of individuals prescribed a neuroleptic develop a rash due to an allergic reaction (Ingersoll & Rak, 2016). Other side effects include (but are not limited to): blurred vision, constipation, sensitivity to the sun, weight gain, and dystonic reactions (Ingersoll & Rak, 2016). A type of dystonic reaction, tardive dyskinesia, is an "abnormal movement of the mouth, lips, and tongue that may be accompanied by involuntary twitching and jerking of muscles" which effects approximately 15% to 20% of individuals on these medications (Ingersoll & Rak, 2016, p. 161). The severity of side effects associated with the traditional antipsychotics led to the second-generation of antipsychotics.

Second-Generation (Atypical) Antipsychotics

Similar to the traditional antipsychotics, second-generation antipsychotics were focused on dopamine, however in combination with serotonin (Marczinski, 2014). Examples of these second-generation medications are loxapine (brand name Loxitane), clozapine (brand name Clozaril), quetiapine (brand name Seroquel), and risperidone (brand name Risperdal; Ingersoll & Rak, 2016). The combination of blocking dopamine and serotonin receptors allows for not only reducing psychotic symptoms but also decreasing impairment in emotional responding, increasing motivation, and decreasing apathy (Marczinski, 2014). While these medications are still being used today, they are also involved with severe side effects that can affect many different systems in the human body (Carpenter & Davis, 2012). It is crucial that counselors working with clients prescribed any antipsychotic continually monitor for side effects and work collaboratively with treatment providers (especially prescribers).

Third-Generation Antipsychotics

The final antipsychotic reviewed is aripiprazole (brand name Abilify) which is sometimes classified as a second-generation antipsychotic (Ingersoll & Rak, 2016). Others consider aripiprazole the beginning of a new class of antipsychotics due to the unique mechanism of action of the medication (Marczinski, 2014). Abilify is classified as a "dopamine system stabilizer" (Ingersoll & Rak, 2016, p. 180) in which the medication utilizes what is known as functional stability to act in selective ways on dopamine receptors, sometimes activating them and sometimes blocking them (Marczinski, 2014). Aripiprazole is generally well-tolerated by individuals with fewer side effects compared to some second-generation antipsychotics (i.e., haloperidol, risperidone; Akhtar & Kahn, 2008). In 2013, the FDA approved a long-acting injectable form of aripiprazole, which would allow individuals to receive one monthly dose (Marczinski, 2014). Despite the advances that have occurred in treating schizophrenia and related psychotic disorders and symptoms, Carpenter and Davis (2012) highlighted the limited progress of innovative treatments that have emerged in the 60 years since chlorpromazine was discovered. However, it is certain that there will continue to be research examining the best ways to treat and medicate people living with psychotic symptoms as our society moves forward. Counselors need to stay up-to-date on these advancements.

MEDICATION-ASSISTED TREATMENT FOR SUBSTANCE USE DISORDERS

Not all individuals who receive MAT are diagnosed with alcohol use disorder (AUD) or opioid use disorder (OUD); some individuals receive MAT for their misuse. This is differentiated in the National Survey on Drug Use and Health (SAMHSA, 2021a) report. In the United States during

2020, approximately 1.16 individuals received MAT for either alcohol or opioid misuse. While this is a large number of individuals, it represents only a fraction of people diagnosed with either AUD (1% or 292,000 people) or OUD (11.2% or 278,000 people). Table 7.6 provides an overview of medications used to treat addictive disorders.

TABLE 7.6 Medications Used in the Treatment of Addictive Disorders

ALCOHOL USE DISORDER	OPIOID USE DISORDER
Disulfiram	Methadone
Naltrexone	Buprenorphine
Acamprosate	Naloxone (prevents overdose)

Source: Created with information from the National Alliance on Mental Illness. (2022). *Mental health medications*. Retrieved from https://www.nami.org/About-Mental-Illness/Treatments/Mental-Health-Medications

MEDICATION-ASSISTED TREATMENT FOR ALCOHOL USE DISORDERS

A limited number of individuals diagnosed with AUD are treated using MAT; however, it is a powerful treatment for those that receive it. Disulfiram was the first medication to receive the FDA's authorization to treat AUD (or alcoholism as it was known at the time) in 1948 (Zindel & Kranzler, 2014). Currently the FDA has approved four medications to treat AUDs: disulfiram, oral naltrexone, long-acting injectable naltrexone, and acamprosate (Kranzler & Soyka, 2018).

Disulfiram

Disulfiram was approved to treat AUD in the late 1940s. The main mechanism of action is that, when combined with alcohol, it produces a number of negative effects (e.g., nausea, sweating, palpitations; Kranzler & Soyka, 2018). The discovery of this was entirely by accident. The chemical compound was being tested in rubber factories as a way to harden rubber, but when the workers left the factory at the end of their shift, some would stop for an alcoholic beverage on their way home only to become ill once alcohol was ingested (Doweiko, 2012). According to Kranzler and Soyka (2018), the reason disulfiram works is less about the side effects occurring and more about the individuals' fear of the side effects, which leads them to avoid alcohol altogether. Disulfiram is not recommended for individuals who are not willing to fully abstain from alcohol because the interaction between disulfiram and alcohol can be deadly (Doweiko, 2012; Kranzler & Soyka, 2018). This medication is not widely used today, one reason being that only 20% of individuals prescribed disulfiram were shown to be in compliance (Doweiko, 2012).

Naltrexone

Naltrexone was initially developed as a treatment for OUD in the early 1980s, but it has since been approved as a treatment for AUD (Ingersoll & Rak, 2016). Two forms of naltrexone are FDA approved: oral and long-acting injectable (Kranzler & Soyka, 2018). Naltrexone works by blocking opioid receptors, mainly the *mu*, which is associated with the reward pathway in the brain (Doweiko, 2012). When the receptor is blocked, the rewarding effects of alcohol that typically occur when dopamine is released do not occur, which leads to reduced alcohol consumption (Kranzler & Soyka, 2018). The long-acting injectable form of naltrexone was developed because, similar to disulfiram, medication compliance rates are very low (Doweiko, 2012). This long-acting form is injected into the individual once per month; however, due to the high cost of the medication its use is rather rare (Doweiko, 2012).

Acamprosate

Acamprosate has been used to treat AUD since the late 1980s (Doweiko, 2012) despite not receiving FDA approval specific to treating AUD until 2002 (Ingersoll & Rak, 2016). Acamprosate focuses on glutamate and GABA receptors which "block some of the rewarding actions of alcohol and limits the 'craving' for alcohol" (Doweiko, 2012, p. 423). There are limited side effects associated with acamprosate (Kranzler & Soyka, 2018). However, like other treatments for AUD, there is limited compliance with the medication among those prescribed the drug (Doweiko, 2012).

Although disulfiram, naltrexone (oral and injectable), and acamprosate are the FDA-approved medications to treat AUD, there are a significant number of other medications being examined to assist in treating AUDs. For example, nalmefene, topiramate, and gabapentin have all been explored as options (Kranzler & Soyka, 2018). Considering the high costs of AUDs in our society, it is almost a guarantee that pharmacological aids will continue to be explored in the coming decades. Zindel and Kranzler (2014) suggested that innovations for treating AUD with medication will involve examining specific genetic and epigenetic profiles and matching prescriptions accordingly.

MEDICATION-ASSISTED TREATMENT FOR OPIOID MISUSE

Dole and Nyswander (1965) described a medical treatment for heroin addiction in the *Journal of the American Medical Association*. Since then, there has been significant research examining the utility of MAT for opioid addiction, and specifically methadone, as Woods and Joseph (2018) claimed that methadone is "the most studied medical treatment or public health issue" (p. 323). Today, there are two main MAT options for treating OUD, including the symptoms of opioid use and withdrawal: methadone and buprenorphine. Naloxone will also be examined due to the important role of this medication in assisting with overdose prevention.

Methadone

Methadone has been a mainstay in the treatment of OUD and withdrawal symptoms for almost half a century (Ingersoll & Rak, 2016). The FDA initially approved it for pain relief and as a cough suppressant, but in 1972 methadone received FDA approval to treat opioid addiction (Rettig & Yarmolinski, 1995). Withdrawing from opioids is a highly undesirable experience, as common side effects include insomnia, diarrhea, high blood pressure, rapid heartbeat, muscle cramps, fever, and chills (Inaba & Cohen, 2007). The fear of experiencing these withdrawal symptoms is often a contributing factor in a user's continued use of opioids (Inaba & Cohen, 2007). Methadone is administered either by a pill, liquid, or a dissolving wafer, and it works by binding to *mu*-opioid receptors which trick the brain to thinking a user is continuing to use an opioid (Ingersoll & Rak, 2016). Methadone is often used as part of a taper process:

> *To minimize the patient's withdrawal distress, physicians will often set up a gradual "taper" program to allow the individual's body to gradually adapt to lower doses of narcotic analgesics, minimizing the physical distress, with the goal being that the patient will eventually discontinue the use of narcotic analgesics.* (Doweiko, 2012, p. 428)

This description used the term "narcotic analgesics," referring to prescription pain relievers, although opioid is the preferred broad term for this classification of substances. The goal as described by Doweiko (2012) is to ultimately taper an individual off of methadone treatment, but because some individuals' opioid use can cause long-term effects on important biological functions, an individual may need to remain on methadone treatment for the long term (Woods & Joseph, 2018).

Buprenorphine

The Drug Addiction Treatment Act of 2000 ushered in a new era of treating addiction by allowing medical physicians to prescribe medications to treat addiction from their office (Woods & Joseph, 2018). Prior to this, an individual was required to attend a specific facility to receive services, such as a methadone clinic. Buprenorphine is a partial opioid antagonist, acting similarly to methadone by binding with opioid receptors; however, buprenorphine is not as strong as methadone or other opioids (SAMHSA, 2022a). Readers interested in learning more about medications used to treat OUDs are referred to SAMHSA's (2021b) free resource, *Treatment Improvement Protocol (TIP) 63: Medications for Opioid Use Disorder*.

Naloxone

Naloxone (brand name Narcan) differs from methadone and buprenorphine in the sense that it is not a medication to prevent the use of opioids or symptoms of opioid withdrawal, but rather it is used to reverse opioid overdoses. According to NIDA (2022), when an opioid user has overdosed, a variety of symptoms can ensue: sedation, pin-point pupils, slow or shallow breathing, vomiting, faint heartbeat, limp arms and legs, pale skin, and purple/blue lips and fingernails. Naloxone can be administered either by injection or a nasal spray. Naloxone works by binding to opioid receptors, which block other opioids (e.g., heroin, morphine, oxycodone; SAMHSA, 2022b). Because it works for a limited time (30 to 80 minutes), another dose may need to be administered (Doweiko, 2012). Naloxone is available in some locations without a prescription due to being distributed by health departments and other community organizations (NIDA, 2022). Free training is available to individuals who suspect they may need to administer naloxone in the future such as medical personnel, first responders, or friends/family members of opioid users at risk for overdose (see getnaloxonenow.org for more information).

THE PSYCHEDELIC RENAISSANCE

Psychedelics are substances that cause disturbances to a user's perception and experiences of reality (Inaba & Cohen, 2007). Psychedelics include a wide variety of substances such as lysergic acid diethylamide (LSD), psilocybin, cannabis, mescaline, and ketamine. While the majority of these substances have been banned in the United States, there is a significant movement in recent years to decriminalize and explore them for therapeutic uses (Belouin & Henningfield, 2018). This movement is identified as a *renaissance*, a revival of sorts, notably growing and expanding upon initial treatment discoveries of psychedelics in the early-mid 20th century. Numerous psychedelics were explored for treatment of psychiatric disorders prior to their prohibition, but eventually these substances were banned for research and treatment purposes in the late 1960s (Belouin & Henningfield, 2018). However, the 21st century has seen a revival of research into these substances for their therapeutic possibilities.

The FDA designated 3,4-methylenedioxy-methamphetamine (MDMA; i.e., "ecstasy") and psilocybin (i.e., "magic mushrooms") as "breakthrough therapies," which allows these substances to be explored for therapeutic uses (Hale, 2020). Specific disorders being researched include AUD, treatment-resistant depression, cancer, acute stress, obsessive-compulsive disorder, and posttraumatic stress disorder (Nutt, 2019). The Multidisciplinary Association for Psychedelic Studies is one organization leading the revival. Interested users are directed to Michael Pollan's (2018) book, *How to Change Your Mind*, or Dr. Ben Sessa's (2013) book, *The Psychedelic Renaissance*. It will be important for all counselors to stay ahead of the research and understand the implications of these psychoactive substances being used as therapeutic agents.

LEGAL AND ETHICAL CONSIDERATIONS

As with all areas of clinical practice, it is crucial that counselors consider the legal and ethical issues involved in psychopharmacology. Specific considerations involve competence as well as legal authority related to medication prescriptions. Each of these are elaborated upon in the following.

COMPETENCE

"Counselors practice only within the boundaries of their competence, based on their education, training, supervised experience, state and national professional credentials, and appropriate professional experience" (ACA, 2014, p. 8). As the *2014 ACA Code of Ethics* indicates, competence is constructed over time in a variety of ways. It is not one isolated training or reading, but a comprehensive process to develop competence. Counselors want to ensure that they are providing counseling services in areas in which they are competent, not only because it is unethical to do otherwise, but because it can harm clients.

In psychopharmacology, counselors need to understand their role and the limits in it. Ingersoll and Rak (2016) recommended that counselors consider their work in a supportive fashion. Counselors can work with clients to help them understand their own relationship with medication and their relationships with the prescribers. Counselors can then utilize the advocacy skills they have developed over time to work collaboratively with clients to help as needed. There are many ways in which counselors can talk with clients about their medications in competent ways; however, there is a clear boundary between supporting clients and advising clients. Problematic behaviors would involve advising a client about a certain medication (particularly if no scholarly resources were consulted), telling a client's doctor which medication to prescribe, or making a recommendation that is counter to the prescribing physician's recommendation. All of these examples involve a counselor practicing out of their boundary of competence.

LEGAL AUTHORITY TO PRESCRIBE

It is crucial that all counselors have familiarity with their scope of practice (i.e., what a counselor is authorized to do in their professional capacity) in the state in which they are licensed to provide counseling. As mentioned previously, professional counselors do not have the legal authority to prescribe medications in the United States (i.e., it is not within the scope of practice). Therefore, consulting with medical prescribers is a fair part of the job when relating to psychopharmacology. Specific ACA (2014) ethical code items that relate to consulting or working collaboratively with other professionals can be found in Section B.3. (Information Shared With Others), item A.3. (Clients Served by Others), and Section D (Relationships With Other Professionals). This is not an exhaustive list of the sections to consult as each ethical dilemma is unique and other sections or code items may apply. Clients need to be informed and provide their written consent for all consultation activities. All of this work is to help provide the client with the best services possible.

CLINICAL CASE ILLUSTRATION AND DISCUSSION

CASE OF OLIVIANNA

Olivianna is a 33-year-old cisgender Latina who has been working with her current counselor for 3 months. Olivianna is single, identifies as polyamorous but is not currently in a relationship. Additionally, after graduating and earning her license as a Certified Public Accountant, she is employed as an accountant with a company she has been with for 10 years. For the past 3 years, she has held the title of senior accountant and oversees the work of four direct reports. Olivianna has done well professionally, owing it to her parents who she says, "showered me with love and support for whatever I wanted to do." Olivianna sought out counseling services this past July due to an overwhelming sense of anxiety that began around the holiday season. She reported, "I thought I was just worrying about the upcoming tax season because I have so much responsibility now. But then tax season started, and I was doing my work well, and my direct reports were doing a great job, but I was still not myself. Then it was June and I was still feeling this way. I was talking to one of my friends who recommended I make an appointment with you." Olivianna experiences the distress by sometimes having "strong feelings like I can't breathe, there is a lot of pressure on my chest" and she reports difficulty sleeping. She reports that some nights she will fall asleep around 11:00 p.m., only to wake up at between 1:00 a.m. and 2:00 a.m. and not be able to fall back asleep for a couple of hours. During the time while awake, she says she is often worrying about what happened at work the day before as well as anticipating problems for the next day.

When her counselor asked how she had been coping with this distress until then, Olivianna reported that she was trying her best to maintain her exercise routine (which she knows helps). She reports doing hot yoga three times a week, and walking her dog every day for 30 minutes or more. She said she has not been going to any of her yoga classes for the past few weeks. She also disclosed an increase in alcohol consumption during this time saying, "I know it's not the best, especially dealing with the headaches in the morning. It started with a glass of wine after work to take the edge off, but lately I've been finishing a whole bottle every couple of nights. I even polish one off by myself on certain Fridays." Olivianna reports that she has never attended counseling in the past, but she recently went to her primary care physician (PCP) because of her difficulties. Her PCP prescribed her 0.5 mg of alprazolam (brand name Xanax) for her to take when she was feeling overwhelmed; this physician also recommended that Olivianna attend counseling.

Olivianna's counselor spends the first session completing a biopsychosocial assessment. Olivianna presented alert and oriented, with appropriate recall of information for the assessment. She was agreeable to the process, with appropriate eye contact; however, she appeared somewhat anxious throughout the interview as evidenced by her twirling her hair and giggling often. The counselor learns that Olivianna met all developmental milestones as expected and exceeded academically. At a young age (sometime in the second or third grade, maybe) she was identified for the Gifted and Talented program at school. This allowed her to take advanced courses in high school which allowed her to graduate one year earlier than expected. Olivianna attended a 4-year college in her hometown, living with her parents during this time. She double majored in accounting and marketing and was active in a business student club on campus in a variety of leadership positions. Olivianna reports a strong social circle, mostly consisting of a group of friends who remained close since junior high school. Olivianna attends work-related functions (mostly happy hours) at least every 3 months. Olivianna reports that she is not currently in a relationship, that she identifies as polyamorous, and she has had a hard time finding someone who understands her so it's "just easier to date casually." Olivianna reports no legal involvement or atypical medical issues. When asked about current medications, Olivianna reiterates the 0.5 mg alprazolam, and says she also takes an oral contraceptive and a vitamin D supplement. She denies any use of medications or other substances, and reports the only drug (besides alcohol) she has ever used is cannabis but "that was years ago, and I didn't like how it made me feel."

CASE DISCUSSION

Olivianna is a client who is receptive and open to the counseling process based on the counselor's first interaction. It is also helpful information to know that Olivianna was compliant with her doctor's recommendation to seek out counseling. These pieces of information provide the counselor with an understanding that Olivianna is motivated and appears committed to the process. There are a few areas that a counselor could hone in on with Olivianna's story, for example:

- Her experience being identified as gifted and talented and any resulting pressure that may have placed on her during childhood and adolescence.
- Her sexual identity and reported difficulty feeling understood by others.
- The pressure from her career and leadership role at work.

However, for the purpose of this discussion we will focus on Olivianna's alcohol consumption and her prescription of alprazolam in relation to this chapter's focus. Olivianna's counselor will want to ask about her new prescription and ask what the doctor may have told her about that. The counselor will also want to know how the decision for alprazolam was made. Alprazolam is a benzodiazepine used to treat anxiety and anxiety disorders; however, it has the potential for dependence. The counselor would want to know if the doctor discussed this addictive potential with Olivianna and what other medications may have been recommended. It is important for Olivianna to know about the addictive potential of this medication, and specifically about the dangers of using it in combination with alcohol (which can significantly increase the sedating effects). Olivianna's counselor will also want to be sure to check in frequently with Olivianna to ask about how often she is taking the medication, including if she is noticing a need to take more to get the same effect (i.e., tolerance). The counselor may also want to have Olivianna sign a release of information so the counselor can consult with the PCP and ensure they are on the same page when working with Olivianna.

Her counselor may also want to consider providing psychoeducation about alcohol. It appears as though Olivianna has been self-medicating her anxiety, and the counselor will want to know how long this has been occurring and if there are any withdrawal concerns occurring. The recommended guideline for a woman Olivianna's age is to drink no more than three standard drinks in one sitting, and no more than seven standard drinks per week (National Institute on Alcohol Abuse and Alcoholism [NIAAA], n.d.). A standard drink of wine (Olivianna's drink of choice) is 5.0 ounces, and there are five standard drinks in a standard 750 mL bottle of wine. Olivianna is exceeding this recommendation on some days when she consumes an entire bottle. A website and 20-page booklet, *Rethinking Drinking: Alcohol and Your Health,* is available for free, details what constitutes risky drinking, and offers suggestions on how to cut down alcohol use (available at https://www.rethinkingdrinking.niaaa.nih.gov). Olivianna's counselor can walk her through the workbook in a session, utilizing counseling skills while providing psychoeducation. Following up regarding her alcohol consumption, along with the medication usage, will be crucial to monitoring Olivianna's progress.

CHAPTER SUMMARY

This chapter provided an overview of psychopharmacology in relation to co-occurring mental and substance use disorders. Common medications for depressive and anxiety disorders, bipolar and related disorders, schizophrenia and other psychotic disorders, as well as MAT for addictive disorders were examined. A brief introduction to the psychedelic renaissance was covered and legal and ethical considerations were discussed. The chapter concluded by studying the case of Olivianna and learning how a counselor may proceed when working with her.

DISCUSSION QUESTIONS

1. The beginning of this chapter explains the debate that exists concerning the integration of pharmacology into mental health treatment. Do you think there is a role that medication should play in the mental health treatment process? Explain your perspective.

2. It is important that counselors understand their role as supportive when talking with clients about medications, and avoid advising clients about medications. What are some actions a counselor may take that would overstep the boundaries in inappropriate ways?

3. As a professional counselor, what will be your plan for monitoring your client's medications? Please consider how you will initially assess for current medications and history, and how often you will check in with the client about their medications (weekly, monthly, etc.).

4. As you read in the chapter, working collaboratively with other professionals (such as medical doctors) is important. To make sure you are prepared for these consultations, practice introducing yourself and explaining your role as the client's counselor for these other professionals.

5. Of all the medications listed here, which ones are you most familiar with, and which are you least familiar with? How will you go about increasing your familiarity?

REFERENCES

Akhtar, N. M., & Khan, A. B. (2008). Aripiprazole (Abilify): A novel atypical antipsychotic medication. *Child & Adolescent Psychopharmacology News, 13*(6), 1–4. https://doi.org/10.1521/capn.2008.13.6.1

American Counseling Association. (2014). *2014 ACA code of ethics*. Retrieved from https://www.counseling.org/docs/default-source/ethics/2014-code-of-ethics.pdf?sfvrsn=2d58522c_4

American Psychiatric Association. (2013). *Diagnostic and statistical manual of mental disorders* (5th ed.). Author.

Anderson, I. M., Ferrier, I. N., Baldwin, R. C., Cohen, P. J., Howard, L., Lewis, G., Matthews, K., McAllister-Williams, R. H., Peveler, R. C., Scott, J., & Tylee, A. (2008). Evidence-based guidelines for treating depressive disorders with antidepressants: A revision of the 2000 British Association of Psychopharmacology guidelines. *Journal of Pscyhopharmacology, 22*(4), 343–396. https://doi.org/10.1177/0269881107088441

Bandelow, B. (2020). Current and novel psychopharmacological drugs for anxiety disorders. In Y.-K. Kim (Ed.) *Anxiety disorders: Rethinking and understanding recent discoveries* (pp. 347–365). Springer.

Belouin, S. J., & Henningfield, J. E. (2018). Psychedelics: Where we are now, why we got here, what we must do. *Neuropharmacology, 142*, 7019. https://doi.org/10.1016/j.neuropharm.2018.02.018

Binder, M. R. (2021). Anticonvulsants: The psychotropic and medically protective drugs of the future. *American Journal of Clinical and Experimental Medicine, 9*(5), 174–182. https://doi.org/10.11648/j.ajcem.20210905.18

Blanco, A., & Blanco, G. (2017). *Medical biochemistry.* Elsevier, Academic Press.

Carpenter, W. T., & Davis, J. M. (2012). Another view of the history of antipsychotic drug discovery and development. *Molecular Psychiatry, 17,* 1168–1173.

Dole, V. P., & Nyswander, M. (1965). A medical treatment for diacetylmorphine (heroin) addiction. *Journal of the American Medical Association, 193*(8), 646–650.

Doweiko, H. E. (2012). *Concepts of chemical dependency* (8th ed.). Brooks/Cole.

Foster, L. H. (2015). Assessment practice in counseling. In D. Capuzzi & D. R. Gross (Eds.), *Introduction to the counseling profession* (6th ed., pp. 291–312). Routledge.

Garakani, A., Murrough, J. W., Freire, R. C., Thom, R. P., Larkin, K., Buono, F. D., & Iosifescu, D. V. (2020). Pharmacotherapy of anxiety disorders: Current and emerging treatment options. *Frontiers in Psychiatry, 11,* 1–21. https://doi.org/10.3389/fpsyt.2020.595584

Hale, V. (2020). *The FDA and psychedelic drug development: Working together to make medicines.* Retrieved from https://maps.org/news/bulletin/the-fda-and-psychedelic-drug-development-working-together-to-make-medicines/

Harris, M., Chandran, S., Chakraborty, N., & Healy, D. (2003). Mood-stabilizers: The archaeology of the concept. *Bipolar Disorders, 5,* 1–7.

Hillhouse, T. M., & Porter, J. H. (2015). A brief history of the development of antidepressant drugs: From monoamines to glutamate. *Experimental and Clinical Psychopharmacology, 23*(1), 1–21. https://doi.org/10.1037/a0038550

Hunt, A. (2011, February 23). *Georgia foster kids medicated at high rates.* The Atlanta Journal-Constitution. Retrieved from https://www.ajc.com/news/local/georgia-foster-kids-medicated-high-rates/utg0rXkCA0asjfaEYycC7N/

Inaba, D. S., & Cohen, W. E. (2007). *Uppers, downers, all arounders: Physical and mental effects of psychoactive drugs* (6th ed.). CNS Publications.

Ingersoll, E., & Rak, C. (2016). *Psychopharmacology for mental health professionals: An integrative approach* (2nd ed.). Cengage.

Kaut, K. P. (2011). Psychopharmacology and mental health practice: An important alliance. *Journal of Mental Health Counseling, 33*(3), 196–222.

Kranzler, H. P., & Soyka, M. (2018). Diagnosis and pharmacotherapy of alcohol use disorder: A review. *Journal of the American Medical Association, 320*(8), 815–824. https://doi.org/10.1001/jama.2018.11406.

López-Muñoz, F., Ucha-Udabe, R., & Alamo, C. (2005). The history of barbiturates a century after their clinical introduction. *Neuropsychiatric Disease and Treatment, 1*(4), 329–343.

Luke, C. (2016). *Neuroscience for counselors and therapists: Integrating the sciences of mind and brain.* Sage.

Luo, Y., Kataoka, Y., Ostinelli, E. G., Cipriani, A., & Furukawa, T. A. (2020). National prescription patterns of antidepressants in the treatment of adults with major depression in the US between 1996 and 2015: A population representative survey based analysis. *Frontiers in Psychiatry, 11.* https://doi.org/10.3389/fpsyt.2020.00035

Marczinski, C. A. (2014). *Drug use, misuse, and abuse: Psychopharmacology in the 21st century.* Wiley.

Murray, T. L. (2011). The role of psychopharmacology in mental health: A response to Kaut (2011). *Journal of Mental Health Counseling, 33*(4), 283–294.

National Alliance on Mental Illness. (2022). *Mental health medications.* Retrieved from https://www.nami.org/About-Mental-Illness/Treatments/Mental-Health-Medications

National Center for Health Statistics. (2019). *Health, United States.* Table 39. Hyattsville, MD. Retrieved from https://www.cdc.gov/nchs/data/hus/2019/039-508.pdf

National Institute on Alcohol Abuse and Alcoholism. (n.d.). *Rethinking drinking: Alcohol and your health.* Retrieved from https://www.rethinkingdrinking.niaaa.nih.gov/

National Institute on Drug Abuse. (2020). *Drugs, brain, and behavior: The science of addiction.* NIH Publication No. 20-DA-5605. National Institutes of Health, U.S. Department of Health and Human Services. Retrieved from https://nida.nih.gov/publications/drugs-brains-behavior-science-addiction/drugs-brain

National Institute on Drug Abuse. (2022). *Naloxone drug facts.* Retrieved from https://nida.nih.gov/download/23417/naloxone-drugfacts.pdf?v=8b748408194dff241c227cf6c7c9d04e

National Institute of Mental Health. (2022). *Major depression.* Retrieved from https://www.nimh.nih.gov/health/statistics/major-depression#:~:text=Figure%201%20shows%20the%20past,8.4%25%20of%20all%20U.S.%20adults.

Nijensohn, D. E., Savastano, L. E., Kaplan, A. D., & Laws, E. R. (2012). New evidence of prefrontal lobotomy in the last months of the illness of Eva Perón. *World Neurosurgery, 77*(3/4), 583–590. https://doi.org/10.1016/j.wneu.2011.02.036

Nutt, D. (2019). Psychedelic drugs-a new era in psychiatry? *Dialogues in Clinical Neuroscience, 21*(2), 139–147.

Pollan, M. (2018). *How to change your mind: What the new science of psychedelics teaches us about consciousness, dying, addiction, depression, and transcendence.* Penguin Books.

Ramachandraih, C. T., Subramanyam, N., Bar, K. J., Baker, G., & Yeragani, V. K. (2011). Antidepressants: From MAOIs to SSRIs and more. *Indian Journal of Psychiatry, 53*(2), 180–182. https://doi.org/10.4103/0019-5545.82567

Ratts, M. J., Toporek, R. L., & Lewis, J. A. (2010). *ACA advocacy competencies: A social justice framework for counselors.* American Counseling Association.

Rettig, R. A., & Yarmolinsky, A. (1995). *Federal regulation of methadone treatment.* National Academies Press. Retrieved from https://www.ncbi.nlm.nih.gov/books/NBK232108/pdf/Bookshelf_NBK232108.pdf

Sessa, B. (2013). *The psychedelic renaissance: Reassessing the role of psychedelic drugs in 21st century psychiatry and society.* Muswell Hill Press.

Shim, I. H., Woo, Y. S., Kim, M.-D., & Bahk, W.-M. (2017). Antidepressants and mood stabilizers: Novel research avenues and clinical insights for bipolar depression. *International Journal of Molecular Sciences, 18*, 1–18. https://doi.org/10.3390/ijms18112406

Substance Abuse and Mental Health Services Administration. (2020). *Substance use disorder treatment for people with co-occurring disorders: Treatment Improvement Protocol Series 42.* SAMHSA Publication No. PEP20-02-01-004. Retrieved from https://store.samhsa.gov/sites/default/files/SAMHSA_Digital_Download/PEP20-02-01-004_Final_508.pdf

Substance Abuse and Mental Health Services Administration. (2021a). *Key substance use and mental health indicators in the United States: Results from the 2020 National Survey on Drug Use and Health* (HHS Publication No. PEP21-07-01-003, NSDUH Series H-56. Rockville, MD. https://www.samhsa.gov/data/sites/default/files/reports/rpt35325/NSDUHFFRPDFWHTMLFiles2020/2020NSDUHFFR1PDFW102121.pdf

Substance Abuse and Mental Health Services Administration. (2021b). *Treatment improvement protocol 63: Medications for opioid use disorders.* Retrieved from https://store.samhsa.gov/sites/default/files/SAMHSA_Digital_Download/PEP21-02-01-002.pdf

Substance Abuse and Mental Health Services Administration. (2022a). *Buprenorphine.* Retrieved from https://www.samhsa.gov/medication-assisted-treatment/medications-counseling-related-conditions/buprenorphine

Substance Abuse and Mental Health Services Administration. (2022b). *Naloxone.* Retrieved from https://www.samhsa.gov/medication-assisted-treatment/medications-counseling-related-conditions/naloxone

Toporek, R. L., & Daniels, J. (2018). *American counseling association advocacy competencies (updated 2018).* Retrieved from https://www.counseling.org/docs/default-source/competencies/aca-advocacy-competencies-updated-may-2020.pdf?sfvrsn=f410212c_4

Wen, P. (2010, December 12). A legacy of unintended side effects. *The Boston Globe.* Retrieved from http://archive.boston.com/news/local/massachusetts/articles/2010/12/12/with_ssi_program_a_legacy_of_unintended_side_effects/

Woods, J. S., & Joseph, H. (2018). From narcotic to normalizer: The misperception of methadone treatment and the persistence of prejudice and bias. *Substance Use & Misuse, 53*(2), 323–329. https://doi.org/10.1080/10826084.2017.1400068

Zindel, L. R., & Kranzler, H. P. (2014). Pharmacotherapy of alcohol use disorders: Seventy-five years of progress. *Journal of Studies on Alcohol and Drugs, Supp. 17,* 79–88.

CHAPTER 8

INTEGRATING MINDFULNESS-BASED PRACTICES IN THE TREATMENT OF CO-OCCURRING DISORDERS

REGINALD W. HOLT AND JOHN PAULSON

LEARNING OBJECTIVES

After reading this chapter, you will be able to:
- Recognize mindfulness and its characteristics.
- Distinguish the primary mindfulness-based programs used in mental health and addiction treatment settings.
- Explain how mindfulness is an effective intervention for the treatment of various co-occurring disorders (CODs).
- Summarize the ethical responsibility of counselors being practitioners of mindfulness themselves if they include mindfulness as a treatment intervention within their clients' plans of care.

INTRODUCTION

The term *mindfulness* is an English word for a term in the Pali language called *sati*, or *smrti* in Sanskrit, which generally translates as "remembering." The term conveys a type of attention involving remembering to be present to the unfolding of each passing moment "just as it is" in relation to thoughts, emotions, physical sensations, or other sensory-based experiences (e.g., sights, sounds, smells). Watching awareness close enough for long enough, however, reveals that this type of mindful attention rarely takes place as a natural occurrence. Attention habitually wanders away from the present moment and primarily focuses on reviewing the past as well as contemplating the future. The wandering of the human mind inherently occurs and routinely interrupts focused attention; however, problems can especially arise when individuals are not aware that the mind has wandered and subsequently pulls them away from the here-and-now of the present moment. Many contemporary mindfulness practitioners refer to these times as operating in "automatic pilot" mode (Bowen et al., 2011, 2021; Segal et al., 2018; Teasdale et al., 2014). An issue with being on automatic pilot occurs when habitual patterns of labeling, evaluating, comparing, and judging internal and external experiences happen too extensively to where individuals are driven by their thoughts and judgments about these experiences rather than mindfully being aware of and effectively relating to them moment by moment. The automatic pilot mode contributes to mind states where the person becomes driven by cognitive ruminations, obsessive thinking, and problem-solving attempts. When such habitual patterns are accompanied by attachment or aversion, then individuals struggle against their experiences and unduly create suffering. Cultivating mindfulness helps shift the perspectives on labeling, evaluating, and judging so that individuals are not as caught up in these experiences; therefore, they do not act in unhelpful ways in response to them, and, in doing so, they may act to the circumstances of the moment from a spacious place of clarity (McCown et al., 2011; Sears, 2014).

Because the practice of mindfulness sharpens the skill of being aware of inner and outer experiences as they occur (e.g., external stimuli, physical sensations, emotions, thoughts) as well as influences how these experiences are responded to, reactions that create or prolongs distress may be avoided. In light of these capabilities, it is not surprising that the integration of mindfulness-based approaches in counseling has evolved over the past 40 years. Different researchers and clinicians have offered several and varying definitions and descriptions of mindfulness, which has led to disagreements about whether they are referring to or describing the same experience or

TABLE 8.1 **Mindfulness: A Step-by-Step Definition and Description**

\	MINDFULNESS
A process of...	Helps us to see and reminds us that our experiences are an ongoing process, ever changing moment-to-moment. This helps to counteract when we tend to get over-identified with or "stuck" in certain experiences.
Paying attention in a particular way...	Cultivating and strengthening a capacity of awareness called concentration, which allows us to: 1. Focus—maintain attention on an experience or object of awareness (e.g., breath at contact point) at the exclusion of other experiences. 2. Refocus—being able increasingly to notice when awareness moves off of or away from the object of awareness and then guiding it back to the object of awareness.
To the present moment...	Attending to actual, lived moment-to-moment experience, as opposed to thinking about or conceptualizing experience, trying to change it or make it different than what it is.
Intentionally and purposefully...	Requires a sense of effort, especially at first, since that natural state of awareness is to go away, to seek novelty or distraction, to get bored and want something different. It also conveys connecting with a sense of intent for the practice—we are practicing to help ourselves find and develop new ways to deal with challenges so that we will suffer less, which ultimately benefits ourselves and others.
Without judgment.	Trying to allow and be with experiences as they are without identifying with experiences, getting caught up in or resisting them, contending with them, trying to force or change them, and without labeling, comparing, criticizing, evaluating and judging them (bringing an open, spacious, allowing attention to the moment and not judging what is in our awareness or our self).

Source:: Definition of mindfulness adapted from Kabat-Zinn, J. (2003). Mindfulness-based interventions in context: Past, present, and future. *Clinical Psychology: Science and Practice, 10,* 144–156.

process (Hartelius, 2015; McCown et al., 2011). Despite the variation and debate, the most commonly agreed upon description for contemporary mindfulness research and clinical application comes from Dr. Jon Kabat-Zinn, the primary progenitor of mindfulness applications in modern day healthcare. He described mindfulness as an awareness that arises through the process of the paying attention in an intentional, nonjudgmental way to the present moment (Kabat-Zinn, 2003; McCown et al., 2011). Embodying mindfulness, therefore, allows the practitioner to be openly receptive to each passing moment as it appears and eventually subsides while not striving for pleasurable experiences to remain and unpleasant experiences to go—mindfulness "simply knows and accepts" (Shapiro & Carlson, 2009, p. 5).

HISTORICAL ORIGINS OF MINDFULNESS

BUDDHISM

While some researchers and clinicians de-emphasize the sociocultural and historical origins of mindfulness practice, others are increasingly acknowledging and exploring the origins of these approaches from within the Buddhist tradition and the potential additional behavioral health applications of other aspects of Buddhist psychology (Feldman & Kuyken, 2019; Mulligan, 2017; Tirch et al., 2016). More than 2,500 years ago, Buddhism was established after Prince Siddhartha Gautama attained enlightenment and became the Buddha (Gach, 2009; Harvey, 1990). The word "Buddha," which is derived from the Sanskrit root "budh," is understood to mean awakened (Gach, 2009) and enlightened (Harvey, 1990).

After many years of contemplation and meditation, Siddhartha achieved enlightenment while sitting under a Bodhi tree (Harvey, 1990), which led to his thesis on the origin of suffering as well as the path to alleviate human suffering: "I teach one thing and one thing only, suffering and the end of suffering" (Gach, 2009, p. 77). The Buddha taught that feelings, thoughts, and perceptions are known as they arise, as they linger, and as they come to an end (Bodhi, 2002). A "tool for observing how the mind creates suffering moment by moment" (Siegel et al., 2009, p. 26), mindfulness, thus, empowers people to remain anchored while intentionally paying attention to what is happening in each passing moment as they accept and relate to the here-and-now experience. In light of this offering, mindfulness-based skills lend counselors an empirically supported intervention where acceptance of thoughts, feelings, and behaviors is emphasized rather than the traditional medical model's focus on diagnosing and treating pathology (Dryden & Still, 2006).

SUFFERING: ITS CAUSES AND THE PATH TO ITS ALLEVIATION

Even though it is quite natural for people to desire comfort and be free from distress, pain will unfailingly occur throughout life. Unsurprisingly, pain occurs when humans experience sickness, aging, and death. Pain transforms into suffering when its cause is viewed to be steadfast and unending; it is further deepened when attempts are made to circumvent discomfort by cleaving to what is considered pleasant and/or avoiding those things considered unpleasant. In order to experience relief from suffering, people must recognize that their circumstances are not "uniquely personal, unchangeable, or generalized to all aspects of life" and "no matter what the situation, one has the freedom to choose how to perceive and understand it" (Yahne & Miller, 1999, p. 225).

Suffering has been defined as a "form of unhealth" (Miller & Thoresen, 1999, p. 4); therefore, it is a common reason why clients seek help through counseling services. An inherent characteristic of the counseling profession is to help individuals who experience pain related to various forms of distress (e.g., emotional, physical, cognitive). And despite the diverse theories and interventions utilized by counseling practitioners, pain can be softened when counselors help their clients transform the manner in which they relate to their internal and external stressors. Although people share a universal characteristic of wanting to avoid pain and suffering, Siegel et al. (2009) indicated that, when individuals attempt to elude their problems, they bypass self-understanding and acceptance while inadvertently intensifying emotional and behavioral distress. Going further, those who strive to avoid pain unknowingly sidestep the profound learning opportunity that is afforded through the process of being with whatever is happening in each passing moment (Rubin, 1996). That is to say, when clients are able to accept painful situations and work through suffering, they can expect "greater knowledge, openness, sensitivity, compassion, and passion" (Rubin, 1996, p. 91) to be an outcome. Bearing in mind these assertions, mindfulness-based counseling strategies are merited considering they help clients effectively recognize, accept, be with, relate to, and respond to whatever is happening moment-to-moment while minimizing the intensification of pain and suffering.

THE PRACTICE OF MINDFULNESS

Practicing mindfulness entails engaging in formal and informal exercises (Germer, 2013). *Formal* meditation involves training the mind to sustain attention on the chosen meditative object as the individual observes and examines the operation of the mind (Germer, 2013). Formal mediation is usually associated with sitting or lying stationary for a certain amount of time while specifically focusing on either the breath, thoughts, physical sensations, or sounds that occur in the internal or external environment as each noticed experience appears and eventually subsides. And, when the mind wanders and gets caught up in its content, the mindful practitioner notices this occurrence and then gently returns awareness to the object of meditation (Germer, 2013). *Informal* practices, however, involve intentionally being mindful while engaging in routine daily activities—the mindful practitioner is aware and observant of whatever is occurring in the moment. Examples include noticing emotions, thoughts, sounds, smells, or physical sensations while moving the body, taking a shower, washing the hands, or eating a meal. Regardless of formal meditation or informal practices, it is important for counselors to recognize that mindfulness is not a technique to induce relaxation or a pathway to achieve a higher state of consciousness. Rather, it is a disciplined practice to notice and investigate how the mind works while cultivating the ability to accept our experiences in an open, compassionate, and nonjudgmental way (Germer, 2013).

MINDFULNESS-BASED THERAPIES

Researchers have investigated meditation for several decades, and mindfulness has been incorporated into a multitude of counseling settings and treatment approaches. Considering the ever-growing body of research, publications, and popularity of incorporating mindfulness skills into counseling services, a comprehensive examination is beyond the scope of this chapter. Abridged descriptions of the major adaptations and applications of mindfulness into contemporary counseling will, however, be offered. The main psychotherapeutic mindfulness-based modalities include: (a) mindfulness-based stress reduction (MBSR; Kabat-Zinn, 1990, 2013), (b) dialectical behavior therapy (DBT; Linehan, 1993), (c) acceptance and commitment therapy (ACT; Hayes et al., 1999, 2016), (d) mindfulness-based cognitive therapy (MBCT; Segal et al., 2002, 2018), and (e) mindfulness-based relapse prevention (MBRP) for addictive behaviors (MBRP; Bowen et al., 2011, 2021).

MINDFULNESS-BASED STRESS REDUCTION

Dr. Jon Kabat-Zinn, founding director of the Stress Reduction Clinic and Professor of Medicine Emeritus at the University of Massachusetts Medical School, is the eminent leader who introduced mindfulness into the healthcare environment. Kabat-Zinn believed the skills and perspectives he gained from studying meditation and yoga could be applied in medical settings for the treatment of health conditions such as chronic pain and stress-related disorders. As a result, in 1979 he developed a formalized and structured 8-week curriculum of mindfulness-related practices known as mindfulness-based stress reduction (MBSR). The primary objectives of MBSR involve helping clients cultivate a nonjudgmental awareness of emotions, cognitions, and sensations as they occur in the here-and-now, let go of ruminations about the past and/or anxieties about the future, and increase understanding of their habitual patterns of ineffectively reacting to stress (Shapiro et al., 2005). And, ideally through these practices, enhanced coping skills are developed vis-à-vis fully accepting whatever is happening in the present moment.

The MBSR program involves participants meeting weekly for 2 to 2-1/2 hours and one 8-hour day to receive instruction on exercises, such as mindfulness of the breath and bodily sensations, eating, walking, and gentle movements and stretches, that they will then practice on daily basis (Baer, 2003; Kabat-Zinn, 1990; Praissman, 2008; Shapiro & Carlson, 2009). Starting in the late 1970s, Kabat-Zinn began offering the MBSR curriculum to groups diagnosed with chronic pain at the University of Massachusetts Medical Center. He believed mindfulness practices could help those suffering by increasing insight into how they noticed and paid attention to their pain and related emotions, as well as learn ways to respond to the discomfort so that the pain was not further amplified. Kabat-Zinn indicated mindfulness is accomplished through the process of "assuming the stance of an impartial witness to your own experience" (1990, p. 33), and through this lens of "moment-to-moment awareness" (p.11), mindfulness-based practices allow individuals to understand that pain is transient. When this is realized, an enhanced sense of control is achieved and suffering is ultimately lessened, if not alleviated. In the decades since Kabat-Zinn first developed MBSR, it has been extensively researched and implemented to help those with a wide variety of physical conditions and mental disorders, as well as used to promote emotional well-being in the general population (Kabat-Zinn, 2013; Stahl & Goldstein, 2019).

DIALECTICAL BEHAVIOR THERAPY

Developed by Marsha Linehan (1993), dialectical behavior therapy (DBT) is an evidence-based psychotherapy program created in service of her effort to help individuals distraught by frequent and intense emotion dysregulation, impulsivity, and suicidality that disrupted their sense of self, relationships in life, and general ability to function. These cognitive and behavioral experiences have most commonly constituted the diagnosis of borderline personality disorder (BPD), which historically presented significant challenges for behavioral healthcare providers working with this diagnostic population.

DBT was one of the first therapeutic interventions to intentionally and formally integrate mindfulness into a standardized treatment program. A modified form of cognitive behavioral therapy (CBT), DBT integrates the concepts of acceptance and change while blending mindfulness-based practices with modern psychological treatments (Linehan, 1993). Based upon her own study of Zen Buddhism, Linehan made mindfulness skills a key component of DBT due to its applicability in helping individuals with intense inner experiences learn how to stay present and to adaptively respond to distressing situations. According to Linehan (1993), the goal of DBT's skills training is for the client "to learn and refine skills in changing behavioral, emotional, and thinking patterns associated with problems in living that are causing misery and distress" (p. 144). In order to bypass habitual, dysfunctional reactions and ultimately enhance the overall quality of life, DBT clients are trained to mindfully be in the here-and-now while observing their experiences without judgment, maintaining present moment awareness of whatever is arising, and responding effectively to inner and external disturbances (Rizvi et al., 2009).

DBT's structured and comprehensive treatment program consists of individual therapy, group skills training, phone coaching, and supportive services offered by a team of providers involved in the client's care. Group skills intervention modules within DBT focus on topics such as distress tolerance, emotion regulation, interpersonal effectiveness, and mindfulness skills. In addition, an integral characteristic of DBT emphasizes dialectics or the balance and synthesis of opposing forces. Although DBT encompasses behavioral interventions for distress tolerance, emotion regulation, and interpersonal effectiveness, a core component of DBT involves learning and practicing the mindfulness skill of nonjudgmentally observing thoughts, emotions, and sensations as they occur (Linehan, 1993). Mindfulness training, therefore, is integrated within DBT's curriculum as this skill allows clients to recognize, accept, and tolerate strong emotions while disrupting ineffective and potentially harmful reactions.

From its beginning, the effectiveness of DBT in the treatment of BPD has been validated through a large collection of empirical studies (Shapiro & Carlson, 2009). And, although the main therapeutic application of DBT has been for clients diagnosed with BPD, DBT and components of its treatment modules are now widely utilized and adapted to a variety of presentations, including mood, anxiety, eating, and substance use disorders (Pederson, 2015; Van Dijk, 2012). Counselors-in-training and counseling practitioners interested in DBT are encouraged to review the many published studies examining DBT's role in the treatment of mental health conditions and addictive behaviors.

ACCEPTANCE AND COMMITMENT THERAPY

Psychologist and researcher Steven C. Hayes began developing ACT in the 1980s in an effort to refine the CBT assumptions that had become dominant. ACT and other mindfulness-based approaches discussed in this section are often referred to as "third wave" CBT: The first wave refers to classic behavior therapy and the second wave being traditional CBT. Hayes took issue with aspects of CBT that attempted to challenge experiences and actively tried to change and eliminate them (Hayes et al., 2016; Luoma et al., 2017). Examples include the necessity to get rid of uncomfortable physical sensations before being able to engage in action or the need to challenge and change the specific content of self-talk to improve mood and functioning. Hayes and others observed that efforts to resist and battle with these experiences often made them worse. They proposed that instead of changing the content or "form" of the experiences, individuals could learn to modify the "function" of their relationship and response to these experiences (Hayes et al., 2016; Luoma et al., 2017).

ACT proposes a general model of psychological problems in that people develop understandable yet unworkable and inflexible ways of reacting to inner distressful experiences that lead them to try and avoid such experiences. Their life then becomes predominantly fixated on trying to eliminate such experiences, and, in doing so, they cease to engage with aspects of their lives that they find meaningful. ACT focuses on attempting to decrease experiential avoidance while increasing one's psychological flexibility to increase involvement in values-based actions. Mindfulness practices are a central component of ACT to help individuals recognize and acknowledge their experiences without repeating patterns of experiential avoidance (Hayes et al., 2016; Luoma et al., 2017).

Similar to other CBT theories where emotions are affected by cognitions and clients attempt to change their mood by challenging their negative thoughts, ACT also supports the view that individuals may influence their lives through the use of language. A core difference of ACT is rather than altering the mood through debating dysfunctional and illogical thoughts, ACT places emphasis on the nonjudgmental observation and acceptance of thoughts as they are in the present moment while changing behaviors in the service of chosen values (Fletcher & Hayes, 2005; Shapiro & Carlson, 2009). *Cognitive fusion*, a term within ACT, purports that individuals view thoughts as absolute truths that dictate their emotional and behavioral responses. Through the process of *cognitive defusion*, however, clients are encouraged to view thoughts for what they are (not what they say they are) and, in so doing, the credibility of the thoughts is reduced (Fletcher & Hayes, 2005). To illustrate, an objective of ACT is to help clients see thoughts, feelings, and behaviors as being separate from the person experiencing them (Baer, 2003; Shapiro & Carlson, 2009) such that the thought "I'm a failure" becomes "I'm having the thought that I'm a failure" (Shapiro & Carlson, 2009, pp. 56–57).

ACT promotes a nonjudgmental acceptance of what is being experienced, including seeing thoughts as fleeting occurrences. When this occurs, clients are no longer attached to and influenced by language, hence "psychological flexibility" (Fletcher & Hayes, 2005, p. 319) is achieved and the ability to have a meaningful life is supported. Fletcher and Hayes (2005) summarized a growing number of studies demonstrating the effectiveness of ACT for the treatment of depression, substance abuse, psychosis, and anxiety, including improved functioning among individuals treated in medical settings.

MINDFULNESS-BASED COGNITIVE THERAPY

The interest in mindfulness-based treatments emerged among healthcare professionals after the publication of Kabat-Zinn's (1990) book, *Full Catastrophe Living: Using the Wisdom of Your Body and Mind to Overcome Pain, Stress and Illness*, as well as research outcomes citing the efficacy of MBSR (Shapiro & Carlson, 2009). Because of the growing interest, variations of MBSR for the treatment of mental health disorders soon developed. In the late 1990s and early 2000s psychologists Zindel Segal, Mark Williams, and John Teasdale adapted the MBSR curriculum for individuals with recurrent major depressive disorder. Like Kabat-Zinn's observation that individuals with chronic pain who struggle against their experience inadvertently and unintentionally intensify distress and hamper coping, Segal et al. (2002) also noticed a similar theme for individuals with recurrent episodes of major depression. Most explanations for the onset of depressive episodes suggested that experiencing significant negative circumstances led to the onset of depressive episodes, especially subsequent ones. Segal et al.'s research, however, found that the more episodes of depression someone had, the less it seemed to take to trigger additional episodes. They postulated that those with recurrent depressive episodes become more sensitive to experiences of low mood, and, when they occur, individuals with a history of recurrent depression are more likely to cognitively worry about and respond to those symptoms in ways that intensify them and lead to further depressive episodes (Segal et al., 2018).

Known as MBCT, their model was inspired by the need to develop an efficacious intervention designed to prevent relapse among clients diagnosed with major depression (Segal et al., 2002; Teasdale et al., 2000). Segal, Williams, and Teasdale integrated aspects of CBT with the practices of the MBSR curriculum and first offered the program in a structured, 8-week group therapy format to individuals who had previously received treatment for major depression and were currently in remission. A primary focus of CBT is to help individuals recognize how negative thoughts and maladaptive beliefs influence and strengthen depressive mood states; however, emotions can be improved when distorted thoughts are disputed and corrected. Similar yet distinct from traditional CBT strategies, MBCT provided an alternate method for the treatment of depression. In MBCT, clients develop awareness of their cognitive patterns, but rather than refuting the negative thoughts (like in CBT), clients allow their thoughts to appear and then pass by. Thoughts are seen as fleeting events that are separate from the clients themselves and are not always true indicators of reality (Baer, 2003; Shapiro & Carlson, 2009). When individuals are informed that "thoughts are not facts" (Germer, 2005, p. 125), clients are able to mindfully notice them as they come and go instead of debating them via traditional CBT methods. This process, therefore, allows clients to view thoughts as transitory entities rather than being transformed into ruminative patterns.

Teasdale et al.'s (2000) seminal research described MBCT as an effective treatment preventing relapse in people diagnosed with recurrent depression. Their research found that individuals who completed MBCT were at lower risk of future depressive episodes. Since their original findings with depression, MBCT has developed into its own treatment approach and is now utilized in both individual and group interventions for a multitude of mental health conditions (Segal et al., 2018; Teasdale et al., 2014).

MINDFULNESS-BASED RELAPSE PREVENTION

Individuals in early stages of abstinence often experience challenges to avoid returning to active substance use, especially when they experience distress from strong emotions and interpersonal conflicts. As with chronic pain and depression, individuals in early abstinence often react to this distress in ways that amplify it, which leads to the need for relief that often takes the form of resuming substance use. Integrating conventional relapse prevention strategies with core components of MBSR and MBCT, Sarah Bowen, Neha Chawla, and the late Alan Marlatt developed MBRP (Bowen et al., 2011, 2021), an 8-week group therapy aimed at the prevention and management of relapse for addictive behaviors after completing an initial phase of substance use treatment.

Designed to reinforce sobriety and sustain longer-term recovery, MBRP educates clients on how to recognize individual triggers, habitual patterns, and automatic pilot reactions when experiencing urges and cravings for substances. When triggered to use, clients practice pausing, observing, considering their options, and then responding effectively to whatever is transpiring in the present moment. Ultimately, these skills allow clients to be liberated from dysfunctional patterns that influence relapse and ongoing substance use. A primary mindfulness technique within MBRP is known as "urge surfing" (Bowen et al., 2011, pp. 60–63, 66–67). Urge surfing is designed to help clients develop the skill of nonjudgmentally noticing the rise and fall of cravings and urges. This exercise offers clients a strategy to mindfully notice that cravings and urges are like ocean waves: They emerge, crest, and eventually recede. This generates insight that a choice exists to stay fully present until cravings and urges subside versus automatically reacting upon their initial arrival. Another hallmark mindfulness-based exercise in the MBRP curriculum is "SOBER breathing space" (Bowen et al., 2011, pp. 84–85, 89–90). Through the meditative practice of *Stopping*, *Observing*, *Breathing*, *Expanding*, and *Responding*, clients step out of automatic pilot mode and create the space to bypass habitual patterns of reacting to high-risk or stressful situations as well as cravings and urges to use.

A pilot efficacy trial of MBRP was conducted by the research team at the University of Washington's Addictive Behaviors Research Center (Bowen et al., 2009). According to these researchers, outcomes of this randomized pilot trial were encouraging and supported the initial efficacy of MBRP and the theoretical underpinnings from which it was developed (Bowen et al., 2009, 2011). Through MBRP, clients are offered a cost-effective alternative to traditional relapse prevention strategies by fusing established relapse prevention interventions with mindfulness meditation practices (Witkiewitz et al., 2005). In the initial publication of the clinician's manual, the developers of MBRP acknowledged that future research is desired to examine the strengths, limitations, and the potential need to adapt MBRP for specific populations in various settings (Bowen et al., 2011). Since then, there appears to be a body of literature supporting the use of mindfulness-based strategies in the treatment of substance use disorders as well as co-occurring negative mood states and emotional dysregulation (Sancho et al., 2018; Vadivale & Sathiyaseelan, 2019).

AUGMENTING THE TREATMENT OF CO-OCCURRING MENTAL AND SUBSTANCE USE DISORDERS WITH MINDFULNESS-BASED THERAPIES

Fortunately, the utility of mindfulness as a counseling intervention has garnered attention among many investigators over the last few decades, so there is a vast amount of empirical research to be considered. As previously mentioned, this chapter is not written to include an exhaustive review of published research studies examining the application of mindfulness in the field of counseling; hence, counselors are encouraged to consider the references contained within as a recommended reading list—a place to begin. The main diagnostic categories that are addressed via select published research studies, systematic reviews, and meta-analyses investigating the efficacy of mindfulness-based counseling strategies, include mood, anxiety and obsessive-compulsive, trauma- and stressor-related, schizophrenia spectrum, and substance use disorders.

MOOD DISORDERS

As described earlier, MBCT was originally adapted from MBSR by Teasdale et al. (2000). MBCT is an 8-week structured curriculum that combines the mindfulness practices of MBSR with CBT skills to help individuals with recurrent major depression to minimize or avoid future relapses of depressive episodes. Teasdale et al.'s original study (2000) evaluated the effectiveness of MBCT by involving 145 individuals who had recovered from their most recent depressive episode. Participants were randomly assigned to either a treatment-as-usual relapse prevention group or to the MBCT group; they were then followed for 60 weeks after the completion of services. These researchers found that individuals with a history of three or more major depressive episodes who completed the MBCT relapse prevention group were nearly 30% less likely to have a subsequent relapse of major depression compared to those who completed the treatment-as-usual group (Teasdale et al., 2000). Since Teasdale et al.'s original work, the application of MBCT has expanded beyond relapse prevention for depression and numerous subsequent studies have supported the effectiveness of MBCT as an intervention for both those in remission from depression and for those experiencing acute depression (Goldberg et al., 2019; Lenz et al., 2016; Thimm & Johnsen, 2020).

ACT has been utilized for the treatment of depression and has proven effective in multiple studies at reducing depression immediately following treatment and for up to 3 months post-treatment (Zettle, 2007). Despite positive findings, the use of ACT for the treatment of depression seems to be more robust for individuals with milder forms of depression as opposed to those who have more moderate or severe presentations (Bai et al., 2020). Additional high-quality research, therefore, is needed to determine ACT's efficacy as well as its sustained effects for individuals with moderate to severe depression, including those who are adolescents (Bai et al., 2020).

MBCT has also been adapted and applied to the treatment of bipolar disorder (Deckersbach et al., 2014) and has demonstrated benefit for reducing symptoms of depression and anxiety for those with bipolar disorder while also improving emotion regulation capacities (Chu et al., 2018; Lovas & Schuman-Olivier, 2018; Xuan et al., 2020). Given the prevalent role of emotion dysregulation difficulties in depressive and bipolar disorders, DBT skills training has also been successfully utilized for these conditions with promising outcomes (Marra, 2005; Van Dijk, 2012). A study by Harley and associates (2008) assessed the benefits of a 16-week DBT skills group for adults receiving outpatient treatment for depression whose condition had not positively responded to antidepressants. Participants were randomly assigned to the skills group or to a wait list. Those completing the DBT skills training demonstrated reductions in depression both on self-report measures and in blind evaluator ratings. Going further, Van Dijk and colleagues (2013) developed and evaluated the effectiveness of a 12-week DBT-based psychoeducation group for individuals diagnosed with either bipolar I or II disorders who were not experiencing acute mania. Compared to those in the wait list, the individuals who completed the DBT groups experienced reductions in depression symptoms, improved emotion regulation, and had fewer hospital contacts and psychiatric admissions.

ANXIETY AND OBSESSIVE-COMPULSIVE DISORDERS

In addition to mood disorders, MBCT has also been adapted for the treatment of both anxiety (Orsillo & Roemer, 2011) and obsessive-compulsive disorders (OCD; Didonna, 2019). MBCT has been found to be effective with a variety of anxiety conditions (Ghahari et al., 2020; Haller et al., 2021) and with OCD—both as relapse prevention once individuals have successfully completed an initial course of CBT-based therapy and as its own initial, standalone intervention (Baskaya et al., 2021; Külz et al., 2019; Mathur et al., 2021; Selchen et al., 2018). ACT-based treatment for anxiety (Eifert & Forsyth, 2005) has also demonstrated significant benefits for the treatment of anxiety-related conditions (Coto-Lesmes et al., 2020; Swain et al., 2013) and for obsessive-compulsive spectrum disorders (Bluett et al., 2014; Krafft et al., 2022). While less formally developed for anxiety disorders, DBT skills are also often used with anxiety difficulties and to augment other CBT and exposure-based interventions (Fitzpatrick et al., 2020; Welch et al., 2010). Even when not utilizing the curriculum of a structured program, aspects of MBSR, MBCT, and ACT have demonstrated benefit in reducing anxiety as well as increasing a sense of self-compassion and improving the perspective on quality of life. Despite these promising outcomes, questions about the methodical rigor of studies and their modest effect sizes, especially compared to other treatments such as CBT, have been raised (Liu et al., 2021; Norton et al., 2015).

TRAUMA AND STRESSOR-RELATED DISORDERS

Comparable to being utilized to minimize relapse following initial treatment and stabilization for depression, MBCT has also been applied in the same way as a relapse prevention strategy after trauma treatment for those recovering from posttraumatic stress disorder (PTSD; Sears & Chard, 2016). MBCT has shown benefits in reducing overall PTSD symptoms, including decreasing intrusive thoughts and recollections, avoidance behaviors, arousal symptoms, and negative mood states such as depression, anxiety, and overall stress (Jasbi et al., 2018; King et al., 2013). ACT has also been applied for the treatment of PTSD and trauma-related difficulties and has been found to reduce PTSD symptoms, suicidal ideation, and substance use while increasing engagement and retention in services (Walser & Westrup, 2007). When integrating ACT for PTSD, however, it is typically added to other established trauma approaches or utilized after first-line treatments have not been successful (Meyer et al., 2018; Phillips et al., 2020).

Given the connection among trauma, complex trauma, PTSD, and borderline personality, it is quite understandable that DBT has also been explored as a treatment for trauma-related conditions and difficulties even if recipients of services do not have a diagnosis of BPD. This is especially true for the use of DBT coping skills and integrating DBT principles and techniques into other established trauma treatments (Bohus et al., 2020; Görg et al., 2019; Harned et al., 2021). In fact, this combined approach led to the development of the DBT Prolonged Exposure (DBT PE) protocol for treating PTSD (Harned, 2022), especially for individuals with comorbid conditions, suicidality, and other problematic behaviors. The DBT PE is a three-stage program that first uses standard DBT to stabilize behavior and then applies adapted prolonged exposure approaches and relapse prevention strategies to address trauma-related difficulties.

In addition to those therapies mentioned in this section, there are additional resources available for counselors-in-training and practicing counselors interested in learning more about combining mindfulness practices and trauma treatment. *Mindfulness-Oriented Interventions for Trauma: Integrating Contemplative Practices* (Follette et al., 2015) is an edited book that contains a wealth of knowledge covering topics such as: (a) foundational information regarding contemplative practices and trauma, (b) adaptation of contemplative approaches in trauma counseling, (c) neurobiological and somatic issues for trauma populations, and (d) special applications of mindfulness-informed counseling for various groups experiencing trauma (e.g., veterans, survivors of childhood trauma). A recent addition to the library of clinical books discussing the integration of mindfulness in the treatment of trauma is Dr. David Treleaven's text (2018), *Trauma-Sensitive Mindfulness: Practices for Safe and Transformative Healing*. Topics covered in the text are organized within two main categories: (a) the foundations of trauma-sensitive mindfulness, and (b) the five principles of trauma-sensitive mindfulness. Endorsed by Jon Kabat-Zinn and other notable experts in the field of contemplative practices (Treleaven, 2022a), Treleaven also offers a two-part comprehensive training program on the use of trauma-sensitive mindfulness, which includes distinguished guest faculty such as Tara Brach, PhD and Rick Hanson, PhD (Treleaven, 2022b).

SCHIZOPHRENIA-SPECTRUM AND OTHER PSYCHOTIC DISORDERS

Perhaps the mindfulness-based intervention with the widest application and research evidence for its use with psychosis is ACT (O'Donoghue et al., 2018). For individuals with psychosis, ACT has been shown to be helpful to lower lengths of hospitalization, lessen the severity of positive and negative symptoms of psychosis, reduce reports of depression and anxiety, and improve psychosocial functioning (Jansen et al., 2020; Yildiz, 2020). While ACT has been the most notable formal treatment model utilized with psychosis, other approaches have also included mindfulness skills as part of their interventions for psychosis and have also integrated mindfulness into other treatments (most commonly CBT) with similar positive results (Hodann-Caudevilla et al., 2020; Li et al., 2021).

SUBSTANCE USE DISORDERS

As previously discussed, the most prominent adaptation of mindfulness-based interventions for the treatment of addictive disorders has been mindfulness-based relapse prevention (MBRP; Bowen et al., 2011, 2021). The 8-week MBRP protocol has consistently demonstrated efficacy across multiple studies in reducing the frequency of substance use, reducing relapse, increasing service retention, and decreasing symptoms of craving, depression, and anxiety (Grant et al., 2017; Ramadas et al., 2021). While not a structured, multiweek program like MBRP, ACT has also been shown to be effective in helping individuals to reduce and discontinue their substance use and to respond to experiences and values-based behaviors in more psychologically flexible ways (Carvalho et al., 2021; Ii et al., 2019; E. B. Lee et al., 2015).

Considering the prevalence of emotion dysregulation, impulsivity, and engagement in harmful behaviors characteristic of BPD, DBT has been used successfully to decrease substance use, suicidality, and nonsuicidal self-injury, and to improve treatment retention and social functioning in individuals with BPD and co-occurring substance use disorders, especially for those diagnosed with opioid use disorder as well as polysubstance dependence (Dimeff & Linehan, 2008; N. K. Lee et al., 2015). Conversely, those with substance use disorders who do not have a co-occurring diagnosis of BPD can experience impulsivity and emotion dysregulation, and engage in self-harm behaviors; therefore, DBT skills have also been successfully utilized in treatment for these individuals (Platter & Cabral, 2012; Warner & Murphy, 2022).

Although mindfulness-based interventions that adapt practices and approaches from established therapies seem to be generally effective for the treatment of substance use and addictive disorders, some researchers have questioned how significant the benefits are, especially when compared to conventional CBT-based interventions and/or traditional 12-step programs (Bautista et al., 2019; Chiesa & Serretti, 2014; Giannelli et al., 2019; Sancho et al., 2018). Regardless of whether mindfulness-based approaches are formally incorporated into the plan of care, ongoing involvement in community-based mutual support groups (e.g., Alcoholics Anonymous and Narcotics Anonymous)—especially following completion of formal treatment—is often seen as an integral aspect of minimizing relapse and maintaining longer-term recovery. And, considering the reported efficacy and widespread integration of mindfulness into counseling, it stands to reason that mindfulness-based recovery support groups have developed in recent years and are becoming increasingly available. These include Recovery Dharma (n.d.), Refuge Recovery (n.d.), and Yoga Twelve-Step Recovery (Y12SR; n.d.). Individuals seeking recovery from substance addiction through services integrating contemplative practices may now choose one of these programs as either a complement or an alternative to traditional 12-step programs.

AUGMENTING THE COUNSELOR AS A PROFESSIONAL AND AS A PERSON

Growing attention has also been given to not only how mindfulness practices can be applied in the treatment of behavioral health and substance use concerns, but also on how they positively impact the therapeutic relationship as well as the counselor's professional and personal well-being (Hick & Bien, 2008; Pollak et al., 2014). Aspects of mindfulness, including fostering a nonjudgmental and compassionate approach to one's inner experiences and outer circumstances, and a focus on the alleviation of suffering while also promoting personal growth and wellness, are consistent with the core values of the counseling profession and other allied helping disciplines (Boone, 2014;

Reilly, 2016). Because practicing mindfulness aids in reducing anxiety, stress, emotional reactivity, and judgmental attitudes while increasing compassion, empathy, therapeutic presence, attending behaviors, and counselor self-care, it has led to the inclusion of mindfulness being covered in direct practice courses (Gockel, 2015; Gockel & Deng, 2016; Thomas, 2017), counselor education textbooks (Holt, 2018, 2019, 2021), as well as with interns completing clinically focused graduate field placements (Fulton & Cashwell, 2015; Lee & Himmelheber, 2016). In fact, mindfulness practices have also been found to reducing burnout and compassion fatigue among graduate interns during field placements (Decker et al., 2015; Testa & Sangganjanavanich, 2016) while even having the potential to enhance their perspective on the quality of their lives in the presence of experiencing the intense, stressful, and challenging circumstances of completing graduate courses and field education simultaneously (Bonifas & Napoli, 2014).

LEGAL AND ETHICAL CONSIDERATIONS

There are important limitations and ethical considerations concerning the counselor's competent use of mindfulness-based interventions. The wide popularity and proliferation of mindfulness has led to public and professional confusion over what it is and what it is not, as well as allegations that the benefits of mindfulness have been exaggerated (Rosenbaum & Magid, 2016; Sears 2021). Others have questioned the rapid dissemination of mindfulness in the literature, criticisms of the rigor of mindfulness research (including modest to minimal effect sizes), and the apparent lack of attention that has been given to possible contraindications or adverse effects of mindfulness-based interventions (Van Dam et al., 2018).

Two of the most prominent considerations for counselors practicing ethically concern (a) attention to diversity and individual preference issues in treatment and (b) developing competency with mindfulness-based interventions. While mindfulness-based interventions now have significant scientific support for their contemporary utilization in behavioral health services for a multitude of mental health and addiction concerns, there is no denying their sociohistorical origins in Eastern wisdom traditions generally, and the Buddhist tradition specifically. While contemplative practices exist in most all religious and secular spiritual traditions and practices, and there is no need for clients to identify as Buddhists in order to engage in mindfulness training, some clients will find such approaches off-putting or inconsistent with their values and preferences. For those of particular religious beliefs and traditions, the practices might seem to conflict with their faith commitments, and for individuals who see themselves as averse to anything that seems "spiritual," they might find the practice to be offensive. While there are secular ways to introduce and discuss the practices with clients that explain their context and utility in clinical services, ultimately, if a client is unwilling to attempt to engage in such interventions, then it is important for counselors to appreciate their choices and preferences, and then collaboratively adapt services and interventions to meet the treatment needs of clients (Sears, 2015, 2021).

The other important ethical issue concerns the competent use of mindfulness skills and mindfulness-based interventions in counseling. A common concern about incorporating mindfulness-based strategies into counseling is a debate over the qualifications of the counseling practitioner (Kostanski & Hassed, 2008), which may result in the potential to inflict harm if the practice of mindfulness is unskillfully taught and practiced (Shapiro & Carlson, 2009). To correct erroneous beliefs and avert harmful actions, counselors are advised to avoid the unsystematic use of mindfulness unless they obtain appropriate training from qualified and reliable sources. Thus, interested counselors should explore and access the many high-quality resources (Brandsma, 2017;

McCown et al., 2011; Piet et al., 2015), training programs, and institutes that are available for clinicians to learn how to effectively combine mindfulness with counseling. The following is a concise but not exhaustive list of skills-training resources for the various mindfulness-based programs.

TABLE 8.2 **Training Provider Resources for Mindfulness-Based Therapies**

PROGRAM	PROVIDER	WEBSITE
MBSR	Brown University School of Professional Studies	https://professional.brown.edu/certificate/mindfulness
	University of California–San Diego Mindfulness-Based Professional Training Institute	https://cih.ucsd.edu/mbpti/mbsr-overview
DBT	Psychwire	https://psychwire.com/linehan
ACT	Praxis Continuing Education	https://act.courses/signup/
	Psychwire	https://psychwire.com/harris
MBCT	MBCT.com	https://www.mbct.com/mbct-instructor-training-workshops/
	University of California–San Diego Mindfulness-Based Professional Training Institute	https://cih.ucsd.edu/index.php/mbpti/mbct-mindfulness-based-cognitive-therapy-teacher-training-intensive
MBRP	MBRP: Treatment for Addictive Behaviors	https://mindfulrp.com/for-clinicians
	University of California–San Diego Mindfulness-Based Professional Training Institute	https://cih.ucsd.edu/mbpti/mbrp-mindfulness-based-relapse-prevention
TSM	David Treleaven, PhD	https://davidtreleaven.com/online-training/

ACT, acceptance and commitment therapy; DBT, dialectical behavior therapy; MBCT, mindfulness-based cognitive therapy; MBRP, mindfulness-based relapse prevention; MBSR, mindfulness-based stress reduction; TSM, trauma-sensitive mindfulness.

While becoming proficient in the use of mindfulness-based interventions is a vast and ongoing process, there are some foundational aspects of developing such competency. Except for MBSR, which is not considered a psychotherapeutic intervention and does not require trained facilitators to possess an advanced degree in either counseling or related therapeutic disciplines, most applications for mindfulness-based interventions are in the context of therapy, therefore necessitating that the provider be a trained clinician with general therapeutic competencies. Mindfulness skills can also be introduced and facilitated by generalist practitioners and paraprofessionals who offer basic coping skills training. Because successfully applying and implementing mindfulness-based interventions and programs in an intentional, structured, and clinically useful manner connotes their integration into a broader scope and plan of therapy, this necessitates providers be formally educated and trained therapists. Such competency includes recognizing when other approaches might be more clinically indicated over mindfulness-based interventions. Not everyone who presents for counseling will need or benefit from mindfulness. Mindfulness-oriented practitioners need to be familiar with a variety of interventions and approaches and choose plans of care that are the most indicated for clients' needs and wishes (Paulson, 2018; Sears, 2015).

Included within the requirements of competent counselors is the ability to skillfully and successfully integrate mindfulness into counseling. Clinicians utilizing mindfulness as part of the services they are providing need to have a solid functional understanding of the purpose and utility of mindfulness; they need to be able to conduct proper screenings, offer psychoeducation, and teach mindfulness skills to clients. This must be conducted in a meaningful way that provides an understandable rationale for making mindfulness part of counseling. Successfully facilitating mindfulness-based skills includes doing so during sessions, structuring practice outside of sessions, and assisting clients in recognizing and addressing challenges commonly encountered as part of practice. As with all therapeutic competencies, it is important for counselors using mindfulness-based interventions to receive ongoing continuing education and clinical supervision (Paulson, 2018; Sears, 2015). Counselors are directed to specific chapters within Germer et. al's book, *Mindfulness and Psychotherapy* (2013), that offer valuable information on mindfulness as clinical training (Fulton, 2013), practical ethics (Morgan, 2013), teaching mindfulness in therapy (Pollak, 2013), and considerations when introducing mindfulness into trauma therapy (Briere, 2013).

Perhaps the most important aspect of counselors developing competency with mindfulness-based interventions is for counselors to maintain their own personal, ongoing mindfulness practice. Doing so is important because it helps the counselor to directly see and experience the application and its usefulness in their own lives. Counselors will be better able to help clients recognize and respond to challenges they are experiencing with the practice because the counselor has had to experience and work with those as well. Most importantly, when counselors then integrate mindfulness into therapy, they can do so from a place of experiential perspective, knowledge, and wisdom (Paulson, 2018; Sears, 2015).

CLINICAL CASE ILLUSTRATION AND DISCUSSION

CASE OF MIKE

Mike, a 39-year-old single, biracial, cisgender male, is currently on parole and living in a sober-living house. Mike started participating in a MBRP group after completing 12 weeks of an intensive outpatient program (IOP) where he received treatment for alcohol use disorder, cannabis use disorder, major depressive disorder, and generalized anxiety disorder. In addition to attending the MBRP groups for addiction recovery, he is also meeting concurrently with a therapist in individual therapy to continue addressing his challenges related to his mental health issues. Beyond formal treatment, Mike is also attending two community-based mutual support groups in town where he resides: Alcoholics Anonymous meetings several days each week along with a Recovery Dharma meeting that was recently established in the area. Although Mike has maintained abstinence from alcohol and marijuana since he entered IOP, he continues to struggle with cravings and urges to use. These are especially strong when he spends time visiting family and friends in his former neighborhood while on a day pass from the sober-living house. He also struggles with his urges whenever his symptoms of anxiety and depression intensify; these especially occur when he experiences conflicts with his parents, sister, and Michelle, his most recent girlfriend.

He says that sometimes it is hard to engage in the mindfulness practices in the sober-living house because "it is so loud with people always around, and some of them even make fun at me for doing that 'weird meditation' stuff." Regardless, Mike remained committed and regularly practices mindfulness skills by streaming audio recordings and listening through headphones. "I do the practices lying in my bed because then it doesn't look as conspicuous if I am sitting on a meditation cushion as I practice."

In the MBRP groups, Mike has been identifying his triggers to craving and developing plans for how to respond to those without using. This has included working with the MBRP "urge surfing" exercise in group. While sometimes challenging, this particular skill has been very helpful. In the past when experiencing urges and before IOP and MBRP, Mike would try to do whatever he could to battle and make them go away. He would try to suppress the urges and force them out of his mind: "I would tell myself that they were bad and wrong and try to push them away, but it only seemed to make them push back harder. Not only would they not go away, but they would get stronger until they just overwhelmed me and I would eventually use again." He states that he is beginning to be able to acknowledge the presence of these experiences "without struggling with them as much … without judging them as bad or seeing myself as being bad or weak for having them." In fact, he says that the aspect of mindfulness practice of trying not to judge the experiences or himself has helped him deal better with his troubling, uncomfortable physical sensations, emotions, and thoughts. "I don't judge them or me as much. It's like the practice has made me a bit more patient and compassionate. I don't get so worked up or fly off the handle as quickly as I used to."

CASE DISCUSSION

In this scenario Mike is engaging in MBRP as it was originally developed—as a relapse prevention program following the completion of an earlier level of treatment. While researchers and clinicians have successfully adapted MBRP and similar curricula to be a first-line treatment approach, there can still be a good case made for it being used as a phase-two aftercare. Individuals who have achieved and maintained abstinence while completing an initial phase of treatment may be better prepared to work with identifying their triggers and high-risk situations as well as have better stability of external and internal resources to consistently and successfully engage in the mindfulness practices during and in between the MBRP weekly group sessions.

An important aspect of mindfulness illustrated by Mike's description of "urge surfing" and his experience of cravings has to do with how he responds to them. It is quite natural for people to experience uncomfortable distress and then try to "get rid" of those experiences; they end up struggling with and fighting against the unwanted experiences in anticipation of eliminating them. Unfortunately, this reaction tends to amplify the experiences and prolongs the individual's contact with them, making the individual more prone to impulsively act on them in unproductive and harmful ways. Mindfulness helps the person to notice and acknowledge the experience of the moment from a less judgmental, receptive space, which then enhances their ability to response to their experiences and circumstances in more productive and healthier ways.

Something important for counselors utilizing mindfulness-based interventions to be aware of and respond to are challenges individuals are likely to face engaging in the practices outside of counseling sessions. In this scenario, Mike has encountered difficulties practicing at his sober-living halfway house due to the noise and chaos of the setting and due to receiving criticism and discouragement from other residents. Through experimenting he has also found that his practice goes better if he is lying down and listening to audio records guiding him through the practices.

While such issues are common for individuals trying to engage in mindfulness practices while incarcerated or in halfway house settings, they are not unique to those circumstances. People often encounter difficulties trying to integrate the practices into their busy lives and daily schedules, somewhere in between (or during) work, taking care of screaming children, and trying to get ready for the next day. Some people find it very helpful to listen to audio records with scripts guiding them through the practice, while others find that to be a distraction. The key is to help individuals identify the times, places, and postures in which they are most likely to practice.

CHAPTER SUMMARY

Having problems and experiencing pain are an integral part of the human condition. When individuals believe their efforts at managing the challenges of life are inadequate, then feelings of depression, anxiety, anger, and helplessness will follow (Kabat-Zinn, 1990). Moreover, when problematic and distressing events occur that are viewed to be beyond the individual's immediate control, unpleasant mood and behavioral states are further set in motion. This impact is additionally aggravated when people attempt to escape emotional and physical pain by ingesting mind-altering substances or engaging in pleasure-seeking activities. Not only is this avoidance-based coping strategy an ineffective approach of dealing with unpleasant and painful experiences in life, it counterproductively deepens the suffering from the primary problem that the individual is attempting to alleviate or escape.

The efficacy of mindfulness-based counseling strategies for the treatment of mood, anxiety, obsessive-compulsive, trauma-and stressor-related, schizophrenia spectrum, and substance use disorders have been presented through an abridged description of published research studies, including systematic reviews and meta-analyses. Despite the well-earned place that mindfulness now has in the counseling profession, it is important for counselors to understand that it is not a cure-all remedy that will miraculously make disappear whatever clients are labeling as unpleasant or unwanted. What mindfulness can offer clients, however, is the ability to intentionally "work with the very stress and pain" that life brings forth, which, in turn, will paradoxically promote greater health and well-being (Kabat-Zinn, 1990, p. 2). Mindfulness-based counseling practices help clients notice their experience with more clarity and immediacy, accept all experiences (including the unwanted ones) as part of the overall human condition, recognize they can have these experiences without automatically reacting in habitual and problematic ways, and realize they can cope effectively in a manner that allows them to lead a life of meaning consistent with their values. By integrating mindfulness-based counseling approaches in the treatment of co-occurring mental and substance use disorders, clients may experience the liberation that is offered by co-existing and accepting whatever is happening during each transitory moment of life.

The late psychiatrist Viktor Frankl (1992) emphasized a belief in the freedom and power of the individual to choose one's attitude in the face of suffering, which is illustrated in a quote that is widely attributed to him:

Between stimulus and response, there is a space.
In that space lies our freedom and power to choose our response.
In our response lies our growth and our happiness. (Pattakos, 2010, p. vi)

Mindfulness creates a space that allows one to choose to respond more skillfully to the circumstances of their life, including those whose lives are especially challenging and overwhelming. In support of Frankl's position, clients with CODs who receive and practice mindfulness may pause, take sanctuary, and enhance their ability to effectively respond to whatever arises moment-by-moment. And, ideally, when consistently employed, mindfulness practices may offer clients some refuge from co-occurring mental health and addiction symptomatology.

DISCUSSION QUESTIONS

1. What is your overall reaction to utilizing mindfulness-based interventions in the treatment of CODs?
2. Do you have any concerns or hesitations about incorporating mindfulness-based services into counseling practice? Please explain your answer.
3. Identify, describe, and discuss the advantages as well as the limitations of utilizing mindfulness-based interventions in the *general* practice of counseling compared to its *specific* use in the integrated treatment of co-occurring mental and substance use disorders.
4. Identify/describe/discuss at least two key aspects of developing competency with the utilization and application of mindfulness-based interventions into counseling practice.
5. Of the related yet different mindfulness-based therapies discussed in this chapter (mindfulness-based stress reduction, mindfulness-based cognitive therapy, mindfulness-based relapse prevention, acceptance and commitment therapy, dialectical behavior therapy), which one do you find the most interesting? Please explain your answer.

REFERENCES

Baer, R. (2003). Mindfulness training as a clinical intervention: A conceptual and empirical review. *Clinical Psychology: Science and Practice, 10*(2), 125–143. https://doi.org/10.1093/clipsy.bpg015

Bai, Z., Luo, S., Zhang, L., Wu, S., & Chi, I. (2020). Acceptance and Commitment Therapy (ACT) to reduce depression: A systematic review and meta-analysis. *Journal of Affective Disorders, 260*, 728–737. https://doi.org/10.1016/j.jad.2019.09.040

Başkaya, E., Özgüç, S., & Tanrıverdi, D. (2021). Examination of the effectiveness of mindfulness-based cognitive therapy on patients with obsessive-compulsive disorder: Systematic review and meta-analysis. *Issues in Mental Health Nursing, 42*(11), 998–1009. https://doi.org/10.1080/01612840.2021.1920652

Bautista, T., James, D., & Amaro, H. (2019). Acceptability of mindfulness-based interventions for substance use disorder: A systematic review. *Complementary Therapies in Clinical Practice, 35*, 201–207. https://doi.org/10.1016/j.ctcp.2019.02.012

Bluett, E. J., Homan, K. J., Morrison, K. L., Levin, M. E., & Twohig, M. P. (2014). Acceptance and commitment therapy for anxiety and OCD spectrum disorders: An empirical review. *Journal of Anxiety Disorders, 28*(6), 612–624. https://doi.org/10.1016/j.janxdis.2014.06.008

Bodhi, B. (2002). *The connected discourses of the Buddha: A translation of the Samyutta Nikaya* (2nd ed.). Wisdom Publications.

Bohus, M., Kleindienst, N., Hahn, C., Müller-Engelmann, M., Ludäscher, P., Steil, R., Fydrich, T., Kuehner, C., Resick, P. A., Stiglmayr, C., Schmahl, C., & Priebe, K. (2020). Dialectical behavior therapy for posttraumatic stress disorder (DBT-PTSD) compared with cognitive processing therapy (CPT) in complex presentations of PTSD in women survivors of childhood abuse: A randomized clinical trial. *JAMA Psychiatry, 77*(12), 1235–1245. https://doi.org/10.1001/jamapsychiatry.2020.2148

Bonifas, R. P., & Napoli, M. (2014). Mindfully increasing quality of life: A promising curriculum for MSW students. *Social Work Education, 33*(4), 469–484. https://doi.org/10.1080/02615479.2013.838215

Boone, M. S. (2014). *Mindfulness and acceptance in social work: Evidence-based interventions and emerging applications* (M. S. Boone (Ed.)). New Harbinger Publications.

Bowen, S., Chawla, N., Collins, S., Witkiewitz, K., Hsu, S., Grow, J., Clifasefi, S., Garner, M., Douglass, A., Larimer, M. E., & Marlatt, G. A. (2009). Mindfulness-based relapse prevention for substance use disorders: A pilot efficacy trial. *Substance Abuse, 30*(4), 295–305. https://doi.org/10.1080/08897070903250084

Bowen, S., Chawla, N., & Marlatt, G. A. (2011). *Mindfulness-based relapse prevention for addictive behaviors: A clinician's guide* (1st ed.). The Guilford Press.

Bowen, S., Chawla, N., Grow, J., & Marlatt, G.A. (2021). *Mindfulness-based relapse prevention for addictive behaviors: A clinician's guide* (2nd ed.). The Guilford Press.

Brandsma, R. (2017). *The mindfulness teaching guide: Essential skills & competencies for Teaching mindfulness-based interventions*. New Harbinger.

Briere, J. (2013). Mindfulness, insight, and trauma therapy. In C. Germer, R. Siegel, & P. Fulton (Eds.), *Mindfulness and psychotherapy* (pp. 208–224). (2nd ed.). The Guilford Press.

Carvalho Maia, M. F., Ferreira dos Santos, B., Costa de Castro, L., Tiago Vieira, N. S., & Santos da Silveira, P. (2021). Acceptance and commitment therapy and drug use: A systematic review. *Paideia (0103863X), 31*, 1–10. https://doi.org/10.1590/1982-4327e3136

Chiesa, A., & Serretti, A. (2014). Are mindfulness-based interventions effective for substance use disorders? A systematic review of the evidence. *Substance Use & Misuse, 49*(5), 492–512. https://doi.org/10.3109/10826084.2013.770027

Chu, C.-S., Stubbs, B., Chen, T.-Y., Tang, C.-H., Li, D.-J., Yang, W.-C., Wu, C.-K., Carvalho, A. F., Vieta, E., Miklowitz, D. J., Tseng, P.-T., & Lin, P.-Y. (2018). The effectiveness of adjunct mindfulness-based intervention in treatment of bipolar disorder: A systematic review and meta-analysis. *Journal of Affective Disorders, 225*, 234–245. https://doi.org/10.1016/j.jad.2017.08.025

Coto-Lesmes, R., Fernández-Rodríguez, C., & González-Fernández, S. (2020). Acceptance and Commitment Therapy in group format for anxiety and depression. A systematic review. *Journal of Affective Disorders, 263*, 107–120. https://doi.org/10.1016/j.jad.2019.11.154

Decker, J. T., Brown, J. C., Ong, J., & Stiney-Ziskind, C. A. (2015). Mindfulness, compassion fatigue, and compassion satisfaction among social work interns. *Social Work & Christianity, 42*(1), 28–42.

Deckersbach, T., Hölzel, B., Eisner, L., Lazar, S. W., & Nierenberg, A. A. (2014). *Mindfulness-based cognitive therapy for bipolar disorder*. Guilford Press.

Didonna, F. (2019). *Mindfulness-based cognitive therapy for OCD: A treatment manual*. The Guilford Press.

Dimeff, L. A., & Linehan, M. M. (2008). Dialectical behavior therapy for substance abusers. *Addiction science & clinical practice, 4*(2), 39–47.

Dryden, W., & Still, A. (2006). Historical aspects of mindfulness and self-acceptance in psychotherapy. *Journal of Rational-Emotive & Cognitive-Behavioral Therapy, 23*(1), 3–28. https://doi.org/10.1007/s10942-006-0026-1

Eifert, G. H., & Forsyth, J. P. (2005). *Acceptance & commitment therapy for anxiety disorders: A practitioner's treatment guide to using mindfulness, acceptance, and values-based behavior change strategies*. New Harbinger Publication.

Feldman, C., & Kuyken, W. (2019). *Mindfulness: Ancient wisdom meets modern psychology*. The Guilford Press.

Fitzpatrick, S., Bailey, K., & Rizvi, S. L. (2020). Changes in emotions over the course of dialectical behavior therapy and the moderating role of depression, anxiety, and posttraumatic stress disorder. *Behavior Therapy, 51*(6), 946–957. https://doi.org/10.1016/j.beth.2019.12.009

Fletcher, L., & Hayes, S. (2005). Relational frame theory, acceptance and commitment therapy, and a functional analytic definition of mindfulness. *Journal of Rational-Emotive & Cognitive-Behavioral Therapy, 23*(4), 315–336. https://doi.org/10.1007/s10942-005-0017-7

Follette, V. M., Briere, J., Rozelle, D., Hopper, J. W., & Rome, D. I. (2015). *Mindfulness-oriented interventions for trauma: Integrating contemplative practices*. The Guilford Press.

Frankl, V. (1992). *Man's search for meaning: An introduction to logotherapy* (4th ed.). Beacon Press.

Fulton, C. L., & Cashwell, C. S. (2015). Mindfulness-based awareness and compassion: Predictors of counselor empathy and anxiety. *Counselor Education & Supervision, 54*(2), 122–133. https://doi.org/10.1002/ceas.12009

Fulton, P. R. (2013). Mindfulness as clinical training. In C. Germer, R. Siegel, & P. Fulton (Eds.), *Mindfulness and psychotherapy* (pp. 59–75). (2nd ed.). The Guilford Press.

Gach, G. (2009). *The complete idiots guide to Buddhism*. (3rd ed.). Alpha Books.

Germer, C. K. (2005). Teaching mindfulness in therapy. In C. Germer, R. Siegel, & P. Fulton (Eds.), *Mindfulness and psychotherapy* (pp. 113–129). The Guilford Press.

Germer, C. K. (2013). Mindfulness: What is it? What does it matter? In C. Germer, R. Siegel, & P. Fulton (Eds.), *Mindfulness and psychotherapy* (pp. 3–35). (2nd ed.). The Guilford Press.

Ghahari, S., Mohammadi-Hasel, K., Malakouti, S. K., & Roshanpajouh, M. (2020). Mindfulness-based cognitive therapy for Generalised anxiety disorder: A systematic review and meta-analysis. *East Asian Archives of Psychiatry, 30*(2), 52–56. https://doi.org/10.12809/eaap1885

Giannelli, E., Gold, C., Bieleninik, L., Ghetti, C., & Gelo, O. C. G. (2019). Dialectical behaviour therapy and 12-step programmes for substance use disorder: A systematic review and meta-analysis. *Counselling & Psychotherapy Research, 19*(3), 274–285. https://doi.org/10.1002/capr.12228

Gockel, A. (2015). Teaching note—practicing presence: A curriculum for integrating mindfulness training into direct practice instruction. *Journal of Social Work Education, 51*(4), 682–690. https://doi.org/10.1080/10437797.2015.1076275

Gockel, A., & Deng, X. (2016). Mindfulness training as social work pedagogy: Exploring benefits, challenges, and issues for consideration in integrating mindfulness into social work education. *Journal of Religion & Spirituality in Social Work, 35*(3), 222–244. https://doi.org/10.1080/15426432.2016.1187106

Goldberg, S. B., Tucker, R. P., Greene, P. A., Davidson, R. J., Kearney, D. J., & Simpson, T. L. (2019). Mindfulness-based cognitive therapy for the treatment of current depressive symptoms: A meta-analysis. *Cognitive Behaviour Therapy, 48*(6), 445–462. https://doi.org/10.1080/16506073.2018.1556330

Görg, N., Böhnke, J. R., Priebe, K., Rausch, S., Wekenmann, S., Ludäscher, P., Bohus, M., & Kleindienst, N. (2019). Changes in trauma-related emotions following treatment with dialectical behavior therapy for posttraumatic stress disorder after childhood abuse. *Journal of Traumatic Stress, 32*(5), 764–773. https://doi.org/10.1002/jts.22440

Grant, S., Colaiaco, B., Motala, A., Shanman, R., Booth, M., Sorbero, M., & Hempel, S. (2017). Mindfulness-based relapse prevention for substance use disorders: A systematic review and meta-analysis. *Journal of Addiction Medicine, 11*(5), 386–396. https://doi.org/10.1097/ADM.0000000000000338

Haller, H., Breilmann, P., Schröter, M., Dobos, G., & Cramer, H. (2021). A systematic review and meta-analysis of acceptance- and mindfulness-based interventions for DSM-5 anxiety disorders. *Scientific Reports, 11*(1), 1–13. https://doi.org/10.1038/s41598-021-99882-w

Harley, R., Sprich, S., Safren, S., Jacobo, M., & Fava, M. (2008). Adaptation of dialectical behavior therapy skills training group for treatment-resistant depression. *Journal of Nervous and Mental Disease, 196*(2), 136–143. https://doi.org/10.1097/NMD.0b013e318162aa3f

Harned, M. S. (2022). *Treating trauma in dialectical behavior therapy: The DBT prolonged exposure protocol (DBT PE)*. The Guilford Press.

Harned, M. S., Schmidt, S. C., Korslund, K. E., & Gallop, R. J. (2021). Does adding the dialectical behavior therapy prolonged exposure (DBT PE) protocol for PTSD to DBT improve outcomes in public mental health settings? A pilot nonrandomized effectiveness trial with benchmarking. *Behavior Therapy, 52*(3), 639–655. https://doi.org/10.1016/j.beth.2020.08.003

Hartelius, G. (2015). Body maps of attention: Phenomenal markers for two varieties of mindfulness. *Mindfulness, 6*(6), 1271–1281. https://doi.org/10.1007/s12671-015-0391-x

Harvey, P. (1990). *An introduction to Buddhism: Teachings, history and practice*. Cambridge University Press.

Hayes, S. C., Strosahl, K. D., & Wilson, K. G. (1999). *Acceptance and commitment therapy: An experiential guide to behavior change* (1st ed.). The Guilford Press.

Hayes, S. C., Strosahl, K. D., & Wilson, K. G. (2016). *Acceptance and commitment therapy: The process and practice of mindful change* (2nd ed.). The Guilford Press.

Hick, S. F., & Bien, T. (Eds.). (2008). *Mindfulness and the therapeutic relationship*. The Guilford Press.

Hodann-Caudevilla, R. M., Díaz-Silveira, C., Burgos-Julián, F. A., & Santed, M. A. (2020). Mindfulness-based interventions for people with schizophrenia: A systematic review and meta-analysis. *International Journal of Environmental Research and Public Health, 17*(13). https://doi.org/10.3390/ijerph17134690

Holt, R. W. (2018). Mindfulness-informed personal abstinence challenge and group processing. In J. Jordan, B. Perkins, & R. Lee (Eds.), *Handbook of experiential teaching in counselor education: A resource guide for counselor educators* (pp. 231–235). CreateSpace Independent Publishing.

Holt, R. W. (2019). Connecting with others: Countering social bias with a compassion-based practice. In M. Pope, M. Gonzalez, E. Cameron, & J. S. Pengelinan (Eds.), *Social justice and advocacy in counseling: Experiential activities for teaching* (pp. 342–346). Routledge/Taylor & Francis.

Holt, R. W. (2021). Mindfulness: A vehicle to pass through substance use craving and navigate the addiction recovery course. In R. Miller & E. Beeson (Eds.), *Neuroeducation: Practical translations of neuroscience in counseling and psychotherapy* (pp. 125–131). Cognella.

Ii, T., Sato, H., Watanabe, N., Kondo, M., Masuda, A., Hayes, S. C., & Akechi, T. (2019). Psychological flexibility-based interventions versus first-line psychosocial interventions for substance use disorders: Systematic review and meta-analyses of randomized controlled trials. *Journal of Contextual Behavioral Science, 13*, 109–120. https://doi.org/10.1016/j.jcbs.2019.07.003

Jansen, J. E., Gleeson, J., Bendall, S., Rice, S., & Alvarez-Jimenez, M. (2020). Acceptance- and mindfulness-based interventions for persons with psychosis: A systematic review and meta-analysis. *Schizophrenia Research, 215*, 25–37. https://doi.org/10.1016/j.schres.2019.11.016

Jasbi, M., Sadeghi Bahmani, D., Karami, G., Omidbeygi, M., Peyravi, M., Panahi, A., Mirzaee, J., Holsboer-Trachsler, E., & Brand, S. (2018). Influence of adjuvant mindfulness-based cognitive therapy (MBCT) on symptoms of post-traumatic stress disorder (PTSD) in veterans - results from a randomized control study. *Cognitive Behaviour Therapy, 47*(5), 431–446. https://doi.org/10.1080/16506073.2018.1445773

Kabat-Zinn, J. (1990). *Full catastrophe living*. Delacorte Press.

Kabat-Zinn, J. (2003). Mindfulness-based interventions in context: Past, present, and future. *Clinical Psychology: Science and Practice, 10*, 144–156. https://doi.org/10.1093/clipsy/bpg016

Kabat-Zinn, J. (2013). *Full catastrophe living: Using the wisdom of your body and mind to face stress, pain, and illness*. Bantam.

King, A. P., Erickson, T. M., Giardino, N. D., Favorite, T., Rauch, S. A. M., Robinson, E., Kulkarni, M., & Liberzon, I. (2013). A Pilot Study of Group Mindfulness-Based Cognitive Therapy (Mbct) for Combat Veterans with Posttraumatic Stress Disorder (Ptsd). *Depression & Anxiety (1091–4269), 30*(7), 638–645. https://doi.org/10.1002/da.22104

Kostanski, M., & Hassed, C. (2008). Mindfulness as a concept and a process. *Australian Psychologist, 43*(1), 15–21. https://doi.org/10.1080/00050060701593942

Krafft, J., Petersen, J. M., & Twohig, M. P. (2022). Acceptance and commitment therapy for obsessive-compulsive and related disorders. In E. A. Storch, J. S. Abramowitz, & D. McKay (Eds.), *Complexities in obsessive-compulsive and related disorders: Advances in conceptualization and treatment.* (pp. 352–369). Oxford University Press. https://doi.org/10.1093/med-psych/9780190052775.003.0019

Külz, A. K., Landmann, S., Cludius, B., Rose, N., Heidenreich, T., Jelinek, L., Alsleben, H., Wahl, K., Philipsen, A., Voderholzer, U., Maier, J. G., & Moritz, S. (2019). Mindfulness-based cognitive therapy (MBCT) in patients with obsessive-compulsive disorder (OCD) and residual symptoms after cognitive behavioral therapy (CBT): A randomized controlled trial. *European Archives of Psychiatry and Clinical Neuroscience, 269*(2), 223–233. https://doi.org/10.1007/s00406-018-0957-4

Lee, E. B., An, W., Levin, M. E., & Twohig, M. P. (2015). An initial meta-analysis of acceptance and commitment therapy for treating substance use disorders. *Drug and Alcohol Dependence, 155*, 1–7. https://doi.org/10.1016/j.drugalcdep.2015.08.004

Lee, J. J., & Himmelheber, S. A. (2016). Field education in the present moment: Evaluating a 14-week pedagogical model to increase mindfulness practice. *Journal of Social Work Education, 52*(4), 473–483. https://doi.org/10.1080/10437797.2016.1215274

Lee, N. K., Cameron, J., & Jenner, L. (2015). A systematic review of interventions for co-occurring substance use and borderline personality disorders. *Drug & Alcohol Review, 34*(6), 663–672. https://doi.org/10.1111/dar.12267

Lenz, A. S., Hall, J., & Bailey Smith, L. (2016). Meta-analysis of group mindfulness-based cognitive therapy for decreasing symptoms of acute depression. *Journal for Specialists in Group Work, 41*(1), 44–70. https://doi.org/10.1080/01933922.2015.1111488

Li, Y., Coster, S., Norman, I., Chien, W. T., Qin, J., Ling Tse, M., & Bressington, D. (2021). Feasibility, acceptability, and preliminary effectiveness of mindfulness-based interventions for people with recent-onset psychosis: A systematic review. *Early Intervention in Psychiatry, 15*(1), 3–15. https://doi.org/10.1111/eip.12929

Linehan, M. M. (1993). *Cognitive-behavioral treatment of borderline personality disorder*. The Guilford Press.

Liu, X., Yi, P., Ma, L., Liu, W., Deng, W., Yang, X., Liang, M., Luo, J., Li, N., & Li, X. (2021). Mindfulness-based interventions for social anxiety disorder: A systematic review and meta-analysis. *Psychiatry Research, 300*, N.PAG. https://doi.org/10.1016/j.psychres.2021.113935

Lovas, D. A., & Schuman-Olivier, Z. (2018). Mindfulness-based cognitive therapy for bipolar disorder: A systematic review. *Journal of Affective Disorders, 240*, 247–261. https://doi.org/10.1016/j.jad.2018.06.017

Luoma, J. B., Hayes, S. C., & Walser, R. D. (2017). *Learning ACT: An acceptance & commitment Therapy skills training manual for therapists* (2nd ed.). Context Press.

Marra, T. (2005). *Dialectical Behavior Therapy in private practice: A practical and comprehensive guide*. New Harbinger Publications.

Mathur, S., Sharma, M. P., Balachander, S., Kandavel, T., & Reddy, Y. C. J. (2021). A randomized controlled trial of mindfulness-based cognitive therapy vs stress management training for obsessive-compulsive disorder. *Journal of Affective Disorders, 282*, 58–68. https://doi.org/10.1016/j.jad.2020.12.082

McCown, D., Reibel, D., & Micozzi, M. S. (2011). *Teaching mindfulness: A practical guide for clinicians and educators*. Springer.

Meyer, E. C., Walser, R., Hermann, B., Bash, H., DeBeer, B. B., Morissette, S. B., Kimbrel, N. A., Kwok, O., Batten, S. V., Schnurr, P. P., La Bash, H., & Kwok, O.-M. (2018). Acceptance and commitment therapy for co-occurring posttraumatic stress disorder and alcohol use disorders in veterans: Pilot treatment outcomes. *Journal of Traumatic Stress, 31*(5), 781–789. https://doi.org/10.1002/jts.22322

Miller, W., & Thoresen, C. (1999). Spirituality and health. In W. Miller (Ed.), *Integrating spirituality into treatment* (pp. 3–18). American Psychological Association.

Morgan, S. P. (2013). Practical ethics. In C. Germer, R. Siegel, & P. Fulton (Eds.), *Mindfulness and psychotherapy* (pp. 112–132). (2nd ed.). The Guilford Press.

Mulligan, B. A. (2017). *The dharma of modern mindfulness: Discovering the Buddhist teachings at the heart of mindfulness-based stress reduction*. New Harbinger Publications.

Norton, A. R., Abbott, M. J., Norberg, M. M., & Hunt, C. (2015). A systematic review of mindfulness and acceptance-based treatments for social anxiety disorder. *Journal of Clinical Psychology, 71*(4), 283–301. https://doi.org/10.1002/jclp.22144

O'Donoghue, E. K., Morris, E. M. J., Oliver, J. E., & Johns, L. C. (2018). *ACT for psychosis recovery: A practical manual for group-based interventions using acceptance and commitment therapy*. Context Press/New Harbinger Publications.

Orsillo, S. M., & Roemer, M. (2011). *The mindful way through anxiety: Break free from chronic worry and reclaim your life*. The Guilford Press.

Pattakos, A. (2010). *Prisoners of our thoughts: Victor Frankl's principles for discovering meaning in life and work* (2nd ed.). Berrett-Koehler Publishers.

Paulson, J. (2018). Developing competence with mindfulness-based interventions: Guidelines for clinical social workers. *Journal of Sociology and Social Work, 6*(1), 1–6.

Pederson, L. D. (2015). *Dialectical behavior therapy: A contemporary guide for practitioners*. Wiley Blackwell.

Phillips, M. A., Chase, T., Bautista, C., Tang, A., & Teng, E. J. (2020). Using acceptance and commitment therapy techniques to enhance treatment engagement in veterans with posttraumatic stress disorder. *Bulletin of the Menninger Clinic, 84*(3), 264–277. https://doi.org/10.1521/bumc.2020.84.3.264

Piet, J., Fjorback, L., & Santorelli, S. (2015). What is required to teach mindfulness effectively in MBSR and MBCT? In E. Shonin, W. V. Gordon & M. D. Griffiths (Eds.), *Mindfulness and Buddhist-derived approaches in mental health and addiction* (pp. 61–83). Springer.

Platter, B. K., & Cabral, O. (2012). *Integrating dialectical behavior therapy with the Twelve Steps: A program for treating substance use disorders*. Hazelden.

Pollak, S. M. (2013). Teaching mindfulness in therapy. In C. Germer, R. Siegel, & P. Fulton (Eds.), *Mindfulness and psychotherapy* (pp. 133–147). (2nd ed.). The Guilford Press.

Pollak, S. M., Pedulla, T., & Siegel, R. D. (2014). *Sitting together: Essential skills for mindfulness-based psychotherapy*. The Guilford Press.

Praissman, S. (2008). Mindfulness-based stress reduction: A literature review and clinician's guide. *Journal of the American Academy of Nurse Practitioners*, 20(4), 212–216. https://doi.org/10.1111/j.1745-7599.2008.00306.x

Ramadas, E., Lima, M. P. de, Caetano, T., Lopes, J., & Dixe, M. dos A. (2021). Effectiveness of mindfulness-based relapse prevention in individuals with substance use disorders: A systematic review. *Behavioral Sciences (2076-328X)*, 11(10), 133. https://doi.org/10.3390/bs11100133

Recovery Dharma. (n.d.). *Recovery Dharma: Using Buddhist practices and principles to recover from addiction*. https://recoverydharma.org/

Refuge Recovery. (n.d.) *Refuge Recovery: A Buddhist path to recovering from addiction*. https://www.refugerecovery.org/

Reilly, B. (2016). Mindfulness infusion through CACREP standards. *Journal of Creativity in Mental Health*, 11(2), 213–224. https://doi.org/10.1080/15401383.2016.1139482

Rizvi, S., Welch, S., & Dimidjian, S. (2009). Mindfulness and borderline personality disorder. In F. Didonna (Ed.), *Clinical handbook of mindfulness* (pp. 245–257). Springer.

Rosenbaum, R. M., & Magid, B. (2016). *What's wrong with mindfulness and what isn't: Zen perspectives*. Wisdom Publications.

Rubin, J. (1996). *Psychotherapy and Buddhism*. Plenum Press.

Sancho, M., De Gracia, M., Rodríguez, R. C., Mallorquí-Bagué, N., Sánchez-González, J., Trujols, J., Sánchez, I., Jiménez-Murcia, S., & Menchón, J. M. (2018). Mindfulness-based interventions for the treatment of substance and behavioral addictions: A systematic review. *Frontiers in Psychiatry*, 9. https://doi.org/10.3389/fpsyt.2018.00095

Sears, R. W. (2014). *Mindfulness: Living through challenges and enriching your life in this moment*. Wiley Blackwell.

Sears, R. W. (2015). *Building competence in mindfulness-based cognitive therapy: Transcripts and insights for working with stress, anxiety, depression, and other problems*. Routledge.

Sears, R. W. (2021). *Myths of mindfulness*. Sequoia Books.

Sears, R. W., & Chard, K. M. (2016). *Mindfulness-based cognitive therapy for posttraumatic stress disorder*. Wiley Blackwell.

Segal, Z., Williams, J., & Teasdale, J. (2002). *Mindfulness-based cognitive therapy for depression: A new approach to prevent relapse* (1st ed.). The Guilford Press.

Segal, Z., Williams, M., & Teasdale, J. (2018). *Mindfulness-based cognitive therapy for depression* (2nd ed.). The Guilford Press.

Selchen, S., Hawley, L. L., Regev, R., Richter, P., & Rector, N. A. (2018). Mindfulness-based cognitive therapy for OCD: Stand-alone and post-CBT augmentation approaches. *International Journal of Cognitive Therapy*, 11(1), 58–79. https://doi.org/10.1007/s41811-018-0003-3

Shapiro, S., & Carlson, L. (2009). *The art and science of mindfulness*. American Psychological Association.

Shapiro, S., Astin, J., Bishop, S., & Cordova, M. (2005). Mindfulness-based stress reduction for health care professionals: Results from a randomized trial. *International Journal of Stress Management*, 12(2), 164–176. https://doi.org/10.1037/1072-5245.12.2.164

Siegel, R., Germer, C., & Olendzki, A. (2009). Mindfulness: What is it? Where did it come from? In F. Didonna (Ed.), *Clinical handbook of mindfulness* (pp. 17–35). Springer.

Stahl, B., & Goldstein, E. (2019). *A mindfulness-based stress reduction workbook* (2nd ed.). New Harbinger.

Swain, J., Hancock, K., Hainsworth, C., & Bowman, J. (2013). Acceptance and commitment therapy in the treatment of anxiety: A systematic review. *Clinical Psychology Review*, 33(8), 965–978. https://doi.org/10.1016/j.cpr.2013.07.002

Teasdale, J., Williams, M., & Segal, Z. (2014). *The mindful way workbook: An eight-week program to free yourself from depression and emotional distress*. The Guilford Press.

Teasdale, J., Williams, M., Soulsby, J., Segal, Z., Ridgeway, V., & Lau, M. (2000). Prevention of relapse/recurrent in major depression by mindfulness-based cognitive therapy. *Journal of Consulting and Clinical Psychology*, 68(4), 615–623. https://doi.org/10.1037/0022-006X.68.4.615

Testa, D., & Sangganjanavanich, V. F. (2016). Contribution of mindfulness and emotional intelligence to burnout among counseling interns. *Counselor Education & Supervision*, 55(2), 95–108. https://doi.org/10.1002/ceas.12035

Thimm, J. C., & Johnsen, T. J. (2020). Time trends in the effects of mindfulness-based cognitive therapy for depression: A meta-analysis. *Scandinavian Journal of Psychology, 61*(4), 582–591. https://doi.org/10.1111/sjop.12642

Thomas, J. T. (2017). Brief mindfulness training in the social work practice classroom. *Social Work Education, 36*(1), 102–118. https://doi.org/10.1080/02615479.2016.1250878

Tirch, D., Silberstein, L. R., & Kolts, R. L. (2016). *Buddhist psychology and cognitive-behavioral therapy: A clinician's guide.* The Guilford Press.

Treleaven, D. A. (2018). *Trauma-sensitive mindfulness: Practices for safe and transformative healing.* W. W. Norton & Company.

Treleaven, D. A. (2022a). *What experts are saying about trauma-sensitive mindfulness (TSM).* David Treleaven. Retrieved June 30, 2022, from https://davidtreleaven.com/.

Treleaven, D. A. (2022b). *The complete trauma-sensitive mindfulness training: A two-part comprehensive program designed for mindfulness practitioners.* David Treleaven. Retrieved June 30, 2022, from https://davidtreleaven.com/online-training/

Vadivale, A. M, & Sathiyaseelan, A. (2019). Mindfulness-based relapse prevention: A meta-analysis. *Cogent Psychology, 6,* Article: 1567090. https://doi.org/10.1080/23311908.2019.1567090

Van Dam, N. T., van Vugt, M. K., Vago, D. R., Schmalzl, L., Saron, C. D., Olendzki, A., Meissner, T., Lazar, S. W., Kerr, C. E., Gorchov, J., Fox, K. C. R., Field, B. A., Britton, W. B., Brefczynski-Lewis, J. A., & Meyer, D. E. (2018). Mind the hype: A critical evaluation and prescriptive agenda for research on mindfulness and meditation. *Perspectives on Psychological Science, 13*(1), 36–61. https://doi.org/10.1177/1745691617709589

Van Dijk, S. (2012). *DBT made simple: A step-by-step guide to dialectical behavior therapy.* New Harbinger.

Van Dijk, S., Jeffrey, J., & Katz, M. R. (2013). A randomized, controlled, pilot study of dialectical behavior therapy skills in a psychoeducational group for individuals with bipolar disorder. *Journal of Affective Disorders, 145*(3), 386–393. https://doi.org/10.1016/j.jad.2012.05.054

Walser, R., & Westrup, D. (2007). *Acceptance & commitment therapy for the treatment of post-traumatic stress disorder & trauma-related problems: A practitioner's guide to using mindfulness & acceptance strategies.* New Harbinger Publications.

Warner, N., & Murphy, M. (2022). Dialectical behaviour therapy skills training for individuals with substance use disorder: A systematic review. *Drug and Alcohol Review, 41*(2), 501–516. https://doi.org/10.1111/dar.13362

Welch, S. S., Osborne, T. L., & Pryzgoda, J. (2010). Augmenting exposure-based treatment for anxiety disorders with principles and skills from dialectical behavior therapy. In D. Sookman & R. L. Leahy (Eds.), *Treatment resistant anxiety disorders: Resolving impasses to symptom remission.* (pp. 161–197). Routledge/Taylor & Francis Group.

Witkiewitz, K., Marlatt, G. A., & Walker, D. (2005). Mindfulness-based relapse prevention for alcohol and substance use disorders. *Journal of Cognitive Psychotherapy: An International Quarterly, 19*(3), 211–228. https://doi.org/10.1891/jcop.2005.19.3.211

Xuan, R., Li, X., Qiao, Y., Guo, Q., Liu, X., Deng, W., Hu, Q., Wang, K., & Zhang, L. (2020). Mindfulness-based cognitive therapy for bipolar disorder: A systematic review and meta-analysis. *Psychiatry Research, 290,* N.PAG. https://doi.org/10.1016/j.psychres.2020.113116

Yahne, C., & Miller, W. (1999). Evoking hope. In W. Miller (Ed.), *Integrating spirituality into treatment* (pp. 217–233). American Psychological Association.

Yildiz, E. (2020). The effects of acceptance and commitment therapy in psychosis treatment: A systematic review of randomized controlled trials. *Perspectives in Psychiatric Care, 56*(1), 149–167. https://doi.org/10.1111/ppc.12396

Yoga Twelve-Step Recovery. (n.d.). *Y12SR: Sustainable Recovery.* https://y12sr.com/#

Zettle, R. D. (2007). *ACT for depression: A clinician's guide to using acceptance and commitment therapy in treating depression.* New Harbinger Publications.

SECTION III

DIAGNOSTIC CONSIDERATIONS

CHAPTER 9

CO-OCCURRING DEPRESSIVE AND SUBSTANCE USE DISORDERS

SARA W. BAILEY

LEARNING OBJECTIVES

After reading this chapter, you will be able to:
- Describe *Diagnostic and Statistical Manual of Mental Disorders, Fifth Edition* (*DSM-5*; American Psychiatric Association) diagnostic criteria for depressive disorders and substance use disorders (SUDs).
- Identify the similarities and differences between diagnostic criteria for depressive disorders and SUDs.
- Apply holistic assessment and diagnosis protocols for co-occurring depressive and substance use disorders.
- Recognize the influence of cultural identities on diagnosis, treatment, and outcomes for clients who live with co-occurring depressive and substance use disorders.

INTRODUCTION

People travel through life like ships sailing on a mercurial sea: We voyage through calm waters, gentle swells, powerful tides, and savage gales. While navigating our voyage, we utilize various resources that are available to us. Those resources may provide a stabilizing ballast (e.g., mindfulness, connection with others) when in challenging waters or threaten our safe passage (e.g., risky substance use) through turbulent seas. When safe passage is threatened, occasional feelings of sadness, disinterest, and depressed mood are not uncommon in response to life's challenges, and, for most individuals, substance use does not result in disordered use. However, when coping mechanisms are either insufficient to match the need for solace or begin to endanger wellness, a situational response to distress may lead to debilitating and life-threatening storms of depression and substance use disorders.

DEPRESSIVE DISORDERS: *DSM-5* DIAGNOSTIC CRITERIA AND DESCRIPTION

Minor, transient emotional upsets resulting from situational inconveniences (e.g., spilling coffee in the car, running late to work) are part of the human experience. Clinically significant depression, however, lingers and represents marked distress and disruption to normal function. The constellation of depressive symptoms includes low mood, disinterest, irritability, somatic (body-oriented) symptoms, and thoughts of suicide (American Psychiatric Association [APA], 2013). Diagnostic criteria for all the *Diagnostic and Statistical Manual of Mental Disorders, Fifth Edition* (*DSM-5*; APA, 2013) depressive disorders (often described as mood disorders) include feelings of sadness, irritability, or emptiness, *and* somatic and cognitive changes leading to disruptions in normal functioning.

DISRUPTIVE MOOD DYSREGULATION DISORDER

The addition of disruptive mood dysregulation disorder to the *DSM-5* represented a new diagnosis (APA, 2013) in response to concerns that children up to 12 years of age were being misdiagnosed with bipolar disorder. Diagnostic criteria for disruptive mood dysregulation disorder include severe, recurrent outbursts of temper inconsistent with age-related development that occur three or more times a week on average. For diagnosis, these outbursts must have begun before the age of 10; must have been present for 12 or more months, with no periods of 3 consecutive months or more without outbursts; and severe irritability must be present most days, and is clearly noticeable by others (APA, 2013).

MAJOR DEPRESSIVE DISORDER

Depression is ubiquitous. One in five people is likely to experience at least one episode of major depressive disorder (MDD) during their lifetime (Hasin et al., 2018). With a diagnosis of MDD using *DSM-5* criteria (APA, 2013), symptoms are persistent (lasting 2 or more weeks) and distressing, representing a departure from normal functioning. In addition to depressed mood and/or loss of interest or pleasure, diagnostic criteria include a minimum of four (out of nine) additional symptoms (e.g., sleep disturbance, feelings of guilt, suicidal ideation).

Those living with MDD are at increased risk for suicide; approximately 14% of those diagnosed with MDD have attempted suicide at least once, and as many as 46.7% of those experiencing MDD reported wanting to die while experiencing a depressive episode (Hasin et al., 2018).

PERSISTENT DEPRESSIVE DISORDER

Also known as dysthymia, diagnosis of persistent depressive disorder (PDD) in adults is appropriate when depressive symptoms have been unrelenting for a period of 2 years or more (1 year or more for children and adolescents). PDD may be preceded by major depression, and those with a PDD diagnosis are more likely to develop MDD. Compared to MDD, a diagnosis of PDD is associated with a higher risk for substance use disorders (SUDs), anxiety disorders, and other psychiatric disorders (APA, 2013).

PREMENSTRUAL DYSPHORIC DISORDER

Affecting approximately 2% to 6% of menstruating women annually, premenstrual dysphoric disorder (PMDD) is notable in its presentation with symptoms developing during the days preceding menses and relenting around the time menses begins (APA, 2013). Diagnosis of PMDD requires the presence of symptoms (e.g., irritability, mood lability) during most menstrual cycles during the past year, and, as with other depressive disorder diagnoses, symptoms must be significant enough to disrupt functioning (APA, 2013). Premenstrual symptoms may be treated

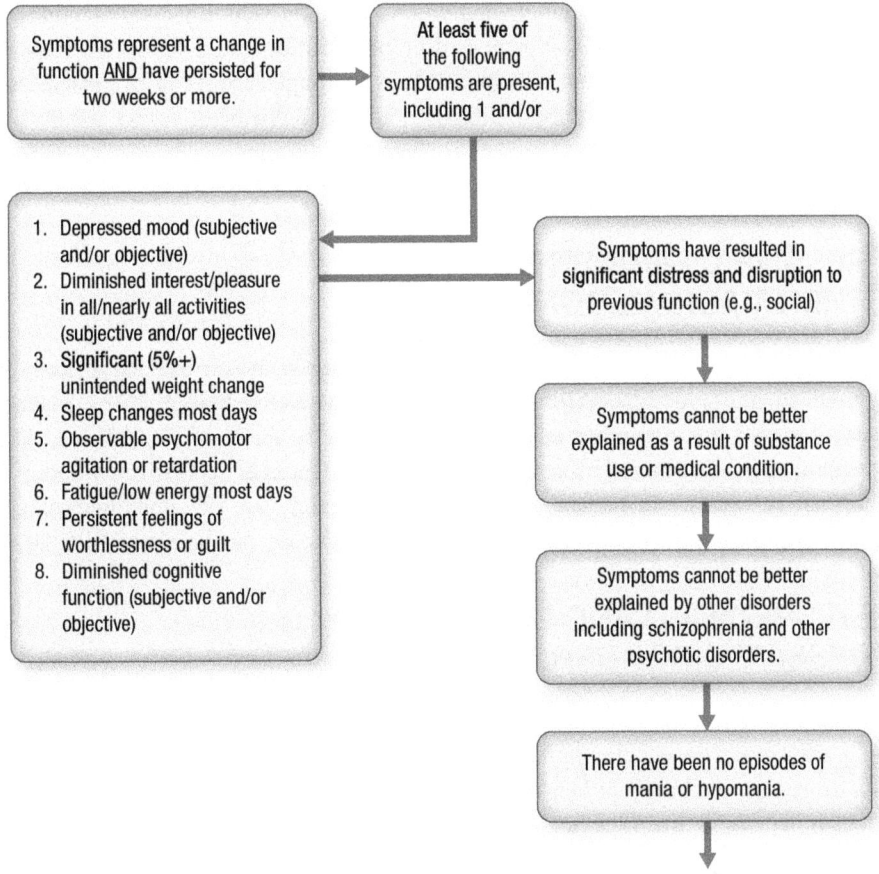

SEVERITY/COURSE SPECIFIER

Mild: little more than minimum symptom required to diagnose; manageable distress; minor impairment
Moderate: number of symptoms, symptom intensity, and impairment between "mild" and "severe"
Severe: greater number of symptoms; symptom intensity is unmanageable; marked interference with functioning
Partial remission: either full diagnostic criteria are no longer met or a period <2 months without significant symptoms from previous depressive episode
Full remission: no significant symptoms for the past 2+ months

When recording diagnosis, specify (in order) if single or recurrent episode, severity/psychotic remission spcifiers, and any additional specifiers (with: anxious distress, mixed features, melancholic features, atypical features, mood-congruent psychotic features, mood-incongruent psychotic features, catatonia, peripartum onset, season pattern).

FIGURE 9.1 Diagnostic Criteria for Major Depressive Disorder.
Source: *Diagnostic and Statistical Manual of Mental Disorders, Fifth Edition* (DSM-5; American Psychiatric Association, 2013, pp. 160–162).

with exogenous hormones (Hantsoo & Epperson, 2015). When depressive symptoms develop in conjunction with such treatment, a diagnosis of substance-/medication-induced depressive disorder may be appropriate (APA, 2013).

SUBSTANCE-/MEDICATION-INDUCED DEPRESSIVE DISORDER

A diagnosis of substance-/medication-induced depressive disorder is made when depressive symptoms can be directly tied to substance/medication use, develop within 1 month of substance/medication use, and persist beyond the physiologic effects of a substance/medication (APA,

2013). For this diagnosis, the substance/medication being ingested, injected, or inhaled must be capable of producing symptoms of depressed mood and must cause significant reduction in interest and pleasure in most activities (APA, 2013). A thorough account of *all* substances being taken (e.g., over the counter, prescription, illicit), a clear timeline of substance/medication use and symptoms, and a keen understanding of the effects of substances/medications being taken is critical in determining this diagnosis.

DEPRESSIVE DISORDER DUE TO ANOTHER MEDICAL CONDITION

Depressive symptoms may also arise from a medical condition such as stroke, Parkinson's disease, hypothyroidism, and traumatic brain injury (APA, 2013; McKee & Brahm, 2016). Diagnosis of depressive disorder due to another medical condition may be made when there is a clear link between physical changes caused by a medical condition and onset of depressive symptoms (APA, 2013). If there is evidence to suggest that depressive symptoms are explained by both another medical condition and substance/medication use, both diagnoses may be given (APA, 2013).

OTHER SPECIFIED AND UNSPECIFIED DEPRESSIVE DISORDERS

Primary differences among the various depressive disorders have to do with timing of *symptom onset* (e.g., PMDD); *duration of symptoms* (e.g., PDD); and *etiology* (e.g., substance/medication-induced depressive disorder). When client's symptoms fail to meet the specific criteria for a particular depressive disorder, a diagnosis of "other specified depressive disorder" (e.g., short-duration depressive episode, recurrent brief episode) or "unspecified depressive disorder" (e.g., when there is insufficient information for a more thorough assessment) may be made. There are seven additional specifiers, including *with anxious distress* and *with atypical features*, that may be included to clarify diagnosis (Figure 9.1).

For all depressive disorders, including those deemed as unspecified, proper assessment and diagnosis are essential first steps for counselors to intervene effectively. When a depressive disorder is accompanied by a co-occurring SUD, the potential for negative outcomes increases. Careful assessment of clients for co-occurring symptoms of depression and substance use affords them the best chance for improved functioning.

SUBSTANCE USE DISORDERS: *DSM-5* DIAGNOSTIC CRITERIA AND DESCRIPTION

Although a diagnosis of SUD is substance specific, shared diagnostic criteria across all 10 SUDs in the *DSM-5* (APA, 2013) include: (a) taking the substance more frequently or in greater amounts than intended, (b) an unsuccessful desire to reduce or eliminate substance use, and (c) continued substance use despite psychosocial consequences. As with depressive disorders, for a diagnosis of a SUD, symptoms must be distressing enough to affect normal functioning.

Both depressive disorders and SUDs are characterized as *mild*, *moderate*, or *severe*, depending on number of symptoms and intensity of distress for depressive disorders and number of diagnostic criteria with SUDs. Even when full diagnostic criteria for a co-occurring depressive disorder and SUD are unmet, clients who present to counseling with subclinical depressive symptoms and co-occurring *risky* substance use/substance misuse (such as using illicit drugs and/or binge drinking) represent an opportunity for encouraging reduction or cessation of substance use (known as *secondary prevention*) for those already engaged in it (Centers for Disease Control and Prevention [CDC], 2021a; Daniels-Witt et al., 2017). By addressing potential risks to health and well-being related to depressive symptoms and/or problematic substance use, counselors may inspire clients to modify current lifestyle factors to reduce the likelihood of devastating outcomes.

PREVALENCE, STATISTICS, AND DEMOGRAPHICS

ADULTS

Culturally sensitive counselors must seek to understand their clients in context, considering their clients' constellation of cultural identities and recognizing the interrelatedness and prevalence of depression, substance use, and SUDs across various populations. Between 2017 and 2018 in the United States, approximately 7.2% of adults aged 18 or older experienced one or more major depressive episodes (2 or more weeks of depressed mood/disinterest, coupled with additional *DSM-5* diagnostic criteria for any depressive disorder); of this group, 64% experienced severe impairment (Substance Abuse and Mental Health Services Administration [SAMHSA], 2019). Prevalence was higher for individuals between the ages of 18 and 25, those reporting two or more races, and for females (SAMHSA, 2019). The lifetime prevalence of MDD is nearly 21%, with females reporting depressive symptoms at a rate 1.5 times that of males (Hasin et al., 2018).

During the same period, between 2017 and 2018, approximately 8.4% of adults aged 18 or older in the United States had a SUD (SAMHSA, 2020a). Across all populations, disordered alcohol use remains the most prevalent of substance use concerns (SAMHSA, 2019, 2020c). In 2018, approximately 5.4% of the population 12 years or older in the United States had an alcohol use disorder (AUD), compared to approximately 3% of those with any other SUD (SAMHSA, 2019).

In 2019, prior to the COVID-19 pandemic, approximately 18.5% of adults in the United States reported experiencing depressive symptoms; some reporting experiencing mild depressive symptoms that failed to meet diagnostic criteria, and others reporting more severe depressive symptoms (Villarroel & Terlizzi, 2020). According to the National Center for Health Statistics, between April 2020 and March 2021, rates of reported depression in the United States were positively correlated ($r = .92$) with rates of COVID-19 cases, ranging from 23.5% to 30.2% of respondents reporting depressive symptoms in the 7 days prior to survey response (CDC, 2021b). Counselors must attend to an array of contextual factors, including geopolitical shifts such as the COVID-19 pandemic, when assessing and counseling their clients.

Across populations, SUDs are highly comorbid with depressive disorders (National Institute on Drug Abuse [NIDA], 2020; Szaflarski et al., 2017). In 2018, 21% of adults who had a SUD also experienced a major depressive episode (SAMHSA, 2019). Of those with a *lifetime* diagnosis of MDD, approximately 57% also experienced a SUD (Hasin et al., 2018). There appear to be higher rates of co-occurring depressive and SUDs for those born in the United States compared to those who immigrated to the United States who share similar cultural/national heritage backgrounds (Szaflarski et al., 2017). There appears to be a greater prevalence of depression for non-Hispanic Black (9.2%), non-Hispanic White (7.9%), and Hispanic (8.2%) individuals compared to non-Hispanic Asian (3.1%) individuals (Brody et al., 2018). Members of American Indian and Native Alaskan communities, and those who report two or more races, appear to be especially burdened by SUDs (16.1% and 11.9%, respectively) compared to White individuals (7.5%; Lynch et al., 2019). Despite the paucity of research addressing the needs of people within the LGBTQ+ community, risk for depression and SUDs for this population appears to be between double and quadruple that of their cisgender, heterosexual peers (Wanta et al., 2019).

ADOLESCENTS

Between 2017 and 2018 in the United States, approximately 13.3% of adolescents between 12 and 17 years of age experienced one or more major depressive episodes (MDEs; 2 or more weeks of depressed mood/disinterest, coupled with additional *DSM-5* diagnostic criteria for any depressive disorder); of this group, 71% experienced severe impairment (SAMHSA, 2019). During the same period, approximately 3.8% of adolescents between 12 and 17 had a SUD (SAMHSA, 2020a). In 2018, compared to adolescents who did not experience an MDE in the previous year, those who did were more likely to use illicit drugs (32.7% vs. 14%), smoke cigarettes (6.1% vs. 2.1%), or engage in binge drinking (8.5% vs. 4.1%; SAMHSA, 2019). In 2018, approximately 1.5% of adolescents between 12 and 17 had a co-occurring MDE and SUD (SAMHSA, 2019).

There appear to be some overlapping risk factors for depressive disorders and SUDs, including genetic vulnerability, temperament, the presence of other mental health disorders, and exposure to trauma (NIDA, 2020). Notably, higher numbers of adverse childhood experiences (ACEs; e.g., psychological, physical, sexual abuse; substance abuse in household; incarceration of household members) have been correlated with exponentially higher risk of negative outcomes (CDC, 2019; McDonald, 2020). There is a graded dose/response relationship between the number of ACEs and the risk for SUDs, depression, and suicide attempts in adolescents and adults (CDC, 2019; Felitti et al., 1998). Exposure to ACEs can threaten a child's sense of stability and safety, and can disrupt neurodevelopment, leading to impairment of social, cognitive, and emotional development (CDC, 2019).

Counselors must be especially attuned for depressive symptoms and substance use in their adolescent clients. *Primary prevention* for co-occurring depressive and SUDs involves increasing awareness of the risks of depressive disorders and SUDs in their clients before such disorders develop (Daniels-Witt et al., 2017). This may include screening for depression and substance use in children and adolescents, even before evidence of depression or substance use emerges. Early primary prevention strategies are potentially life-saving. Untreated depression in those under the age of 18 may contribute to development of SUDs (Kessler et al., 2007), and the risks of adolescent substance use are especially grave. For example, those who start drinking alcohol before their 15th birthday are as much as five times more likely to develop an AUD than those who wait until young adulthood to start drinking (CDC, 2020). In addition to sharing psychoeducation with their younger clients, by normalizing conversations about mental health, specifically depression and substance use, counselors offer adolescent clients the chance to build awareness and to develop health-promoting strategies that may last well into their adult years (CDC, 2020).

OVERLAPPING RISKS, GREATER SEVERITY, AND POORER OUTCOMES

Co-occurring depressive disorders and SUDs are linked with increased severity and poorer outcomes, including risk for suicide, other psychiatric disorders, and disordered functioning. Although the bidirectional relationship between SUDs and depressive symptoms may complicate a counselor's diagnostic strategies and treatment approaches, counselors must expect, assess for, and treat co-occurring depressive disorders and SUDs in their clients. Tragically, almost half of adults aged 18 or older diagnosed with a co-occurring depressive and SUD receive *no* treatment (SAMHSA, 2020b).

ASSESSMENT AND DIAGNOSTIC CONSIDERATIONS

Clients living with a co-occurring depressive disorder and a SUD present with diverse histories, cultural identities, and symptom severity. A combination of biological and environmental factors may predict greater *likelihood* for developing depression and using substances, but ultimately, holistic, multidimensional assessments (rather than algorithms), provide clients with the best care. A holistic, multidimensional assessment of a client's depression and substance use will likely involve both *formal* and *informal* tools and procedures occurring throughout the therapeutic relationship, from the intake session to conclusion of services. A wellness-based, comprehensive approach to assessment and diagnosis recognizes life satisfaction as dynamic and multidimensional, involving physical, emotional, spiritual, social, occupational, environmental, financial, and intellectual factors (Swarbrick, 2006). The American Society of Addiction Medicine (ASAM) Criteria (Mee-Lee et al., 2013) offers a useful framework for planning and conducting a comprehensive biopsychosocial assessment across six dimensions of wellness and may be especially useful for counselors' assessment of clients with co-occurring depressive disorders and SUDs (Drymalski & Nunley, 2018). Additionally, assessing a client's stage of change (Prochaska & Velicer, 1997) allows counselors to better match treatment with the needs of each individual.

ESTABLISHING THE CLIENT/COUNSELOR RELATIONSHIP

Person-centered assessment and diagnosis support client autonomy and elicit client engagement and growth. For person-centered, culturally sensitive counselors, standard intake forms are fashioned with cultural sensitivity and use accessible language, therefore serving as a bridge between the client and the counselor. Initial demographics forms and assessment tools can be useful in informing a more comprehensive, engaging interview, but the most critical step in any counseling relationship begins with client/counselor connection, whether in an office or virtually (i.e., telebehavioral health). Rapport building, counselor empathy, humility, and authenticity demonstrate a counselor's sincere interest in their client. By attending, gently inquiring, inviting clients to speak their truth and tell their story *their way* without oppressive directives, boundaries, or shame, counselors co-create a collaborative therapeutic environment.

STRUCTURING THE INTAKE

Recognizing the possibility of co-occurring depressive disorders and SUDs in their clients, counselors engage in thorough assessment procedures for both, including formal depression and substance use screening tools within the intake paperwork. Tucked between the medical history and insurance information forms, such instruments may seem rather mundane to clients filling out required forms. Inclusion of these assessment instruments into standard paperwork helps introduce and normalize conversations about mental health and substance use; counselors can also use these tools to inform further assessment.

Once initial paperwork is completed, counselors can use the information as a point of reference, continuing to assess their clients by inviting them to describe themselves, their current mood, and their primary goals for treatment. Counselors must assess their client for current safety (e.g., suicide, risk of violence toward others) and, if needed, enlist additional collateral resources (e.g., supportive family members, other healthcare professionals) to support the safety of their clients and those around them. Inviting clients to describe their current and past depressive symptoms and substance use helps inform the counselor's *and* the client's understanding of the relationship between substance use and depressive symptoms. Open-ended invitations (e.g., "*Describe your mood ... Tell me about a time when you had thoughts of suicide ... Talk to me about your substance use*"), rather than a binary approach (e.g., "*Are you depressed? ... Are you having thoughts of suicide? ... Do you drink or use drugs?*") communicate to the client that there is no "right" or "wrong" answer to the counselor's inquiries.

EXAMINING THE ETIOLOGY AND SORTING THROUGH THE SYMPTOMS

Depressive and SUD symptoms are often interrelated. As clients seek respite from distress, they may feel stuck in a feedback loop of depressive symptoms, substance use to alleviate those symptoms, withdrawal symptoms that exacerbate depressive symptoms, and recurrent use of substances. By understanding the risks of devastating outcomes for untreated co-occurring depression and SUDs, counselors attend to the constellation of symptoms affecting their clients' lives with compassion and clarity.

Clients living with co-occurring depression and SUDs may be reluctant or may lack the energy or desire to look within themselves and risk unmasking past trauma and current regret. Understanding the ubiquity of trauma, culturally sensitive counselors employ a trauma-informed approach, recognizing client reluctance as a possible sign of self-protection and *not* resistance. Joining with clients as reflective co-investigators, counselors explore their clients' current needs, risk and protective factors, symptoms, and goals for counseling. The relationship between biopsychosocial factors and risk for depression and a SUD requires counselors to attend to contextual considerations such as economic factors, race, gender identity, sexuality, and age (SAMHSA, 2020b).

To determine if depressive symptoms are due to a substance or another medical condition, counselors will consider the onset of depressive symptoms within a carefully constructed timeline of depressive symptom onset, substance use, and medical condition progression. With the client's written consent, this may entail interdisciplinary collaboration with medical providers to carefully assess the relationship between depression and intoxication, withdrawal symptoms, acute medical events (e.g., stroke), and chronic disease (e.g., Parkinson's disease). When depressive symptoms emerge prior to or in conjunction with symptoms of SUDs and do not appear to be caused by substances or other medical conditions, conducting a *functional analysis* of the relationship between depressive symptoms and substance use allows the client to reflect on their feelings, thoughts, and behaviors in context, and provides the counselor with critical information with which to make accurate diagnoses. The following questions may be helpful in initiating a functional analysis, understanding the history of depressive symptoms and substance use, and teasing apart antecedents related to current distress:

- *Which of the current symptoms are the most distressing?*
- *When did these symptoms begin?*
- *How have past symptoms changed over time?*
- *What biopsychosocial events (e.g., physical changes, environmental factors) preceded current symptoms?*
- *How is this similar to or different from previous symptom presentation?*
- *How has substance use influenced or been influenced by depressive symptoms?*
- *How have depressive symptoms influenced or been influenced by substance use?*
- *What behaviors have provided relief?*
- *What behaviors have exacerbated symptoms?*

SCREENING AND ASSESSMENT TOOLS

An array of validated formal screening and assessment tools for depression and substance misuse are freely available and simple to administer by counselors and/or self-administered by clients. For the purposes of this chapter, a few of the free primary instruments are identified and briefly described; however, counselors are encouraged to review the comprehensive list of resources provided by SAMHSA (2020b).

PATIENT HEALTH QUESTIONNAIRE-9

The Patient Health Questionnaire-9 (PHQ-9; Kroenke et al., 2001) is a free, nine-item, self-administered screening tool for depressive symptoms that is available in online and paper formats. The nine items are correlated with *DSM-5* diagnostic criteria, and can be used to establish diagnosis of depressive disorders and symptom severity (Kroenke et al., 2001). Items are self-scored from "0" (not at all) to "3" (nearly every day). Higher scores indicate more severe depression, and question 9 screens for suicide risk, which is an essential query in all comprehensive assessments. The PHQ-9 can be completed and scored in approximately 10 minutes.

CLINICALLY USEFUL DEPRESSION OUTCOME SCALE

The Clinically Useful Depression Outcome Scale (CUDOS; Zimmerman et al., 2008) is a free, 18-item, self-administered scale that assesses a client's depression symptoms and symptom impacts on psychosocial functioning over the previous 7 days. This scale may be especially effective as a weekly check-in assessment due to its brevity. Items are scored using a 5-point Likert scale ("0" not at all true, to "4" almost always true). The CUDOS aligns well with *DSM-5* diagnostic criteria, although using the CUDOS as a diagnostic tool must be done over the course of 2 weeks, as *DSM-5* diagnostic criteria for depressive disorders include symptoms lasting 2 weeks or more (APA, 2013).

HAMILTON DEPRESSION RATING SCALE

The Hamilton Depression Rating Scale (HAM-D; Hamilton, 1960), a free, 21-item, clinician-administered assessment, was designed to be used with individuals already diagnosed with depression and can be useful in measuring symptoms during treatment over time. Items include both those correlating with *DSM-5* diagnostic criteria and those of paranoia, derealization, and obsessional symptoms (Hamilton, 1960). Items are scored using either a 5-point ("0" absent, to "4" severe) or 3-point ("0" absent, to "2" clearly present) scale. The HAM-D may be administered and scored in approximately 20 minutes.

CAGE-AID SUBSTANCE MISUSE SCREENING TOOL

Designed as a brief, initial screening for substance misuse, the four-item CAGE-AID (Cut down, Annoyed, Guilty, Eye-opener-Adapted to Include Drugs; Brown & Rounds, 1995) tool is simple to administer and offers counselors the opportunity to open a conversation about substance use. Endorsement of one or more items in the four-item tool indicates a need for further assessment for SUDs. Its simplicity and ease of use is useful in a variety of settings, as the four items are easy to remember and lend themselves well to insertion into conversations about general health.

ALCOHOL USE DISORDERS IDENTIFICATION TEST (AUDIT)

The 10-item Alcohol Use Disorders Identification Test (AUDIT; Babor et al., 2001) assesses for amount and frequency of alcohol use, indicators of alcohol dependence, and problems associated with alcohol. This free assessment may be administered as part of a structured or semi-structured clinician interview or by clients themselves. It is freely available in printed (Babor et al., 2001) and electronic versions (e.g., Saunders, n.d.). Each response is scored from "0" to "4" and score totals are correlated with risk from low to severe. A score of 8 or more indicates harmful alcohol use.

NIDA-MODIFIED ASSIST

The freely-available NIDA-Modified ASSIST (NM ASSIST; NIDA, 2012) may help counselors explore a client's use of alcohol, tobacco, and prescription and illegal drugs. Eight questions assess the client's use, desire to use, and negative ramifications of use for a variety of target substances (e.g., cocaine, inhalants, hallucinogens). Ranging from lower risk to high risk, counselors tally a *Substance Involvement Score* that not only helps guide them as they make diagnostic determinations and develop treatment plans, it also enhances the client's insight and understanding of their own individual risk factors.

OTHER STRATEGIES AND CONSIDERATIONS

Formal and informal screening and assessment tools, understanding mood and substance use over time, and engaging in functional analysis can be useful in a counselor's assessment and diagnostic process. Informal and nonstandardized screening and assessment strategies for depression and substance use can be initiated in many ways, including offering an open-ended invitation such as, *"Tell me about your mood?"* or *"Describe your use of alcohol and other substances."* The binary *"Do you feel depressed?"* or *"Do you drink or use drugs?"* suggests a good and bad paradigm, thus offering clients the opportunity to evade or avoid (whether willfully or unknowingly) by answering with a simple, *"No."*

For clients who have never talked about their depression or their substance use before, engaging in the assessment process guided by a compassionate counselor may spark a corrective experience. One strategy for counselors to elicit client "buy in" is to invite them to offer a self-score outside of the mathematical scoring of a formal instrument:

> *"You just completed the PHQ-9. A total score of 0 means you have no symptoms of depression, and a total score of 27 suggests that depression is a big part of your life right now. Thinking about how you have been feeling over the last couple of weeks, what do you think your score is? What does that number mean to you?"*

Allowing clients to self-reflect and evaluate *themselves* bolsters client self-efficacy and supports a collaborative approach to assessment, providing clients the chance to make meaning out of assessment results.

Formal assessments also give clinicians and clients the opportunity to monitor changes over time with readministration. However, clients may be reluctant or lack the awareness to respond accurately to formal assessments. For example, a client who does not measure out their evening "nightcap" might respond *"Never"* to the AUDIT question #3, *"How often do you have five or more drinks on one occasion?"* (Babor et al., 2001). The client may be unaware that their favorite 9-ounce tumbler holds *six* standard 1½ ounce servings of alcohol.

With formal assessment results in hand, the clinical interview provides counselors the opportunity to continue a holistic client assessment. To support collaborative assessment and well-informed diagnosis, counselors engage clients in information gathering and meaning making in order to get a *complete* picture before foreclosing on a diagnosis. For example, for a client who uses heroin, a central nervous system depressant, in increasing amounts over a period of 2 years, with depressive symptoms developing over the past 2 months, an incomplete assessment might lead a counselor to perceive depression *because* of heroin use instead of occurring concurrently with substance use. Teasing apart the tangled strands of behavior, history, and environmental factors is a task requiring focus, collaboration, and counselor humility. In collaboration with the client, and consulting with other medical and mental health professionals, counselors are better able to successfully assess, diagnose, and treat their clients.

ASSESSMENT AND DIFFERENTIAL DIAGNOSTIC DELIBERATIONS

For clients with depressive symptoms and risky substance use behaviors that do not meet diagnostic criteria, counselors must remain focused on the client's level of distress and disordered functioning. A client who has lost interest in previously enjoyable activities and is using a substance more frequently may not meet the full diagnostic criteria for a co-occurring depression disorder and SUD, but distress in any capacity associated with depressive symptoms and substance use must be addressed by counselors. Intervening early to prevent symptoms of a disease or disorder from becoming worse, *secondary prevention* (Daniels-Witt et al., 2017) can be a powerful part of a holistic assessment and treatment protocol for clients.

A client does not have to demonstrate the full spectrum of *DSM-5* diagnostic criteria to benefit from focused treatment for their distressing symptoms. For some clients, although their substance use does not meet the criteria for a SUD diagnosis, it may negatively affect mood and interfere with therapeutic depressive disorder treatment progress. For others, although a diagnosis of a SUD seems clear, increasing symptoms of depression must *not* be immediately discounted as withdrawal symptoms. Integrating psychoeducation on risks of depression and SUDs may be useful for clients with subclinical symptomatology as well as those whose symptoms are more clinically significant. By investing in client awareness and working with clients to move toward more optimal functioning, counselors support client wellness.

For clients under medical care for other health concerns, interactions between physical health, prescribed medications, mood, and the effects of other substance use must be considered as part of an ongoing, holistic assessment throughout the counseling relationship. Additionally, vitamin deficiencies are associated with behavioral disorders and substance abuse—symptoms of depression may manifest due to insufficient levels of vitamins B6, B9, and B12, while a poor diet combined with excessive alcohol use negatively affects vitamins A, B2, and C levels (Ramsey & Muskin, 2013). Physiologic and psychosocial effects of conditions such as diabetes and cardiovascular disease, and the medications used in treating them, may increase the likelihood of developing depression or a SUD, as well as potentially enhance the negative effects of substance use (McKee & Brahm, 2016). Medications prescribed for certain heart problems, such as beta-blockers and calcium-channel blockers, may lead to depressive symptoms (Jha et al., 2019). Individuals living with SUDs may be at much greater risk of chronic diseases such as cancers, cardiovascular disease, and chronic pain (Bahorik et al., 2017). Combining opiate pain management with medications for depression such as selective serotonin reuptake inhibitors (SSRIs) may reduce the opiates' effectiveness, potentially leading clients to use more of the medications, leading to potentially life-threatening serotonin syndrome (Parthipan et al., 2019). Combining prescribed opiate pain medications with alcohol or other depressants (such as benzodiazepines) could lead to devastating consequences, including increased risk of falls, respiratory crisis, and death (Bahorik et al., 2017; Tori et al., 2020).

Conducting holistic biopsychosocial assessments helps counselors untangle physical symptoms, medical conditions, prescribed medications, mood, and substance use. Working collaboratively with the client, the counselor can establish accurate diagnoses and develop effective treatment planning. It must be noted that without client engagement in this process, gaps in the counselor's understanding of the client may, at best, lead to missed opportunities to provide care, and, at worst, put the client at risk for potentially life-altering outcomes.

TREATMENT MODALITIES

Individuals living with co-occurring depression and SUDs are diverse in matters of cultural identity, life roles, symptom severity, biopsychosocial history, and motivation for change. Working with clients using a holistic, wellness-based approach aligns with the counseling profession's commitment to prevention, diversity, and lifelong wellness (American Counseling Association [ACA], 2014). Treatment needs are as varied as client presentations, and treatment planning and interventions should be conducted within these contexts. From brief interventions (BIs) to medication assisted treatment (MAT), from outpatient services to medically managed intensive inpatient services (Mee-Lee et al., 2013), counselors must be prepared to engage in flexible, person-centered treatment planning and service delivery in collaboration with their clients *and* in consultation with other professionals. Select items on the menu of treatment options that counselors may consider when working with clients who have co-occurring depressive disorders and SUDs are reviewed.

BRIEF INTERVENTIONS

BIs range from standalone, 15-minute, bedside counseling interventions in the emergency department to several weeks of group or individual counseling interventions. Examples of BIs include motivational interviewing (MI) techniques and skill-building interventions while integrating cognitive behavioral therapy (CBT), solution-focused therapy, and psychodynamic approaches (SAMHSA, 1999). Although BIs are flexible, six elements remain consistent using the FRAMES model presented by Miller and Sanchez (1994):

1. Individual **F**eedback regarding risk or impairment;
2. **R**esponsibility for change belongs to the client;
3. The counselor offers **A**dvice regarding change;
4. Counselors offer clients a **M**enu of possible treatment and self-help options;
5. Counselors relate to clients with **E**mpathy; and
6. Counselors engender **S**elf-efficacy and empowerment in their clients.

BIs may involve enhancing motivation to change by using MI, a collaborative, evocative approach to counseling that honors each client's autonomy and recognizes their ability to enact change (Miller et al., 2019). Using this approach, counselors elicit change talk by asking open-ended questions that invite the client to reflect on their reasons, ability, desire, and commitment to change. "*How would you like your relationship with your kids to be different?*" invites the client to consider their desires for change. "*How do you think you'll solve this problem?*" invites clients to consider steps they might take. Counselors attend to language reflective of client ambivalence. When a client states, "*My drinking isn't making my depression worse. I just wish my kids would stop scowling when I drink*," a counselor might reflect, "*You wish your kids saw you in a different light.*" By reflecting, affirming, and sometimes amplifying client change talk, counselors evoke client awareness and motivation for change by tapping into what their clients already know but have not yet explored.

WELLNESS-PROMOTING STRATEGIES

Developing wellness-promoting coping strategies can help individuals living with depression and SUDs regain a sense of autonomy and control as they are supported in their movement toward better health. Feelings of guilt and shame are common in individuals living with co-occurring depressive disorders and SUDs, and skills-building approaches may help clients feel more empowered to maintain positive health practices, reduce or eliminate substance use, and manage distressing symptoms of depression. CBT and dialectical behavior therapy (DBT) approaches may be especially useful to clients interested in developing coping skills regarding cravings, emotional regulation, and cognitive distortions (e.g., "*I'll always be an addict. I don't deserve to be happy.*"). Helping clients regain awareness of their emotional responses to stressors by using mindfulness practices, worksheets, journaling, and other means of intentional self-exploration may feel grounding and offer clients a sense of stability and power in their own recovery. Helping clients identify triggers for depressive episodes or substance use builds awareness and supports client self-efficacy.

For clients living with co-occurring depressive disorders and SUDs, whether changing substance use or unpacking trauma histories, change is hard. It is easy for the transition process toward a new normal to feel out of control. DBT practices (e.g., practicing wise mind, ACCEPTS model; Linehan, 2014) may help clients withstand the emotional and physical discomfort that accompanies withdrawal or abstinence from substances and deep exploration into self. Counselors are well served to integrate mindfulness practices into their work with clients.

MEDICATION-ASSISTED TREATMENT

When MAT, such as methadone and buprenorphine, is provided in conjunction with ongoing counseling, this combination of services offers many clients the best chance to remain engaged in treatment (SAMHSA, 2020b). Although counseling is effective in treating clients with depression, a comprehensive treatment approach may also include antidepressant medications such as SSRIs and serotonin-norepinephrine reuptake inhibitors (SNRIs; SAMHSA, 2020b). Some of these medications and their brand names (SMI Adviser, 2019) include:

- **SSRIs:** Fluoxetine (Prozac), sertraline (Zoloft), citalopram (Celexa), escitalopram (Lexapro)
- **SNRIs:** Venlafaxine (Effexor), duloxetine (Cymbalta), desvenlafaxine (Pristiq)

There remains evidence for increased risk of suicidal thoughts in clients starting treatment with antidepressant medications (e.g., SSRIs, SNRIs), particularly in clients between the ages of 18 and 24 (Bielefeldt et al., 2016). Regular assessment for suicidal thoughts and behaviors, normalized in the intake session and integrated into every session thereafter, is part of ongoing holistic assessment and treatment. Counselors must maintain strong partnerships with medical providers to stay abreast of new developments in psychotropic medications and develop a collaborative referral network of professionals in the community to support their clients. Additionally, if a potential medical concern arises during the therapeutic process, counselors promote their clients' wellness by recommending client consultation with medical professionals. Clients who wish to engage in more intensive inpatient treatment are best supported by counselors who are aware of such resources and work collaboratively with treatment partners.

BIOPSYCHOSOCIAL APPROACHES

Individuals living with co-occurring depressive disorders and SUDs often experience concurrent psychosocial difficulties and socioeconomic stressors. A practical, realistic, and collaborative approach to the counseling relationship affords clients the opportunity to recognize strengths, areas for growth, and develop strategies that are tailored to their needs while linking them to additional resources that may support their path toward wellness. Counselors committed to culturally sensitive, holistic therapeutic approaches will develop strong partnerships within a broad network of community partners to support clients needing assistance with employment, housing, food, education, and legal matters. In addition, counselors may offer clients resources regarding alternative treatment strategies to support continued movement toward wellness.

ADJUNCT SERVICES

Alternative therapies such as yoga, eye movement desensitization and reprocessing therapy, mindfulness, acupuncture, and equine therapy may be part of a comprehensive menu of services for effective client care. For some clients, group counseling interventions and mutual-help support groups such as Alcoholics Anonymous (Alcoholics Anonymous World Services, 2021) and Narcotics Anonymous (Narcotics Anonymous World Services, 2021), as well as more secular options such as SMART Recovery (2021) and LifeRing Secular Recovery (2020), may be useful. These groups may provide some clients much desired collegial support and peer accountability. The National Alliance on Mental Illness (2021) offers online and face-to-face support group options for individuals living with mental illness. For some clients, building community with others who are living with depressive disorders and SUDs can support their recovery. For others, such groups may not be an ideal fit. Counselors should be knowledgeable about local and online support groups to offer their clients a full menu of options.

HARM REDUCTION, CRISIS MITIGATION, AND STIGMA MANAGEMENT

Attending to client safety also includes recognizing health risks such as the physiologic dangers of binge use and overdose, the risks of bacterial infections from intravenous drug use, and communicable disease transmission via shared needles. Addressing practical safety considerations may include overdose education, client access to naloxone (SAMHSA, 2020b), needle exchanges, and establishing emergency protocols.

Helping clients diagnosed with depressive disorders and SUDs put safeguards in place *before* a crisis occurs supports their self-efficacy and reinforces hope. Despite the mixed research on the value of safety plans as a deterrent to suicide, as part of a person-centered therapeutic approach, counselors who help clients establish a safety framework of accessible community supports are promoting client wellness. Along with hotlines, emergency contacts, and local agencies, free and low-cost apps and websites offer on-demand support for clients at times of acute distress. Examples of these resources include the *Stanley-Brown Safety Plan* app (Two Penguins Studio, 2013); the Hazelden Betty Ford's *Thought for the Day* website (2021); and the *I Am Sober* app (*2021*).

Structural stigma in mental health and addiction treatment sustains barriers between clients and appropriate services (National Academies of Sciences, Engineering, and Medicine [NASEM], 2016). Counselors must understand the devastating impact of systemic disparity and stigmatizing language, and must educate themselves regarding person-first language. However, counselors must not serve as "language police" for their clients. When a client blames themselves for being depressed or describes themselves as an "addict," or a "drunk," counselors may feel pulled by their own culturally conscious training to classify such language as harmful. Correcting or "schooling" clients to describe themselves in less stigmatizing terms may inadvertently condemn clients to silence. Culturally sensitive counselors use person-first language, clearly demonstrating the belief that all clients have inherent value, that co-occurring disorders (CODs) are treatable, and that all clients deserve care. By approaching the work with humility, counselors remain open to client-initiated correction (e.g., *"I'm an addict. It's how I see myself. It's how I talk about myself in meetings. Why won't you say it?"*). By being open to such correction, counselors demonstrate a willingness to grow and work collaboratively *with* their clients.

Clients in treatment for co-occurring depression and SUDs are likely to return to risky behaviors (e.g., abandoning wellness practices, binge drinking) many times before the desired change becomes more permanent. Despite setbacks in treatment progression, counselors who offer a nonjudgmental therapeutic presence bolster client long-term success and optimal well-being.

LEGAL AND ETHICAL CONSIDERATIONS

Despite the lack of a diagnostic serum test for depression or a SUD, blood and urine are often tested for substances as part of a complete medical assessment or for conditions of employment. In all institutions that receive federal funding, *42 CFR Part 2* (SAMHSA, 2020a) provides additional protections from clinical information related to client substance use from being used in ways that put client welfare in undue danger. Even so, reluctance to discuss substance use is understandable considering societal stigma toward individuals with SUDs. Healthcare professionals may be especially concerned about healthcare privacy related to substance use for fear of the risks to licensure and professional standing should their substance use or SUD come to light (Kunyk et al., 2016). Similarly, although 20% or more of adults may experience depressive episodes during their lifetimes, stigma around depression remains and creates an unnecessary and sometimes lethal barrier to effective treatment (NASEM, 2016).

Legal implications of substance use include ramifications of being charged with impaired driving, criminal possession of illegal substances, threats to professional licensure (Kunyk et al., 2016), and the racial imbalance in arrest, citation, and incarceration rates for substance possession (Nellis, 2016). Clients may be court mandated to receive SUD counseling, and although this may prove beneficial to clients and society (Hatchel et al., 2019), if clients conflate the legal censure resulting from substance misuse with a coercive therapeutic environment, establishing a collaborative counseling relationship may be difficult.

Many legal and ethical considerations related to providing counseling for clients with co-occurring depression and SUDs extend across all diagnostic criteria. In any ethical or legal conundrum, counselors must calmly assess the situation and engage established ethical guidelines and decision-making models (ACA, 2014; Forester-Miller & Davis, 2016). Consultation with all collateral parties, as well as collaborating with clients themselves, is essential. Within the therapeutic relationship, clients may disclose difficult truths (e.g., suicidal or homicidal thoughts or behaviors, abuse or neglect of minors or vulnerable adults). Such revelations, although unsettling, provide counselors with opportunities to safeguard the well-being of clients and others. For many who live with depressive disorders and SUDs, families, friends, and colleagues may have grown weary of the frequent crises and calls for help. As a counselor, sitting with clients in their pain and taking necessary steps to protect the welfare of clients and others may be shocking to clients accustomed to people turning their heads and closing their hearts.

Any client disclosure can spark profound growth and healing when shared within a person-centered, collaborative, therapeutic counseling relationship. There are instances, however, when counselors may be ethically and/or legally mandated to report client disclosures, specifically regarding cases of child or elder abuse or neglect, threats of harm toward an identified other or others, and suicidal ideation. Clearly explaining the limits of confidentiality as part of intake is an essential step in establishing a collaborative counseling relationship.

Acting on legal and ethical mandates to break confidentiality may threaten a client's autonomy (e.g., involuntary admission into a psychiatric inpatient unit following suicidal ideation or behavior). When faced with the decision to break confidentiality in order to protect the health and safety of the client or others, counselors must engage in clear communication and thoughtful consultation with both the client and other professionals. The risk of fractured counselor/client relationships may cause counselors to hesitate to break confidentiality, but such a fracture pales in comparison to the potential risks for injury or death if confidentiality is not broken and preventable harm to self or others occurs.

CLINICAL CASE ILLUSTRATION AND DISCUSSION

CASE OF XAVIER

Until recently, Xavier (a 48-year-old Black, straight, cisgender male whose preferred pronouns are he/him/his) seemed to be thriving professionally and personally. Six months after a cycling accident and surgery to repair his shattered kneecap, Xavier's friends and family were growing increasingly concerned about his mood and his drinking. Being a hospital pharmacist, Xavier was aware of the risk of addiction to opioid-based medications, and he was against using prescribed opiates for his pain. He had witnessed colleagues who had been censured or who had lost their licenses due to opiate addiction.

Despite his reluctance to take opiates, Xavier was in a lot of pain. To lessen his discomfort and to help him sleep, Xavier began taking a nightly shot of whiskey. When the pain wouldn't subside and sleep remained restless and elusive, Xavier slowly increased his drinking until he began taking a full 9-ounce tumbler of whiskey with him to bed every night. Concerned that Xavier might be drinking at a dangerous level, his wife, Gayle, suggested that he cut back. Although Xavier promised he would, he did not, explaining, *"You just don't get how much pain I'm in."*

Although Xavier believed himself to be functioning reasonably well at work (despite frequent hangovers), his coworkers noticed that since his accident, Xavier seemed to be moving in slow motion. Before the accident, Xavier had been the life of the party. Since then, Xavier refused invitations to social events and family outings, in spite of his family's urging. His three children (ages 8, 10, and 12) also noticed a change in their normally fun-loving father, and one day the oldest asked his mother, "*Why is dad so depressed?*" At Gayle's insistence, Xavier made an appointment with Tobias, a 41-year-old Peruvian-American cisgender male licensed professional counselor to talk about what was going on.

At the intake session, Xavier was neatly dressed and appeared attentive as he sat down in Tobias's office, but Tobias noticed that Xavier seemed to move and speak very slowly and with great effort. Xavier cleared his throat and shifted in his chair when Tobias invited him to explain what he hoped to get from counseling. Several seconds passed before Xavier began to answer. "*Before my accident, I guess I was just happy. I didn't really think about it. When the car ran me off the road that night, I had no idea how my life would change. That life seems very far away now.*" Xavier cast his eyes downward. "*I guess I want to get my life back, you know?*" Tobias allowed the silence to remain for a few seconds, waiting for Xavier to continue, which ultimately, he did.

Xavier described the pain and inconvenience of surgery and 6 weeks of physical rehab while continuing to go to work every day and manage his family responsibilities. "*I'm a hospital pharmacist. I know about addiction. We see it all the time in our patients, and I've seen it in my colleagues at the hospital. I wasn't going to be hooked on opiates. I was in pain and not sleeping, so I started taking a couple of sips of whiskey before bed.*" Xavier explained that within a couple of weeks, a few sips a few nights a week became a couple of shots every night. "*When I've been sad in the past, like after my brother died, exercise helped a lot. But now, I feel stuck.*" Tobias noted Xavier's experiences with sadness, his current sleep disturbance, his slow rate of speech, and his depressed mood. Exercise, Xavier's go-to coping strategy, seemed off the table for now. Tobias wondered if this were true or if Xavier's symptoms of depression were making it more difficult to engage in any form of physical activity, not just vigorous exercise.

On Tobias's invitation, Xavier explained that he started drinking in college, and before the accident, that he drank one or two drinks containing alcohol one or two nights a week. "*I'm a social drinker, maybe a beer with a friend or a couple of drinks at a party.*" He denied current use of other substances, reporting some experimentation with marijuana and cocaine in pharmacy school but nothing since graduation. As with all his clients, Tobias engaged in a suicide risk assessment by inquiring, "*Xavier, tell me about any past or current thoughts of suicide.*" Xavier denied current suicidal thoughts, but said that he did think about suicide when he was 24 years old and his brother died. Tobias invited Xavier to walk him through that time, describing how he managed those thoughts. Xavier explained that at the time he trained harder with his cycling team and connected with family for support. Tobias recognized that past suicidal thoughts or behaviors increased Xavier's current risk for suicide. Tobias assessed protective factors including Xavier's relationships and his professional identity. Xavier explained, "*I've been pretty down at work, but being a pharmacist is my calling. I love being a dad, but lately I feel like a lousy father. Gayle, my wife, is a treasure. She's worried about me, which is why I called you.*"

Tobias wanted to be sure that he understood Xavier's story, and he also wanted Xavier to know that his story mattered. Tobias began, "*It sounds like you're having a rough time of it right now. You have a job you love, and a family you cherish. After your accident, it's been harder to enjoy your life. The things you used to do to help you feel better, or to even feel normal, now seem out of reach. You've been trying to figure out a way to feel less pain and to sleep better, and so you've been drinking more than you used to. I wonder if we might unpack that a little more to make sure we both get a clear picture of how to move toward reaching your goals.*"

Xavier felt comfortable enough to continue, and he and Tobias explored his alcohol use. Xavier explained that occasionally he woke up feeling "*hungover,*" and that starting about noon every workday, *"when my knee starts to swell,"* he starts thinking about the relief he would get from his nighttime whiskey. *"I'm drinking more now than I ever have, and I know it's not helping my mood or my energy level, but I don't think I have a drinking problem,"* Xavier explained. Tobias understood that talking about substance use could be difficult, and did not attempt to argue or convince Xavier that he might be mistaken. Xavier explained, *"Sometimes when the pain gets to me, I fill my tumbler so I don't have to walk back downstairs for a refill, and most of the time when I wake up in the morning, it's empty."* Tobias gathered more detailed information about the timing and the quantity of Xavier's alcohol use, and made a note to offer some psychoeducation regarding the risks of alcohol intoxication and the risks of complicated withdrawal. Later in the intake session, Tobias and Xavier talked about risky drinking, using the NIAAA "Rethinking Drinking" resources to frame the discussion. Xavier seemed receptive to that information.

CASE DISCUSSION

Tobias believed a diagnosis of MDD (moderate severity) was likely. Xavier's depressive symptoms had lasted for over a month, he felt sad and disinterested much of the time, and family and coworkers had commented on his change in affect. He continued to have trouble sleeping, reported low energy levels, and indicated that he felt as if he was letting his family down (guilt). He denied current thoughts of suicide. His depressive symptoms had significantly impaired his functioning, he did not report episodes of mania or hypomania, and his depression could not be better explained by other disorders.

Tobias believed that Xavier's increased alcohol use was in response to his depressive symptoms. Increased use might be complicating things, but at this point Tobias suspected that Xavier might also meet the diagnostic criteria for moderate AUD. Xavier was spending a lot of time thinking about drinking. He was using alcohol to cope. He experienced mild withdrawal symptoms (hangover), and sometimes he drank more than he intended, despite understanding its potentially negative impact on his mood and his energy.

Tobias believed that a co-occurring diagnosis of MDD and AUD, both of moderate severity, was likely appropriate. Because Xavier reached out for help and indicated a desire for things in his life to change, Tobias anticipated Xavier would engage in the therapeutic process and would have the power to return to better functioning. Tobias believed that Xavier was somewhere between the *contemplative* and *preparation* stages of change.

Following their intake session, Tobias counseled Xavier for several months. Tobias advised Xavier to see his primary care physician to rule out organic causes for his depressive symptoms and his orthopedic surgeon to rule out any lingering knee dysfunction. There were no related medical disorders, and Xavier's surgeon recommended he ride a stationary bicycle 20 minutes a day to build up his endurance. After a couple of months, Xavier reported to Tobias that, *"Just sweating again feels great."*

Using a CBT approach, Tobias invited Xavier to keep a thought record and to question distressing thoughts. He also suggested that Xavier work with his wife, Gayle, to improve sleep hygiene. Xavier had told Tobias that he did not believe he was addicted to alcohol, and although Tobias was very direct in offering psychoeducation about the risks of alcohol use for someone experiencing depressive symptoms, Xavier was adamant that he did not need to quit alcohol altogether, stating, *"My neighbor is in AA. That's way too rigid for me."* Tobias was well aware of the potentially lethal risks of complicated alcohol withdrawal, and was upfront and open in the conversation with Xavier. Tobias told Xavier that signs of a potentially risky withdrawal from alcohol included tremors, increased heart rate, sweating, and hallucinations. Per his recollection, Xavier denied having ever experienced such symptoms.

In Tobias's office, Xavier explained that in preparation for his first counseling session with Tobias, that he had abstained from alcohol the night before. Recognizing the value of harm reduction for an individual who is not interested in or willing to cease substance use, Tobias introduced Xavier to the idea of "sobriety sampling," in which Xavier would experiment with not drinking for a set period. Xavier was relieved that Tobias did not insist that complete abstinence was the only way, and Xavier agreed to do an experiment and not drink for 3 weeks. Although at their session the following week, he reported a couple of "slips," Xavier described sleeping better and feeling more like himself. Xavier reported, *"I really do feel better, but I miss the occasional beer or shot. I'm going to experiment with drinking only on the weekends."* Two months of further experimentation with drinking and then abstaining, plus several late-night conversations with Gayle, led Xavier to recognize that at least at this phase of his life as he was rebuilding his physical health and restoring his relationships with family and friends, he would not drink. Tobias affirmed this decision, encouraging Xavier to continue to be open with his wife and honest with his healthcare providers.

Growing more confident, Xavier continued to take risks and reached out to colleagues and to his family for support when he experienced depressive symptoms. Xavier began journaling and continued to use some of the resources Tobias had shared when they began their counseling relationship. Learning these new coping mechanisms boosted Xavier's mood. Within 6 months of beginning counseling, Xavier reported that his depressive symptoms had diminished and that he felt more focused and more interested in his normal activities. Xavier continued to check in with Tobias less frequently as he continued to develop more health-promoting behaviors. He even returned to road cycling, which felt like coming back home.

For clients living with co-occurring depressive disorders and SUDs, culturally sensitive, trauma-informed counseling care may provide a calming force in a sea of uncertainty. Like Tobias, approaching such work within the framework of person-centered, holistic, collaborative assessment, diagnosis, and treatment affords clients like Xavier the best chance of re-establishing equilibrium and moving toward optimal wellness.

The first and most important step toward improved functioning for clients like Xavier is the establishment of the therapeutic alliance between client and counselor. Counselor empathy, humility, and authenticity set the stage for trust within a collaborative therapeutic environment. Using first-person language and treating the client and not just the client's symptoms afford the client the most corrective environment for exploration, healing, and growth.

Next, engaging standardized and more informal assessments, counselors begin to examine a client's history, including timeline and etiology of symptoms, in order to determine the most accurate and useful diagnosis and treatment plan. Woven into such a multidimensional assessment strategy is attention to safety, including risks of overdose, complicated withdrawal, and suicide. Determining best treatment approaches should be undertaken in collaboration with clients and in consultation with other professionals. A flexible approach to treatment may include modalities such as BIs, CBT, MAT, and adjunct therapies such as yoga and mindfulness. Counselors further support clients when they develop collaborative relationships within the larger community in order to link clients with services outside of counseling such as medical care, housing, and legal assistance.

CHAPTER SUMMARY

In this chapter, the diagnostic criteria, prevalence, assessment, treatment, and legal and ethical implications of co-occurring depressive disorders and SUDs were explored using a person-centered, collaborative, multidimensional approach to care. Specifically, the diagnostic considerations for co-occurring depressive disorders and SUDs included an overview of the co-occurring mental disorder, the unique aspects of how that particular disorder interplays with various addictive disorders, and how these concurrent processes impact the individual. While integrating a concise review of the *DSM-5* criteria, deliberations for assessing and diagnosing the co-occurring depressive disorders and SUDs were discussed. Additionally, considerations for ruling-out other disorders beyond the primary disorder(s), including any potential comorbid medical condition, were incorporated.

Culturally sensitive counselors must remain aware of stigma and structural barriers to mental health and SUD treatment. Working with community stakeholders on the local, regional, and national levels to increase awareness of and access to all forms of mental health and substance-related care aligns with the counseling profession's emphasis on professional advocacy. Primary prevention strategies such as speaking about depressive disorders and substance use at local school and civic events is one way to advocate for the profession and to advocate for greater awareness and understanding of risks, protective factors, and available prevention and treatment resources in the community. Additionally, counselors must remain active and curious learners, seeking out updated information about the prevalence of depressive disorders and SUDs, innovative prevention and treatment strategies, local and national regulations, and sociocultural and geopolitical phenomena. Counselors must stay connected to their communities and stay current in their knowledge and connected in their ongoing professional and personal development.

Co-occurring depressive disorders and SUDs present clients and counselors with a complicated set of symptoms, but within a collaborative, supportive counseling relationship, the client's progress toward healing may be fostered. Not all clients will respond as enthusiastically as Xavier. In some cases, depressive disorders coupled with SUDs result in devastating physical, psychological, and relational consequences; therefore, making a return to previous function seem unlikely. Person-centered counselors understand that *all* clients have the potential for growth and that movement toward wellness is possible (even if it is slow and nonlinear), and that counselors have a privileged role to play in support of that growth for all their clients, regardless of the diagnosis.

DISCUSSION QUESTIONS

1. The term "depression" is used in many contexts. After reading the chapter, how would you describe depressive disorders to a friend who is not a mental health professional?

2. People living with depressive disorders sometimes use substances to help alleviate distressing symptoms. How might you engage in conversation with a client who tells you, "I feel so much better when I use my substance. You'd better not be telling me I need to stop."

3. There is no blood or laboratory test to diagnose depression or a SUD, and when using the *DSM-5* diagnostic criteria to determine the presence of a co-occurring depressive disorder and SUD, a fair amount of clinical judgment comes into play. Recognizing these diagnostic limitations, think about how a misdiagnosis (false positive) or a missed diagnosis (false negative) could occur, then consider ways you can reduce that likelihood when working as a counselor.

4. What are your beliefs about recovery from (a) depressive disorders, (b) SUDs, and (c) co-occurring depressive disorders and SUDs? On a 1 to 10 scale, how confident are you that people who live with a co-occurring depressive disorder and a SUD can truly achieve optimal wellness? On that same scale, how confident are you that you are ready to work with individuals living with a co-occurring depressive disorder and SUD? How might you work to improve both ratings?

5. Some have argued that only those who are in long-term recovery from addiction are qualified to counsel clients with SUDs. What are your beliefs about this? Do you think the same is true for depressive disorders? Why or why not?

REFERENCES

Alcoholics Anonymous World Services. (2021). *Welcome to alcoholics anonymous.* https://www.aa.org/

American Counseling Association. (2014). *ACA code of ethics.* https://www.counseling.org/knowledge-center

American Psychiatric Association. (2013). *Diagnostic and statistical manual of mental disorders* (5th ed.). https://doi.org/10.1176/appi.books.9780890425596

American Society of Addiction Medicine. (n.d.). *About The ASAM Criteria.* Retrieved February 21, 2022, from https://www.asam.org/asam-criteria/about-the-asam-criteria

Babor, T. F., Higgins-Biddle, J. C., Saunders, J. B., & Monteiro, M. G. (2001). *AUDIT: The alcohol use disorders identification test: Guidelines for use in primary care* (2nd ed.). https://apps.who.int/iris/bitstream/handle/10665/67205/WHO_MSD_MSB_01.6a.pdf?sequence=1&isAllowed=y

Bahorik, A. L., Satre, D. D., Kline-Simon, A. H., Weisner, C. M., & Campbell, C. I. (2017). Alcohol, cannabis, and opioid use disorders, and disease burden in an integrated health care system. *Journal of Addiction Medicine, 11*(1), 3–9. https://doi.org/10.1097/ADM.0000000000000260

Bielefeldt, A. A., Danborg, P. B., & Gøtzsche, P. C. (2016). Precursors to suicidality and violence on antidepressants: Systematic review of trials in adult healthy volunteers. *Journal of the Royal Society of Medicine, 109*(10). 381–392. https://doi.org/10.1177/0141076816666805

Brody, D. J., Pratt, L. A., & Hughes, J. P. (2018). *Prevalence of depression among adults aged 20 and over: United States, 2013–2016.* NCHS Data Brief, no 303. National Center for Health Statistics. https://www.cdc.gov/nchs/data/databriefs/db303.pdf

Brown, R. L., & Rounds, L. A. (1995). Conjoint screening questionnaires for alcohol and other drug abuse: Criterion validity in a primary care practice. *Wisconsin Medical Journal, 94,* 135–140.

Centers for Disease Control and Prevention. (2019). *Preventing adverse childhood experiences: Leveraging the best available evidence.* National Century for Injury Prevention and Control. https://www.cdc.gov/violenceprevention/pdf/preventingACES.pdf

Centers for Disease Control and Prevention. (2020). *Substance use screening and intervention implementation guide: No amount of substance use is safe for adolescents.* https://www.cdc.gov/ncbddd/fasd/features/teen-substance-use.html

Centers for Disease Control and Prevention. (2021a). *Alcohol and public health.* U.S. Department of Health & Human Services. https://www.cdc.gov/alcohol/faqs.htm#bingeDrinking

Centers for Disease Control and Prevention. (2021b). *Anxiety and depression: Household pulse survey.* National Center for Health Statistics. https://www.cdc.gov/nchs/covid19/pulse/mental-health.htm

Daniels-Witt, Q., Thompson, A., Glassman, T., Federman, S., & Bott, K. (2017). The case for implementing the levels of prevention model: Opiate abuse on American college campuses. *Journal of American College Health, 65*(7), 518–524. https://doi.org/10.1080/07448481.2017.1341900

Drymalski, W. M., & Nunley, M. R. (2018). Sensitivity of the ASAM Criteria to psychiatric need. *International Journal of Mental Health & Addiction, 16,* 617–629. https://doi.org/10.1007/s11469-017-9801-8

Felitti, V. J., Anda, R. B., Nordenberg, D., Williamson, D. F., Spitz, A. M., Edwards, V., Koss, M. P., & Marks, J. S. (1998). Relationship of childhood abuse and household dysfunction to many of the leading causes of death in adults: The Adverse Childhood Experiences (ACE) Study. *American Journal of Preventive Medicine*, *14*(4), 245–258. https://doi.org/10.1016/S0749-3797(98)00017-8

Forester-Miller, H., & Davis, T. E. (2016). *Practitioner's guide to ethical decision making*. https://www.counseling.org/docs/default-source/ethics/practioner-39-s-guide-to-ethical-decision-making.pdf

Hamilton, M. (1960). A rating scale for depression. *Journal of Neurology, Neurosurgery, and Psychiatry*, *23*, 56–62. https://jnnp.bmj.com/content/23/1/56

Hantsoo, L., & Epperson, C. N. (2015). Premenstrual dysphoric disorder: Epidemiology and treatment. *Current Psychiatry Reports*, *17*(11), 87. https://doi.org/10.1007/s11920-015-0628-3

Hasin, D. S., Sarvet, A. L., Meyers, J. L., Saha, T. D., Ruan, W. J., Stohl, M., & Grant, B. F. (2018). Epidemiology of adult DSM-5 major depressive disorder and its specifiers in the United States. *JAMA Psychiatry*, *75*(4). 336–345. https://jamanetwork.com/journals/jamapsychiatry/fullarticle/2671413

Hatchel, H., Vogel, T., & Huber, C. G. (2019). Mandated treatment and its impact on therapeutic process and outcome factors. *Frontiers in Psychiatry*, *10*(219), 1–8. https://doi.org/10.3389/fpsyt.2019.00219

I Am Sober LLC. (2021). *I Am Sober* [Mobile app]. App Store. https://apps.apple.com/us/app/i-am-sober/id672904239

Jha, M. K., Qamar, A., Vaduganathan, M., Charney, D. S., & Murrough, J. W. (2019). Screening and management of depression in patients with cardiovascular disease. *Journal of the American College of Cardiology*, *73*(14), 1827–1845. https://doi.org/10.1016/j.jacc.2019.01.041

Kessler, R. C., Angermeyer, M., Anthony, J. C., deGraaf, R., Demyttenaere, K., Gasquet, I., de Girolamo, G., Gluzman, S., Gureje, O., Haro, J. M., Kawakami, N., Karam, A., Levinson, D., Medina Mora, M. E., Oakley Browne, M. A., Posada-Villa, J., Stein, D. J., Adley Tsang, C. H., Aguilar-Gaxiola, S., . . . Üstün, T. B. (2007). Lifetime prevalence and age-of-onset distributions of mental disorders in the World Health Organization's World Mental Health Survey Initiative. *World Psychiatry: Official Journal of the World Psychiatric Association (WPA)*, *6*(3), 168–76.

Kroenke, K., Spitzer, R. L., & Williams, J. B. (2001). The PHQ-9: Validity of a brief depression severity measure. *Journal of General Internal Medicine*, *16*(9), 606–613. https://doi.org/10.1046/j.1525-1497.2001.016009606.x

Kunyk, D., Inness, M., Reisdorfer, E., Morris, H., & Chambers, T. (2016). Help seeking by health professionals for addiction: A mixed studies review. *International Journal of Nursing Studies*, *60*, 200–215. https://doi.org/10.1016/j.ijnurstu.2016.05.001

LifeRing Secular Recovery. (2020). *About LifeRing*. https://lifering.org/

Linehan, M. M. (2014). *DBT skills training manual* (2nd ed.). Guilford Press.

Lynch, V., Clemans-Cope, L., & Winiski, E. (2019). *Prevalence of substance use disorder and interventions of unhealthy substance use among parents by race and Hispanic origin in the United States, 2015-2017*. Urban Institute. https://www.urban.org/research/publication/prevalence-substance-use-disorder-and-interventions-unhealthy-substance-use-among-parents-race-and-hispanic-origin-united-states-2015-2017

McDonald, M. J. (2020). Adverse childhood experience and substance use disorder: Exploring connections and trauma informed care. *International Journal of Child Development & Human Development*, *13*(4), 383–387.

McKee, J., & Brahm, N. (2016). Medical mimics: Differential diagnostic considerations for psychiatric symptoms. *Mental Health Clinician*, *6*(6), 289–296. https://doi.org/10.9740/mhc.2016.11.289

Mee-Lee, D., Shulman, G. D., Fishman, M. J., Gastfriend, D., Miller, M. M., & Provence, S. M. (Eds.). (2013). *The ASAM Criteria: Treatment criteria for addictive, substance-related, and co-occurring conditions* (3rd ed.). American Society of Addiction Medicine.

Miller, W. R., Forcehimes, A. A., & Zweben, A. (2019). *Treating addiction: A guide for professionals*. The Guilford Press.

Miller, W. R., & Sanchez, V. C. (1994). Motivating young adults for treatment and lifestyle change. In G. S. Howard & P. E. Nathan (Eds.), *Alcohol use and misuse by young adults* (pp. 55–81). University of Notre Dame Press.

Narcotics Anonymous World Services. (2021). *Welcome to www.NA.org*. https://na.org/

National Academies of Sciences, Engineering, and Medicine. (2016). *Ending discrimination against people with mental and substance use disorders: The evidence for stigma change*. The National Academies Press. https://doi.org/10.17226/23442

National Alliance on Mental Illness. (2021). *About NAMI*. https://www.nami.org/About-NAMI

National Institute on Drug Abuse. (2012). *Resource guide: Screening for drug use in general medical settings*. https://nida.nih.gov/sites/default/files/resource_guide.pdf

National Institute on Drug Abuse. (2020). *Common comorbidities with substance use disorders research report*. https://www.drugabuse.gov/publications/research-reports/common-comorbidities-substance-use-disorders/why-there-comorbidity-between-substance-use-disorders-mental-illnesses

Nellis, A. (2016). *The color of justice: Racial and ethnic disparities in state prisons*. The Sentencing Project. https://www.sentencingproject.org/publications/color-of-justice-racial-and-ethnic-disparity-in-state-prisons/

Parthipan A., Banerjee I., Humphreys K., Asch S. M., Curtin C., Carroll I., & Hernandez-Boussard T. (2019). Predicting inadequate postoperative pain management in depressed patients: A machine learning approach. *PLoS ONE, 14*, Article e0210575. https://doi.org/10.1371/journal.pone.0210575.

Prochaska, J. O., & Velicer, W. F. (1997). The transtheoretical model of health behavior change. *American Journal of Health Promotion, 12*(1), 38–48. https://doi.org/10.4278/0890-1171-12.1.38.

Ramsey, D., & Muskin, P. R. (2013). Vitamin deficiencies and mental health: How are they linked? *Current Psychiatry, 12*(1), 37–43.

Saunders, J. B. (n.d.). *AUDIT: Alcohol use disorders identification test*. Retrieved from https://auditscreen.org/

SMART Recovery. (2021). *There's life beyond addiction*. https://www.smartrecovery.org/

SMI Adviser. (2019). *Antidepressants - Medication fact sheets*. https://smiadviser.org/knowledge_post/antidepressants-medication-fact-sheets

Substance Abuse and Mental Health Services Administration. (1999). *Brief interventions and brief therapies for substance abuse*. In Treatment Improvement Protocol (TIP) Series, No. 34. https://www.ncbi.nlm.nih.gov/books/NBK64947/

Substance Abuse and Mental Health Services Administration. (2019). *Key substance use and mental health indicators in the United States: Results from the 2018 National Survey on Drug Use and Health* (HHS Publication No. PEP19-5068, NSDUH Series H-54). Center for Behavioral Health Statistics and Quality. https://www.samhsa.gov/data/

Substance Abuse and Mental Health Services Administration. (2020a). *Key substance use and mental health indicators in the United States: Results from the 2019 National Survey on Drug Use and Health* (HHS Publication No. PEP20-07-01-001, NSDUH Series H-55). Center for Behavioral Health Statistics and Quality. https://www.samhsa.gov/data/

Substance Abuse and Mental Health Services Administration. (2020b). *Fact sheet: SAMHSA 42 CFR Part 2 revised rule*. https://www.samhsa.gov/newsroom/press-announcements/202007131330

Substance Abuse and Mental Health Services Administration. (2020c). *Substance use disorder treatment for people with co-occurring disorders*. Treatment Improvement Protocol (TIP) Series, No. 42. https://store.samhsa.gov/sites/default/files/SAMHSA_Digital_Download/PEP20-02-01_004.pdf

Swarbrick, M. (2006). A wellness approach. *Psychiatric Rehabilitation Journal, 29*(4), 311–314.

Szaflarski, M., Bauldry, S., Cubbins, L. S., & Meganathan, K. (2017). Nativity, race-ethnicity, and dual diagnosis among US adults. *Research in the Sociology of Healthcare, 35*, 171–191. https://www.ncbi.nlm.nih.gov/pmc/articles/PMC5685548/

Tori, M. E., Larochelle, M. R., & Naimi, T. S. (2020). Alcohol or benzodiazepine co-involvement with opioid overdose deaths in the United States, 1999-2017. *JAMA Network Open, 3*(4), 1–11. https://doi.org/10.1001/jamanetworkopen.2020.2361

Two Penguins Studio. (2013). *Stanley-Brown Safety Plan* [Mobile app]. App Store. https://apps.apple.com/us/app/safety-plan/id695122998

Villarroel, M. A., & Terlizzi, E. P. (2020). Symptoms of depression among adults: United States, 2019. *NCHS Data Brief (No. 379)*. National Center for Health Statistics. https://www.cdc.gov/nchs/products/databriefs/db379.htm

Wanta, J. W., Niforatos, J. D., Durbak, E., Viguera, A., & Altinay, M. (2019). Mental health diagnoses among transgender patients in the clinical setting: An all-payer electronic health record study. *Transgender Health, 4*(1), 313–315. https://doi.org/10.1089/trgh.2019.0029

Zimmerman, M., Chelminski, I., McGlinchey, J. B., & Posternak, M. A., (2008). A clinically useful depression outcome scale. *Comprehensive Psychiatry, 49*, 131–140. https://doi.org/10.1016/j.comppsych.2007.10.006

CHAPTER 10

CO-OCCURRING BIPOLAR AND SUBSTANCE USE DISORDERS

NEDELJKO GOLUBOVIC, LAUREN FLYNN, ALEXIS ISAAC, AND SAUNDRA M. TABET

LEARNING OBJECTIVES

After reading this chapter, you will be able to:
- Recognize risk factors associated with co-occurring bipolar disorder and substance use disorders (SUDs).
- Identify presenting symptoms and make appropriate diagnostic impressions.
- Compare and apply relevant screening and assessment tools.
- Employ pertinent ethical and legal standards when addressing these co-occurring disorders (CODs).
- Identify effective treatment approaches.

INTRODUCTION

Bipolar disorder (BD) is one of the psychiatric issues most likely to co-occur with substance use disorders (SUD; Hunt et al., 2016). Conservative estimates indicate that up to 50% of persons diagnosed with a BD also will experience a SUD at some point in their lifetimes (Substance Abuse and Mental Health Services Administration [SAMHSA], 2016). In addition to the high prevalence rates, the co-occurrence of BD and SUD also increases already severe symptoms and high-risk factors associated with each disorder (Hunt et al., 2016). For example, individuals with BD who use alcohol or illicit substances have higher rates of hospitalizations, lower rates of remissions during hospitalizations, higher rates of mixed episodes, rapid mood cycling, persistent mood symptoms while in treatment, and are more likely to respond poorly to medications (Sonne & Brady, 2002).

Although counselors are starting to better understand the impact co-occurring BD and SUD have on clients, and research is improving treatment options available to persons who struggle with these issues, a full understanding of the relationship between these two disorders remains limited. Several theories have been proposed to explain the high rates of co-existence between BD and SUD; however, the nature of the correlation between these disorders is yet to be well understood. The first of the possible explanations proposed that individuals with BD use substances to self-medicate and counteract undesirable symptoms associated with the disorder

(Rowland & Marwaha, 2018). Examples of substances serving as means of self-medication include the use of central nervous system stimulants, such as cocaine to counter depressive symptoms, or heroin, a central nervous system depressant, to offset symptoms of mania. Conversely, an alternative theory suggested that persons with BD may use substances (e.g., methamphetamine) to accentuate desirable symptoms of mania and prolong the pleasurable state (Bizzarri et al., 2007). In addition to these two theories that described the use of substances as a reaction to (or the result of) BD, hypotheses that proposed SUD to be the preceding disorder also have been offered. These explanations typically are built on the notion that psychiatric symptoms are triggered or induced by drug consumption (Swann, 2010). However, despite these efforts to account for BD and SUDs co-occurrence in terms of causation, the nature of these disorders' relationship is likely bidirectional and influenced by a multitude of complex factors. Thus, in this chapter, the focus is on exploring the intricate impact the co-occurrence of these disorders has on clients, examine associated risk factors, consider relevant assessment and screening implications, and review effective treatment strategies.

BIPOLAR DISORDER: *DSM-5* DIAGNOSTIC CRITERIA AND DESCRIPTION

Although BD is most likely first diagnosed in early adulthood, onset in childhood or later adulthood may also occur (American Psychiatric Association [APA], 2013). This disorder is characterized primarily by repeated manic, hypomanic, or depressive episodes. These episodes often are separated by periods of stable mood during which presenting symptoms fall below the diagnostic threshold. Based on the presenting issues, persons who are experiencing BD would be diagnosed with one of the two subtypes: (a) *bipolar I disorder* (BD-I) or (b) *bipolar II disorder* (BD-II). The term *"bipolar spectrum"* oftentimes is used in the professional literature as a broader, more encompassing expression for BD. Bipolar spectrum, in addition to BD-I and BD-II, also encompasses subthreshold BD (or BD-NOS; Hunt et al., 2016; Merikangas et al., 2011).

BD-I is differentiated by full manic episodes that are more severe than the hypomanic episodes that characterize BD-II. Depressive symptoms in BD-I and BD-II are not distinguishably different; however, an episode of depression is not required to make a diagnosis of BD-I, while it is necessary for BD-II diagnosis. For this reason, BD-II is no longer considered to be the "milder" condition of the two subtypes (APA, 2013). Finally, a subthreshold diagnosis of either *other specified* or *unspecified* is given to persons who do not meet the full criteria for a specific bipolar and related disorder (APA, 2013). Examples of *other specified* presentations include: (a) short-duration hypomanic episodes (2–3 days); (b) hypomanic episodes with insufficient symptoms and major depressive episodes; (c) hypomanic episode without prior major depressive episode; and (d) short-duration cyclothymia (less than 22 months; APA, 2013, p. 148).

These diagnostic subtypes tend to be stable over time (Culpepper, 2014). That is, if a client is diagnosed with a BD-II, they are unlikely to experience significant changes in presenting symptoms that would require an alteration of their diagnosis to BD-I. Additionally, it is important to note that although we are categorizing BD in terms of subtypes, counselors should not expect homogeneous presentations for clients who are diagnosed with each subtype. Rather, it is critical to remember that there are significant variations in the rates at which the mood episodes alternate, the duration, and the symptom severity across individuals diagnosed with BD. We explore each diagnostic subtype further in the following.

BIPOLAR I DISORDER

A diagnosis of BD-I requires at least one lifetime manic episode (APA, 2013). To meet the criteria for this diagnosis, the manic episode must not result from substance use, medications, or other physical or mental illnesses. Although nonessential for a BD-I diagnosis, depressive episodes and hypomanic episodes also may occur in conjunction with a manic episode. A manic episode is a severe mood disturbance that results in significant impairments in functioning. The range of mood disturbances during a manic episode could vary. Still, the most distinguishable symptoms are periods of an uncharacteristically elevated or irritable mood that persist for at least 1 week at a time. During these periods, affected individuals will experience heightened energy, reduced need for sleep, and increased goal-focused behaviors.

In addition to these behavioral changes, individuals experiencing a manic episode also will encounter at least three of the following changes: (a) boosted self-esteem, (b) racing thoughts, (c) difficulty paying attention, (d) heightened goal-directed activities, (e) increased involvement in pleasurable activities (e.g., sexual activity or excessive spending), and (f) appear unusually talkative (APA, 2013). A person having a manic episode may also experience psychotic features, including delusions and hallucinations. The severity of impairments a person may experience during a manic episode could necessitate hospitalization in order to prevent harm to self or others (APA, 2013).

A client experiencing a manic episode may present in the following manner: The client's rate of speech is likely to be exceptionally high, and they could talk continuously and loudly without regard for others. Their emotional expression and body language may be greatly exaggerated, and they could experience an inflated sense of self-importance. For example, the client could express an intent to become a writer and produce a novel within a short period without prior experience or training in this area. Additionally, they may also engage in impulsive or risky behaviors such as extensive gambling, uncharacteristically frequent or unprotected sexual encounters, and unplanned career changes.

BIPOLAR II DISORDER

The essential diagnostic features of BD-II include at least one lifetime *hypomanic episode* and at least one lifetime *major depressive episode* (APA, 2013). And, just like BD-I, neither the hypomanic nor the depressive episodes could be due to the effects of substance use, medications, or other physical or mental illnesses if a diagnosis of BD-II is to be considered.

A hypomanic episode has a similar symptom criterion as a manic episode; however, the length of the episode is shorter (i.e., at least 4 days of persistent symptom presentation compared to at least 1 week), and the presenting issues do not result in severe functional impairment or require hospitalization. It is important to note that a person diagnosed with BD-II is not likely to enter treatment during a hypomanic episode; instead, they are more likely to complain of the depressive symptoms or persistent mood changes that characterize the disorder (APA, 2013). Additionally, they may not even view periods of hypomania as distressing; they might report interpersonal and professional issues resulting from unpredictable emotional states and erratic behavior.

The presence of at least one major depressive episode is also required if a diagnosis of BD-II is to be contemplated. A depressive episode is characterized by a despondent mood that results in a notable change in functioning and a reduced interest in previously enjoyable activities during a period of 2 or more weeks. In addition to these features, a depressive episode requires the occurrence of five or more of the following symptoms: (a) significant weight changes, (b) notable changes in sleep patterns, (c) observable restlessness or sluggishness, (d) loss of energy, (e) unwarranted feelings of guilt and worthlessness, (f) poor concentration, and (g) persistent thoughts of death or suicide (APA, 2013). It is important to point out that an individual with BD-II is likely to display symptoms typical of major depressive disorder; however, they also will report distinguishing frequent mood changes indicative of BD.

Bipolar Disorder Severity and Specifications

The severity of BD-I and BD-II symptoms could vary considerably, and for diagnostic purposes, are categorized as *mild, moderate,* or *severe* (APA, 2013). A person experiencing a *mild* episode would exhibit a few symptoms, if any, beyond the baseline diagnostic criteria. These symptoms would result in minor impairments that are troublesome but manageable. An individual with a *moderate* episode would experience a functional impairment that would cause a noticeable disturbance of their daily functioning. Finally, a person experiencing a *severe* episode would be significantly more distressed, and the level of impairment would be unmanageable for them. Hence, the number of symptoms associated with a severe episode is far beyond the level necessary to meet the disorder's criteria.

In addition to the level of severity, two other significant diagnostic specifications to consider are the presence of *mixed features* and *rapid cycling*. Mixed features refer to the simultaneous occurrence of depressive and manic or hypomanic symptoms. An example of an episode containing mixed features is a depressive episode that also includes racing thoughts and a diminished need for sleep. Rapid cycling pertains to frequent alternating of mood episodes. This specification requires at least four mood episodes that meet the criterion for a manic, hypomanic, or depressive episode in the previous 12 months. Additional specifiers to consider when working with this population are *melancholic features, anxious distress, mood-congruent psychotic features, mood-incongruent psychotic features, catatonia, peripartum onset,* and *seasonal pattern atypical features* (APA, 2013, p. 135).

PREVALENCE, STATISTICS, AND DEMOGRAPHICS
BIPOLAR DISORDERS

Before examining prevalence rates of co-occurring bipolar and substance use disorders (SUDs) and exploring the significance of impact their co-existence could have, it is important to first acknowledge the pervasiveness of a BD itself. BD ranks as the fifth most frequently occurring mental health disorder (0.6%) among the world's population (Ritchie & Roser, 2018), and is preceded in prevalence by anxiety (4.0%), depression (3.0%), alcohol use disorders (1.0%), and drug use disorders (1.0%) When comparing the occurrence of BD in the entire world with the rates seen within the United States, the numbers are even more alarming. The United States has the highest rates of BD (Rowland & Marwaha, 2018)—it is estimated more than one in 20 people in the United States is diagnosed with BD during their lifetime, and more than one in 50 people has this disorder in a 12-month period (Merikangas et al., 2011).

CO-OCCURRING BIPOLAR AND SUBSTANCE USE DISORDERS

When starting to examine the prevalence for co-occurring BD and SUD closer, it is important to note that comorbidity rates for BD and SUD are among the highest for co-occurring disorders

(CODs; Merikangas et al., 2011; Rowland & Marwaha, 2018); these statistics have remained stable over the last two decades (APA, 2013; Cerullo & Strakowski, 2007; SAMHSA, 2016). It is estimated that between 30% and 50% of persons diagnosed with a BD will have a coexisting SUD during their lifetimes (APA, 2013; SAMHSA, 2016), while up to 25% are expected to develop a SUD within a 12-month period (SAMHSA, 2016). More specifically, the *Diagnostic and Statistical Manual of Mental Disorders, Fifth Edition* (*DSM-5*; APA, 2013) noted that 50% of individuals with BD-I and 37% of persons with BD-II would experience a SUD during their lifetime.

Risk Factors

A diagnosis of a BD also increases the risk of developing a SUD. It is estimated that persons who have a BD are three times more likely to develop nicotine and alcohol dependence, and five times more likely to develop a dependency to an illicit drug than individuals who do not have this diagnosis (Salloum & Brown, 2017; Swendsen et al., 2010). Although the general risk of developing a SUD for persons diagnosed with BD is well established, the data on risk rates associated with specific types of BD disorders are inconsistent. The results from some studies suggest diagnostic severity on the BD spectrum may impact the risk of developing a co-occurring SUD (Grant et al., 2016; Hunt et al., 2016; Merikangas et al., 2011). These findings indicated the greatest rates of comorbidity were associated with more severe presentations (i.e., BD-I), and the lowest prevalence was noted in individuals with subthreshold BD (Grant et al., 2016; Merikangas et al., 2011). Conversely, the results from a large meta-analysis found little difference in risk between BD-I and BD-II in the lifetime rates of SUD (Hunt et al., 2016). Despite these inconsistent findings on the risk rates across different subtypes of BD disorders, it is essential to remember that research findings consistently indicate that persons diagnosed with BD are at an increased risk of developing a SUD (Hunt et al., 2016; Messer et al., 2017).

Risk factors for developing co-occurring BD and SUD also are influenced by demographic characteristics. A meta-analysis on the prevalence of comorbid BD and SUD in clinical settings found that, of persons diagnosed with BD, males have two times higher rates of lifetime alcohol use disorder (AUD). It is important to note women diagnosed with BD also experience AUDs. Nearly 20% of women diagnosed with BD report lifetime AUDs (Di Florio et al., 2014). Additionally, persons of North American or European descent have the highest co-occurring BD and AUD rates, while prevalence rates were the lowest for individuals of Asian descent (Di Florio et al., 2014). Persons diagnosed with BD report higher rates of drug use and dependence, including cannabis, cocaine, and amphetamines (Hunt et al., 2016). Hunt and colleagues (2016) suggest males diagnosed with BD also face increased risk of SUDs (i.e., AUDs and drug use disorders) compared to females diagnosed with BD. Comorbidity of BD and SUD is also higher for people who have started experiencing symptoms at a younger age (i.e., less than 18 years) and those who have increased hospitalization rates (Hunt et al., 2016; Joshi & Wilens, 2009).

Now that the general prevalence rates and risk factors have been examined, implications for specific types of SUD that are most commonly associated with BD are explored. The most frequently co-occurring SUD is alcohol, followed by cannabis and tobacco (Cerullo & Strakowski, 2007; Salloum & Brown, 2017). In the next section, we review each of these substances.

Alcohol

Alcohol is the most misused substance by people diagnosed with BD. AUD is more prevalent in BD than in any other mood disorder, and AUD is twice as likely to co-occur in people with BD than in those with unipolar depression (Sonne & Brady, 2002). A meta-analysis of co-occurring BD and SUD found that 42% of individuals with BD reported alcohol use. Additionally, persons who had an AUD were at four times greater risk of developing BD (Hunt et al., 2016). Individuals with BD and AUD experienced higher suicidality rates and were less likely to seek clinical treatment (Oquendo et al., 2010). Sonne and Brady (2002) found that symptoms of BD could be triggered (or emerge) during the course of chronic alcohol intoxication or withdrawal, and that alcohol use could lead to worsening BD symptoms.

Cannabis and Other Illicit Substances

Cannabis use is highly prevalent among individuals with BD, second only to alcohol. Previous studies have shown that between 38% and 48% of individuals with BD engaged in cannabis use (Etain et al., 2012; Frank et al., 2007). Outcomes of the *2020 National Survey on Drug Use and Health* found the prevalence of cannabis use in adults with any mental illness to be 32.8%, compared to 14.6% of adults without mental illness (SAMHSA, 2021). Although cannabis use has not shown the same high correlation to suicidality, hospitalization, and negative treatment outcomes as other substances, individuals with BD who use cannabis are at increased risk of developing nicotine dependence, AUD, drug use disorders, and antisocial personality disorder as compared to those without cannabis use disorder (Lev-Ran et al., 2013). Additionally, a systematic review of BD and SUD literature found that 17% of individuals with BD used illegal substances, 11% of which reported using cocaine (Hunt et al., 2016). Some studies have even found a stronger association between BD and illicit drug use than alcohol or cannabis use, noting that individuals with BD were five times more likely to use illicit substances (Hunt et al., 2016).

Tobacco

Persons with BD are two to three times more likely to start smoking tobacco (Heffner et al., 2011). Additionally, these individuals are less likely to initiate and maintain smoking abstinence than people without BD (Heffner et al., 2011). People with diagnosed BD face added challenges in attempting smoking cessation, such as chronic mood dysregulation, high prevalence of alcohol and drug use, and more severe nicotine dependence (Heffner et al., 2011). Results of international and national studies suggested that tobacco use may be an important risk factor for higher rates of suicide attempts (Icick et al., 2019; Schaffer et al., 2015) and adverse treatment outcomes in persons with BD (Graff et al., 2008). An additional component that is important to consider with tobacco use is its role as a secondary risk factor. Tobacco use is a risk factor for some of the most frequent causes of death in the United States (e.g., cancer, cardiovascular, cerebrovascular, and respiratory diseases; Heffner et al., 2011). Because these secondary effects of tobacco use in co-occurring disorders are overlooked frequently, the impact this substance has is often underestimated.

ASSESSMENT AND DIAGNOSTIC CONSIDERATIONS

BD is one of the most misdiagnosed mental health disorders, and persons with BD often do not receive an accurate diagnosis until a decade after they begin experiencing symptoms (Atkins, 2014). Additionally, due to a wide range of presenting symptoms associated with BD, assessment and diagnosis could be complex and challenging. Therefore, it is critical to examine contextual factors that might influence assessment and diagnostic procedures and contribute to the lack of accurate and timely BD diagnosis.

EXAMINING FOR MENTAL, SUBSTANCE USE, AND MEDICAL COMORBIDITIES

To start, it is important to consider other common mental health and medical comorbidities since these conditions are likely to exacerbate symptom severity as well as increase the risks of developing SUD (Salloum & Brown, 2017). The most frequently documented mental health comorbidities include anxiety disorders, posttraumatic stress disorder (PTSD), attention deficit/hyperactivity disorder (ADHD), conduct disorder, and personality disorders (Atkins, 2014; Messer et al., 2017). The co-existence of these disorders could make it particularly challenging to discriminate presenting issues appropriately and increase the risk of misdiagnosis. Additionally, the co-existence of another mental health disorder could present a secondary risk factor for developing a SUD. For example, the likelihood of stimulant, sedative, and opioid use disorders increases when individuals with BD have a comorbid anxiety disorder (Goodwin et al., 2002). Assessment and diagnosis are even further complicated when considering that SUDs themselves could represent a risk factor for developing other co-occurring disorders. That is, the presence of an anxiety disorder in individuals with BD is reported to be more common when a SUD is occurring (Baethge et al., 2005). As a result of these intricacies, it is critical for counselors to conduct thorough assessment procedures and consider all relevant factors.

Regarding medical conditions, clients diagnosed with BD are at a higher risk of having cardiovascular disorders, respiratory disorders, diabetes, hypothyroidism, and sleep apnea (Patel et al., 2018; Rowland & Marwaha, 2018). Although counselors are not expected to diagnose or treat medical conditions, it is important to consider how these issues might affect a client's mental health and/or addiction treatment. When completing the initial screening procedures and the more comprehensive assessment protocols, working collaboratively with an integrated treatment team and/or the primary care physician is encouraged. When appropriate, referrals to medical specialists should also be presented to the client.

The co-occurrence of a bipolar and SUD could further complicate diagnosis because some effects of substance use could mimic, distort, and conceal symptoms of BD (Atkins, 2014). For example, stimulants (e.g., cocaine, methamphetamine) could mirror symptoms of mania: increased energy, decreased need for sleep, and heightened productivity (Ming et al., 2018). Stimulants also may be used to counteract episodes of depression, creating difficulties in accurately identifying these symptoms. Additionally, sedatives or depressive substances, such as alcohol, cannabis, and heroin, may distort or conceal symptoms of mania and hypomania, or mimic depressive symptoms during stable periods between mood episodes (Ming et al., 2018).

Additionally, SUD appears to impact the onset and severity of BD symptoms (Hunt et al., 2016). Several studies suggested that, when compared to individuals with BD who do not use substances, persons with co-occurring BD and SUD have more prolonged and frequent mood episodes, higher rates of rapid cycling and mixed episodes, more hospitalizations, and earlier onset of symptoms (Cerullo & Strakowski 2007; Nery et al., 2013; Swann, 2010; Tolliver & Hartwell, 2012). Two meta-analyses also identified that individuals with BD who have a history of alcohol and other SUDs have elevated risk levels for suicidality (Cerullo & Strakowski, 2007; Messer et al., 2017). For individuals with BD, suicidality is most likely to occur within the context of a depressive episode, and a greater number of depressive episodes increases the probability of suicide attempts (Oquendo et al., 2010). Also, depressive episodes occur more frequently and have a longer duration for individuals with comorbid BD and SUD (Cerullo & Strakowski, 2007; Tohen et al., 2003).

Finally, people with BD are less likely to seek treatment when in a manic or hypomanic state than during a depressive episode (Atkins, 2014). Those with BD might not consider mania or hypomania episodes as abnormal; instead, they may view manic and hypomanic symptoms of increased energy, a diminished need for sleep, and heightened productivity as times when they felt well (Atkins, 2014). Manic and hypomanic states may even be experienced as pleasurable for individuals with BD, leading them to engage in stimulant use in an attempt to prolong or intensify sensations. A person in a state of mania can resemble someone intoxicated or in a state of withdrawal, resulting in difficulty differentiating symptoms of the underlying illness (Atkins, 2014). Several studies have shown the potential for the use of substances, especially stimulants, to predict the onset of a manic episode (Frank et al., 2007; Gold et al., 2018); however, this pattern has not been observed universally.

SCREENING AND ASSESSMENT TOOLS

The *Structured Clinical Interview for DSM-5* (SCID-5; APA, 2013), a semi-structured interview guide, is recommended for counselors to use as a framework for screening and assessing clients. The SCID-5 includes interview questions corresponding to *DSM-5* criteria and, for most presenting problems, is typically administered within 45 and 120 minutes. This approach provides the most complete and comprehensive evaluation of clients' presenting issues and provides direction for a *DSM-5* diagnosis. The assessment tools offered in the remainder of this section can all be administered using the SCID-5 as a grounding interview approach. Assessment and screening for co-occurring BD and SUD, as assessment for any mental health condition, should include a battery of instruments and procedures to create a complete and thorough understanding of clients' presenting issues with consideration of all other principal contextual factors.

Additionally, careful attention should be given to the length of abstinence from mood-altering substances before developing a formal diagnostic assessment to allow time for acute intoxication and withdrawal symptoms to alleviate (Quello et al., 2005). Nallet and colleagues (2013) as well as Salloum and Brown (2017) highlighted commonly used approaches when assessing and screening for co-occurring BD and SUD, which can include any combination of the SCID-5 (APA, 2013), the Bech-Rafaelsen Mania Rating Scale (MAS; Bech et al., 1979), the *Mood Disorder Questionnaire* (MDQ; Hirschfeld et al., 2000), and the *Psychiatric Research Interview for Substance and Mental Disorders for DSM-5* (PRISM-5; Hasin et al., 1996). Table 10.1 provides a summary of the commonly used BD and SUD assessment and screening tools. Please note that this table does not represent an exhaustive list of assessment and screening tools; rather, it is a succinct review of instruments frequently used and referenced in the literature.

In addition to assessment and screening considerations for clients who meet the diagnostic criteria, it is essential to note that clients below the diagnostic threshold for BD also face increased risk for a co-occurring SUD compared to clients without BD (Merikangas et al., 2011). A unique challenge working with this population is that the symptomatology of substance use/abuse may mimic BD presentation. For instance, the use of central nervous system stimulants may produce manic-like symptoms, and the withdrawal from substances may produce depression-like symptoms. Conversely, the use of central nervous system depressants may induce depression-like symptoms, and the withdrawal process may increase agitation and anxiety (SAMHSA, 2016).

Although beyond the scope of this chapter, counselors should consider behavioral addictions beyond substance use when screening clients with BD for co-occurring diagnoses. In a comprehensive systemic review, BD was found to have high co-occurrence with problematic gambling, kleptomania, compulsive buying, compulsive sexual behavior, and problematic internet use (Varo et al., 2019). Similar to SUD, the presence of behavioral addictions with a BD was found to impact prognosis and increase the severity of overall presentation negatively (Varo et al., 2019).

TABLE 10.1 **Assessment Tools**

ASSESSMENT MEASURE	BRIEF OVERVIEW OF ASSESSMENT MEASURE
Composite International Diagnostic Interview (CIDI): Bipolar Disorder Screening Scale	The Composite International Diagnostic Interview Bipolar Disorder Screening Scale (CIDI; Kessler et al., 2006) is a structured clinical interview with a strong discriminatory ability to identify bipolar disorder. The CIDI consists of two stem questions. The first is targeting distinct periods of elevated, expansive, or persistently abnormal mood, and the second targeting symptoms of mania. If one of the stem questions is answered affirmatively, respondents are directed to answer a series of nine questions related to diagnostic criterion B of the *DSM-5*.
Bech-Rafaelsen Mania Rating Scale (MAS)	The Bech-Rafaelsen Mania Rating Scale (MAS; Bech et al., 1979) is a clinician administered and rated brief clinical interview. This instrument consists of 11 items that are rated on a five-point scale (0, "not present" to 4, "severe") and addresses classic manic symptoms including elevated mood, irritability, sleep, increased activity, talkativeness, flight of ideas, self-esteem, noise level, and sexual interest.
Mood Disorder Questionnaire (MDQ)	The Mood Disorder Questionnaire (MDQ; Hirschfeld et al., 2000) is a pencil-and-paper, self-report measure which screens for lifetime bipolar spectrum disorders. The MDQ is considered both a sensitive and specific measure, and includes 13 questions related to *DSM-5* criteria, as well as items targeting level of impairment, risk factors, and duration of symptoms. Seven or more "yes" answers warrant more in-depth assessment for a possible bipolar diagnosis.
Young Mania Rating Scale (YMRS)	The Young Mania Rating Scale (YMRS; Young et al., 1978) is a brief clinical interview used to assess the severity of manic states. This 11-item scale can be used by a trained clinician to assess the severity of manic states based on the client's subjective experience over the past 48 hours. Each item is rated based on the severity of presentation. Created for research purposes, this scale is appropriate only to measure the severity of manic states, and not as a diagnostic tool. Although originally developed for use with adult patients, the YMRS has been adapted for adolescent use as well.
Psychiatric Research Interview for Substance and Mental Disorders for DSM-5 (PRISM-5)	The Psychiatric Research Interview for Substance and Mental Disorders for DSM-5 (PRISM-5; Hasin et al., 1996) is a semi-structured, computer-based diagnostic interview. This tool is appropriate for use when conducting psychiatric diagnoses with clients who use substances, as it specifically targets co-occurring occurrences. The PRISM-5 assess both *DSM-IV* and *DSM-5* substance use disorder criteria and *DSM-5* psychiatric criteria for past 12-month and lifetime prevalence.

TREATMENT MODALITIES

When discussing treatment modalities for co-occurring BD and SUD, it is vital to start with an acknowledgment that no "gold standard" treatment model has been established. That is, no single agreed-upon method that is superior to others has been developed thus far. Regardless, researchers have invested significant efforts in developing effective treatment options for persons with co-existing BD and SUD over the last 30 years. Both group and individual treatment modalities, in conjunction with pharmacotherapy, have been shown helpful in alleviating symptoms and improving overall functioning for individuals who have these co-occurring disorders (Grande & Vieta, 2015). Before specific treatment modalities are examined, a review of the major theoretical rationales that have guided the delivery of treatment for persons with co-occurring disorders is given.

THREE MODELS FOR TREATING CO-OCCURRING DISORDERS

It is imperative to consider these theoretical rationales as they provide an overall framework (and create limitations) for treatment of persons with co-occurring BD and SUD. Individuals who are treated for these co-existing disorders most likely receive treatment according to one of the following models: (a) sequential, (b) parallel, or (c) integrated (Morisano et al., 2014).

The *sequential model* assumes a hierarchical approach to treatment. Disorders are treated in order of perceived importance (determined based on the symptom acuity and disruptive impact), and each disorder is treated exclusively from the other. Although, according to the sequential approach, the most acute disorder is addressed first, the model overlooks the complex nature of the co-occurring disorder (Morisano et al., 2014).

Converse to the sequential model, under the *parallel model*, both disorders are addressed at the same time. But a critical component is that each disorder is treated by a different provider (typically a specialist for that disorder). The parallel approach's advantage is that it offers specialized treatment; however, different clinicians could have inconsistent approaches, and clients could receive conflicting messages (Torrens et al., 2012).

Finally, the *integrated model* is focused on treating both disorders simultaneously, and one counselor provides the care. The main advantage of the integrated approach acknowledges the complexity of these issues and is sensitive to clients' acute needs (Horsfall et al., 2009). Now that these theoretical frameworks have been introduced, specific treatment modalities are reviewed.

INTEGRATED GROUP THERAPY

Integrated group therapy (IGT) is an evidence-based treatment for persons with co-occurring BD and SUD (Weiss & Smith Connery, 2011). This approach is considered one of the most effective treatments designed explicitly for these disorders. The essence of IGT lies in the emphasis on addressing both disorders simultaneously. While clients attend IGT, they are taught to consider themselves as having one disorder: *bipolar substance abuse* (Weiss & Smith Connery, 2011). This approach operates on a belief that unless clinicians consider the symptoms of *both* disorders in unison, they will not be able to effectively address their clients' concerns and help them improve. This attitude is further reflected in the three guiding principles of IGT (Weiss & Smith Connery, 2011):

1. Symptoms of BD and SUD are highly interactive, and their impact on clients' lives should be considered as one complex disorder.

2. There are significant parallels between the two disorders when it comes to recovery and relapse.

3. A clear strategy must be developed for improving outcomes for both disorders simultaneously.

This approach is based theoretically on cognitive behavior theory (CBT). As such, it focuses on thoughts and behaviors that are recovery oriented and focused on preventing relapse of mood disruption and substance use (Weiss & Smith Connery, 2011). CBT principles are integrated throughout IGT, and clients are expected to examine their thought processes and behavioral patterns continuously. Some examples of the CBT techniques that are actively used in IGT sessions are: (a) symptom monitoring; (b) connecting thoughts to symptoms, mood, and behavior; (c) thought distortions and the use of evidence gathering; and (d) skills training and behavioral problem solving (Weiss & Smith Connery, 2011).

Finally, the IGT approach outlines five major goals that counselors need to consider when working with persons who are diagnosed with co-occurring BD and SUD. The first two goals are focused on adherence to treatment, which includes (a) *abstinence from drug use*, and (b) *following the medication regimen* prescribed for the management of BD and/or SUD. The next two goals are focused on helping clients obtain tangible skills that will be useful in their recovery. These include teaching clients (c) *symptom recognition skills*, and (d) *relapse prevention* and *mood stabilizing techniques*. Finally, the last goal aims to help clients (e) *enhance other aspects of life functioning*, including but not limited to interpersonal relationships, anger management, and so on (Weiss & Smith Connery, 2011).

INTEGRATED MOTIVATIONAL INTERVIEWING AND COGNITIVE BEHAVIORAL THERAPY

Integration of motivational interviewing (MI) and CBT for co-occurring BD and SUD treatment was introduced by Jones and colleagues (2011). This approach was adapted from an integrated model used successfully in treating persons with psychosis and substance use issues (Barrowclough et al., 2007). Integration of MI and CBT was shown effective in helping clients manage symptoms associated with both disorders, increasing clients' engagement and internal motivation, and improving their overall functioning (Jones et al., 2011).

This intervention aims to address issues related to both disorders and the combined effect they have on clients' lives by strategically utilizing a combination of MI and CBT techniques (Jones et al., 2011). For example, MI techniques are heavily used during the early stages to engage clients and help them consider immediate concerns and central life goals. MI is also used to help clients explore the impact of their co-occurring disorders on the primary goals and priorities in their lives. Additionally, MI techniques are used to increase clients' commitment toward change and explore potential barriers in this process. Following these initial processes, counselors use various CBT techniques to resolve symptoms clients were experiencing. For example, counselors utilize psychoeducation to (a) inform clients about their disorder and presenting symptoms, (b) review medication adherence techniques to help clients maintain their course of treatment, and (c) assess high-risk behaviors to help clients prevent relapse. During this "intervention phase," counselors often use MI skills when issues with clients' ambivalence, motivation, and engagement are present (Jones et al., 2011).

In addition to the utility MI and CBT integration offers, an additional advantage of this model is that it gives counselors a prodigious level of freedom to tailor the treatment to clients' unique set of circumstances. This approach is not prescriptive and does not demand strict adherence to a predetermined protocol; rather, it provides an overall structure and suggestions on how these two evidence-based approaches could be integrated to assist clients in overcoming issues associate with co-occurring BD and SUD (Jones et al., 2011).

LEGAL AND ETHICAL CONSIDERATIONS
GENERAL REMINDERS

Considering all the factors regarding co-occurring BD and SUD discussed thus far, it is noticeable that these comorbid disorders pose a unique set of ethical and legal considerations. But before these specific implications are discussed, two broader perspectives relevant to the counseling profession must be reviewed. First, all counselors should adhere to the American Counseling Association (ACA, 2014) *Code of Ethics* and embody the meta-ethical principles of *autonomy*, *nonmaleficence*, *beneficence*, *justice*, *fidelity*, and *veracity* in all professional decisions. Second, counselors are responsible for understanding and upholding all relevant state and federal laws pertaining to counseling practice. Keeping these principles in mind, the key ethical considerations pertinent to working with this population are addressed in the remainder of this section.

ETHICAL AND LEGAL CONSIDERATIONS RELATED TO SUICIDE RISK

One of the most significant considerations when working with clients diagnosed with co-occurring BD and SUD is the risk of suicide. Researchers generally agree that both BD and SUD increase the overall risk of suicide attempts and completed suicide (Fazel et al., 2010; Icick et al., 2019; Pompili et al., 2013). Compared to other mental health conditions, BD has the highest lifetime prevalence of suicide attempts and completed suicides (Icick et al., 2019). It is estimated the risk for suicide attempts is 20 to 30 times greater for individuals diagnosed with BD than for the general population (Pompili et al., 2013). Additionally, the results from a large cross-sectional study indicated that persons diagnosed with BD who smoke tobacco were at an increased risk for suicide attempts (Icick et al., 2019).

ETHICAL AND LEGAL CONSIDERATIONS RELATED TO VIOLENCE RISK

Co-occurring BD and SUD also are associated with increased rates of violence. A large longitudinal study found an increased risk of violent crime convictions for persons diagnosed with BD, and this risk is nearly tripled when SUD comorbidity is present (Fazel et al., 2010). The results of this study suggested that substance use likely mediates the association between violence and BD. That is, BD alone does not increase the risk for violence, but the presence of a co-occurring SUD increases the risk for violent behavior. Increased risk-taking behavior and impulsivity, prevalent in both BD and SUD, may also be connected to increased rates of violence reported as well, although a bidirectional and environmental etiology may partially explain the rates of violence within this population (Alnıak et al., 2016; Fazel et al., 2010). Given the increased risk of harm to self and others, intentional suicide and homicide screening and safety planning are critical when working with persons diagnosed with co-occurring BD and SUD.

ETHICAL AND LEGAL CONSIDERATIONS RELATED TO ASSESSMENT, DIAGNOSIS, AND TREATMENT

Another important consideration for working with this population is (mis)diagnosis of BD and SUD. Merikangas and colleagues (2011) found that clients with BD are often misdiagnosed or only receive treatment related to common comorbidities (e.g., anxiety disorders, SUDs). This potential lack of recognition of BD related symptoms could lead to inappropriate or less effective treatment. Additionally, many effects of substance use could either mimic, accentuate, or mask BD symptoms, therefore making it more difficult to appropriately diagnose clients' issues and develop an effective treatment plan. It is imperative that counselors can appropriately assess, diagnose, and treat both BD and SUD disorders to serve this especially vulnerable population ethically.

CLINICAL CASE ILLUSTRATION AND DISCUSSION

CASE OF ROBERT

Robert K. is a 26-year-old, biracial, single, cisgender male who presented for treatment at his parents' insistence. Robert is not motivated to seek help, but his parents threatened to stop their financial support and force Robert to leave his childhood home if he did not seek immediate help. Robert shared that his parents are concerned with his drinking, mood swings that sometimes get violent, and an inability to maintain steady employment. The tipping point for his parents' concern was the most recent incident when he was fired from his job of 2 years due to a verbal altercation with his supervisor and then subsequently attending a "party" that resulted in Robert not returning home or answering his parent's phone calls for over 60 hours.

Robert shared that he started experiencing his "issues" at the beginning of high school. He remembers feeling "really sad and tired all of a sudden" and lacked the motivation to do anything "for a long time" during his first semester. Robert stated that during that time he stopped talking to most of his friends and quit his high school track and field team that he joined shortly before his symptoms started. He also reported it was difficult to go to sleep at night, and he had a hard time paying attention in classes. He shared that his parents believed his symptoms were related to his transition to high school and offered him financial incentives to start doing better at school. He said his feelings of sadness and lack of motivation went away "for a while" but remembers being very irritable and anxious "for no reason" toward the end of his freshman year. Although his issues with concentration and sleep persisted through this period, he disclosed experiencing bursts of energy that lasted for days. Despite liking these periods because he could catch up on all his schoolwork and household chores, Robert stated these emotional and physical states had a downside. He was irritable and consistently got into altercations with peers at school, which led to multiple after-school detentions and one out-of-school suspension. He reported that he saw his primary care physician during this period who diagnosed him with ADHD and prescribed a psychotropic medication regimen of Adderall® 5 mg twice a day (i.e., amphetamine/dextroamphetamine). Robert, however, believed the medication was not very helpful because he continued to experience mood disturbances, anxiety, sleep issues, and academic challenges; therefore, he stopped taking it soon after it was initially prescribed.

Robert disclosed that he started drinking alcohol during his second year of high school. He shared that he has not gone more than a couple of days without an alcoholic drink in the past 5 to 6 years. Robert stated that he primarily drinks alcohol to help him go to sleep and numb all the negativity he is experiencing consistently; he shared that alcohol helps him calm his anxiety too. He reported that most days, he consumes about "a fifth" (750 mL) of hard liquor. He reported typically starting to drink around noon and continues drinking until he "passes out." When asking about the use of other drugs, he disclosed smoking tobacco (i.e., one pack of cigarettes; 20 cigarettes, approximately 22 to 36 mg of nicotine) daily since he was 18. He also shared that he periodically snorts cocaine. He revealed that he only has the urge to use cocaine during periods when he has a lot of energy and can at times exceed consuming over 2 grams in a few days.

Robert said that cocaine helps him concentrate during those times and allows him to stay in this energized state longer. However, he shared that he experiences a more severe state of sadness and depression following "party time" when cocaine is included. He also shared that he is more likely to get irritable when using cocaine, and he often gets into physical fights when in this state.

CASE DISCUSSION

When considering an initial treatment plan for Robert, there is an important range of factors to examine. Issues relevant to co-occurring BD and SUDs, as well as general considerations related to working with Robert, are identified and briefly discussed.

Screening, Assessment, and Diagnosis

The first step in creating a treatment plan is appropriate assessment and diagnosis. This step is particularly imperative in Robert's case considering how prevalent misdiagnosis is with co-occurring BD and SUD. Also, a thorough assessment of risk factors associated with these disorders, including suicide, is needed. Specifically, the counselor is recommended to use the *Psychiatric Research Interview for Substance and Mental Disorders for DSM-5* (PRISM-5; Hasin et al., 1996). The PRISM-5 is a semi-structured diagnostic interview appropriate for use when conducting psychiatric diagnoses with clients who use substances, as it specifically targets co-occurring occurrences. As such, the counselor must finally consider the relationship between these disorders in Robert's case and how they jointly affect his overall well-being.

Level of Care and Treatment Interventions

It is important for the counselor to work with Robert in determining the appropriate level of care and treatment modalities. The counselor should always strive for the least restrictive level of care; however, the counselor also needs to consider the level of support Robert will need to address symptoms associated with both disorders. The counselor could use the American Society for Addiction Medicine (ASAM) level of care assessment criteria to determine an appropriate setting (Mee-Lee, 2013). Also, the counselor should consider whether Robert would benefit from participation in group counseling (e.g., IGT).

Psychoeducation on co-occurring BD and SUD should be presented to Robert early on in this process. Being diagnosed with a co-occurring disorder may be confusing or scary for Robert. It is essential for the counselor to provide pertinent information and demystify co-occurring conditions and treatment needs. This will be achieved, in part, when the counselor helps Robert understand the correlational relationship between BD and SUD. Additionally, the counselor should create a list of resources available for Robert and answer any specific questions he may have.

The counselor may consider a referral for psychiatric assessment and education on medication adherence. Common psychiatric medications prescribed for the treatment of bipolar and related disorders often include a combination of a mood stabilizer (e.g., lithium, carbamazepine, divalproex sodium, lamotrigine) and an antipsychotic (e.g., aripiprazole, chlorpromazine, olanzapine, risperidone; Vieta et al., 2018). It would be vital to refer Robert for a psychiatric examination to determine if medically assisted treatment would be appropriate. Significant research evidence indicates that pharmacotherapy effectively manages mood disturbance of BD, and medical treatment may be needed to manage Robert's withdrawal process from alcohol (Grande & Vieta, 2015). Additionally, it is essential for the counselor to utilize psychoeducational strategies to help Robert understand the reasons for medication use and how this treatment could aid in his recovery.

Preliminary Treatment Plan

It is vital for the counselor to actively include Robert when establishing treatment objectives and goals. During this stage, the counselor could use MI techniques to help Robert explore the impact present symptoms have on his life and determine what is important for him moving forward. The counselor should work with Robert to determine *short-term* (0–3 months), *intermediate* (4–6 months), and *long-term* (after 6 months) goals. While it is crucial this step occurs with client input and agreement, here are a few ideas for goals:

1. Short-Term Goals:
   a. Complete psychological testing to assess the nature and impact of mood problems and substance use.
   b. Participate in a medical and psychiatric evaluation to assess the effects of substance abuse and potential pharmacological treatment (i.e., psychiatric medication).
   c. Withdraw from mood-altering substances, stabilize physically and emotionally, and then establish a supportive recovery plan.
   d. Verbalize an understanding of the cognitive, physiologic, and behavioral components of BD and SUD and their treatment.
2. Intermediate Goals:
   a. Develop healthy cognitive patterns and beliefs about self and the world that lead to alleviation and help prevent the relapse of manic/hypomanic and depressive episodes.
   b. Acquire the necessary behavioral and cognitive coping skills to establish sobriety from all mood-altering substances.
3. Long-Term Goals:
   a. Normalize energy level and return to baseline usual activities, appropriate judgment, stable mood, more realistic expectations, and goal-directed behavior.
   b. Achieve sustained recovery; be free from the use of all mood-altering substances.
   c. Implement and maintain a daily schedule and routine that support mood stabilization and mitigates substance use.

Psychoeducation Needs

The psychoeducation process should also include a focus on helping Robert identify warning signs of an impending mood episode. If the onset of a mood disorder is identified early, actions can often be taken to lessen the severity of an episode. Common indicators of an incoming mood episode are: (a) change in sleep patterns; (b) significant change in mood (e.g., overly happy, really sad, irritable); (c) behavioral changes (e.g., getting in verbal or physical altercations, withdrawing from friends); and (d) changes in thought and speech patterns.

Community Resources and Support Systems

Counselors may want to work with Robert on finding peer support groups. It would be helpful for Robert to connect with others who are also diagnosed with co-occurring disorders. This can be an additional resource and point of support for Robert. Also, it can aid Robert in establishing a social group that would be supportive of his recovery efforts. Dual Recovery Anonymous (DRA) is a support group grounded in the tenets of 12-step organizations that may be a possibility for Robert (Dual Recovery Anonymous World Network Inc., n.d.).

Daily Routines Impacting Overall Health and Well-Being

Robert and his counselor can work on goals to establish healthy sleep hygiene. Considering Robert's difficulties with sleep that persist in both his depressive and manic mood episodes, this issue must be addressed. Additionally, as previously mentioned, sleep disturbance can be one of the leading indicators of an incoming mood episode. The counselor could utilize CBT techniques to help Robert establish a nighttime routine, including consistent bedtime, that will assist him in regulating his sleep.

The counselor will want to work with Robert in developing daily routines that will help him regulate his mood and mitigate his substance use. The counselor should utilize CBT techniques to help Robert establish a sustainable schedule. The schedule should be comprehensive and cover all his work and family obligations as well as leisure activities. Keeping a record or maintaining a journal of his sleep, mood, and behavior patterns will be helpful for both Robert and the counselor to track potential "red flags" as well as monitor progress.

Concluding Considerations

Robert presents with symptoms consistent with co-occurring BD and SUD. Specifically, he exhibits an abnormally and persistently elevated mood with at least three symptoms of BD (e.g., mood disturbances [happy, sad, irritable], decreased need for sleep, distractibility, impulsivity) and poly-substance abuse (i.e., alcohol, tobacco, and cocaine). It is recommended that the counselor first assess for co-occurring BD and SUD to determine the appropriate level of care and treatment modalities. In addition to treatment selection, the counselor should also refer Robert for a full medical and psychiatric evaluation to assist in substance withdrawal symptoms and the potential need for psychiatric medication. Within treatment, counselors can utilize psychoeducation, MI techniques, CBT, and IGT.

CHAPTER SUMMARY

Within the chapter, *DSM-5* diagnostic criteria, prevalence rates, screening and assessment methods, and treatment implications were reviewed. Comorbidity of bipolar disorder and SUDs is characterized by significant mood disturbances and exacerbated substance use. The co-occurrence of these two disorders increases the complexity of assessing, diagnosing, and treating persons affected, thereby impacting bipolar and SUDs risk factors and treatment outcomes. Because the relationship between co-occurring bipolar and SUDs is a complex one, counselors should be skilled in the practices of screening and assessing, diagnosing, and treatment planning when working with this high-risk population.

DISCUSSION QUESTIONS

1. In what ways does substance use impact diagnosis of BD?
2. What presenting symptoms would someone who is in an active manic state exhibit?
3. What current and past symptoms would you look for when assessing someone for BD-II?

4. Why might someone with BD experience hypomanic or manic symptoms as nonproblematic, or even pleasurable?
5. How do the sequential, parallel, and integrated models of treatment differ?
6. Considering the sequential, parallel, and integrated models of treatment, identify which you would choose as your model for treatment (be sure to include a clinical rationale when explaining your answer).

REFERENCES

Alnıak, I., Erkıran, M., & Mutlu, E. (2016). Substance use is a risk factor for violent behavior in male patients with bipolar disorder. *Journal of Affective Disorders*, *193*, 89–93. https://doi.org/10.1016/j.jad.2015.12.059

American Counseling Association. (2014). *ACA code of ethics*. Alexandria, VA.

American Psychiatric Association. (2013). *Diagnostic and statistical manual of mental disorders* (5th ed.). https://doi.org/10.1176/appi.books.9780890425596

Atkins, C. (2014). *Co-occurring disorders: Integrated assessment and treatment of substance use and mental disorders*. PESI Publishing & Media.

Baethge, C., Baldessarini, R. J., Khalsa, H. M., Hennen, J., Salvatore, P., & Tohen, M. (2005). Substance abuse in first-episode bipolar I disorder: Indications for early intervention. *The American Journal of Psychiatry*, *162*(5), 1008–1010. https://doi.org/10.1176/appi.ajp.162.5.1008

Barrowclough, C., Haddock, G., Lowens, I., Allott, R., Earnshaw, P., Fitzsimmons, M., & Nothard, S. (2007). Psychosis & drug and alcohol problems. In A. Baker, & R. Velleman (Eds.), *Clinical handbook of co-existing mental health and drug and alcohol problems* (pp. 241–265). Routledge.

Bech, P., Bolwig, T. G., Kramp, P., & Rafaelsen, O. J. (1979). The Bech-Rafaelsen Mania Scale and the Hamilton Depression Scale: Evaluation of homogeneity and inter-observer reliability. *Acta Psychiatrica Scandinavica*, *59*(4), 420–430. https://doi.org/10.1111/j.1600-0447.1979.tb04484.x

Bizzarri, J. V., Sbrana, A., Rucci, P., Ravani, L., Massei, G. J., Gonnelli, C., Spagnolli, S., Doria, M. R., Raimondi, F., Endicott, J., Dell'Osso, L., & Cassano, G. B. (2007). The spectrum of substance abuse in bipolar disorder: Reasons for use, sensation seeking and substance sensitivity. *Bipolar Disorders*, *9*(3), 213–220. https://doi.org/10.1111/j.1399-5618.2007.00383.x

Cerullo, M. A., & Strakowski, S. M. (2007). The prevalence and significance of substance use disorders in bipolar type I and II disorder. *Substance Abuse Treatment, Prevention, and Policy*, *2*, 29. https://doi.org/10.1186/1747-597X-2-29

Culpepper, L. (2014). The diagnosis and treatment of bipolar disorder: decision-making in primary care. *The Primary Care Companion for CNS Disorders*, *16*(3), Article PCC.13r01609. https://doi.org/10.4088/PCC.13r01609

Di Florio, A., Craddock, N., & van den Bree, M. (2014). Alcohol misuse in bipolar disorder: A systematic review and meta-analysis of comorbidity rates. *European Psychiatry: The Journal of the Association of European Psychiatrists*, *29*(3), 117–124. https://doi.org/10.1016/j.eurpsy.2013.07.004

Dual Recovery Anonymous World Network Inc. (n.d.). *Dual Recovery Anonymous (DRA)*. http://draonline.org/

Etain, B., Lajnef, M., Bellivier, F., Mathieu, F., Raust, A., Cochet, B., Gard, S., M'Bailara, K., Kahn, J. P., Elgrabli, O., Cohen, R., Jamain, S., Vieta, E., Leboyer, M., & Henry, C. (2012). Clinical expression of bipolar disorder type I as a function of age and polarity at onset: Convergent findings in samples from France and the United States. *The Journal of Clinical Psychiatry*, *73*(4), e561–e566. https://doi.org/10.4088/JCP.10m06504

Fazel, S., Lichtenstein, P., Grann, M., Goodwin, G. M., & Långström, N. (2010). Bipolar disorder and violent crime: New evidence from population-based longitudinal studies and systematic review. *Archives of General Psychiatry*, *67*(9), 931–938. https://doi.org/10.1001/archgenpsychiatry.2010.97

Frank, E., Boland, E., Novick, D. M., Bizzarri, J. V., & Rucci, P. (2007). Association between illicit drug and alcohol use and first manic episode. *Pharmacology Biochemistry and Behavior*, *86*(2), 395–400. https://doi.org/10.1016/j.pbb.2006.11.009

Gold, A. K., Peters, A. T., Otto, M. W., Sylvia, L. G., Magalhaes, P., Berk, M., Dougherty, D. D., Miklowitz, D. J., Frank, E., Nierenberg, A. A., & Deckersbach, T. (2018). The impact of substance use disorders on recovery from bipolar depression: Results from the Systematic Treatment Enhancement Program for Bipolar Disorder psychosocial treatment trial. *The Australian and New Zealand journal of psychiatry*, 52(9), 847–855. https://doi.org/10.1177/0004867418788172

Goodwin, R. D., Stayner, D. A., Chinman, M. J., Wu, P., Tebes, J. K., & Davidson, L. (2002). The relationship between anxiety and substance use disorders among individuals with severe affective disorders. *Comprehensive Psychiatry*, 43(4), 245–252. https://doi.org/10.1053/comp.2002.33500

Graff, F. S., Griffin, M. L., & Weiss, R. D. (2008). Predictors of dropout from group therapy among patients with bipolar and substance use disorders. *Drug and Alcohol Dependence*, 94(1-3), 272–275. https://doi.org/10.1016/j.drugalcdep.2007.11.002

Grande, I., & Vieta, E. (2015). Pharmacotherapy of acute mania: monotherapy or combination therapy with mood stabilizers and antipsychotics? *CNS drugs*, 29(3), 221–227. https://doi.org/10.1007/s40263-015-0235-1

Grant, B. F., Saha, T. D., Ruan, W. J., Goldstein, R. B., Chou, S. P., Jung, J., Zhang, H., Smith, S. M., Pickering, R. P., Huang, B., & Hasin, D. S. (2016). Epidemiology of DSM-5 drug use disorder: Results from the National Epidemiologic Survey on alcohol and related conditions-III. *JAMA psychiatry*, 73(1), 39–47. https://doi.org/10.1001/jamapsychiatry.2015.2132

Hasin, D. S., Trautman, K. D., Miele, G. M., Samet, S., Smith, M., & Endicott, J. (1996). Psychiatric Research Interview for Substance and Mental Disorders (PRISM): Reliability for substance abusers. *The American Journal of Psychiatry*, 153(9), 1195–1201. https://doi.org/10.1176/ajp.153.9.1195

Heffner, J. L., Strawn, J. R., DelBello, M. P., Strakowski, S. M., & Anthenelli, R. M. (2011). The co-occurrence of cigarette smoking and bipolar disorder: Phenomenology and treatment considerations. *Bipolar Disorders*, 13(5-6), 439–453. https://doi.org/10.1111/j.1399-5618.2011.00943.x

Hirschfeld, R. M., Williams, J. B., Spitzer, R. L., Calabrese, J. R., Flynn, L., Keck, P. E., Jr., Lewis, L., McElroy, S. L., Post, R. M., Rapport, D. J., Russell, J. M., Sachs, G. S., & Zajecka, J. (2000). Development and validation of a screening instrument for bipolar spectrum disorder: The Mood Disorder Questionnaire. *The American Journal of Psychiatry*, 157(11), 1873–1875. https://doi.org/10.1176/appi.ajp.157.11.1873

Horsfall, J., Cleary, M., Hunt, G. E., & Walter, G. (2009). Psychosocial treatments for people with co-occurring severe mental illnesses and substance use disorders (dual diagnosis): A review of empirical evidence. *Harvard Review of Psychiatry*, 17(1), 24–34.

Hunt, G. E., Malhi, G. S., Cleary, M., Lai, H. M., & Sitharthan, T. (2016). Prevalence of comorbid bipolar and substance use disorders in clinical settings, 1990-2015: Systematic review and meta-analysis. *Journal of Affective Disorders*, 206, 331–349. https://doi.org/10.1016/j.jad.2016.07.011

Icick, R., Melle, I., Etain, B., Ringen, P. A., Aminoff, S. R., Leboyer, M., Aas, M., Henry, C., Bjella, T. D., Andreassen, O. A., Bellivier, F., & Lagerberg, T. V. (2019). Tobacco smoking and other substance use disorders associated with recurrent suicide attempts in bipolar disorder. *Journal of Affective Disorders*, 256, 348–357. https://doi.org/10.1016/j.jad.2019.05.075

Jones, S. H., Barrowclough, C., Allott, R., Day, C., Earnshaw, P., & Wilson, I. (2011). Integrated motivational interviewing and cognitive-behavioral therapy for bipolar disorder with comorbid substance use. *Clinical Psychology and Psychotherapy*, 18, 426–437.

Joshi, G., & Wilens, T. (2009). Comorbidity in pediatric bipolar disorder. *Child and Adolescent Psychiatric Clinics of North America*, 18(2), 291-viii. https://doi.org/10.1016/j.chc.2008.12.005

Kessler, R. C., Akiskal, H. S., Angst, J., Guyer, M., Hirschfeld, R. M., Merikangas, K. R., & Stang, P. E. (2006). Validity of the assessment of bipolar spectrum disorders in the WHO CIDI 3.0. *Journal of Affective Disorders*, 96(3), 259–269. https://doi.org/10.1016/j.jad.2006.08.018

Lev-Ran, S., Le Foll, B., McKenzie, K., George, T. P., & Rehm, J. (2013). Bipolar disorder and co-occurring cannabis use disorders: Characteristics, co-morbidities and clinical correlates. *Psychiatry Research*, 209(3), 459–465. https://doi.org/10.1016/j.psychres.2012.12.014

Mee-Lee, D. (2013). *The ASAM criteria: Treatment criteria for addictive, substance-related, and co-occurring conditions* (3rd ed.). The Change Companies.

Merikangas, K. R., Jin, R., He, J. P., Kessler, R. C., Lee, S., Sampson, N. A., Viana, M. C., Andrade, L. H., Hu, C., Karam, E. G., Ladea, M., Medina-Mora, M. E., Ono, Y., Posada-Villa, J., Sagar, R., Wells, J. E., & Zarkov, Z. (2011). Prevalence and correlates of bipolar spectrum disorder in the world mental health survey initiative. *Archives of General Psychiatry, 68*(3), 241–251. https://doi.org/10.1001/archgenpsychiatry.2011.12

Messer, T., Lammers, G., Müller-Siecheneder, F., Schmidt, R. F., & Latifi, S. (2017). Substance abuse in patients with bipolar disorder: A systematic review and meta-analysis. *Psychiatry Research, 253*, 338–350. https://doi.org/10.1016/j.psychres.2017.02.067

Ming, M., Coles, A. S., & George, T. P. (2018). Understanding and treating co-occurring bipolar disorder and substance use disorders. *Psychiatric Times, 35*(9). Retrieved from https://www.psychiatrictimes.com/view/understanding-and-treating-co-occurring-bipolar-disorder-and-substance-use-disorders

Morisano, D., Babor, T. F., & Robaina, K. A. (2014). Co-occurrence of substance use disorders with other psychiatric disorders: Implications for treatment services. *Nordic Studies on Alcohol and Drugs, 31*(1), 5–25.

Nallet, A., Weber, B., Favre, S., Gex-Fabry, M., Voide, R., Ferrero, F., Zullino, D., Khazaal, Y., & Aubry, J. M. (2013). Screening for bipolar disorder among outpatients with substance use disorders. *European Psychiatry: The Journal of the Association of European Psychiatrists, 28*(3), 147–153. https://doi.org/10.1016/j.eurpsy.2011.07.004

Nery, F. G., Hatch, J. P., Monkul, E. S., Matsuo, K., Zunta-Soares, G. B., Bowden, C. L., & Soares, J. C. (2013). Trait impulsivity is increased in bipolar disorder patients with comorbid alcohol use disorders. *Psychopathology, 46*, 145–152. https://doi.org/10.1159/000336730

Oquendo, M. A., Currier, D., Liu, S. M., Hasin, D. S., Grant, B. F., & Blanco, C. (2010). Increased risk for suicidal behavior in comorbid bipolar disorder and alcohol use disorders: Results from the National Epidemiologic Survey on Alcohol and Related Conditions (NESARC). *The Journal of Clinical Psychiatry, 71*(7), 902–909. https://doi.org/10.4088/JCP.09m05198gry

Patel, R. S., Virani, S., Saeed, H., Nimmagadda, S., Talukdar, J., & Youssef, N. A. (2018). Gender differences and comorbidities in U.S. adults with bipolar disorder. *Brain Sciences, 8*(9), 168. https://doi.org/10.3390/brainsci8090168

Pompili, M., Gonda, X., Serafini, G., Innamorati, M., Sher, L., Amore, M., Rihmer, Z., & Girardi, P. (2013). Epidemiology of suicide in bipolar disorders: A systematic review of the literature. *Bipolar Disorders, 15*(5), 457–490. https://doi.org/10.1111/bdi.12087

Quello, S. B., Brady, K. T., & Sonne, S. C. (2005). Mood disorders and substance use disorder: A complex comorbidity. *Science & Practice Perspectives, 3*(1), 13–21. 10.1151/spp053113

Ritchie, H., & Roser, M. (2018). *Mental health*. Our World in Data. Retrieved from https://ourworldindata.org/mental-health

Rowland, T. A., & Marwaha, S. (2018). Epidemiology and risk factors for bipolar disorder. *Therapeutic Advances in Psychopharmacology*, 251–269. https://doi.org/10.1177/2045125318769235

Salloum, I. M., & Brown, E. S. (2017). Management of comorbid bipolar disorder and substance use disorders. *The American Journal of Drug and Alcohol Abuse, 43*(4), 366–376. https://doi.org/10.1080/00952990.2017.1292279

Schaffer, A., Isometsä, E. T., Tondo, L., H Moreno, D., Turecki, G., Reis, C., Cassidy, F., Sinyor, M., Azorin, J. M., Kessing, L. V., Ha, K., Goldstein, T., Weizman, A., Beautrais, A., Chou, Y. H., Diazgranados, N., Levitt, A. J., Zarate, C. A., Jr., Rihmer, Z., . . . Yatham, L. N. (2015). International society for bipolar disorders task force on suicide: Meta-analyses and meta-regression of correlates of suicide attempts and suicide deaths in bipolar disorder. *Bipolar Disorders, 17*(1), 1–16. https://doi.org/10.1111/bdi.12271

Sonne, S. C., & Brady, K. T. (2002). Bipolar disorder and alcoholism. *Alcohol Research & Health, 26*(2), 103–108.

Substance Abuse and Mental Health Services Administration. (2016). An introduction to bipolar disorder and co-occurring substance use disorders. *Advisory, 15*(2). Retrieved from https://store.samhsa.gov/product/Advisory-An-Introduction-to-Bipolar-Disorder-and-Co-Occurring-Substance-Use-Disorders/SMA16-4960

Substance Abuse and Mental Health Services Administration. (2021). *Key substance use and mental health indicators in the United States: Results from the 2020 National Survey on Drug Use and Health* (HHS Publication Np. PEP21-07-01-003, NSDUH Series H-56). Center for Behavioral Health Statistics and Quality, Author. Retrieved from https://www.samhsa.gov/data/sites/default/files/reports/rpt35325/NSDUHFFRPDFWHTMLFiles2020/2020NSDUHFFR1PDFW102121.pdf

Swann, A. C. (2010). The strong relationship between bipolar and substance-use disorder. *Annals of the New York Academy of Sciences, 1187*(1), 276–293. https://doi.org/10.1111/j.1749-6632.2009.05146.x

Swendsen, J., Conway, K. P., Degenhardt, L., Glantz, M., Jin, R., Merikangas, K. R., Sampson, N., & Kessler, R. C. (2010). Mental disorders as risk factors for substance use, abuse and dependence: Results from the 10-year follow-up of the National Comorbidity Survey. *Addiction, 105*(6), 1117–1128. https://doi.org/10.1111/j.1360-0443.2010.02902.x

Tohen, M., Zarate, C., Hennen, J., Khalsa, H., Strakowski, S., Gebre-Medhin, P., Salvatore, P., & Baldessarini, R. (2003). The McLean-Harvard first-episode mania study: Prediction of recovery and first recurrence. *American Journal of Psychiatry, 160*(12): 2099–2107. https://doi.org/10.1176/appi.ajp.160.12.2099.

Tolliver, B. K., & Hartwell, K. J. (2012). Implications and strategies for clinical management of co-occurring substance use in bipolar disorder. *Psychiatric Annals, 42*(5), 190–197. https://doi.org/10.3928/00485713-20120507-07

Torrens, M., Rossi, P. C., Martinez-Riera, R., Martinez-Sanvisens, D., & Bulbena, A. (2012). Psychiatric co- morbidity and substance use disorders: Treatment in parallel systems or in one integrated system? *Substance Use and Misuse, 47*(8-9), 1005–1014.

Varo, C., Murru, A., Salagre, E., Jiménez, E., Solé, B., Montejo, L., Carvalho, A. F., Stubbs, B., Grande, I., Martínez-Arán, A., Vieta, E., & Reinares, M. (2019). Behavioral addictions in bipolar disorders: A systematic review. *European Neuropsychopharmacology: The Journal of the European College of Neuropsychopharmacology, 29*(1), 76–97. https://doi.org/10.1016/j.euroneuro.2018.10.012

Vieta, E., Berk, M., Schulze, T. G., Carvalho, A. F., Suppes, T., Calabrese, J. R., Gao, K., Miskowiak, K. W., & Grande, I. (2018). Bipolar disorders. *Nature reviews. Disease primers, 4*, Article 18008. https://doi.org/10.1038/nrdp.2018.8

Weiss, R. D., & Smith Connery, H, (2011). *Integrated group therapy for bipolar disorder and substance abuse.* Guilford Press.

Young, R. C., Biggs, J. T., Ziegler, V. E., & Meyer, D. A. (1978). A rating scale for mania: Reliability, validity and sensitivity. *The British Journal of Psychiatry, 133*, 429–435. https://doi.org/10.1192/bjp.133.5.429

CHAPTER 11

CO-OCCURRING ANXIETY AND OBSESSIVE-COMPULSIVE DISORDERS AND SUBSTANCE USE DISORDERS

GERI MILLER, DOMINIQUE S. HAMMONDS, EMILY PROCTOR, AND MILLER A. FAW

LEARNING OBJECTIVES

After reading this chapter, you will be able to:

- Explain the overall interaction between the mental health disorders of anxiety, obsessive-compulsive, and substance use disorders (SUDs).
- Discuss the philosophical perspective presented of working with clients dually diagnosed with anxiety, obsessive-compulsive, and SUDs.
- Develop general assessment and treatment approaches that can be used in working with clients dually diagnosed with anxiety, obsessive-compulsive, SUDs.
- Demonstrate an understanding of the legal and ethical implications/considerations of working with clients dually diagnosed with anxiety, obsessive-compulsive, and SUDs.

INTRODUCTION

"Fear is like a candle flame."

—G. Miller (2021)

This quote, made by the first author, acknowledges the human condition of fear as we face our existential realities. All of us live with fear, and, like a candle flame, the fear can "light our way" *if* it is contained in a holder that keeps it upright. However, for individuals who have untreated anxiety and/or obsessive-compulsive disorders, this "candle flame" of fear (that is *not* contained in a candle holder) is out of control and can be destructive to the candle and what is around it (e.g., their loved ones, their level of functioning, their lives). Staying with this metaphor, the individual may try to create their own "candle holder" to hold it in place by using substances. This use, when it becomes a disorder, only serves to make the "candle of fear" more unbalanced and out of control (e.g., more destructive). Thus, the complicated struggle of two or more disorders serves to "fuel" the shared "flame." This chapter, therefore, is dedicated to the brave individuals who struggle with anxiety and substance use, as well as their loved ones who suffer with them, as they attempt to find their way while struggling with two disorders that feed off each other. Counselors can serve as "candle holders," assisting them in finding a balanced way of living with their existential reality.

The co-occurrence of mental disorders is common in substance use disorder (SUD) clients (Veach & Moro, 2018). Overall, the 2019 National Survey on Drug Use and Health found co-occurring mental illness and SUDs in the past year occurring in 3.8% of the United States adult population (Substance Abuse and Mental Health Services Administration [SAMHSA], 2020). Miller et al. (2019) reported that SUD clients are twice as likely to struggle with anxiety, mood, conduct, or antisocial disorders, and that their occurrence increases with the severity of the clients' substance use disorder and the number of drugs they use. For example, with obsessive-compulsive disorder (OCD), researchers have found: (a) When compared with the general population, OCD is associated with higher rates of substance abuse (Blom et al., 2011; Mancebo et al., 2009; McAnally, 2017); and (b) there is increased suicidality risk with this co-occurring disorder (Gentil et al., 2009).

Miller (2021) provided an overall summary of this population in a review of the literature: The strong relationship between substance use and mental illness is a combination of several components such as the individual's lifestyle, biology, psychology, or social/causal experiences and other contextual factors (e.g., childhood abuse, limited social support, heredity). Problematic substance use may stem from impaired judgment or, as is the case with anxiety, be a result of self-medicating the anxiety. Additionally, the substance misuse and abuse may cause psychiatric symptoms of the co-occurring disorder (COD); a "kindling" effect has been described by other authors (Miller et al., 2019) where certain drugs can trigger a mental disorder making the client vulnerable to further/more severe episodes. For example, the vulnerability to a psychotic episode may be present (and unknown) in the client and when the client takes a hallucinogenic drug the first psychotic episode is triggered (Miller et al., 2019). This episode may increase the risk of further psychotic episodes which is known as the "kindling" effect (Miller et al., 2019).

In comparison with other psychiatric patients, those individuals with co-occurring mental illness and SUDs have tendencies to be more: (a) suicidal/homicidal/impulsive, (b) intelligent, (c) likely to binge use substances, and (d) manipulative (Miller, 2021). With this impulsivity, there are higher rates of relapse, violence, and hospitalization. These individuals may have begun using substances as a way of self-medicating. When at a treatment center, they have high drop-out rates and return to their typically precarious social networks. Thus, co-occurring diagnoses require professional teamwork with the tenets of honesty, communication, and trust operating between professional care providers. This is in sharp contrast to the history of the two fields of substance abuse and mental health treating the issues separately rather than collaborating with one another. Therefore, collaboration and teamwork must occur among healthcare providers.

CONCEPTUALIZING ANXIETY

In order to facilitate such collaboration, a shared understanding of the relationship between these disorders of substance use and mental health needs to begin with a philosophical discussion of anxiety and the addictive process. Historically, Tillich (1952) stated there are three types of anxiety: (a) the anxiety of fate and death (*the anxiety of death*), (b) the anxiety of emptiness and meaninglessness (*the anxiety of meaninglessness*), and (c) the anxiety of guilt and condemnation (*the anxiety of condemnation*). Therefore, counselors need to understand the client's anxiety to effectively treat anxiety rather than simply managing its symptoms.

Another helpful historical framework in understanding the client's experience of anxiety is as follows. Anxiety is experienced when the security pattern of the client has been threatened, and neurotic anxiety is when the anxiety is inappropriate to the level of danger because of inner conflict (May, 1979). Metaphorically, then, anxiety is a like a fever that indicates there is something off balance in the individual (May, 1979). If a client has been diagnosed with a generalized anxiety disorder (GAD), it is important for the counselor to understand the specific manifestations of the disorder while concurrently exploring the historical and contextual factors contributing to the disorder.

Symptoms can also develop as defensive structures to cope with contextual actual threats (e.g., early childhood vulnerability, war), and, in these cases, the symptoms have a purpose of self-protection. For example, the COVID-19 pandemic has increased anxiety in the general public (Sammons, 2020). It has altered sleep patterns for many individuals, and sleep disturbances are known to increase mental health problems (Abrams, 2021). With regard to using substances to cope with stress and emotions related to the pandemic, 13% of Americans reported starting or increasing their use of substances (Abramson, 2021b). Diagnostically, the pandemic has both initiated and exacerbated OCD, fears/phobias related to health and contamination, as well as social anxiety and hoarding (Abramson, 2021a). Generalized anxiety, resulting from isolation, stress, and uncertainty, is a current issue affecting many people around the world due to the global pandemic (Phillips, 2021). Also, in terms of drug overdoses during the early months of the pandemic, 2020 showed an increase of 18% when compared to the same time frame in 2019 (Abramson, 2021b). Therefore, in order to effectively assess and treat anxiety, OCD and SUDs, the counselor needs to examine these disorders within the context of the COVID-19 pandemic to determine if they were present prior to the pandemic, as well as how the pandemic exacerbated the disorder(s).

As such, examining the relationship between the disorders from a sociocultural perspective may be helpful. One such model is Cushman's (1990) empty self theory as shown in Figure 11.1.

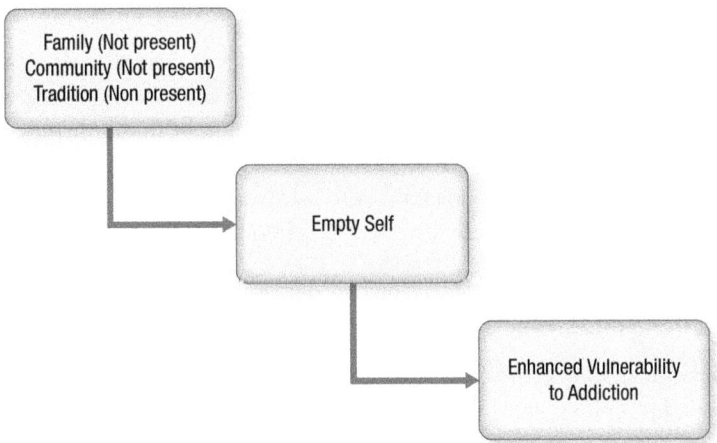

FIGURE 11.1 The Addictive Process Modeled by Cushman's (1990) Empty Self Theory (Sociocultural Model).
Source: Adapted from Cushman, P. (1990). Why the self is empty: Toward a historically situated psychology. *American Psychologist, 45*(5), 599–601.

In this model, individuals experience a loss of family, community, and tradition that provides shared meaning in their lives—a loss due to industrialization, urbanization, and secularism. This loss results in an empty self where there are specific psychological boundaries, an internal locus of control, and a desire to manipulate the external world for personal ends. When an individual in this state engages in substance use, it likely means that the person is using the substances to stop the feelings of alienation, fragmentation, worthlessness, and confusion.

Kemp (2018) expanded on this model describing addiction as "...pain intolerance, a pleasure pursuit, and dealing with life alienation and ambiguity" (as cited in Miller, 2021, p. 19). This model ties together, then, the relationship between anxiety disorder, OCD, and SUDs. Through the loss of family, community, and tradition, the person feels empty and anxious and then attempts to fill up the emptiness and end the anxieties related to existence through the use of substances. Additional contextual stressors (e.g., COVID-19) may exacerbate and accelerate this process.

ANXIETY AND OBSESSIVE-COMPULSIVE DISORDERS: *DSM-5* DIAGNOSTIC CRITERIA AND DESCRIPTION

The co-occurrence of mental health disorders and SUDs makes the process of this work challenging because of the convoluted and interactive nature of the disorders in terms of diagnosing and developing treatment plans. Since the *Diagnostic and Statistical Manual of Mental Disorders, Fifth Edition* (*DSM-5*; American Psychiatric Association [APA], 2013) has numerous anxiety-related disorders and SUDs (see the following), the sheer number of possible diagnoses can be overwhelming, confusing, and challenging for the counselor. Additionally, symptoms of anxiety may be related to substance use withdrawal and vice versa, anxiety symptoms may result in substance use to reduce anxiety. Also, because the disorders interact with one another and they fluctuate in intensity, the assessment and treatment plans are labor intensive because they need to be constantly monitored. For example, the counselor needs to continually check the *DSM-5* criteria as well as assess the effectiveness of the treatment plan by examining the accuracy of the diagnoses and the appropriateness of the treatment plan.

There are numerous anxiety disorders in the *DSM-5*. Each of these disorders involves the experiencing of fear and/or anxiety by the individual. "*Fear* is the emotional response to real or perceived imminent threat, whereas *anxiety* is the anticipation of future threat" (APA, 2013, p. 189). Anxiety disorders are identified in the following, or additionally as an other-specified or unspecified anxiety disorder. The two mental health lists (e.g., anxiety disorder, OCD) have some disorders noted by an asterisk (*); these disorders *may* frequently co-occur with SUDs.

ANXIETY DISORDERS

- **Separation anxiety disorder:** an individual experiences inappropriate distress when separated from their attachment figure(s)
- **Selective mutism:** an individual fails to speak in situations that it would normally be expected; however they do speak in other situations
- ***Specific phobia:** an individual has a specific fear or anxiety of a specific object(s) or situation(s)
- ***Social anxiety disorder (social phobia):** an individual is distressed by social situation(s) in which they may be negatively critiqued

- ***Panic disorder:** an individual has unexpected panic attacks which lead to constant worry of future panic attacks
- ***Agoraphobia:** an individual has distress about being in specific situations (e.g., being in a crowd, using public transportation) due to concerns about the inability to escape the situation
- ***Generalized anxiety disorder:** an individual experiences consistent and excessive concern, as well as physical symptoms (e.g., restlessness, fatigue) about various life domains (e.g., work, school)
- **Anxiety disorder due to another medical condition:** an individual experiences anxiety as a result of another medical diagnosis

OBSESSIVE-COMPULSIVE DISORDERS

The *DSM-5* obsessive-compulsive and related disorders are as follows, with the addition of those due to another medical condition, other-specified, and unspecified:

- **Other specified obsessive-compulsive and related disorder**
- **Unspecified obsessive-compulsive and related disorder**
- ***Obsessive-compulsive disorder:** an individual experiences obsessions and/or compulsions

According to the APA (2013), "*obsessions* are recurrent and persistent thoughts, urges, or images that are experienced as intrusive or unwanted, whereas *compulsions* are repetitive behaviors or mental acts that an individual feels driven to perform in response to an obsession or according to rules that must be applied rigidly" (p. 235).

- ***Body dysmorphic disorder:** an individual is consumed by perceived deficits in their physical appearance that are non- or minimally existent to others
- ***Hoarding disorder:** an individual is compelled to keep personal possessions regardless of their value
- **Trichotillomania:** also known as "hair-pulling disorder"
- **Excoriation disorder:** also known as "skin-picking disorder"

SUBSTANCE-RELATED AND ADDICTIVE DISORDERS

These overall areas require specifiers such as severity, intoxication, withdrawal, remission, controlled environment, perceptual disturbances, and so on. Substance-related and addictive disorders fall into the areas of:

- **Alcohol**
- **Caffeine**
- **Cannabis**
- **Hallucinogens**
- **Inhalants**
- **Opioids**
- **Sedatives/hypnotics/anxiolytics**

- **Stimulants**
- **Tobacco**
- **Other** (or unknown substance-related disorders)
- **Non-substance-related disorders** (e.g., gambling)

In summary, exploring the specific diagnostic criteria for each of these disorders (e.g., anxiety disorders, obsessive-compulsive disorders and related disorders, and substance-related and addictive disorders) is outside the scope of this chapter. Rather, the counselor is encouraged to become familiar with the *DSM-5* (APA, 2013) for these disorders through coursework, trainings, readings, supervision, and consultation. Counselors need to be trained in the use of the *DSM-5* manual, and then supervised in the application of the diagnoses to use them in the best interest of the client. While this area is explored further in the assessment section, the counselor is encouraged to follow this process:

1. Assess the symptoms presented.
2. Gather relevant biopsychosocial, familial, and medical history related to the symptoms.
3. Examine precipitating and contributing factors.
4. Refer to the *DSM-5* (APA, 2013) to determine if the criteria for a diagnosis is met.
5. Follow the guidelines as outlined in the section of assessment and diagnostic considerations.

PREVALENCE, STATISTICS, AND DEMOGRAPHICS

In this section, the prevalence, statistics, and demographics of SUDs co-occurring with anxiety and obsessive-compulsive disorders, as they relate to SUDs, are discussed. There are approximately 9.5 million adults that have co-occurring mental and substance use disorders, which represents about 3.8% of the U.S. adult population (SAMHSA, 2020). Outside of populations with SUDs, OCD occurs at a rate of 1.6% to 2.3% (SAMHSA, 2016). Per a National Comorbidity Survey (Smith & Randall, 2012), a person with GAD is 4.6 times likely to be diagnosed with an alcohol-related disorder. Additionally, those with social anxiety are 2.8 times as likely, and those with panic disorder are 2.2 times as likely, to have substance-related concerns (Smith & Randall, 2012).

Through knowledge of the prevalence, statistics, and demographics, counselors can understand both their biases as well as the vulnerability or protective factors of their clients. The prevalence of anxiety in minority groups is important for counselors to know and examples of some of the available information follow. According to the National Institute of Mental Health (2017), 31.1% of adults will experience some form of anxiety in their lifetime, with current anxiety diagnoses being around 19.1%. Women reported experiencing anxiety disorders more often than men (23.4% vs. 14.3%, respectively). A total of 31.9% of adolescents had an anxiety disorder putting them more at risk than the adult population. The LGBT+ population is 2.5 times more likely to be diagnosed with and experience anxiety, depression, and/or SUD (APA, 2017).

The prevalence, statistics, and demographics underscore the importance of carefully assessing for CODs. For example, clients presenting with SUDs may have anxiety or a related condition rather than OCD (Brady et al., 2013). The most common diagnoses presenting for treatment are GAD, panic disorder, and posttraumatic stress disorder (PTSD), in that order (Brady et al., 2013). OCD, while still prevalent, is less robust than the other three disorders (Brady et al., 2013).

ASSESSMENT AND DIAGNOSTIC CONSIDERATIONS

CO-OCCURRING ANXIETY AND SUBSTANCE USE ETIOLOGICAL PARADIGMS

Vorspan et al. (2015) explained three models that may assist the counselor in understanding the association between anxiety concerns and substance use issues:

1. Shared vulnerability factors model,
2. Self-medication model, and
3. Substance-induced model.

The *shared vulnerability factors model* (Carson, 2011) examines an individual's vulnerabilities to various psychopathologies (e.g., mood disorders) and correlates them with a person's cognitive protective factors (e.g., intelligence). Using this model, correlations between pathologies and protective factors indicate that artistic/creative people have an increased susceptibility to substance abuse and psychopathologies (e.g., mood disorders).

The *self-medication model* suggests that individuals with psychopathologies, such as anxiety disorders, are at a higher risk to develop dependencies on substances due to their need to cope, live with, and medicate their disorder. This model illustrates that the underlying illness (like an anxiety disorder or OCD) leads an individual to experiment with alcohol, drugs, and related substances fostering dependence.

Lastly, the *substance-induced model* proposes that the use of a substance has intensified or brought out a mental health disorder, such as anxiety. This model suggests that the substances in which the individual is partaking functions as a catalyst for co-occurring mental illnesses.

BUILDING AN INTEGRATED TEAM TO INFORM THE DIAGNOSTIC PROCESS

As stated in the introduction, because of the complicated, potentially intense interaction of CODs, a teamwork approach is required where there is honesty, communication, and trust among the healthcare providers. When the variables are aligned, a *true* integrated healthcare approach is demonstrated. The manner in which a counselor sets up this team may be determined by the setting in which a formal team already exists (e.g., inpatient care), or a team needing to be organized by the counselor through a network of consultants (e.g., licensed clinical professional counselor working in private practice).

This team of healthcare professionals needs to have as few as possible and as many as necessary individuals working together. Each professional provides a *visual lens* necessary to ensure the best interests of the client are met in the assessment process from a holistic, interactive view by working together (Miller, 2021). Each *lens* may propose diagnoses that need to be ruled out. For example, a medical professional may recommend that the symptoms of a GAD be examined in relation to the medication(s) taken by the client to ensure the diagnosis of a GAD is accurate and not caused solely (or partially) by the medication prescribed. Such integrated care means that the diagnoses and treatments are coordinated from mental health, substance abuse, and primary care perspectives to clarify the client's accurate diagnoses, thereby allowing the treatment process to effectively meet the needs of the client (Miller, 2021). Additionally, on a regular basis, including during the treatment process, such screening for all the professional areas involved (e.g., mental health, substance abuse, primary care) needs to be conducted. The constant and ongoing monitoring of the diagnoses is why it is noted in the *DSM-5* section of this chapter that the screening and assessment practices, which are then followed by the treatment planning procedures, are all labor-intensive processes.

Because the counselor has to work quite earnestly with this population, it may be helpful for the counselor to work on a team to share the load in the assessment process. The number and type of professionals on the team is built on the minimum of one professional from mental health services, one from addiction recovery treatment, and another from the primary care profession. Additional number/emphasis of professionals to add into the treatment team is guided by the client's presenting problem/symptoms. An example in this context is a client who has OCD: The counselor may want to include an OCD expert in the consultant network to make sure these concerns are being adequately addressed in the assessment of the substance use diagnosis.

Keep in mind that while this is the recommended ideal plan for client care, the reality for the individual counselor may be a lack of time, energy, and possibly the finances, to create this plan with each client. If this is the case, what should a counselor do? One of the ways the counselor may approach this is to have releases signed by the client to consult with experts in their area of struggle (e.g., mental health, addiction, primary care) and create time to reach out to each of these consultants. Another option is for the counselor (with the assistance of a supervisor or experienced colleague) to set up a team consisting of a network of professionals with whom to consult. Finally, if a counselor who determines their client requires multiple services beyond the counselor's or the treatment setting's capabilities, they may make a referral to a more comprehensive treatment setting.

OTHER CONSIDERATIONS FOR THE ASSESSMENT AND TREATMENT OF CLIENTS

Individual practitioners can also integrate an assessment of the co-occurring mental and substance use issues as described in Figure 11.2 (Miller, 2021, p. 87):

This figure may serve as an anchoring "map" for the counselor who needs to determine the type of treatment that will best serve the client. The components of a *broad screening assessment* are outlined in item 1, *anchoring questions* the counselor can ask are listed in item 2, and the *care quadrants* that simply rank each disorder (e.g., mental health, addiction) as less/more in terms of severity are illustrated in item 3.

With regard to the ongoing assessment process as it relates to treatment, Miller (2021) suggested some basic behavioral characteristics for which the counselor may want to monitor within an addiction treatment setting: Clients may become (a) more agitated during the treatment process, (b) "troublesome" or challenging to work with for the counselor and staff, and (c) scapegoats for others (e.g., counselors, professionals, staff, clients). Some basic behavioral characteristics of possible SUDs in various mental health settings include: (a) physiological-related ones (i.e., neurologic difficulties, withdrawal symptoms, or medication-seeking behaviors); (b) noncompliance with medication; and (c) a number of treatment failures.

Finally, the National Institute on Drug Abuse (NIDA, 2018) outlined some of the barriers faced by individuals with CODs obtaining treatment. A significant barrier to treatment falls in the realm of socioeconomic status. Such barriers relate to lack of monetary means to pay for treatment, having little to no insurance coverage, or not having time because of employment restraints. The second most common reason for not receiving treatment for a SUD and comorbid anxiety relates to fear (NIDA, 2018). This fear encompasses social perceptions, confidentiality,

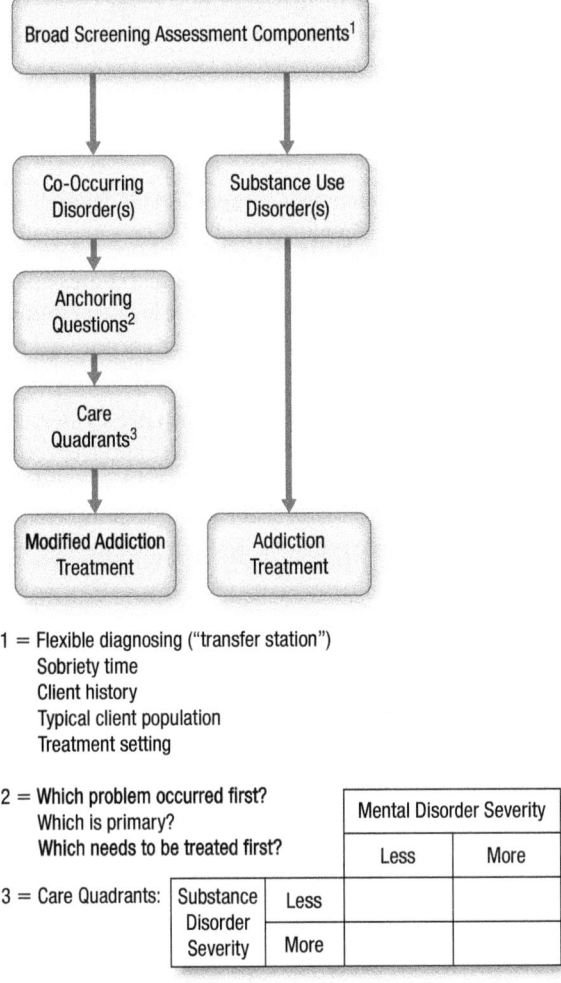

FIGURE 11.2 Broad Screening Assessment Components.
Source: Miller, G. (2021). *Learning the language of addiction counseling*, 5 ed. Copyright © 2021 by John Wiley & Sons, Inc. All rights reserved. Reprinted with permission.

and an alarm about being hospitalized. Mental health disorders and SUDs both carry a stigma that can prevent or inhibit clients seeking treatment. Counselors working with this population need to be aware of these barriers as they assess and refer clients to treatment.

SCREENING AND ASSESSMENT TOOLS

As stated in the *DSM-5* section, the numerous anxiety-related disorders, OCD and related disorders, and substance-related and addictive disorders can be overwhelming, confusing, and challenging for the counselor. Because of these factors, the number of screening and assessment tools available to the counselor can equally be overwhelming, confusing, and challenging. As a result, it is suggested that counselors use broad screening assessment instruments appropriate for the population of the clientele, both in the areas of mental health disorders (e.g., anxiety, obsessive-compulsive) and SUDs. All websites noted in the following have information regarding the reliability and the validity of the instruments.

Screening Instruments

Some broad screening instruments for anxiety disorders and OCDs are:

- **Kessler Psychological Distress Scale** (K10; Kessler, n.d.): A 10-item self-report screening tool with scores that range from 10 to 50. The scores are explained and must be followed through with a primary care helper. Surface level questions may need additional clarification after some answers. Potential users are encouraged to review the copyright information for accessing and implementing the instrument.
- **Generalized Anxiety Disorder (GAD) Questionnaire IV** (GAD-Q-IV; Newman et al., 2002): A 9-item screening tool from the Anxiety and Depression Association of America (ADAA). The information page on the ADAA.org website informs the instrument is a self-report questionnaire that should be completed by the individual and then shared with a primary care provider. The instrument is accessible on the ADAA's website.
- **Generalized Anxiety Disorder 7-Item Scale** (GAD-7; Spitzer et al., 2006): The GAD-7 is an initial screening tool that contains 7 items with a numbered anxiety severity scoring tool. Potential users are encouraged to review the copyright information for accessing and implementing the instrument.
- **OCD Screening Tool** (Anxiety and Depression Association of America [ADAA], 2021): A 21-item tool. The ADAA website provides instructions to answer the questions and then print the form to take to their primary care provider. The instrument is accessible on the ADAA's website.

Some broad screening instruments for SUDs are:

- **Alcohol, Smoking, and Substance Involvement Screening Test** (ASSIST, 2010): An 8-item tool developed for the World Health Organization (WHO). Detailed information regarding the ASSIST is accessible on WHO's website.
- **Alcohol Use Disorders Identification Test** (AUDIT, 2001): A 10 question tool that screens for dangerous patterns of alcohol use, the AUDIT is available in both clinical and self-report versions. Detailed information regarding the AUDIT is accessible and available in various languages on WHO's website.

Assessment Instruments

If the results of the broad screening assessment instruments indicate a mental health disorder and/or a SUD, the counselor can then follow up with a specific assessment instrument appropriate for the indicated diagnosis. Common anxiety measures include the State-Trait Anxiety Inventory (STAI; Spielberger et al., 1983), the Beck Anxiety Inventory (BAI; Beck & Steer, 1993), or the Multidimensional Anxiety Questionnaire (MAQ; Reynolds, 1999). Assessments to explore OCD include the Yale-Brown Obsessive-Compulsive Scale (Y-BOCS; Goodman et al., 1989), which also has a youth version, or the Maudsley Obsessional-Compulsive Inventory (Hodgson & Rachman, 1977). SUD assessments include the Global Appraisal of Individual Needs (GAIN; Chestnut Health Systems, 2021) or the Addiction Severity Index (ASI; McLellan et al., 2006). Counselors can become familiar with these or more specific instruments they anticipate using through readings, trainings, workshops, and websites (Miller, 2021).

In summary, when using either broad or specific mental health and SUD assessment instruments, the counselor is encouraged to:

1. Determine typical diagnoses presented by the client population through consultation with a review of the literature and consultation with experienced mental health counselors/supervisors and SUD counselors/supervisors.
2. Decide on a broad assessment instrument(s) in both areas (mental health, SUD) to use based on typical diagnoses presented by the client population.
3. Decide on a specific assessment instrument(s) to use in both areas (mental health, SUD) based on the broad assessment instruments chosen.
4. Be prepared to repeat this process (steps 2 and 3) when atypical symptoms/diagnoses present themselves in each area.

TREATMENT MODALITIES

As reviewed in the introduction, Kemp's (2018) philosophical, theoretical approach to addiction is presented in this section because of its impact on treatment in general, and, specifically, to the CODs of mental health and SUDs. In terms of SUD treatment, Kemp described the person with an addiction as someone who uses substances to handle their pain and suffering, which results in the person living in a world without meaning and being alienated from others. The person's behaviors may include withdrawal from the world, little contact with others that is genuine, physical inactivity, excessive participation in passive leisure activities, and a monotonous lifestyle. The obsessive cycle of addiction leads to a chaotic lifestyle that lacks concern for long-term consequences. Recovery from the addiction means the opposite of the active SUD: finding meaning, being connected with others, engaging with the world, having genuine connection with others, being physically active, participating less in passive leisure activities, and having an alive, interesting lifestyle. Counselors can assist clients by helping them explore who they are without substances in their lives and establish a lifestyle that has shared meaning through family, community, and tradition. This philosophical, theoretical approach is portrayed in Figure 11.3.

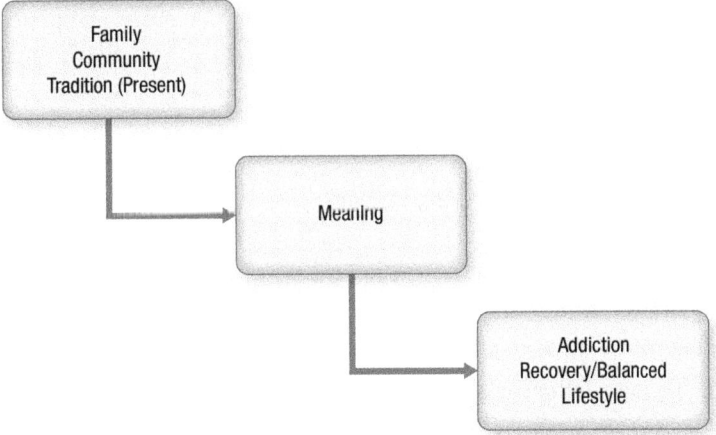

FIGURE 11.3 Addictive Recovery Modeled by Cushman's (1990) Empty Self Theory (Sociocultural Model).
Source: Adapted from Cushman, P. (1990). Why the self is empty: Toward a historically situated psychology. *American Psychologist, 45,* 599–611.

Kemp's perspective may be enhanced in a client who experiences similar struggles with the mental health disorder as well as a SUD. This client may have additional suffering and struggles in active addiction in addition to a heightened need for the components necessary for a successful recovery from both. For example, a client that is diagnosed with both GAD and a co-occurring cannabis use disorder may have difficulty maintaining sobriety for any length of time. This is likely because the client was using cannabis to help reduce the GAD symptoms. When this client obtains a period of abstinence, they may feel like they have stepped into an "anxiety minefield" where the anxiety is triggered easily by events that occur in daily living. The counselor may need to help the client find a family, a community, that provides support and meaningful traditions in an *ongoing* manner to help them live with such anxiety. For example, if the client attends a 12-step self-help group regularly, the group may provide the client with a sense of family, community, and traditions. It may also provide a perspective as manifested in slogans, such as "Easy Does It," or "One Day at a Time," that help reduce their anxiety. Such a framework may act as a rudder for the client who needs to find a way to live with the chronic illnesses of mental health disorders and the SUD.

Essentially the counselor is acting like an old-fashioned lighthouse that guides the client to shore while traveling through waters. An important part of the counseling process is helping the client feel cared for, encouraged, and safe. This support needs to extend beyond the counseling room by assisting the client in finding a sense of family, community, and tradition that is helping them again feel cared for, encouraged, and safe. At its core is the question to the client: "What keeps your 'spirit' alive?" or "What keeps you going?" Helping them find the activities, people, places that offer them an oasis, a sanctuary from the issues with which they struggle (e.g., mental health, SUDs) and encouraging them to have as much as possible of those experiences in their lives. These areas will help them stay in balance by offering others' perspectives, breaking up their struggles with humor, play, love, and stories that can help them in living day-to-day and provide them with hope.

EVIDENCE-BASED PRACTICE

Evidence-based practice (EBP) involves integrating the best research available with clinical expertise anchored in the context of the client's characteristics, culture, and preferences (Miller, 2021). Miller et al. (2019) presented the following 10 EBPs that can be used with anxiety disorders, OCDs, and SUDs:

- Motivational interviewing,
- Brief interventions,
- Contingency management,
- Community reinforcement,
- Behavioral coping skills,
- Working with significant others,
- Strengthening relationships,
- Mutual self-help groups,
- Medications in treatment, and
- Meditation and mindfulness.

ASPECTS AND ADJUNCTS TO COUNSELING

While integrated treatment for CODs is recommended, many counselors may not be working in such settings (Miller, 2021). Therefore, the following overall aspects of counseling may be adapted by making modifications to work with this population in their clinical setting. These counseling aspects include (Miller, 2021):

- Case management,
- Client education,
- Supportive counseling,
- Family therapy,
- Group therapy,
- Specific therapeutic approaches (e.g., cognitive behavioral therapy, dialectical behavior therapy),
- Crisis intervention,
- Relapse-prevention approaches, and
- Residential treatment.

Modifications to treatment include but are not limited to (Miller, 2021):

- Longer time frame for abstinence,
- Psychotropic medication,
- Psychiatric support,
- Counseling/confrontational style (e.g., less confrontive),
- Screening for substance use, and
- Self-help groups (e.g., Double Trouble, Dual Diagnosis Anonymous, Dual Recovery Anonymous).

All of these treatment approaches need to be adjusted to the unique needs connected to both the specific mental health disorder and the SUD. This means the counselor needs to be clear about the diagnoses for each disorder and their interaction as evidenced in the individual client to develop an effective treatment plan. For example, asking the client, *"What symptoms concern you?"* can assist the counselor in gathering information about how the disorders idiosyncratically impact *that* client (Wilson, 2021). The counselor then needs to help the client *imbed* the treatment plan into their life (Wilson, 2021).

Finally, the counselor needs to consistently monitor the effectiveness of the treatment plan in assisting the client in being symptom free from both disorders and revising the treatment plan based on new information regarding the client's dual recovery process. The counselor needs to be aware, however, that there may be limitations in modifying treatment. For example, Barthwell (2016) noted that accepted guidelines are lacking for clinical testing that identifies and treats substance use.

LEGAL AND ETHICAL CONSIDERATIONS

Legal and ethical practice is central to counseling; however, it is of particular importance in the treatment of co-occurring anxiety disorders/OCDs and SUDs due to the complex nature of diagnosis and treatment. Touchstones for legal and ethical practice in the field of counseling are the *DSM-5* (APA, 2013), the American Counseling Association *Code of Ethics* (ACA, 2014), and national and state guidelines.

DSM-5

The *DSM-5*, released as a follow-up to the fourth edition text revision published 13 years earlier, made several updates that impacted substance use treatment. Counselors working with these clients need to stay abreast of the knowledge in order to work ethically and effectively with clients. These changes can be categorized as changes in class, substance, disorder, and criteria. The updated section describes a wide range of SUDs on a continuum of severity rather than maintaining the categorization system used in the previous edition of the manual that delineated substance use from substance abuse. Similarly, diagnostic criteria that once identified dependence and abuse now includes the designations of mild, moderate, and severe. Notably, gambling disorder is now officially recognized in the substance use and addictive disorder chapter. In general, major changes aim to update nomenclature and categorization and to clarify and remove potentially stigmatizing terms such as abuse, dependence, and addiction.

AMERICAN COUNSELING ASSOCIATION CODE OF ETHICS

While the current edition of the ACA Code of Ethics (2014) did not make substantial changes regarding substance use treatment, several codes may bear particular significance in the context of co-occurring substance use and anxiety disorder treatment. These include: A.2.e. (mandated clients), A.4.b. (personal values), A.7.a. (advocacy), C.2.b. (new specialty areas of practice), C.5. (nondiscrimination), and D.1.c. (interdisciplinary teamwork; Doyle, 2019). Doyle (2019) highlighted the counselor's responsibility to the client, rather than the legal entity or referring agency, in the case of mandated clients. Counselors may inappropriately disclose treatment details to individuals representing the referring entity or other adjunct services. This can easily happen due to the presence of a perceived power dynamic in which one may incorrectly assume that counselors must prioritize the needs of the system over the needs of the client. Instead, counselors must serve as advocates and act in their client's best interest.

Standard A.4.b. reminds counselors they are expected to be aware of their own personal values and guard against imposing those values onto their clients. This may be particularly important when assessing their clients' substance use history and linking biopsychosocial demographics to conceptualization, diagnosis, and even the counselor's personal beliefs about how all of these factors interact. For example, unacknowledged biases related to type of substance used or method of intake may be reflected in more severe diagnoses or recommendations for higher levels of treatment that are not clinically indicated.

Standard A.7.a. further explores counselors' responsibilities to their clients. In addition to acting in their clients' best interest, counselors are expected to advocate for their clients, which includes helping them navigate systemic barriers to treatment and goal attainment. How counselors help clients navigate systemic barriers to care may look different depending on the system and the difficulty; however, it is a collaborative process that engages and empowers the client.

Standards C.2.b. (new specialty areas of practice) and D.1.c. (interdisciplinary teamwork), although housed in different sections of the Code of Ethics (ACA, 2014), reference counselor-related expectations. Counselors are expected to receive appropriate training for new specialty areas of practice and refrain from practicing without proper coursework, training, and supervision. For example, counselors experienced with treating opioid use disorder may not be as skilled in the treatment of cannabis use disorder. This is particularly important given the complexity of CODs and the knowledge needed to competently provide services to this population. It is important to be aware of one's own skills, recognize areas for improvement, remain open to feedback, and seek clinical consultation and/or supervision. In some cases, counselors may work with interdisciplinary teams to collaboratively treat clients and use the lens of diverse treatment providers to improve treatment outcomes; however, it will be important to centralize the counseling needs of the client and act in a manner that emphasizes the role of the counselor.

Standard C.5. communicates the counselor's expectation of nondiscriminatory practice with respect to race/ethnicity, gender, sexual orientation, ability status or other identity actors. Doyle (2019) stated that SUDs can be considered a disability, and clients presenting with substance use should not be refused services because they are "too difficult" or "not ready for a change" (p. 2). The shared theme among these divergent codes is that they are of an ethical nature and have an indirect, but definite impact, on the treatment of addiction, anxiety disorders, and OCDs. A brief discussion of additional considerations for the legal and ethical treatment of co-occurring anxiety and SUDs is included in the following.

COUNSELOR COMPETENCE

Counselors are uniquely challenged to be in tune with their mind, body, beliefs, and behaviors as it pertains to their professional practice. Commonly, the individual personhood of a counselor is viewed as the "tool" that underscores the change process in therapy. Counselors can negatively affect the counseling relationship through the absence of properly "tuning in" to the self and the impact of one's beliefs, values, behaviors, and abilities on the counseling relationship.

Self-Awareness

Awareness of one's internal experience in the moment can be particularly pertinent to the treatment of CODs. Carl Rogers, the creator of person-centered counseling, theorized that there are six conditions that are both necessary and sufficient to the counseling relationship and supporting the client on their journey toward reaching their best selves (Rogers, 1951). Notably, according to Rogers (1951), counselor attitudes make up three core conditions: (a) *congruence*, (b) *unconditional positive regard*, and (c) *empathy*. Essentially, the counselor should be able to allow the client to connect to their unique personhood as well as believe that the client is a good human deserving of empathy, regardless of the client's choices. Counselors treating clients who use substances are likely to encounter experiences that challenge their beliefs and values; therefore, they must continuously engage in the self-reflection process to ensure that they are acting in ways that facilitate client growth rather than inhibit it.

Perhaps the clearest means of describing this potential roadblock can be viewed through the lens of the psychodynamic principle of countertransference. Countertransference occurs when the counselors engage in the "process of seeing themselves in their clients, overidentifying with their clients, or of meeting their needs through their clients" (Corey, 2009, p. 22). This is why insight about one's beliefs about clients who use substances, awareness of individual reactions to clients who relapse, and recognition of over identifying with client successes and missteps on the lifelong journey toward sobriety are all necessary components of counselor self-awareness.

Burnout

Beyond awareness of one's beliefs, values, and reactions, counselors should also attune to their sense of emotional and physical health and satisfaction with life—essentially their wellness. An overwhelmed counselor is more likely to make mistakes that endanger the client's welfare as well as put their professional license in jeopardy. Burnout becomes an issue of counselor competence, as a counselor who is not impaired has a greater awareness of when they are approaching a point when their current state of being may begin to negatively impact their work. Addiction counselors may work in challenging, fast-paced, stressful, and resource-deficient environments—a recipe for burnout.

Boundaries and Dual Relationships

As Rogers (1951) suggested, genuineness, congruence, and the development of an authentic human connection is the most powerful component of the counseling intervention. Clients working toward self-actualization and in close relationship with a stable and congruent figure dedicated to supporting their growth can be facilitative; however, counselors need to be aware that this can easily lead to blurred boundaries. For example, good rapport over time can be perceived as less professional and more like friendship, especially from the perspective of a client in a state of incongruence.

What if a counselor also struggles with substance use? Shared connection and common experiences in substance use treatment is common, as many clinicians enter the field as peer recovery specialists having had their own history with substance use. While this alone is not unethical or cause for legal concern, additional implications for treatment highlight the increased potential for dual relationships, particularly in small towns or rural areas. There may be limited community support groups and the counselor and client may have encountered one another in different treatment settings. Counselors can navigate these challenges by establishing clear boundaries and having open discussions with clients during the informed consent process about how to handle shared treatment circles and other dual relationships, as well as seeking support from supervisors and/or peers.

Specifically, dual relationship issues have been raised with regard to *peer support experts* that have been called the fastest growing U.S. addiction professional (Miller, 2021). Peer-based recovery support experts are nonprofessionals (as inherently acknowledged by the definition of their role) who provide nonclinical support to clients by using their shared experiences to support others who have similar challenges. Dual relationship issues can readily arise when the peer support expert role shifts to a professional role (e.g., certification, licensure) related to mental health and/or addiction treatment. They need consistent, attentive supervision to assist them in establishing clear boundaries with their clients. For example, a peer support with an anxiety disorder and a SUD may be working with a mental health agency client who has similar issues. When the peer support expert registers with a SUD board, the peer support expert is now under the auspices of a professional in addition to the role of being a supportive nonprofessional. This can be confusing for both individuals, which is why supervision is needed to assist them in keeping their boundaries and roles clear with their clients.

MULTICULTURALISM AND VALUES

Section C.5 of the ACA Code of Ethics (2014) describes counselors' responsibility to be nondiscriminatory in their practice. Counselors need to be aware of their beliefs and biases and their potential impact on clients. Consideration of multiculturalism and values should apply to the individual counseling relationship and to the systems with which the counselor and client engage. The multicultural counseling competencies (Arredondo et al., 1996) provide a framework for how counselors can attend to counselor (a) self-awareness, (b) awareness of their own cultural values and biases, and (c) application of culturally appropriate intervention strategies. The following presents a brief checklist of counselor knowledge, awareness, and skills applicable to COD treatment mapped onto the multicultural counseling competencies:

I. Counselor Awareness of Their Own Cultural Values and Biases
   a. Attitudes and Beliefs
      i. Recognition of how the counselor's cultural background and experiences influence their attitudes about substances and substance users.
   b. Knowledge
      i. Culturally skilled counselors have specific knowledge about their own racial and cultural heritage and how it personally and professionally affects their definitions and biases of normality/abnormality and the process of COD counseling.
      ii. Culturally skilled counselors possess knowledge and understanding about how oppression, racism, discrimination, and stereotyping affect them personally and in their work in the field of COD counseling.
   c. Skills
      i. Culturally skilled counselors are constantly seeking to understand themselves as racial and cultural beings and are actively seeking a nondiscriminatory identity that recognizes and values differences in all aspects of human identity.

II. Counselor Awareness of Client's Worldview
   a. Attitudes and Beliefs
      i. Culturally skilled counselors are aware of their negative and positive emotional reactions toward other racial/ethnic groups and clients diagnosed with CODs that may prove detrimental to the counseling relationship.
   b. Knowledge
      i. Culturally skilled counselors understand how components of identity, such as race, culture, ethnicity, history of substance use, and systemic factors may affect personality formation, vocational choices, manifestation of psychological disorders, help-seeking behavior, the appropriateness of counseling approaches, and the accessibility of adequate treatment resources.
   c. Skills
      i. Culturally skilled counselors should familiarize themselves with relevant research and the latest findings regarding mental health, mental disorders, and substance use that affect various ethnic and racial groups. They should actively seek out educational experiences that enrich their knowledge, understanding, and cross-cultural skills for more effective counseling behavior.

III. Culturally Appropriate Intervention Strategies
   a. Attitudes and Beliefs
      i. Culturally skilled counselors respect clients' religious and/or spiritual beliefs and values, including attributions, taboos, and spiritual/healing aspects of substance use (e.g., peyote), because they affect worldview, psychosocial functioning, and expressions of distress.

b. Knowledge
   i. Culturally skilled counselors are aware of institutional barriers that prevent minorities from using mental health and substance use treatment services.
c. Skills
   i. Culturally skilled counselors are able to exercise institutional intervention skills on behalf of their clients. They can help clients determine whether a "problem" stems from racism or bias in others (the concept of healthy paranoia) so that clients do not inappropriately personalize problems.

CLINICAL CASE ILLUSTRATION AND DISCUSSION

CASE OF SHANNON

Shannon, a White woman who is single, is in her late 30s, has no children, and is unemployed. She describes behaviors that led the counselor to diagnose the following disorders: social anxiety disorder, cannabis use disorder, and alcohol use disorder. Specifically, Shannon says she is often afraid to interact with others in social settings and, therefore, she uses marijuana and alcohol in preparation of entering a social setting. Shannon does say that this is in regard to most social settings, although she is able to go to her best friend's house without experiencing anxiety symptoms. In all other social circumstances, she reports smoking about "half a joint" and a drinking at least two cocktails prior to departing her house.

Shannon's substance use helps reduce her social anxiety; however, once she enters the social setting, she reports having difficulty controlling her use of substances. She stated, "I feel so good when I get there, and I really do not want to lose that feeling, so I keep drinking." She indicates she will drink a maximum of 8 to 10 alcoholic drinks, which frequently results in her experiencing a blackout. After she experiences an alcohol-induced blackout in a social setting, her social anxiety further increases when she plans to go into her next social setting. And this once again results in Shannon self-medicating her anxiety with substances. "I just want this cycle to stop," she reports when she arrives to the counselor's office.

Shannon had previous treatments for her mental health diagnoses separate from her previous treatments for her substance use (e.g., outpatient clinic treatments in combination with 12-step recovery groups). Shannon has never had any counseling, however, where counselors examined the interaction between both mental health and SUD and integrated COD treatment at the same time. Shannon's counselor is committed to treating both issues at the same time.

CASE DISCUSSION

A counselor working with Shannon is encouraged to consider building an integrated treatment team that includes professionals that will support her recovery. A strength of Shannon's is her strong internal awareness as she has articulated her own understanding of the etiology of her COD (i.e., the cycle she reports). This knowledge is incredibly helpful for the counselor to have and to build on. The counselor will want to be particularly considerate about the social anxiety that Shannon reports. For instance, many counselors encourage clients to become actively engaged in a mutual aid community-based support group for SUDs (e.g., Alcoholics Anonymous, Narcotics Anonymous, Refuge Recovery). While these may be beneficial to Shannon due to her alcohol and cannabis use disorders, she will need to be well prepared for handling any anxiety that occurs if she is triggered by being surrounded by other people in a meeting. This is particularly important given her report that any social interaction, of any size, spurs these feelings. The counselor may inquire if Shannon would be willing and able to attend a meeting, talk through the ambivalence Shannon expresses using motivational interviewing techniques (Slagle & Gray, 2007), and perhaps explore if she is willing for her best friend to accompany her.

There cannot be a "one-size-fits-all" approach when treating CODs, as making the referral to a mutual aid recovery group without taking into consideration Shannon's COD would be highly inappropriate. A counselor working with Shannon will need to take a full inventory of her symptoms as well as explore coping strategies that Shannon is willing and able to integrate into her everyday life to combat the social anxiety, thus resulting in a reduction in the substance use. There are many different avenues a counselor may take with Shannon, so reflecting further on the following questions may assist in clarifying the clinical picture and developing the treatment plan:

1. How would the setting in which you practice as a counselor (e.g., private practice, intensive outpatient program, inpatient level of care) impact your work with Shannon regarding assessment and treatment?
2. How might you use Figures 11.1 and 11.2 in the assessment and treatment process that integrates the CODs? [NOTE: Figure 11.1 helps develop an assessment and treatment perspective, and Figure 11.2 helps determine the focus of treatment based on your assessment.]
3. Using Figure 11.3, what formal and/or informal resources might you draw upon to use in your work with Shannon?
4. How would the setting in which you work support and/or inhibit working together as a team?
5. How might you organize a integrated team of professionals while you work with Shannon regarding her co-occurring anxiety and SUDs?

CHAPTER SUMMARY

This chapter provided an overview of the interaction between anxiety disorders, OCDs, and SUDs with the intention of helping counselors as they work within the complicated area of CODs. A philosophical approach of working with this population both in terms of assessment and treatment approaches, as well as legal and ethical implications and considerations, were introduced. More specifically, the chapter integrated content related to the following topics:

- Conceptualizing anxiety;
- *DSM-5* diagnostic criteria and description;
- Prevalence, statistics, and demographics;
- Assessment and diagnostic considerations;
- Screening and assessment tools;
- Treatment modalities; and
- Legal and ethical implications/considerations.

In addition to these important topics, counselors should continually examine the multicultural influences that impact clients struggling with these disorders so they can incorporate these factors into the assessment and treatment process. A synopsis of working with clients with co-occurring anxiety and SUDs was offered with the hope that counselors will obtain additional coursework, trainings, readings, supervision, and consultation that specifically focuses on these disorders. The ongoing education of the counselor should additionally focus on learning about the application of these general concepts to their specific client population. In doing so, counselors will be more competent and clients will be better served.

DISCUSSION QUESTIONS

1. What general or specific concerns do you have in working with this diagnostic population?
2. Describe the general interaction between the anxiety disorder, OCD, and SUDs. Then, describe the interaction among the disorders as they impact both assessment and treatment.
3. What is critical in the process of simultaneously assessing for and treating co-occurring anxiety and substance disorders?
4. What are some of the critical treatment approaches you can use in working with this population based on Kemp's and Cushman's theories and evidence-based practices?
5. Which of the 10 evidence-based practices presented would you consider exploring more and how might you obtain education on them (e.g., coursework, trainings, readings, clinical supervision, consultation)?

REFERENCES

Abrams, Z. (2021). Growing concerns about sleep. *Monitor on Psychology, 52*(4), 30–34.

Abramson, A. (2021a). The ethical imperative of self-care. *Monitor on Psychology, 52*(3), 46–53.

Abramson, A. (2021b). Substance use during the pandemic. *Monitor on Psychology, 52*(2), 22.

American Counseling Association. (2014). *ACA code of ethics.* Retrieved from http://www.counseling.org/docs/ethics/2014-aca-code-of-ethics.pdf

American Psychiatric Association. (2013). *Diagnostic and statistical manual of mental disorders* (5th ed.). https://doi.org/10.1176/appi.books.9780890425596

American Psychiatric Association. (2017). *Mental health disparities: LGBTQ.* Psychiatry.org.

Anxiety & Depression Association of American. (2021). *Screening for obsession-compulsive disorder (OCD).* https://adaa.org/screening-obsessive-compulsive-disorder-ocd

Arredondo, P., Toporek, M. S., Brown, S., Jones, J., Locke, D. C., Sanchez, J., & Stadler, H. (1996). *Operationalization of the multicultural counseling competencies.* AMCD: Alexandria, VA

Barthwell, A. G. (2016). Clinical and public health considerations in urine drug testing to identify and treat substance use. *Substance Use & Misuse, 51*(6), 700–710.

Beck, A. T., & Steer, R. A. (1993). *Beck anxiety inventory manual.* Psychological Corporation.

Blom, R. M., Koeter, M., Den Brink, W. V., De Graaf, R., Ten Have, M., & Denys, D. (2011). Co-occurrence of obsessive-compulsive disorder and substance use disorder in the general population. *Addiction (Abingdon. Print), 106*(12), 2178–2185.

Brady, K. T., Haynes, L. F., Hartwell, K. J., & Killeen, T. K. (2013). Substance use disorders and anxiety: A treatment challenge for social workers. *Social Work in Public Health, 28*, 34, Article 407423, https://doi.org/10.1080/19371918.2013.774675

Carson, S. H. (2011). Creativity and psychopathology: A shared vulnerability model. *The Canadian Journal of Psychiatry, 56*(3), 144–153. https://doi.org/10.1177/070674371105600304

Chestnut Health Systems. (2021). *GAIN instruments.* https://gaincc.org/instruments/

Corey, G., 2009. *Theory and practice of counseling and psychotherapy* (8th ed.) United States of America: Brooks/Cole Cengage Learning.

Cushman, P. (1990). Why the self is empty: Toward a historically situated psychology. *American Psychologist, 45*, 599–611.

Doyle, K. S. (2019). The opioid crisis and ethical considerations for counselors. *Counseling Today.* https://www.counseling.org/docs/default-source/ethics/ethics-columns/ethics_january_2019_opiod-crisis.pdf?sfvrsn=7717552c_2

Gentil, A. F., De Mathis, M. A., Torresan, R. C., Diniz, J. B., Alavargena, P., Conceicao do Rosario, M., Cordioli, A. V., Torres, A. R., & Miguel, E. C. (2009). Alcohol use disorders in patients with obsessive-compulsive disorder: The importance of appropriate dual-diagnosis. *Drug and Alcohol Dependence, 100* (1-2), 173–177.

Goodman, W. K., Price, L. H., & Rasmussen, S. A. (1989). The yale-brown obsessive compulsive scale. I.: Development, use, and reliability. *Archives of General Psychiatry, 46*(11), 1006–1011. https://doi.org/10.1001/archpsyc.1989.01810110048007

Hodgson, R. J., & Rachman, S. (1977). Obsessional-compulsive complaints. *Behavior Research and Therapy, 15*, 389–395.

Kemp, R. (2018). *Transcending addiction: An existential pathway to recovery.* Routledge.

Kessler, R. (n.d.). *Kessler psychological distress scale (K10).* https://www.tac.vic.gov.au/files-to-move/media/upload/k10_english.pdf

Mancebo, M. C., Grant, J. E., Pinto, A., Eisen, J. L., & Rasmussen, S. A. (2009). Substance use disorders in an obsessive-compulsive disorder clinical sample. *Journal of Anxiety Disorders, 23*(4), 429–435.

May, R. (1979). *The meaning of anxiety.* Washington Square Press.

McAnally, H. B. (2017). Opioid dependence risk factors and risk assessment. *Opioid dependence: A clinical and epidemiologic approach,* 233. https://doi.org/10.1007/978-3-319-47497-7_10

McLellan, A. T., Cacciola, J. C., Alterman, A. I., Rikoon, S. H., & Carise, D. (2006). The addiction severity Index at 25: Origins, contributions, and transitions. *American Journal on Addictions, 15*(2), 113–124. https://doi.org/10.1080/10550490500528316

Miller, G. A. (2021). *Learning the language of addiction counseling* (5th ed.). Wiley.

Miller, W. R., Forcehimes, A. A., & Zweben, A. (2019). *Treating addiction: A guide for professionals.* (2nd ed.) Guilford.

National Institute of Mental Health, United States Department of Health and Human Services. (2017, November). *Any anxiety disorder.* https://www.nimh.nih.gov/health/statistics/any-anxiety-disorder#part_155094

National Institute on Drug Abuse. (2018, August 15). *Comorbidity: Substance use and other mental disorders.* Retrieved from https://nida.nih.gov/research-topics/trends-statistics/infographics/comorbidity-substance-use-other-mental-disorders

Newman, M. G., Zuellig, A. R., Kachin, K. E., Constantino, M. J., Przeworski, A., Erickson, T., & Cashman-McGrath, L. (2002). Preliminary reliability and validity of the generalized anxiety disorder questionnaire-IV: A revised self-report diagnostic measure of generalized anxiety disorder. *Behavior Therapy, 33*, 215–233. https://doi.org/10.1016/S0005-7894(02)80026-0

Phillips, L. (2021). How COVID-19 is affecting out fears, phobias and anxieties. *Counseling Today, 63*(9), 36–42.

Reynolds, W. M. (1999). *Professional manual for multidimensional anxiety questionnaire.* Psychological Assessment Resources.

Rogers, C. R. (1951). *Client-centered therapy; its current practice, implications, and theory.* Houghton Mifflin.

Sammons, M. T. (2020). Effects of a pandemic on psychologists and the public. *Journal of Health Service Psychology, 46*(4), 129–131.

Slagle, D. M., & Gray, M. J. (2007). The utility of motivational interviewing as an adjunct to exposure therapy in the treatment of anxiety disorders. *Professional Psychology: Research and Practice, 38*(4), 329–337. https://doi.org/10.1037/0735-7028.38.4.329

Smith, J. P., & Randall, C. L. (2012). Anxiety and alcohol use disorders: Comorbidity and treatment considerations. *Alcohol Research: Current Reviews, 34*(4).

Spielberger, C. D., Gorsuch, R. L., Lushene, R., Vagg, P. R., & Jacobs, G. A. (1983). *Manual for state-trait anxiety inventory.* Consulting Psychologists Press.

Spitzer, R. L., Kroenke, K., Williams, J. B., & Löwe, B. (2006). A brief measure for assessing generalized anxiety disorder: The GAD-7. *Archives of Internal Medicine, 166*(10), 1092–1097.

Substance Abuse and Mental Health Services Administration (SAMHSA). (2016). *Obsessive compulsive disorder and substance use disorders* [Brochure]. https://store.samhsa.gov/sites/default/files/d7/priv/sma16-4977.pdf

Substance Abuse and Mental Health Services Administration (SAMHSA). (2020). *Key substance use and mental health indicators in the United States: Results from the 2019 National Survey on Drug Use and Health.* https://www.samhsa.gov/data/sites/default/files/reports/rpt29393/2019NSDUHFFRPDFWHTML/2019NSDUHFFR090120.htm

Tillich, P. (1952). *The courage to be.* Yale University Press.

Veach, L. J., & Moro, R. R. (2018). *The spectrum of addiction: Evidence-based assessment, prevention, and treatment across the lifespan.* Sage.

Vorspan, F., Mehtelli, W., Dupuy, G., Bloch, V., & Lépine, J. P. (2015). Anxiety and substance use disorders: Co-occurrence and clinical issues. *Current Psychiatry Reports, 17*(2). https://doi.org/10.1007/s11920-014-0544-y

Wilson, R. (2021). Brief strategic treatment of the anxiety disorders. North Carolina Psychological Association *Spring Conference.* Chapel Hill, NC.

World Health Organization. (2001). *The alcohol use disorders identification test: Guidelines for use in primary care.* https://www.who.int/publications/i/item/audit-the-alcohol-use-disorders-identification-test-guidelines-for-use-in-primary-health-care

World Health Organization. (2010). *The alcohol, smoking and substance involvement screening test (ASSIST): Manual for use in primary care.* https://www.who.int/publications/i/item/978924159938-2

CHAPTER 12

CO-OCCURRING SCHIZOPHRENIA AND OTHER PSYCHOTIC DISORDERS AND SUBSTANCE USE DISORDERS

KEITH MORGEN AND KATHERINE WEBER

LEARNING OBJECTIVES

After reading this chapter, you will be able to:

- Identify the *Diagnostic and Statistical Manual of Mental Disorders, Fifth Edition (DSM-5)* symptoms of schizophrenia spectrum and other psychotic disorders.
- Recognize the role of co-occurring substance use disorders on schizophrenia spectrum and other psychotic disorders.
- Evaluate the prevalence rates for co-occurring substance use disorders on schizophrenia spectrum and other psychotic disorders.
- Apply the counseling and assessment content in their work with co-occurring substance use disorders on schizophrenia spectrum and other psychotic disorders.

INTRODUCTION

Co-occurring substance use disorders are often underdetected and undertreated in mental health settings due to a lack of knowledge about co-occurring disorders (CODs) among professionals (Morgen, 2017). This unfortunate reality is clearly problematic for effective care. Considering that substance use disorder (SUD) and substance misuse commonly occurs in people with schizophrenia and other psychotic disorders (Substance Abuse and Mental Health Services Administration [SAMHSA], 2020), there is a need for counselors to be aware of the prevalence rates and needs of clients diagnosed with SUDs alongside co-occurring schizophrenia and other psychotic disorders. Consequently, this chapter will succinctly review the relevant *Diagnostic and Statistical Manual of Mental Disorders, Fifth Edition (DSM-5;* American Psychiatric Association [APA], 2013) diagnostic criteria, prevalence rates and statistics, assessment strategies, diagnostic considerations, treatment modalities, and ethical considerations relevant for clients with co-occurring substance use and schizophrenia and other psychotic disorders. Considering the required brevity to cover all of these concepts, the reader is strongly recommended to use this chapter as merely a starting point to guide a deeper and more detailed review of these concepts via other readings, clinical training, and supervisory discussions.

FIVE DOMAINS OF PSYCHOTIC DISORDERS

The latest edition of the *DSM-5* (APA, 2013) reorganized schizophrenia into schizophrenia spectrum and other psychotic disorders. Psychotic disorders are "defined by abnormalities in one or more of the following five domains: (a) delusions, (b) hallucinations, (c) disorganized thinking/speech, (d) grossly disorganized or abnormal motor behavior, and negative symptoms" (APA, 2013, p. 87). Each of these domains are briefly reviewed.

HALLUCINATIONS

Hallucination is a sensory perception in the absence of external or somatic sensory stimuli. Hallucinations may occur with or without insight into their hallucinatory nature. Furthermore, the hallucination can be unformed (i.e., a nonspecific sensory perception) or formed (i.e., voices speaking commands; APA, 2013; Tandon et al., 2013).

DELUSIONS

Delusions are fixed beliefs based on incorrect or false inferences about reality. Furthermore, these beliefs are maintained despite obvious evidence contradictory to the belief (APA, 2013). Typical delusions include those of persecution (e.g., coworkers conspiring to have you fired) or grandiosity (e.g., false belief you are famous or far more respected than otherwise the reality). Arciniegas (2015) provided a comprehensive review of the common delusions found in psychotic disorders, many of which are identified and described in Table 12.1.

DISORGANIZED THINKING/SPEECH

The APA (2013) explains that disorganized thinking is inferred from the individual's speech. The individual may frequently switch between topics (i.e., derailment) or their answers to specific questions may be completely unrelated to the questions posed (i.e., tangentiality). In some instances, speech may be so severely disorganized that it is nearly incomprehensible and significantly impairs communication (i.e., incoherence or "word salad").

GROSSLY DISORGANIZED OR ABNORMAL MOTOR BEHAVIOR

The APA (2013, p. 88) discusses how these atypical behaviors can present as a childlike "silliness" or "unpredictable agitation." There may also be significant deficits of goal-directed behavior impairing daily functioning. Furthermore, the APA (2013) discusses catatonic behavior as decreased reactivity to the environment. These can present as a simple resistance to instructions, a rigid, or bizarre posture, or a lack of verbal and motor responses (i.e., mutism and stupor).

NEGATIVE SYMPTOMS

Negative symptoms are primarily associated with schizophrenia and less prominent in the other psychotic disorders (APA, 2013). The *DSM-5* (APA, 2013) denotes two prominent types of negative symptoms: (a) diminished emotional expression, which is demonstrated by deficits in facial expression, eye contact, flow of speech, and/or the movements that coincide with emotions

TABLE 12.1 **Common Delusions**

• **Persecutory:** One is being intentionally harmed or such harm is impending (e.g., being followed, tricked, spied on, cheated, or conspired against)
• **Grandiosity:** Conviction that one possesses special powers, talents, or abilities; may also manifest as a belief one is famous or holds a special relationship with a famous person (or deity)
• **Religiosity:** Belief that one is God, the son or daughter of God, or otherwise deific (this is a subtype of grandiosity)
• **Referential:** Belief that objects or events are directed at or are about oneself
• **Thought Control:** Belief that one's thoughts, feelings, or behaviors are externally controlled
• **Thought Insertion:** Belief that thoughts are being inserted into one's mind by an external force(s)
• **Thought Withdrawal:** Belief that thoughts are being deleted from one's mind by an external force(s)
• **Thought Broadcasting:** Belief that one's thoughts are broadcast to others or are heard aloud by others
• **Infidelity:** Belief that spouse/lover is unfaithful
• **Parasitosis:** Belief one is infested with insects, bacteria, mites, or other organisms
• **Negation:** Belief that one is dead or does not exist

Source: Adapted from Arciniegas, D. B. (2015). Psychosis. *CONTINUUM: Lifelong Learning in Neurology, 21*(3), 715–736.

when speaking; and (b) avolition, which is when an individual has little interest in engaging in activities that provide meaning or purpose. Other negative symptoms include *alogia* (i.e., diminished speech output), *anhedonia* (i.e., diminished capacity for experiencing pleasure despite positive stimuli), and *asociality* (i.e., limited interest or engagement with social interactions).

SCHIZOPHRENIA AND OTHER PSYCHOTIC DISORDERS: *DSM-5* DIAGNOSTIC CRITERIA AND DESCRIPTION

SCHIZOPHRENIA

Schizophrenia, and other psychotic disorders, present with positive and negative symptoms within three phases: (a) *prodromal* (i.e., deterioration of functioning); (b) *active* (i.e., presence of symptoms that significantly impair daily functioning); and (c) *residual* (i.e., following active symptoms; similar to the prodromal phase but also with negative psychotic symptoms). During the active phase of the disorder, positive symptoms include delusions, hallucinations, disorganized speech, and grossly disorganized behavior, whereas the negative symptoms, which were previously described, include flattened affect and avolition. The symptoms are experienced continuously over a period of at least 6 months with approximately 1 month of active-phase symptoms, with the remainder of the period manifesting as prodromal and residual symptoms (APA, 2013). Research findings suggest there is a difference between genders regarding the age of symptom onset. In a meta-analysis of 46 studies with 29,218 males and 19,402 females, Eranti et al. (2013) report age of onset (AOO) of symptoms as earlier for males by approximately 1.07 years (95% confidence interval, 0.21 to 1.93 years).

SCHIZOPHRENIFORM DISORDER

The APA (2013) underscores that the symptoms of schizophrenia and schizophreniform disorder are identical and only differentiated by the duration of symptoms and impairment. A schizophreniform disorder diagnosis is only appropriate if there has been an entire episode (i.e., with the prodromal, active, and residual phases as described earlier) that lasted a minimum of 1 month but no more than 6 months. Consequently, effective diagnosis and monitoring includes establishing a well-corroborated timeline of symptom onset and duration.

DELUSIONAL DISORDER

Criteria for this diagnosis are the presence of one or more delusions lasting for at least 1 month. This diagnosis entails the presentation of persistent delusions but without the disorganized and other positive symptoms characteristic of schizophrenia (e.g., hallucinations, odd speech, bizarre behavior). Individuals diagnosed with delusional disorder present as normal until their delusions are triggered. At that point, the individual will commence demonstrating their fixed/false beliefs (APA, 2013).

SCHIZOAFFECTIVE DISORDER

This diagnosis is for individuals who do *not* meet sufficient criteria for either schizophrenia or a mood disorder (e.g., major depressive disorder or bipolar disorder I/II) but have features of both schizophrenia and a mood disorder (APA, 2013). This is critical because both these disorders can present with symptoms associated with the other. For example, it is possible for a counselor to encounter a client who presents with major depressive disorder (typically severe) while experiencing hallucinations. Schizoaffective disorder is a challenging diagnosis due to the presence of symptoms for both schizophrenia and either major depressive disorder or bipolar disorder. The *DSM-5* (APA, 2013) designates two types of schizoaffective disorder: (a) the bipolar type and (b) the depressive type. The *bipolar type* is relevant if a manic episode is part of the symptom presentation (regardless of any major depressive episode). The *depressive type* is relevant if only major depressive episodes are part of the symptom presentation.

BRIEF PSYCHOTIC DISORDER

The APA (2013) indicates that this diagnosis is given to individuals who experience a sudden onset of psychotic symptoms such as hallucinations, delusions, dissociation, or agitation. The onset of symptoms is rapid, where within approximately 2 weeks the individual shifts from a nonpsychotic to a psychotic state. Brief psychotic disorder lasts at least 1 day but no more than a month. After the course of symptoms, the individual returns to their previous level of functioning.

The *DSM-5* (APA, 2013) denotes three types of this disorder. *Brief psychotic disorder with marked stressor(s)*—also called brief reactive psychosis—is appropriate if symptoms occur just after and in response to stressful situations. *Brief psychotic disorder without marked stressor(s)* is appropriate if the psychotic symptoms do not occur immediately after or not in response to stressful situations. And, lastly, *brief psychotic disorder with postpartum onset* is appropriate if the onset of the conditions occurs within 4 weeks following birth.

SUBSTANCE-/MEDICATION-INDUCED PSYCHOTIC DISORDER

This disorder presents with psychotic symptoms (i.e., delusions and/or hallucinations) that are a direct result from the use of medications or substances. Symptoms occur due to substance intoxication or withdrawal. Symptoms must develop during or within 1 month of intoxication by or withdrawal from the substance, and the substance must be capable of producing these symptoms. There are two specifiers associated with this disorder: (a) the designation *with onset during intoxication* for when symptoms develop during the period of intoxication, and (b) the designation *with onset during withdrawal* for when symptoms develop during the period of withdrawal (APA, 2013).

DSM-5 DISORDERS AND *ICD-10-CM* CODING

Sperry and Sperry (2015) emphasized clinicians need to understand the diagnostic criteria for the psychotic disorders; therefore, counselors need to be proficient in using the *DSM-5*. Part of this diagnostic fluency involves the professional counselor bridging the *DSM-5* (the diagnostic manual most frequently used by counselors in the United States) with the *ICD-10-CM* (World Health Organization, 1993) for diagnostic coding, which is included on healthcare billing for third-party reimbursement. The relevant *ICD-10-CM* codes for the *DSM-5* disorders discussed in this chapter are presented in Table 12.2.

TABLE 12.2 **Schizophrenia Spectrum and Other Psychotic Disorders (*ICD-10-CM* Codes)**

• Schizophrenia	F20.9
• Delusional Disorder	F22
• Brief Psychotic Disorder	F23
• Schizophreniform Disorder	F20.81
• Schizoaffective Disorder	
○ Bipolar Type	F25.0
○ Depressive Type	F25.1
• Alcohol-Induced Psychotic Disorder	
○ Use Disorder, Mild	F10.159
○ Use Disorder, Moderate or Severe	F10.259
○ Without Use Disorder	F10.959

(continued)

TABLE 12.2 Schizophrenia Spectrum and Other Psychotic Disorders (*ICD-10-CM* Codes) (*Continued*)

• Cannabis-Induced Psychotic Disorder	
○ Use Disorder, Mild	F12.159
○ Use Disorder, Moderate or Severe	F12.259
○ Without Use Disorder	F12.959
• Phencyclidine-Induced Psychotic Disorder	
○ Use Disorder, Mild	F16.159
○ Use Disorder, Moderate or Severe	F16.259
○ Without Use Disorder	F16.959
• Other Hallucinogen-Induced Psychotic Disorder	
○ Use Disorder, Mild	F16.159
○ Use Disorder, Moderate or Severe	F16.259
○ Without Use Disorder	F16.959
• Inhalant-Induced Psychotic Disorder	
○ Use Disorder, Mild	F18.159
○ Use Disorder, Moderate or Severe	F18.259
○ Without Use Disorder	F18.959
• Sedative/Hypnotic/Anxiolytic-Induced Psychotic Disorder	
○ Use Disorder, Mild	F13.159
○ Use Disorder, Moderate or Severe	F13.259
○ Without Use Disorder	F13.959
• Amphetamine/Other Stimulant-Induced Psychotic Disorder	
○ Use Disorder, Mild	F15.159
○ Use Disorder, Moderate or Severe	F15.259
○ Without Use Disorder	F15.959
• Cocaine-Induced Psychotic Disorder	
○ Use Disorder, Mild	F14.159
○ Use Disorder, Moderate or Severe	F14.259
○ Without Use Disorder	F14.959
• Other (Unknown) Substance-Induced Psychotic Disorder	
○ Use Disorder, Mild	F19.159
○ Use Disorder, Moderate or Severe	F19.259
○ Without Use Disorder	F19.959

PREVALENCE, STATISTICS, AND DEMOGRAPHICS

Schizophrenia and other psychotic symptoms frequently co-occur with SUDs, whether due to withdrawal, substance-induced symptoms, or CODs (Morgen, 2017; SAMHSA, 2020; Tandon & Shariff, 2019). Substance misuse in those diagnosed with schizophrenia or other psychotic disorders contribute to an increased likelihood of poorer health and functional outcomes, including an increased risk for violent behaviors, suicide, housing instability, poor social relationships, cognitive impairment, employment problems, legal difficulties, and reduced antipsychotic medication adherence (Bennett et al., 2017; Drake et al., 2006; Schmitt et al., 2011; Trudeau et al., 2018). Consequently, an understanding of the prevalence of substance use co-occurring with schizophrenia and other psychotic disorders is one of the critical initial steps of formulating effective co-occurring care.

CO-OCCURRING SCHIZOPHRENIA AND SUBSTANCE USE DISORDERS

Recent comprehensive multidecade work by Hunt and colleagues (2018) underscored the interrelationship between schizophrenia and co-occurring substance use disorders via a worldwide study of articles published between 1990 and 2017. Overall, 961 studies (representing 165,811 total participants) were identified, including 123 studies of co-occurring substance use rates for those diagnosed with a schizophrenia spectrum disorder. The overall schizophrenia prevalence for the 71 studies investigating SUDs was 0.417, or 41.7%. Specific findings per each substance are discussed in the following.

ALCOHOL USE DISORDERS

Of the 88 studies reviewed, Hunt and colleagues (2018) found the overall prevalence for alcohol use disorders (AUDs) was 0.243, or 24.3%. These rates mirror other evidence demonstrating the relationship between schizophrenia and substance use as consistent over many years of examination. For instance, dating back over 30 years, Regier et al. (1990) found that 47% of the individuals with schizophrenia spectrum disorder also met the criteria of alcohol use disorder (33.7%) and SUD (27.5%). Furthermore, Mueser et al. (1990) found that between 12% and 50% of those diagnosed with schizophrenia were also diagnosed with alcohol consumption disorder.

ILLICIT DRUG USE

Hunt et al. (2018) found that the overall prevalence for general illicit drug use ($n = 33$ studies reviewed) was 0.275, 27%%, with a significantly higher prevalence in those with a first episode of psychosis as compared to those diagnosed with chronic schizophrenia. Again, these findings by Hunt and colleagues support other work where, for instance, the substance use rate in patients diagnosed with schizophrenia was found to run between 44% and 48% (Margolese et al., 2004; Wobrock et al., 2007).

CANNABIS USE DISORDER

In cannabis use disorders ($n = 69$ studies reviewed), Hunt et al. (2018) found the overall prevalence was 0.262, 26.2% with the prevalence significantly higher for individuals experiencing a first episode of psychosis as compared to those with chronic schizophrenia. Other work also demonstrates the relationship between cannabis and schizophrenia and other psychotic disorders. Studies demonstrate that up to 64% of individuals experiencing a first episode of psychosis have used cannabis, with 30% of these individuals presenting with a cannabis use disorder featuring positive psychotic symptoms and increased disorder severity (Barnes et al., 2006; Oluwoye et al., 2019). In addition, other studies may demonstrate the relationship between cannabis use and psychotic symptoms and psychotic disorders. For instance, Di Forti et al. (2019) sought to elaborate on whether cannabis use is associated with psychotic disorder onset by examining data from 901 patients with first-episode psychosis and 1,237 population controls across 11 sites. Findings underscored daily use of cannabis and the use of high-potency cannabis as the two strongest independent predictors of psychotic disorder onset. The odds of psychotic disorder onset among daily cannabis users were 3.2 times higher than for noncannabis users. The odds of psychotic disorder onset among users of high-potency cannabis were 1.6 times higher than for noncannabis users.

STIMULANT USE DISORDER

Hunt and colleagues (2018) noted that the overall prevalence for stimulant use disorders ($n = 42$ studies reviewed) was 0.073, 7.3%. Other studies also show a relationship between schizophrenia/psychotic disorders and stimulant use. For instance, in a study of 198 methamphetamine users, Hides et al. (2015) demonstrated that a high percentage of methamphetamine users present with a co-occurring psychotic disorder where 51% reported a lifetime psychotic disorder and 80% reported a substance-induced psychotic disorder. In other works, Sara et al. (2015) completed a meta-analysis of 64 studies completed over approximately eight decades that focused on stimulant use and psychosis. These reviewers noticed similar results in that the lifetime or recent stimulant use disorders in 22,500 people with psychosis produced a pooled rate of stimulant use disorder of 8.9%. Furthermore, Wearne and Cornish (2018) found that some methamphetamine users developed a persistent psychotic syndrome similar to schizophrenia.

OPIOID USE DISORDER

Hunt and colleagues (2018) reported that the overall prevalence for opioid use disorders ($n = 20$ studies reviewed) was 0.051, 5.1%, with prevalence rates significantly lower for individuals with recent psychotic disorder onset as compared with cases of chronic schizophrenia. However, the epidemiological data for co-occurring psychosis with opioid use disorder are not as clear as with other disorders, with reported prevalence rates widely varying between 1% and 16% (Maremmani et al., 2011; Westermeyer, 2006).

NICOTINE USE DISORDER

Scott and colleagues (2018) reviewed eight longitudinal studies (seven cohort studies and one case control study) identified as focused on tobacco smoking and psychosis as an outcome. Six of the eight studies found statistically significant and positive associations between tobacco smoking and schizophrenia spectrum disorders symptom onset. This finding (and others like it) are interesting because it starts to craft an alternative narrative as to the relationship between schizophrenia spectrum disorders and tobacco.

Nicotine use by those with schizophrenia spectrum disorders had typically (over the past few decades) been explained as secondary to the schizophrenia spectrum disorders; for example, the use of nicotine as a self-medicating agent to cope with symptoms (MacCabe 2018). However, work such as by Scott and colleagues (2018) and others (e.g., Quigley & MacCabe, 2019) have initiated an alternative explanation that self-medication cannot fully explain the association between tobacco use and schizophrenia spectrum disorders. As of now, the literature seems to reflect that it is still unclear as to whether nicotine does actually increase the risk of psychosis onset, is used as a self-medicating agent, or (likely) some combination of the two along with other yet unspecified factors (e.g., genetic, psychosocial).

ASSESSMENT AND DIAGNOSTIC CONSIDERATIONS

Beyond the presence of a co-occurring schizophrenic or psychotic disorder, symptoms of psychosis can occur during intoxication or withdrawal, or via a substance-induced psychotic disorder. Understanding the differences among these three potential avenues for psychotic symptoms is critical to the diagnostic process. Although an exhaustive review is beyond the scope of this chapter, substance-induced psychotic disorder, as well as psychotic symptoms presenting in intoxication and withdrawal, are discussed.

SUBSTANCE-INDUCED PSYCHOTIC DISORDER

Numerous substances are capable of producing psychotic symptoms resembling a psychotic disorder. The symptoms typically are relatively brief, resolving shortly after cessation of the causative substance. Of greater clinical concern, the substance-induced psychotic symptoms may also facilitate the onset of a co-occurring psychotic disorder. For example, Kendler and colleagues (2019) evaluated 7,606 individuals who had an index registry diagnosis of substance-induced psychotic disorder and assessed their diagnostic evolution over the next 7 years, on average. A good-sized number of the sample (11%) with an index diagnosis of substance-induced psychotic disorder progressed to a diagnosis of schizophrenia. Both the substance type (i.e., cannabis, alcohol) and severity impacted the cumulative hazard progression to a diagnosis of schizophrenia for both cannabis-induced (18%) and alcohol-induced (4.7%) psychotic disorders.

Kendler and colleagues (2019) are not alone in underscoring the potential of a progression from substance-induced psychotic disorder to primary diagnosis of psychotic disorder. Caton et al. (2005) evaluated 386 patients presenting to the emergency department with psychosis and substance use. At follow-up (6 and 12 months later), 319 subjects out of the original 386 were again evaluated with 285 individuals (89%) retaining their baseline diagnostic category; however, 34 individuals (11%) changed from substance-induced psychosis to primary psychosis. Consequently, careful monitoring of the psychotic symptoms is critical for appropriate clinical care.

INTOXICATION AND WITHDRAWAL

The *DSM-5* (APA, 2013) specifically identifies substances such as cannabis, stimulants, and opioids as capable of producing perceptual disturbances (e.g., hallucinations). However, other substances, such as alcohol, are also capable of producing psychotic-type symptoms during intoxication. Of note is that during intoxication, more stimulating substances (e.g., amphetamines and cocaine) are more likely to be associated with substance-induced psychotic disorders (or substance-induced anxiety disorders; Morgen, 2017). Similarly, numerous substances produce symptoms mirroring psychosis during the withdrawal phase (APA, 2013). The substances producing psychotic type symptoms during intoxication and/or withdrawal are presented in Table 12.3.

TABLE 12.3 **Substances Producing Psychotic Symptoms in Intoxication or Withdrawal**

SUBSTANCE	INTOXICATION	WITHDRAWAL
Alcohol	✓	✓
Sedative/hypnotic/anxiolytic	✓	✓
Cannabis	✓	✓
Stimulant (including cocaine)	✓	
Hallucinogens	✓	
Inhalants	✓	

DIAGNOSTIC DECISION-MAKING

Two basic organizing principles, diagnostic history and timing, can assist the counselor to determine the appropriate diagnosis of substance-induced psychotic disorder, co-occurring psychotic disorder, or substance intoxication/withdrawal. Each principle is briefly addressed.

DIAGNOSTIC HISTORY

Understanding the client's full clinical history is critical for a few reasons. First, the presence of an established *DSM-5* schizophrenia spectrum or other psychotic disorder will negate any likelihood of a substance-induced psychotic disorder. Second (and in a related manner), examining for evidence that the individual presents with an undiagnosed *DSM-5* schizophrenia spectrum or other psychotic disorder. If this is the case, then any psychotic symptom presenting in early recovery may be more indicative of the individual no longer using substances that may have kept the psychotic symptoms relatively managed (e.g., heroin). Third, if there is an established *DSM-5* diagnosis of schizophrenia or other psychotic disorder, one must determine if the individual is adhering to their medication regimen. Nonadherence (or inconsistent adherence) to medication can clearly produce psychotic symptoms. Fourth, determine the existence or presence of other diagnoses. For example, the onset of psychotic symptoms related to an established major depressive disorder with psychotic features would explain the presence of psychosis during a period of distress and substance use. The careful counselor diagnostician would recognize that many *DSM-5* disorders beyond schizophrenia spectrum and other psychotic disorders can present with a psychotic/psychotic-like symptom (e.g., paranoia in personality disorder or invasive/distressing thoughts in obsessive-compulsive disorder).

TIMING

When symptoms occur is also a critical piece of diagnostic data. Questions the counselor should consider include: Did the psychotic symptoms present during intoxication or withdrawal, or did they present in a period soon after withdrawal? Such information can inform whether the symptoms best reflect intoxication, withdrawal, or substance-induced causes. Timing is also relevant in regard to the substances used. For instance, alcohol and stimulants both can produce psychotic symptoms during the withdrawal period; however, the onset of withdrawal differs per substance. Alcohol withdrawal (with can produce psychotic symptoms during withdrawal) typically occurs 6 to 24 hours after the last drink. Of note is that heavy drinkers (i.e., those with a *DSM-5* severe AUD) may actually experience withdrawal symptoms by only reducing their daily alcohol intake (as opposed to complete cessation of drinking). Dissimilarly, symptoms of withdrawal for amphetamines typically start about 2 to 4 days after last use, peak in severity at around 7 to 10 days, and subside within 2 to 4 weeks. Cocaine withdrawal symptoms appear within 1 to 2 days after last use, peak in severity at around 4 to 7 days, and subside within 1 to 2 weeks (Breggin, 2013). Knowing the substances used, and the timing of those substances, is critical to understanding the presence of any psychotic symptoms potentially occurring due to withdrawal.

SCREENING AND ASSESSMENT TOOLS

Morgen (2017) provided a comprehensive list of measures relevant to the co-occurring psychiatric and SUDs discipline. Regarding assessment of psychotic symptoms specifically, the crucial component is that the measure captures recent symptomatology. Doing so permits for an accurate assessment as well as provides the clinician the capacity to reassess on a continual basis. Three common measures relevant to psychotic symptoms assessment are discussed within this chapter.

DSM-5 SELF-RATED LEVEL 1 CROSS-CUTTING SYMPTOM MEASURE

The *DSM-5* Level 1 Cross-Cutting Symptom Measure (APA, 2013) is a self-/informant-rated measure consisting of 23 questions that assess 13 psychiatric domains, including (as relevant to this chapter) psychotic thought. Each item examines how the individual has been bothered by the specific symptom(s) during the prior 2 weeks. The two measures specifically examining psychosis are items 12 (*Hearing things other people couldn't hear, such as voices even when no one was around?*) and 13 (*Feeling that someone could hear your thoughts, or that you could hear what another person was thinking?*). Each of these two questions are each scored on a 0 (none) to 4 (severe, nearly every day) scale. If these two scores sum to greater than or equal to 2, further inquiry is warranted with the next tool (APA, 2013).

DSM-5 CLINICIAN-RATED DIMENSIONS OF PSYCHOSIS SYMPTOMS SEVERITY

As discussed, if warranted, the Clinician-Rated Dimensions of Psychosis Symptom Severity can be administered (APA, 2013). This is an 8-item measure assessing various psychotic and related symptoms severity (e.g., delusions, hallucinations, disorganized speech, abnormal psychomotor behavior, negative symptoms, impaired cognition, depression, and mania). The clinician rates symptom severity as experienced by the individual during the past 7 days. Each item on the measure is rated on a 5-point scale (0 = none; 1 = equivocal; 2 = present, but mild; 3 = present and moderate; and 4 = present and severe) with a symptom-specific definition of each rating level (APA, 2013). This tool does not provide a cut-off score for problem severity as this is best used to monitor client's symptoms over time. Counselors are encouraged to use their clinical judgement in interpreting their client's scores and making decisions about treatment foci (APA, 2013).

THE POSITIVE AND NEGATIVE SYNDROME SCALE

Beyond the *DSM-5* assessments, there are numerous other assessments of relevance to the clinician. One common measure is the Positive and Negative Syndrome Scale (PANSS), which is a standardized, clinical interview with strong reliability and validity (Edgar et al., 2014a, 2014b). The PANSS is for use with those diagnosed with schizophrenia and rates the presence and severity of positive and negative symptoms, as well as general psychopathology, within the past week. Of the 30 items, seven are related to positive symptoms, another seven correspond to negative symptoms, and the remaining 16 are specific to general psychopathology symptoms. Symptom severity for each item is rated according to which anchoring points in the 7-point scale (1 = absent; 7 = extreme) best describe the presentation of the symptom (Kay, Fiszbein, & Opler, 1987).

TREATMENT MODALITIES

SAMHSA (2020) underscores both pharmacotherapy and counseling for treatment of co-occurring substance use and schizophrenia spectrum and other psychotic disorders. Effective comprehensive care likely combines both of these approaches. This section covers the basics of pharmacotherapy, cognitive behavioral therapy (CBT), and mindfulness-based interventions for those diagnosed with schizophrenia spectrum and other psychotic disorders.

PHARMACOTHERAPY

Antipsychotic drugs reduce or eliminate symptoms of psychosis. In their review of psychotic disorders, Lieberman and First (2018) noted that all the antipsychotic medications currently prescribed in the United States function by blocking or mitigating dopamine (D2) receptor activity. They are most effective in treating hallucinations, delusions, disorganized thinking, and aggression. Antipsychotic drugs are divided into two groups: (a) first-generation (older/conventional or "typical") antipsychotics and (b) second-generation (newer or "atypical") antipsychotics. Table 12.4 lists the typical and atypical antipsychotic medications along with the longer-lasting injectable antipsychotic medications.

COGNITIVE BEHAVIORAL THERAPY

The evidence for the efficacy of CBT in treating patients with persistent symptoms of schizophrenia has progressed from case studies and uncontrolled trials to methodologically rigorous and controlled trials that include individuals across the schizophrenia spectrum. For example, Tai and Turkington (2009) summarized the results of the CBT studies and concluded the following two points. One, that randomized controlled trials (RCTs) show moderate effect sizes for treating the positive and negative symptoms. Two, that hallucinations and delusions respond to CBT interventions. Tarrier and Haddock (2004) discussed the use of CBT for enhancing coping strategies as a buffer against psychotic decompensation. They reviewed strategies such as focusing on the general process of dealing with psychosis as adversity (psychosis is an example of adversity) as well as behavioral coping skills learned through graded practice and/or rehearsal.

TABLE 12.4 **Typical, Atypical, and Long-Lasting Antipsychotic Medications**

TYPICAL MEDICATIONS
• Haldol (haloperidol)
• Loxitane (loxapine)
• Mellaril (thioridazine)
• Moban (molindone)
• Navane (thiothixene)
• Prolixin (fluphenazine)
• Serentil (mesoridazine)
• Stelazine (trifluoperazine)
• Trilafon (perphenazine)
• Thorazine (chlorpromazine)
ATYPICAL MEDICATIONS
• Abilify (aripiprazole)
• Clozaril (clozapine)
• Geodon (ziprasidone)
• Risperdal (risperidone)
• Seroquel (quetiapine)
• Zyprexa (olanzapine)
LONG-LASTING INJECTABLE MEDICATIONS
• Aripiprazole (Abilify Maintena)
• Aripiprazole lauroxil (Aristada)
• Fluphenazine (Prolixin)
• Haloperidol (Haldol)
• Olanzapine pamoate (Zyprexa Relprevv)
• Paliperidone (Invega Sustenna, Invega Trinza)
• Risperidone (Risperdal Consta)

MINDFULNESS-BASED INTERVENTIONS

Generally defined, mindfulness-based interventions entail an application where the individual becomes more aware of their physical and psychological condition in the present moment. One critical mindfulness-based application for those with psychotic symptoms comes from Chadwick (2006) who developed an application specifically for schizophrenia spectrum disorders to incorporate mindfulness alongside other therapeutic interventions from CBT. These interventions for those with schizophrenia spectrum disorders assist the individual to more effectively engage with distressful psychotic symptoms such as hallucinations and delusions via a reduction in rumination and avoidant behavior. Instead, individuals build skills for a mindful response via permitting the psychotic symptoms to come into awareness for engagement, as compared to prior applications stemming from avoidance and fear (see Chadwick [2006] for further review). Evidence for the effectiveness of mindfulness-based interventions for schizophrenia spectrum disorders comes from Hodann-Caudevilla et al. (2020) who conducted a recent meta-analysis of 10 published studies that included a total of 1,094 participants. This systematic review concluded that mindfulness-based interventions combined with standard interventions facilitate significant improvements in areas such as the severity of overall symptomatology, positive symptoms, and negative symptoms.

LEGAL AND ETHICAL CONSIDERATIONS

Commentary regarding ethical issues in the treatment of schizophrenia and other psychotic disorders predominantly exists in the psychiatry literature (e.g., Beck & Ballon, 2020). However, numerous ethical concepts from psychiatry easily align with the practice of professional counseling in the treatment of co-occurring substance use and schizophrenia and other psychotic disorders. Specifically, the concepts of shared decision-making, autonomy in regard to medication, and the capacity to engage in the treatment informed consent process. These concepts are critical to schizophrenia spectrum disorders for a number of reasons, including the risk of self-harm. Suicide is a major cause of mortality for those with schizophrenia spectrum disorders (e.g., Zaheer et al., 2020). Consequently, an understanding of the interface between mental health and law regarding protective interventions (e.g., commitment) is critical, and each reader is encouraged to examine their state's laws regarding mental health care. SAMHSA (2019) also provides a comprehensive review of the concepts of mental health care, commitment, and legal issues, which is easily available for reference.

SHARED DECISION-MAKING

Hamann et al. (2006) and Hudson et al. (2008) discussed the shared decision-making approach as where the provider offers clients ample information and actively involves them in treatment decisions. Often, this involves the use of directional aids. For example, one directional aid may assist the client in reviewing the pros and cons of a specific treatment scenario (e.g., switching to a different antipsychotic medication). By utilizing the shared decision-making strategy via the directional aid intervention, the client is empowered to play a larger role in the process and the provider further demonstrates the respect for client autonomy.

MEDICATION REFUSAL

Noordsy (2016) emphasized that schizophrenia spectrum disorders treatment heavily focuses on pharmacotherapy (and much more so than for other psychiatric disorders). However, antipsychotic medications typically produce side effects. Too often there exists a conflict between the provider trying to convince the client of the importance of pharmacotherapy while the client would rather engage in an alternative and nonpharmacotherapeutic intervention. The professional counselor cannot prescribe medication, but they may play a role in the discussion process to persuade the client to engage in/continue with pharmacotherapy. Consequently, the professional counselor should engage the client in a thoughtful dialogue regarding pharmacotherapy reluctance so that (similar to shared decision-making discussed previously) the client feels their autonomy respected in the treatment process.

INFORMED CONSENT CAPACITY

The MacArthur Treatment Competence Study (Appelbaum & Grisso, 1995; Grisso & Appelbaum, 1995) examined the abilities of psychiatric inpatients hospitalized for schizophrenia or depression, medically ill inpatients, and healthy, nonhospitalized community controls regarding the ability to make treatment-related decisions. Patients diagnosed with schizophrenia poorly performed on measures of understanding, appreciation, and reasoning as compared to other study groups. Furthermore, the study showed that the overall psychopathology severity was associated with the patient impaired performance on the understanding measure. Nearly 20 years later, Morris and Heinssen (2014) echoed these findings by discussing how requesting informed consent from individuals at elevated risk for psychosis requires clear therapist/patient communication while also likely involving the participation of family members. Professional counselors can adhere to the recommendations of the MacArthur Treatment Competence Study and Morris and Heinssen by coming to the informed consent process with a good understanding of the current functioning of the individual diagnosed with schizophrenia. Furthermore, the professional counselor should work with the individual to secure a release of information authorizing the counselor to speak with healthcare collateral persons (e.g., prescribers, case managers) as well as close family members/significant others (e.g., spouse, parent, partner) so that counseling decisions can be made if/when the individual's psychotic symptom(s) prohibits their effective involvement in their treatment process.

CLINICAL CASE ILLUSTRATION AND DISCUSSION

CASE OF REBECCA

Rebecca is a 24-year-old female MBA student who also works at a grocery store. Rebecca started smoking marijuana approximately 3 years ago. What started as an occasional joint gradually increased to approximately between five and seven joints per day. In addition, what began as recreational use with friends quickly escalated into use to manage daily stressors of school and work. Rebecca believed that she could only manage her stressors with the assistance of cannabis. Though she refused to tell anyone, she was terrified that she could not manage day-to-day life without cannabis. Her boyfriend noticed the increased cannabis use and Rebecca had agreed to cut back on her cannabis use after a lengthy discussion with her boyfriend. Reluctantly, she fully ceased all cannabis use 3 days prior to her hospitalization.

Upon cessation, her friends noticed Rebecca acting oddly. For example, her roommate found her shouting into an empty closet whereas her boyfriend found her pacing and murmuring to herself in her backyard. Rebecca also started hearing an unfamiliar voice whispering that she is a "failure" and "too stupid to be worth living." She told nobody out of fear of being considered crazy. In the hours immediately preceding her hospitalization, she was involved in a verbal altercation with a customer at the grocery store. When a customer asked about the price on a box of cereal, Rebecca became enraged and started screaming and throwing cereal boxes up and down the aisle. When approached by her store manager and a few coworkers, she grabbed a shopping cart and shoved her way through the crowd while shouting that the store employees were trying to kill her. The police were called and 20 minutes later, Rebecca was found in the parking lot hiding under a car while pleading for the voices to stop and that she did not want to be murdered by the store manager.

CASE DISCUSSION

This is a case of acute onset cannabis-induced psychotic disorder following cessation of cannabis. The patient had no prior psychological disorders and there was no personal/family history of psychotic thought. As is typical with substance-induced psychotic disorder, the primary and immediate necessity was to keep Rebecca safe as she was experiencing command auditory hallucinations of a suicidal nature as well as aggressive behaviors and significant paranoia. The stabilization and safety components were achieved via a brief medically managed withdrawal management under physician care. Supportive counseling care using CBT helped Rebecca manage the remaining psychotic symptoms during the course of the withdrawal period and beyond. As is typical, Rebecca's cannabis-induced psychotic symptoms subsided as she remained abstinent from cannabis use. However, counseling (using CBT) continued as Rebecca needed to learn skills to effectively manage stressors without cannabis and/or other substances.

CHAPTER SUMMARY

This chapter was intended to initially review the critical concepts of *DSM-5* diagnostic criteria, prevalence rates and statistics, assessment and diagnostic considerations, assessment tools, treatment modalities, and ethical considerations relevant for clients with SUD alongside co-occurring schizophrenia spectrum and other psychotic disorders. As with all co-occurring substance use and psychiatric disorders, the considerable overlap of symptoms between the intoxication, withdrawal, substance-induced, and co-occurring psychiatric conditions present both diagnostic and treatment challenges. Counselors are encouraged to review all of the materials cited in this chapter (particularly the references noted with an asterisk) for further detailed information beyond the limits and scope afforded this chapter.

DISCUSSION QUESTIONS

1. Considering the other co-occurring substance use disorders reviewed in this book, how do you think the onset and presentation of psychotic symptoms are impacted by the use of multiple substances simultaneously (e.g., alcohol and cocaine, cocaine and heroin)?

2. If substance use and psychotic symptoms can both consist of confused thought, poor memory, and disorganized speech, how would a counselor gather the appropriate clinical data required for effective diagnosis and treatment planning?

3. After reviewing the other chapters, do you see any similarities and dissimilarities with schizophrenia and other psychotic disorders regarding the prevalence rates of various substances and the other psychiatric disorders?

REFERENCES

American Psychiatric Association. (2013). *Diagnostic and statistical manual of mental disorders* (5th ed.). https://doi.org/10.1176/appi.books.9780890425596

Appelbaum, P. S., & Grisso, T. (1995). The MacArthur treatment competence study I: Mental illness and competence to consent to treatment. *Law and Human Behavior, 19*(2), 105–126.

Arciniegas, D. B. (2015). Psychosis. *CONTINUUM: Lifelong Learning in Neurology, 21*(3), 715–736.

Barnes, T. R. E., Mutsatsa, S. H., Mutton, S. B., Watt, H. C., & Joyce, E. M. (2006). Comorbid substance use and age at onset of schizophrenia. *The British Journal of Psychiatry, 188*(3), 237–242.

Beck, N. S., & Ballon, J. S. (2020). Ethical issues in schizophrenia. *Focus: The Journal of Lifelong Learning in Psychiatry, 18*(4), 428–431.

*Bennett, M. E., Bradshaw, K. R., & Catalano, L. T. (2017). Treatment of substance use disorders in schizophrenia. *The American Journal of Drug and Alcohol Abuse, 43*(4), 377–390.

Breggin, P. R. (2013). *Psychiatric drug withdrawal: A guide for prescribers, therapists, patients, and their families*. Springer Publishing Co.

Caton, C. L. M., Drake, R. E., Hasin, D. S., Dominguez, B., Shrout, P. E., Samet, S., & Schanzer, W. B. (2005). Differences between early-phase primary psychotic disorders with concurrent substance use and substance-induced psychoses. *Archives of General Psychiatry, 62*(2), 137–145.

Chadwick P. (2006). *Person-based cognitive therapy for distressing psychosis*. John Wiley & Sons.

Di Forti, M., Quattrone, D., Freeman, T. P., Tripoli, G., Gayer-Anderson, C., Quigley, H., Rodriguez, V., Jongsma, H. E., Ferraro, L., La Cascia, C., La Barbera, D., Tarricone, I., Berardi, D., Szöke, A., Arango, C., Tortelli, A., Velthorst, E., Bernardo, M., Del-Ben, C. M., & Murray, R. M. (2019). The contribution of cannabis use to variation in the incidence of psychotic disorder across Europe (EU-GEI): A multicentre case-control study. *The Lancet Psychiatry, 6*(5), 427–436.

Drake, R. E., McHugo, G. J., Xie, H., Fox, M., Packard, J., & Helmstetter, B. (2006). Ten-year recovery outcomes for clients with co-occurring schizophrenia and substance use disorders. *Schizophrenia Bulletin, 32*(3), 464–473.

Edgar, C. J., Blaettler, T., Bugarski-Kirola, D., Le Scouiller, S., Garibaldi, G. M., & Marder, S. R. (2014a). Reliability, validity and ability to detect change of the PANSS negative symptom factor score in outpatients with schizophrenia on select antipsychotics and with prominent negative or disorganized thought symptoms. *Psychiatry Research, 218*(1–2), 219–224.

Edgar, C. J., Blaettler, T., Bugarski-Kirola, D., Le Scouiller, S., Garibaldi, G. M., & Marder, S. R. (2014b). Validity and utility of the PANSS negative symptoms factor score as a clinical trial outcome. *Schizophrenia Research, 158*(1–3). https://doi.org/10.1016/j.schres.2014.07.037

Eranti, S. V., MacCabe, J. H., Bundy, H., & Murray, R. M. (2013). Gender difference in age at onset of schizophrenia: A meta-analysis. *Psychological Medicine, 43*(1), 155–167.

Grisso, T., & Appelbaum, P. S. (1995). The MacArthur treatment competence study III: Abilities of patients to consent to psychiatric and medical treatments. *Law and Human Behavior, 19*(2), 149–174.

Hamann, J., Langer, B., Winkler, V., Busch, R., Cohen, R., Leucht, S., & Kissling, W. (2006). Shared decision making for in-patients with schizophrenia. *Acta Psychiatrica Scandinavica, 114*(4), 265–273.

*Hides, L., Dawe, S., McKetin, R., Kavanagh, D. J., Young, R. M., Teesson, M., & Saunders, J. B. (2015). Primary and substance-induced psychotic disorders in methamphetamine users. *Psychiatry Research, 226*(1), 91–96.

Hodann-Caudevilla, R. M., Diaz-Silveira, C., Burgos-Julian, F. A., & Santed, M. A. (2020). Mindfulness-based interventions for people with schizophrenia: A systematic review and meta-analysis. *International Journal of Environmental Research and Public Health, 17*, 1–18. https://doi.org/10.3390/ijerph17134690

Hudson, T. J., Owen, R. R., Thrush, C. R., Armitage, T. L., & Thapa, P. (2008). Guideline implementation and patient-tailoring strategies to improve medication adherence for schizophrenia. *The Journal of Clinical Psychiatry, 69*(1), 74–80.

*Hunt, G. E., Large, M. M., Cleary, M., Lai, H. M. X., & Saunders, J. B. (2018). Prevalence of comorbid substance use in schizophrenia spectrum disorders in community and clinical settings, 1990–2017: Systematic review and meta-analysis. *Drug and Alcohol Dependence, 191*, 234–258.

Kay, S. R., Fiszbein, A., & Opler, L. A. (1987). The Positive and Negative Syndrome Scale (PANSS) for schizophrenia. *Schizophrenia Bulletin, 13*(2), 261–276.

Kendler, K. S., Ohlsson, H., Sundquist, J., & Sundquist, K. (2019). Prediction of onset of substance-induced psychotic disorder and its progression to schizophrenia in a Swedish national sample. *The American Journal of Psychiatry, 176*(9), 711–719.

*Lieberman, J. A., & First, M. B. (2018). Psychotic disorders. *The New England Journal of Medicine, 379*(3), 270–280. https://doi.org/10.1056/NEJMra1801490

MacCabe, J. H. (2018). It is time to start taking tobacco seriously as a risk factor for psychosis: Self-medication cannot explain the association. *Acta Psychiatrica Scandinavica, 138*(1), 3–4.

Maremmani, A. G., Dell'Osso, L., Pacini, M., Popovic, D., Rovai, L., Torrens, M., & Maremmani, I. (2011). Dual diagnosis and chronology of illness in treatment-seeking Italian patients dependent on heroin. *Journal of Addictive Diseases, 30*(2), 123–135. https://doi.org/10.1080/10550887.2011.554779

Margolese, H. C., Malchy, L., Negrete, J. C., Tempier, R., & Gill, K. (2004). Drug and alcohol use among patients with schizophrenia and related psychoses: Levels and consequences. *Schizophrenia Research, 67*(2–3), 157–166.

Morgen, K. (2017). *Substance use disorders and addictions.* Sage Publications, Inc.

Morris, S. E., & Heinssen, R. K. (2014). Informed consent in the psychosis prodrome: Ethical, procedural and cultural considerations. *Philosophy, Ethics, and Humanities in Medicine, 9*, Article number: 19. https://doi.org/10.1186/1747-5341-9-19

Mueser, K. T., Yarnold, P. R., Levinson, D. F., Singh, H., Bellack, A. S., Kee, K., Morrison, R. L., & Yadalam, K. G. (1990). Prevalence of substance abuse in schizophrenia: Demographic and clinical correlates. *Schizophrenia Bulletin, 16*(1), 31–56.

Noordsy, D. L. (2016). Ethical issues in the care of people with schizophrenia. *Focus: The Journal of Lifelong Learning in Psychiatry, 14*(3), 349–353.

Oluwoye, O., Monroe, D. M., Burduli, E., Chwastiak, L., McPherson, S., McClellan, J. M., & McDonell, M. G. (2019). Impact of tobacco, alcohol and cannabis use on treatment outcomes among patients experiencing first episode psychosis: Data from the national RAISE-ETP study. *Early Intervention in Psychiatry, 13*(1), 142–146.

Quigley, H., & MacCabe, J. H. (2019). The relationship between nicotine and psychosis. *Therapeutic Advances in Psychopharmacology, 9*, 1–12. https://doi.org/10.1177/2045125319859969

Regier, D. A., Farmer, M. E., Rae, D. S., Locke, B. Z., Keith, S. J., Judd, L. L., & Goodwin, L. (1990). Comorbidity of mental disorders with alcohol and other drug abuse: Results from the Epidemiologic Catchment Area (ECA) study. *Journal of the American Medical Association, 264*, pp. 2511–2518.

Sara, G. E., Large, M. M., Matheson, S. L., Burgess, P. M., Malhi, G. S., Whiteford, H. A., & Hall, W. D. (2015). Stimulant use disorders in people with psychosis: A meta-analysis of rate and factors affecting variation. *Australian and New Zealand Journal of Psychiatry, 49*(2), 106–117.

Schmitt, A., Hasan, A., Gruber, O., & Falkai, P. (2011). Schizophrenia as a disorder of disconnectivity. *European Archives of Psychiatry and Clinical Neuroscience, 261*(Suppl. 2), S150–S154.

Scott, J. G., Matuschka, L., Niemelä, S., Miettunen, J., Emmerson, B., & Mustonen, A. (2018). Evidence of a causal relationship between smoking tobacco and schizophrenia spectrum disorders. *Frontiers in Psychiatry, 9*. Article 607. https://doi.org/10.3389/fpsyt.2018.00607

Sperry, L., & Sperry, J. (2015). Schizophrenia spectrum and other psychotic disorders. In L. Sperry, J. Carlson, J. D. Sauerheber, & J. Sperry (Eds.), *Psychopathology and psychotherapy: DSM-5 diagnosis, case conceptualization, and treatment.*, 3rd ed. (pp. 177–204). Routledge/Taylor & Francis Group.

Substance Abuse and Mental Health Services Administration. (2019). *Civil Commitment and the Mental Health Care Continuum: Historical Trends and Principles for Law and Practice.* Rockville, MD.

*Substance Abuse and Mental Health Services Administration. (2020). *Substance use disorder treatment for people with co-occurring disorders.* Treatment Improvement Protocol (TIP) Series, No. 42. SAMHSA Publication No. PEP20-02-01-004. Rockville, MD: Substance Abuse and Mental Health Services Administration.

Tai, S., & Turkington, D. (2009). The evolution of cognitive behavior therapy for schizophrenia: Current practice and recent developments. *Schizophrenia Bulletin, 35*(5), 865–873.

*Tandon, R., & Shariff, S.M. (2019). Substance-induced psychotic disorders and schizophrenia: Pathophysiological insights and clinical implications. *The American Journal of Psychiatry, 176*(9), 683–684.

*Tandon, R., Gaebel, W., Barch, D. M., Bustillo, J., Gur, R. E., Heckers, S., Malaspina, D., Owen, M. J., Schultz, S., Tsuang, M., Van Os, J., & Carpenter, W. (2013). Definition and description of schizophrenia in the DSM-5. *Schizophrenia Research, 150*(1), 3–10.

Tarrier N, Haddock G. (2004). Cognitive behavioral therapy for schizophrenia. A case formulation approach. In S.G. Hofmann & M.C. Tompson (Eds). *Treating chronic and severe mental disorders. A handbook of empirically supported interventions* (pp. 69–95). New York, NY: Guilford Press.

Trudeau, K. J., Burtner, J., Villapiano, A. J., Jones, M., Butler, S. F., & Joshi, K. (2018). Burden of schizophrenia or psychosis-related symptoms in adults undergoing substance abuse evaluation. *Journal of Nervous and Mental Disease, 206*(7), 528–536.

*Wearne, T. A., & Cornish, J. L. (2018). A comparison of methamphetamine-induced psychosis and schizophrenia: A review of positive, negative, and cognitive symptomatology. *Frontiers in Psychiatry, 9*.

Westermeyer, J. (2006). Comorbid schizophrenia and substance abuse: A review of epidemiology and course. *American Journal on Addictions, 15*(5), 345–355. https://doi.org/10.1080/10550490600860114

Wobrock, T., Sittinger, H., Behrendt, B., D'Amelio, R., Falkai, P., & Caspari, D. (2007). Comorbid substance abuse and neurocognitive function in recent-onset schizophrenia. *European Archives of Psychiatry and Clinical Neuroscience, 257*(4), 203–210.

World Health Organization (WHO). (1993). *The ICD-10 classification of mental and behavioural disorders.* World Health Organization.

Zaheer, J., Olfson, M., Mallia, E., Lam, J. S. H., de Oliveira, C., Rudoler, D., Carvalho, A. F., Jacob, B. J., Juda, A., & Kurdyak, P. (2020). Predictors of suicide at time of diagnosis in schizophrenia spectrum disorder: A 20-year total population study in Ontario, Canada. *Schizophrenia Research, 222*, 382–388.

CHAPTER 13

CO-OCCURRING TRAUMA- AND STRESSOR-RELATED AND SUBSTANCE USE DISORDERS

ELIZABETH H. SHILLING AND YASMIN GAY

LEARNING OBJECTIVES

After reading this chapter, you will be able to:
- Describe the characteristics of co-occurring posttraumatic stress disorder (PTSD) and substance use disorders (SUDs).
- Explain symptoms that overlap between PTSD and substance use withdrawal and intoxication.
- Discuss ethical and legal concerns relevant to co-occurring PTSD and SUDs.
- Identify common psychological and pharmacological treatments for co-occurring PTSD and SUDs.

INTRODUCTION

Trauma, a phenomenon experienced by many individuals over the course of their lifetime, can occur after a single incident or multiple traumatic events. The literature continues to reflect the keen lasting impact such exposure has on a person mentally, physically, emotionally, socially, spiritually, and, in some cases, financially (Substance Abuse and Mental Health Services Administration [SAMHSA], 2014). Frequently, trauma and substance use co-occur. This chapter presents a brief review of the diagnostic criteria for the major trauma- and stressor-related disorders (TSRD), co-occurrence with substance use disorders (SUDs), screening and assessment tools, common treatment strategies, and legal and ethical considerations. The chapter ends with a case illustration and discussion.

TRAUMA- AND STRESSOR-RELATED DISORDERS: *DSM-5* DIAGNOSTIC CRITERIA AND DESCRIPTION

The TSRD section of the *Diagnostic and Statistical Manual of Mental Disorders, Fifth Edition* (*DSM-5*; American Psychiatric Association [APA], 2013) captures disorders that include exposure to a traumatic or stressful event. The major diagnoses within this section are child-specific attachment-related disorders (i.e., reactive attachment disorder and disinhibited social engagement); posttraumatic stress disorder (PTSD); acute stress disorder; and adjustment disorders. The development and inclusion of the TSRD chapter in the *DSM-5* follows research over the last two decades on the impact of stressful and traumatic events on individuals (APA, 2013). The central component of each TSRD is a traumatic event or stressor. Of the aforementioned diagnoses, PTSD is the only mental health issue widely researched, both individually and as it relates to the co-occurrence with SUDs. As such, this chapter focuses on the co-occurrence of PTSD and SUD. In the next section, we briefly review PTSD, and the corresponding diagnostic criteria, etiology, and differential diagnoses.

POSTTRAUMATIC STRESS DISORDER

PTSD is likely the diagnosis within this category with which readers are most familiar. Developed to describe the experiences of war veterans after the Vietnam War, PTSD was initially included in the third edition of the *DSM* (APA, 1980) and listed as an anxiety disorder in both the third- and fourth-revised editions of the *DSM* (APA, 1980; 2000). The diagnosis underwent substantial changes in the fifth edition. Most notably, the diagnosis was moved into the newly created section which this chapter addresses (APA, 2013). PTSD requires a precipitating traumatic event, either through direct exposure, witnessing trauma to someone else, learning of trauma to a relative or close friend, or experiencing repeated or extreme exposure to traumatic event details (APA, 2013). Examples of traumatic events include threatened or actual physical or sexual violence, war, disasters, terrorist attacks, and accidents (including motor vehicle crashes). PTSD shares symptoms with anxiety disorders, depressive disorders, and affective disorders.

As a brief review, the *DSM-5* (APA, 2013) identifies the major symptom categories for PTSD as: (a) intrusive symptoms, (b) avoidant symptoms, (c) mood and cognition symptoms, and (d) arousal and reaction symptoms. When an individual meets the criteria for the PTSD diagnosis, two specifiers may also apply: with dissociative symptoms (i.e., depersonalization or derealization) and with delayed expression (i.e., symptoms not met until 6 months after event). Children 6 years old and younger can be diagnosed with PTSD using slightly adjusted criteria (see the *DSM-5* for more information). Differential diagnoses include adjustment disorders, acute stress disorder, major depressive disorder, personality disorders, dissociative disorders, conversion disorder, psychotic disorders, and traumatic brain injury.

According to the *DSM-5*, the lifetime prevalence rate of PTSD is 8.7% (APA, 2013). Importantly, the majority of individuals who experience a traumatic event do not develop PTSD. Prevalence rates of PTSD vary based on a number of factors, including gender, cultural background, age, and traumatic event. Higher rates of PTSD cluster in select groups, including adults; women; veterans; people in occupations where the risk of traumatic exposures is high such as emergency medical personnel, police, and firefighters; and survivors of rape, genocide, and captivity (APA, 2013; Dworkin et al., 2018; Goldstein et al., 2016; Kilpatrick et al., 2013; Loignon et al., 2020).

Complex Trauma and Complex PTSD

Though not described in the *DSM-5* (APA, 2013), complex trauma is a term widely accepted to describe multiple traumatic experiences that are typically interpersonal, repetitive or ongoing, include physical attack or threatened harm, occur or begin during childhood/adolescence, and, as a result of these factors, are more likely to result in more severe negative outcomes

(Ford & Courtois, 2020). Complex trauma is frequently synonymous with polyvictimization and is associated with an increased risk for revictimization (Ford & Courtois). The age of onset of traumatic experiences, the duration, and the layering, or cumulative effect on development are thought to have a specific impact on survivors of complex trauma. Often survivors of complex trauma present with additional symptoms, above and beyond posttraumatic symptoms, including the following: symptoms related to development including personality, psychosexual, and identity; interpersonal issues; dissociation; emotion dysregulation; and physical health problems (Figley, 2012). In 1992, Judith Herman proposed a complex PTSD diagnosis that would include all of the symptoms experienced by survivors of complex trauma (Herman, 1992). While not recognized in the *DSM-5* (APA, 2013), complex PTSD (CPTSD) is included as a diagnostic category in the International Classification of Diseases, 11th edition (ICD-11; World Health Organization [WHO], 2018). A diagnosis of CPTSD must meet the PTSD criteria plus three additional criteria related to the trauma that are severe, persistent, and cause significant impairment: (a) problems with affect regulation; (b) feeling worthless, shame, guilt or failure; and (c) challenges with relationships (WHO, 2018).

PREVALENCE, STATISTICS, AND DEMOGRAPHICS

Co-occurring PTSD and SUDs are common. Across various populations, individuals with PTSD are roughly two times more likely to have a SUD (Messman-Moore & Bhuptani, 2017). Substance misuse is also common among those with PTSD and is associated with avoidance, numbing, and hyperarousal symptoms. Understanding and attending to PTSD and SUD comorbidity is imperative: Individuals with co-occurring PTSD-SUD have significantly greater symptoms in both disorders, higher rates of additional comorbid mental health diagnoses, greater functional impairment, higher rates of suicide attempts, and worse treatment outcomes (Blanco et al., 2013; Danovitch, 2016; Debell et al., 2014; Hawn et al., 2020; Messman-Moore & Bhuptani, 2017).

According to Danovitch (2016) there are four models to explain how the relationship between PTSD and SUD develops. These models are:

1. The *self-medication model* posits individuals with PTSD use substances to relieve symptoms and thus are more likely to develop problematic use patterns.

2. The *mutual maintenance model* proposes that both PTSD and SUD affect each other bidirectionally, where aspects of each individual disorder reinforce aspects of the other.

3. The *PTSD susceptibility model* proposes that substance use makes individuals more susceptible to PTSD after traumatic events.

4. The *common factors model* hypothesizes that shared factors contribute to greater risk for both PTSD and substance use.

The self-medication model is the most popular; however, while some empirical evidence is supportive, more rigorous empirical evidence is needed (Hawn et al., 2020).

As evidence for the self-medication model, frequently PTSD appears to develop first, with the onset of the SUD following (Hawn et al., 2020; McCauley et al., 2012). This appears to be at least partially due to the severity of PTSD symptoms. Greater avoidance and arousal PTSD symptoms are common among individuals with co-occurring PTSD and SUD (Messman-Moore & Bhuptani, 2017). Individuals with co-occurring PTSD and SUD are more likely to report a history of child maltreatment, a greater number of trauma and childhood adversities, and a greater number of lifetime physical or sexual assault (McCauley et al., 2012). The next sections review common SUDs that co-occur with PTSD.

ALCOHOL USE DISORDERS

The incidence of comorbid PTSD and alcohol use disorders (AUD) is high (Smith & Cottler, 2018): individuals with PTSD are three times more likely to develop an AUD (Grant et al., 2015). Nationally representative studies have demonstrated that individuals with comorbid PTSD-AUD developed PTSD earlier, were more likely to use substances to relieve symptoms, met more AUD diagnostic criteria, and reported greater difficulty in emotion expression and impulsivity (Blanco et al., 2013). Additionally, individuals with comorbid PTSD-AUD are more likely to have a history of childhood maltreatment, an increased prevalence of another psychiatric disorder, and suicide attempts. Individuals with comorbid PTSD-AUD had higher rates of treatment-seeking for AUD, and higher lifetime use of outpatient mental health services and psychotropic medications (Blanco et al., 2013).

Several factors appear to affect the development and consequences of comorbid PTSD-AUD beyond those that affect the development of other co-occurring PTSD-SUDs. Studies have reported that risk factors for comorbid PTSD-AUD differ based on gender. Among men, emotional abuse in childhood is most substantial (Gilpin & Weiner, 2017). For women, risk factors for the development of comorbid PTSD-AUD include rape facilitated by substances, a belief that drinking reduces distress, history of other traumas, and less education (Gilpin & Weiner, 2017). Additionally, comorbid PTSD-AUD tends to result in increased symptoms of both disorders, worse overall physical and mental health, and poorer recovery prognosis. Recent research has highlighted potential mitigating factors related to comorbid PTSD-AUD. In a meta-analysis of PTSD and alcohol misuse, controlling for depression or depressive symptoms resulted in nonsignificant associations between alcohol misuse and PTSD (Debell et al., 2014).

DRUG USE DISORDERS

PTSD is associated with high rates of comorbid drug use disorders (DUDs), including cannabis use disorder (CUD), opioid use disorder (OUD), and nicotine use disorder (NUD). In a national sample, 22.3% of individuals diagnosed with PTSD had a co-occurring DUD (Pietrzak et al., 2011). In a sample of adult patients admitted to outpatient addiction treatment programs ($n = 573$), rates of co-occurring PTSD and use disorders were as follows: heroin use disorder (9.4%), cocaine use disorder (15.9%), and prescription OUD (20.2%; Saunders et al., 2015).

CANNABIS USE DISORDER

Even after accounting for trauma type and frequency, socioeconomic variables, additional SUDs, and co-occurring anxiety and mood disorders, PTSD is associated with an increased likelihood to use cannabis (Gentes et al., 2016). A complicating factor for co-occurring PTSD and CUD is the use of cannabis to treat PTSD. At the time this chapter was written, of the 38 states (including Washington, D.C. and Guam) that have medical cannabis programs, 29 include PTSD as a qualifying condition and five others allow doctors latitude to recommend medical cannabis for any serious medical condition (Federation of State Medical Boards, 2021; Marijuana Policy Project, 2021). While medical cannabis is supported for the treatment of various medical conditions, including PTSD, scientific reviews have found no evidence that cannabinoids are effective in treating depressive or anxiety-related disorders, including PTSD (Hasin, 2018). In a review of the epidemiology of and associated problems with cannabis use, Hasin (2018) also noted that cannabis use is associated with more severe PTSD symptoms and increased alcohol use, and extended use increases the risk of withdrawal symptoms that mimic those of PTSD symptoms, thus exacerbating the overall symptom presentation.

OPIOID USE DISORDER

There is a high comorbidity between opioid misuse, OUD, and PTSD. In research using national samples, individuals with PTSD report significantly higher rates of misuse of opioids as compared to those without PTSD (Hassan et al., 2017), and individuals who abuse opiates have significantly higher rates of PTSD (Bilevicius et al., 2018). National research identified that when individuals with PTSD are exposed to prescription opioids they are at an increased risk to develop OUD, and that comorbid PTSD and OUD results in significantly worse quality of life (Hassan et al., 2017).

One pathway to comorbid PTSD-OUD is through chronic pain. Researchers report high rates of comorbid chronic pain conditions and PTSD in general and in veteran populations (López-Martínez et al., 2019). In a systematic review of studies of individuals with PTSD and chronic noncancer pain, PTSD was associated with OUD, especially with musculoskeletal pain, digestive pain, and nerve pain (Bilevicius et al., 2018). Comorbid PTSD-OUD results in increased addiction symptoms and severity, mental and physical health issues, pain, suicidality, and worse treatment outcomes (Elman & Borsook, 2019).

NICOTINE USE DISORDER

PTSD is associated with substantially higher rates of reported smoking and heavy smoking across multiple populations (Kalman et al., 2005). Heavy smoking (more than 25 cigarettes/day) is associated with higher numbers of PTSD symptoms, especially avoidance, numbing, and hyperarousal symptoms (Kalman et al., 2005). After controlling for sociodemographic characteristics and additional comorbid psychiatric disorders, individuals with any NUD in the past 12 months were 1.27 times more likely to have PTSD, and those individuals who had a severe NUD were 1.5 times more likely to have PTSD (Chou et al., 2016). Trauma exposure and PTSD appear predictive of increased smoking behaviors, including early onset and heavy smoking, as well as the development of an NUD (Chou et al., 2016; Kalman et al., 2005).

GAMBLING DISORDER

The association of PTSD and gambling disorder (GD) is well-established in the literature. Rates of PTSD in individuals reporting a lifetime diagnosis of GD range from 11% to 15% (Kessler et al., 2008), and rates among treatment-seeking gamblers range from 12% to 29% (Najavits et al., 2011). GD and PTSD are predictive of each other across various populations. Comorbid GD and PTSD are associated with greater depressive and anxiety symptoms, higher incidence of additional SUD symptoms, more severe psychiatric symptoms, increased frequency of suicide attempts, and worse overall outcomes (Najavits et al., 2011). The two disorders share similar symptoms and associated symptoms including impulsiveness, suicidality, dissociation, and comorbidity with additional substance use and mental disorders including personality disorders (Najavits et al., 2011), mood disorders, and anxiety disorders (Ledgerwood & Milosevic, 2015). More specifically, evidence supports pathological dissociation as a potential etiological mechanism for the development of comorbid GD and PTSD (Moore & Grubbs, 2021). Child maltreatment is heavily associated with gambling, and pathological dissociation is common among individuals who report histories of child maltreatment (Carr et al., 2020), problem gambling (Rogier et al., 2021), and PTSD (Kratzer et al., 2018). Initial evidence suggests that pathological dissociation may fully mediate the relationship between childhood maltreatment and PTSD (Kratzer et al., 2018), as well as with childhood maltreatment and problem gambling (Imperatori et al., 2017). Thus, one potential mechanism for the development of comorbidPTSD-GD could be pathological dissociation (Moore & Grubbs, 2021).

ASSESSMENT AND DIAGNOSTIC CONSIDERATIONS

Accurately assessing and diagnosing co-occurring PTSD-SUD can be difficult; therefore, counselors should consider the following as they work with clients. Factors that can affect assessment and diagnosis include the skills necessary to assess for a trauma history effectively and appropriately, individual client factors, overlapping symptomology between substance intoxication and withdrawal and PTSD, differential diagnoses, and additional co-occurring mental health disorders. Additionally, a counselor will only be effective and accurate in the assessment and diagnosis process if they account for client-specific cultural factors from the onset and consider how systems of stigma, oppression, and racism intertwine with the client's experiences.

Assessing and diagnosing individuals with complex co-occurring symptom presentations require a thorough understanding of diagnostic criteria, the impact of trauma on developmental and mental and physical health outcomes, substance use and addiction, and trauma-informed and person-centered therapeutic approaches. In a trauma-informed approach, the counselor will attend to the safety of the client, work diligently to create trust and transparency, empower the client through collaboration and mutuality, and attend to cultural and gender specific issues (Centers for Disease Control and Prevention, 2020). Attention to cultural norms related to trauma, definitions of private information, sharing information with strangers, relationship and sexual violence history, and substance use is of utmost importance when assessing and diagnosing both trauma and substance-related disorders. A trauma-informed approach to assessment and diagnosis will help the counselor create a safe space where there is minimal to no risk for re-traumatization. In order to diagnose PTSD, a counselor does not need a client to recount the entirety of a traumatic event: The only thing necessary to know is that the client was exposed to a precipitating traumatic event. The need for cultural consideration is also important when considering cultural experiences and norms related to substance use. For example, not all cultures consider drinking beer as consuming alcohol: If you ask someone (who drinks beer) if they drink alcohol, they may say "no" because ingesting beer is not considered to be a hard alcohol, liquor, or distilled spirit. Therefore, attending to culturally specific differences in attitudes and understanding of substance use is vitally important.

Specifically related to diagnostic criteria, counselors need to be aware that the diagnostic criteria for PTSD and SUD intoxication and withdrawal symptoms overlap, making the assessment and diagnosis process more challenging. Table 13.1 reviews the overlapping symptoms between the intoxication and withdrawal associated with multiple substances of use and PTSD.

PTSD also shares a number of similar symptoms with panic disorder, generalized anxiety disorder, affective disorders, and mood disorders. Further complicating the process, as previously stated, individuals with comorbid PTSD-SUD are more likely to have additional co-occurring mental health disorders. Counselors will benefit from remembering that some clients will present with complex symptomology; therefore, taking time and care during the screening and assessment process will help ensure accurate and appropriate diagnoses.

TABLE 13.1 **Overlapping PTSD and Substance Use-Related *DSM-5* Symptoms**

SUBSTANCE	INTOXICATION EFFECTS	WITHDRAWAL EFFECTS	OVERLAPPING TSRD SYMPTOMS
Alcohol	Inappropriate sexual or aggressive behavior Mood lability Impairment in memory or attention	Autonomic hyperactivity Insomnia Psychomotor agitation Anxiety	Marked physiologic reactions to trauma-related cues Negative alterations in cognitions and mood: memory deficits Alterations in arousal and reactivity: irritability, anger, aggression, insomnia
Cannabis	Anxiety Dysphoria Social withdrawal	Irritability, anger, aggression Nervousness or anxiety Sleep difficulty Restlessness Depressed mood	Alterations in arousal and reactivity: irritability, anger, aggression, insomnia, problems with concentration Negative alterations in cognitions and mood: negative emotional state
Phencyclidine	Assaultiveness Impulsiveness Psychomotor agitation Hypertension or tachycardia	(No withdrawal effects listed in the *DSM-5*)	Marked physiologic reactions to trauma-related cues Alterations in arousal and reactivity: irritability, anger, aggression, insomnia
Other hallucinogens	Anxiety or depression Depersonalization, derealization Tachycardia Sweating, palpitations	(No withdrawal effects listed in the *DSM-5*)	Negative alterations in cognitions and mood: negative emotional state Depersonalization, derealization Marked physiologic reactions to trauma-related cues
Opioids	Apathy, dysphoria Psychomotor agitation Impairment in memory or attention	Dysphoric mood Insomnia Anxiety Restlessness Irritability	Negative alterations in cognitions and mood: negative emotional state Marked physiologic reactions to trauma-related cues Alterations in arousal and reactivity: irritability, insomnia, problems with concentration
Sedatives, hypnotics, anxiolytics	Impairment in memory or attention Behavioral changes including aggressive behavior Mood lability	Autonomic hyperactivity Insomnia Psychomotor agitation	Marked physiologic reactions to trauma-related cues Negative alterations in cognitions and mood: memory deficits Alterations in arousal and reactivity: irritability, anger, aggression, insomnia

(continued)

TABLE 13.1 **Overlapping PTSD and Substance Use-Related *DSM-5* Symptoms (*Continued*)**

SUBSTANCE	INTOXICATION EFFECTS	WITHDRAWAL EFFECTS	OVERLAPPING TSRD SYMPTOMS
Stimulants	Affective blunting Hypervigilance Anxiety, tension, or anger Social withdrawal Tachycardia Psychomotor agitation	Fatigue Insomnia or hypersomnia Psychomotor agitation Dysphoric mood	Negative alterations in cognitions and mood: negative emotional state, detachment/estrangement from others Alterations in arousal and reactivity: irritability, anger, aggression, hypervigilance, insomnia Marked physiologic reactions to trauma-related cues
Tobacco	(No intoxication effects listed in the *DSM-5*)	Irritability, anger Anxiety Difficulty concentrating Restlessness Depressed mood Insomnia	Alterations in arousal and reactivity: irritability, anger, insomnia, problems with concentration Negative alterations in cognitions and mood: memory deficits, negative emotional state
Caffeine	Restlessness Nervousness Insomnia Psychomotor agitation	Dysphoric or depressed mood, irritability Difficulty concentrating	Alterations in arousal and reactivity: irritability, insomnia, problems with concentration Negative alterations in cognitions and mood: negative emotional state

PTSD, posttraumatic stress disorder; TSRD, trauma- and stressor-related disorders.

SCREENING AND ASSESSMENT TOOLS

Trauma-related disorders and SUDs are highly intertwined and present multifaceted circumstances, as individuals exhibit various symptoms that mimic and mask symptoms of other disorders. While clinicians often inquire about the best practice and utilization of instruments and tools to screen and assess for co-occurring disorders, there is no single gold standard screening or assessment tool for co-occurring disorders (CODs; SAMHSA, 2020). Clinicians utilize a variety of screenings tools, instruments, and assessments to capture the historical attributes, presence of symptoms, problem areas, diagnosis, barriers, and stages of change.

Screening

Screening is often the first contact between an individual and a treatment provider, and, as such, should be a clear and concise process that places a considerable emphasis on maintaining sensitivity to the needs of the individual, as well as the larger contextual issues (Fallot & Harris, 2001). Although there is a high prevalence of predisposing trauma conditions among individuals who concurrently have a SUD (McCauley et al., 2012), employing effective screening measures will help providers identify symptoms that are often unrecognized or unaddressed. Examples of screening measures for substance use include the Alcohol Use Disorders Identification Test (AUDIT; J. B. Saunders et al., 1993) and the Drug Abuse Screening Tool (DAST-10; Skinner, 1982). When screening for PTSD, the

Post Traumatic Stress Disorder Symptom Scale-Self Report (PSS-SR; Foa et al., 1993) is one option. Table 13.2 presents additional screening instruments. While mental health providers utilize a variety of screening instruments and tools to detect elements of trauma and substance use, it is imperative that they screen all clients for co-occurring trauma-related disorders and SUDs (SAMHSA, 2020).

ASSESSMENT

Unlike screening, assessment is an ongoing process that determines the nature and extent of the client's historical context, symptomology, and experiences, and guides the appropriate interventions and level of care. When assessing an individual for co-occurring trauma-related disorders and SUDs, no one singular method is recommended over others. There are various effective assessment modalities to collect the information needed to make an appropriate diagnosis and recommendation for service. Using a combination of methods to obtain information is most effective as each approach and measure has its advantages and disadvantages. Table 13.2 presents screening and assessment instruments used to aid in diagnosis of trauma-related disorders and SUDs.

TABLE 13.2 Select Screening and Assessment Instruments for PTSD, SUD, and Co-Occurring PTSD-SUD

INSTRUMENT/TOOLS	DESCRIPTION OF INSTRUMENT	RELEVANT CITATIONS
TRAUMA-RELATED SCREENERS		
PSS-SR	17-item self-report questionnaire	Foa et al., 1993
The PTSD Checklist for *DSM-5*	20-item self-report tool	Blevins et al., 2015
SUBSTANCE USE SCREENERS		
AUDIT	10-item self-report instrument for past year alcohol use. See also, AUDIT-C, a 3-question version	J. B. Saunders et al., 1993
DAST-10	10-item brief screening tool for past year drug use	Skinner, 1982
MAST	25-item alcohol screener. See also, B-MAST, a 10-item version and MAST-G, a version for older adults	Selzer, 1971
ASSIST	8-item survey to explore use of 9 different drugs	WHO ASSIST Working Group, 2002
COMORBID SCREENERS		
DDSI	Screening instrument used to identify comorbidity among substance users	Mestre-Pintó et al., 2014

(continued)

TABLE 13.2 Select Screening and Assessment Instruments for PTSD, SUD, and Co-Occurring PTSD-SUD (*Continued*)

INSTRUMENT/TOOLS	DESCRIPTION OF INSTRUMENT	RELEVANT CITATIONS
SUBSTANCE USE ASSESSMENTS		
ASI	Comprehensive evaluative tool used to identify substance use	McLellan et al., 1980
SASSI-4	Identifies probability of substance use disorders	Miller, 1985; Lazowski & Geary, 2019
TRAUMA-RELATED ASSESSMENTS		
THQ	24-item self-administered questionnaire that explores traumatic lifetime events	Hooper et al., 2011
TAA	17-item self-report trauma assessment that explores stressful life events	Gray et al., 2009

ASI, Addiction Severity Index; ASSIST, Alcohol Smoking and Substance Involvement; AUDIT, Alcohol Use Disorders Identification Test; DAST-10, Drug Abuse Screening Tool; DDSI, Dual Diagnosis Screening Interview; MAST Michigan Alcoholism Screening Test; PSS-SR, Post Traumatic Stress Disorder Symptom Scale-Self Report; PTSD, posttraumatic stress disorder; SASSI-4, Substance Abuse Subtle Screening Inventory; SUD, substance use disorder; TAA, Trauma Assessment for Adults; THQ, Trauma History Questionnaire.

Screening and assessment are critical components when working with individuals who may have co-occurring PTSD-SUD. As established earlier, co-occurring PTSD-SUD will likely result in a more complicated clinical picture; thus, attention to identifying the presence of this co-occurring disorder is the first crucial step to ensuring appropriate and successful treatment. While there is no single recommended method for identifying co-occurring PTSD-SUD through screening and assessment measures, using a combination of approaches is often warranted. Utilizing a trauma-informed approach to the screening and assessment process, with attention to safety, collaboration, empowerment, and cultural factors, will help providers better identify and treat individuals with CODs in a manner that is timely, effective, and tailored to all of their needs (SAMHSA, 2020).

TREATMENT MODALITIES

Despite the high prevalence and correlation between substance use and trauma-related disorders, the development and study of integrated treatment approaches have been slow. Historical approaches to treatment have been a barrier to integrated treatment. The substance use treatment community traditionally defers treatment of trauma-related issues fearing that addressing such would lead to relapse, while providers specializing in trauma view clients with SUDs as too complex or fragile for trauma-focused interventions. Given the complexity and substantial symptomology present in individuals with co-occurring PTSD-SUD, concurrently treating both is necessary for the best possible outcomes. As with screening and assessment, there is no standard method, technique, or treatment intervention for treating individuals with co-occurring substance use and trauma-related disorders. Appropriate and effective treatment interventions may include psychotherapeutic and pharmacotherapeutic treatment, along with other measures such as mutual support groups, while attending to the co-occurrence of both disorders.

PSYCHOTHERAPEUTIC TREATMENT

Both individual and group therapy are appropriate and helpful for co-occurring trauma disorders, stressor-related disorders, and SUDs. As research continues to provide more insight and direction, evidence has emerged for integrated treatment using psychotherapy modalities including cognitive behavioral approaches, eye movement desensitization and reprocessing (EMDR), trauma-focused behavioral interventions, and mindfulness-based interventions. In this section, we focus on various evidence-based psychotherapy treatments appropriate for co-occurring trauma-related disorders and SUDs organized into nonexposure-based treatments and exposure-based treatments.

COGNITIVE BEHAVIORAL THERAPIES

Cognitive behavioral therapy (CBT) is a widely accepted and evidence-based approach to treating substance use and trauma-related disorders (Rawson et al., 2002; Roberts et al., 2010). CBT can be applied as a standalone approach or integrated with other modalities to treat the symptoms and needs of the client, and can be used in individual and group settings. CBT approaches for co-occurring PTSD-SUD include exposure-integrated treatments and nonexposure-integrated treatments.

Exposure-Based Cognitive Behavioral Therapy Treatments of Co-Occurring PTSD and Substance Use Disorders

Great debate has existed over the last few decades about the appropriateness of exposure-based (also referred to as trauma-focused) therapeutic interventions for CODs, which is primarily based on the concern that trauma-focused treatments would cause worsening substance use. Several large reviews of clinical trials of the treatment of co-occurring PTSD and SUD have demonstrated that exposure-based/trauma-focused behavioral and pharmacological interventions are more effective than interventions that are not trauma-focused (Petrakis & Simpson, 2017; Simpson et al., 2017).

One of the more widely researched integrated exposure-based treatments is Concurrent Treatment of PTSD and Substance Use Disorders Using Prolonged Exposure (COPE; Back et al., 2014); Killeen et al., 2011; Mills et al., 2012). COPE is a manualized CBT that combines two highly efficacious therapies: prolonged exposure therapy and relapse prevention for SUD (Back et al., 2014). The COPE treatment consists of twelve 90-minute therapy sessions utilizing CBT and motivational enhancement for both PTSD and SUD: Sessions 1 to 3 set up the treatment process, describe trauma processes and substance use craving, and introduce in vivo exposure (direct exposure to the feared situation) homework. Sessions 4 to 11 include a review of the in vivo exposure homework, and sessions 6 to 11 additionally integrate imaginal exposure (thoroughly imagining and describing the feared situation) practice after the homework review. The focus of the last session, session 12, is reviewing treatment as well as developing after-care plans upon conclusion of services.

Eye Movement Desensitization and Reprocessing

Another example of an exposure-based treatment for co-occurring PTSD-SUD is EMDR (Shapiro, 1989). This specialized form of psychotherapy was developed to treat traumatic memories and associated symptoms of stress using bilateral brain stimulation. Standard EMDR involves asking clients to recall a traumatic event and then focus simultaneously on visual images, negative beliefs, bodily sensations, and emotional responses that are associated with the traumatic memory. This treatment approach has been explored, utilized, and examined extensively. In fact, according to the World Health Organization (WHO, 2013) EMDR is the psychotherapy approach of choice in the treatment of PTSD for children, teenagers, and adults. Several addiction-specific EMDR protocols targeting addiction memory related to craving, triggers, and negative beliefs have been shown to be efficacious in reducing substance use (Kullack & Laugharne, 2016). Furthermore, integrating EMDR with other forms of treatment, including *Seeking Safety*, has shown to be effective in treating co-occurring PTSD-SUD (Brown et al., 2016).

Although EMDR is highly efficacious in treating PTSD and found efficacious in treating addiction specifically, clinicians have been wary of integrating EMDR in the treatment of co-occurring PTSD-SUD. The initial stages of EMDR treatment can cause strong emotional responses from clients that may temporarily result in a greater risk for return to use. Recommendations for using EMDR to treat co-occurring PTSD-SUD include the following: (a) being an experienced addiction and trauma provider or being supervised by an experienced provider; (b) beginning EMDR treatment only after the client has maintained at least 30 days of sobriety; (c) providing extensive education to the client and their support system about trauma and addiction; and (d) attending thoughtfully to safety, support and resources for clients throughout all phases of treatment, but especially in the preparation and initial phases (Brown et al., 2016).

Nonexposure-Based Cognitive Behavioral Therapy Treatments of Co-Occurring PTSD and Substance Use Disorders

An example of a nonexposure-integrated treatment is *Seeking Safety* (Najavits, 2002). Developed by Dr. Lisa Najavits, *Seeking Safety* is a manualized, evidence-based treatment approach designed to explore the connection between the comorbidity of substance use and trauma without going into past memories. It is one of the most widely recognized and studied nonexposure-based treatments for co-occurring PTSD-SUD and consists of an average of twenty-five 60- to 90-minute sessions covering a wide variety of topics such as decreasing risky behaviors, setting boundaries, and coping with substance triggers. *Seeking Safety* offers clients the opportunity to learn more about themselves through the means of psychoeducation, development, and implementation of safe coping skills, and support. This approach can be integrated into both individual and/or group psychotherapy.

Mindfulness-Based Approaches

Mindfulness is a present-centered approach that can be defined as the capacity to maintain nonjudgmental awareness, openness, and acceptance of current experiences, including mental states and aspects of the external world (Boyd et al., 2018). Mindfulness-based interventions include the following: (a) dialectical behavior therapy (DBT; Linehan, 2015); (b) mindfulness-based stress reduction (MBSR; Kabat-Zinn, 2013); (c) mindfulness-based cognitive therapy (MBCT; Segal et al., 2013); (d) acceptance and commitment therapy (ACT; Hayes et al., 2012); and (e) mindfulness-based relapse prevention for addictive behaviors (MBRP; Bowen et al., 2021). Often, mindfulness interventions occur mostly in group settings, as the focus is on the development of skill rather than individual's psychological symptoms (Baer, 2003). The practice of mindfulness is efficacious in significantly reducing a variety of psychological symptoms, including those associated with co-occurring PTSD-SUD (Briere & Scott, 2015). Researchers have found that mindfulness is a significant mediating factor in the relationship between symptoms of PTSD and severity of substance dependence (Bowen et al., 2017). A mindfulness approach, with a focus on acceptance and nonjudgmental support, fosters the individual's ability to become more attuned with their present experience and to learn ways they can break the cyclical pattern of symptoms associated with PTSD-SUD.

PHARMACOTHERAPEUTIC TREATMENT

As previously indicated, individuals with co-occurring PTSD-SUD display a range of symptoms and experiences that may require multiple interventions, including pharmacotherapies. Medications can be helpful in multiple ways: They can provide relief for the intense emotional distress experienced by individuals with comorbid conditions, and they can help mitigate withdrawal symptoms and cravings that may hinder the treatment process. Despite the regular use of evidence-based medications to treat PTSD and available evidence-based medications to treat SUD, few studies have investigated medications to treat the co-occurrence of the two. This section briefly reviews evidence-based pharmacotherapies available for the treatment of PTSD, SUD, and co-occurring PTSD-SUD.

To date, a number of evidence-based medication treatments exist for PTSD. Selective serotonin reuptake inhibitors (SSRIs) are considered a first-line medication treatment for PTSD, with sertraline (Zoloft) and paroxetine (Paxil) being the only medications approved by the Food and Drug Administration (FDA) for this purpose (Briere & Scott, 2015). The efficacy of SSRIs for the treatment of PTSD is somewhat limited, however, and little research has looked at the efficacy of SSRIs with co-occurring PTSD-SUD (Verplaetse et al., 2018). An additional medication that has shown promise in the treatment of PTSD is prazosin (Minipress). And while some hypothesize that prazosin may also work well in treating SUD and co-occurring issues, more research is needed to determine its efficacy.

Naltrexone and disulfiram are the only two FDA-approved medications for the treatment of AUD. Both are effective in reducing alcohol use in individuals with co-occurring PTSD-AUD, while disulfiram appears to also reduce PTSD symptoms (Shorter et al., 2015). One concern about naltrexone is medication adherence. The once monthly injectable version of naltrexone (Vivitrol) can help increase medication adherence. Three medications—methadone, naltrexone, and buprenorphine—are FDA approved for the treatment of OUD. Emerging retrospective research suggests that buprenorphine helps reduce PTSD symptoms in veterans with PTSD and chronic pain, potentially above and beyond SSRIs, and that the combination of buprenorphine and naltrexone is especially effective (Madison & Eitan, 2020). There are no FDA-approved medications for CUD and few studies have investigated medications for CUD or co-occurring PTSD-CUD. Limited pre-clinical and small clinical studies have identified potential promise in medications including buspirone, fluoxetine, lithium, and lofexidine, but more research is critical (Shorter et al., 2015).

Currently, there are no contraindications for combining FDA-approved medications for PTSD and SUD as treatment for co-occurring PTSD-SUD (Shorter et al., 2015). Additionally, pre-clinical animal studies have demonstrated that a number of medications may be helpful in treating co-occurring PTSD-SUD, with some clinical trials showing promising support as well (Shorter et al., 2015; Verplaetse et al., 2018). More research is needed to identify appropriate pharmacotherapies for co-occurring PTSD-SUD. While the development of pharmacotherapies is crucial, the combination with psychotherapy is an effective course of treatment in relieving distressing symptoms and improving functioning among individuals with co-occurring PTSD-SUD.

LEGAL AND ETHICAL CONSIDERATIONS

Legal and ethical issues can arise at any point during the therapeutic process and are not unique to co-occurring PTSD-SUD; however, clinicians need to be thoughtful about several specific areas when working with individuals with co-occurring PTSD-SUD. These considerations include duty to report, boundaries, privacy and confidentiality, scope of practice, and treating minors. Providers need to be aware that disclosure of abuse may occur during screening and assessment and need to be prepared to respond appropriately based on legal and ethical guidelines.

Additionally, traumatic experiences often result in trust issues and safety-related concerns for clients. As such, establishing appropriate boundaries and transparently sharing these with clients with co-occurring PTSD-SUD is an essential component of developing and maintaining a trusting, safe therapeutic relationship. Breeches of confidentiality, inappropriate conduct, and other violations of trust can further harm individuals who already have histories of trauma (SAMHSA, 2014). As evident, the treatment requirements for individuals with co-occurring PTSD-SUD are significant and a counselor should consider whether this treatment is within their scope of practice and refer out if it is not.

The final major legal and ethical area to consider is providing therapeutic services to minors. When working with minors, clinicians have to balance the responsibility to parent/guardians and the trust and relationship with the minor. Some states permit minors to consent to SUD treatment without parental consent, which can cause various issues. This may present a challenge if, for example, the provider learns during the course of substance use treatment that there is co-occurring PTSD and compounding traumatic experiences that involve the parent and/or guardian.

CLINICAL CASE ILLUSTRATION AND DISCUSSION

CASE OF KRYSTAL

Krystal, a 38-year-old, bisexual Black woman, lives with her partner in an urban area where she works as a real estate agent. She was admitted to the local hospital for burn injuries to over 19% of her body after falling into an outdoor fire pit during a party. She was admitted with a high blood alcohol level of 0.21, consistent with roughly six standard-sized alcoholic beverages in the previous hour. Her resulting injuries are substantial and require weeks of inpatient hospital treatment. In addition to the medical providers, her hospital treatment team includes a dually licensed clinical mental health counselor and addiction specialist.

Initially, Krystal is unable to participate in therapy due to the severity of her injuries. The counselor, however, is able to identify the potential risk for alcohol withdrawal and recommends to the treatment team that Krystal be placed on an alcohol withdrawal monitoring protocol, such as the Clinical Institute Withdrawal Assessment Alcohol Scale Revised (CIWA-AR), to ensure that she receives an appropriate assessment. Krystal begins to experience withdrawal symptoms during the first 3 days of her hospitalization, including nausea, sweating, psychomotor agitation, increased hand tremor, and anxiety—all of which further complicate her treatment. The medical team utilizes the medication gabapentin (Neurontin) to treat Krystal's withdrawal symptoms.

The counselor is able to initiate rapport building and initial support during the second week of Krystal's admission. Utilizing a trauma-informed approach, the counselor considers cultural factors that may impact Krystal's experience in the hospital and her view of counselors and the medical team. During the rapport building and initial support sessions, the counselor learns that

Krystal has a history of trauma and substantial alcohol use that began in her teens. After the treatment team determines that Krystal is more stable and better able to cope with pain, the counselor conducts a more detailed evaluation that includes administering the AUDIT and the PTSD Checklist.

Krystal reports consuming about one to two standard-sized bottles of wine (i.e., 750 mL) every day for at least the past year. And, at times, she drinks even more when attending a party or after experiencing particularly stressful conflicts with family members. After completing a comprehensive assessment, her counselor determines that Krystal meets the following *DSM-5* diagnostic criteria for AUD-moderate:

1. Persistent or unsuccessful efforts to cut down or control alcohol use;
2. Craving;
3. Recurrent use resulting in a failure to fulfill major role obligations at work, school, or home;
4. Recurrent alcohol use in situations in which it is physically hazardous; and
5. Withdrawal.

In addition to her progressive and problematic use of alcohol, Krystal shares that she witnessed the death of her mother in a motor vehicle crash 2 years ago. Upon further examination, Krystal reported experiencing symptoms that are congruent with a diagnosis of PTSD:

1. Distressing memories and dreams,
2. Dissociation,
3. Efforts to avoid distressing memories,
4. Persistent negative beliefs about the world,
5. Feelings of shame,
6. Irritability, and
7. Problems sleeping.

Based on the results of the additional assessments and the information the counselor learned in the rapport-building sessions, it is clear that Krystal meets the criteria for co-occurring PTSD and AUD-moderate. The counselor develops a treatment plan which addresses treatment while Krystal remains in the hospital and plans for treatment after discharge. During Krystal's remaining weeks of hospitalization, the counselor focuses on introducing and practicing CBT skills for coping with pain, stress, and cravings. Additionally, the counselor introduces medications as a treatment option and Krystal agrees that they would be helpful. After consultation with her medical team, her physician prescribes prazosin (Minipress) and naltrexone.

CASE DISCUSSION

Important considerations for initial steps in Krystal's counseling include alcohol withdrawal, the traumatic nature of burn injuries and an associated risk for the development of PTSD, the hospital treatment required for burn injuries, and awareness that historical racism in the medical field may result in treatment disparities for Krystal. The counselor takes note of the potential for Krystal to have issues trusting the medical team because of historical racism in the medical field toward Black Americans, as well as the need to attend to the potential for a trauma history outside of the burn accident. As a result, the counselor carefully attends to issues of safety, trust, and empowerment with Krystal, in addition to assessing for acute stress symptoms. Black Americans are more likely to have their pain under-recognized and under-treated, to experience less effective medical treatment, and to receive generally poorer quality of healthcare (Smedley et al., 2003). Cultural factors may also affect how an individual conceptualizes alcohol and drinking, so the counselor attends to the screening and assessment process carefully to ensure Krystal's description of her drinking patterns and history is clearly understood.

Krystal's injuries pose a unique challenge for treatment after her hospital discharge. The severity of her injuries and the healing process are additional stressors that can lead to substantial isolation, negatively affect the treatment process, and exclude Krystal from intensive outpatient mental health treatment while she heals. These unique factors, plus the complexity of a co-occurring PTSD-AUD diagnosis, lead the counselor to recommend continued psychopharmacologic treatment; involvement in support groups for AUD, burn injuries, and trauma; involvement of supportive family; and outpatient sessions with the hospital counselor. Krystal agrees that, given her injuries and the stress associated with them, a combination of outpatient counseling, support groups, family support, and medication is the best solution for her as she heals. Upon discharge, the counselor uses a combination of the *Seeking Safety* treatment protocol and mindfulness-based approaches with Krystal. The counselor and Krystal also acknowledge that ongoing assessment is critical for Krystal and, that once she is physically stable enough, a higher level of care may be necessary.

CHAPTER SUMMARY

One of the new chapters in the *DSM-5* (APA, 2013), TSRD, includes several diagnoses related to traumatic or stressful events. Of these, PTSD is the most critical as it relates to co-occurring TSRD and SUDs. PTSD is more likely to co-occur with SUDs and the resultant clinical presentation is complex. Individuals with co-occurring PTSD-SUD have an increased risk of developing more severe PTSD and SUD symptoms, experiencing higher rates of suicidality, and encountering additional co-occurring mental health issues. Important considerations for screening and assessment are integrating a trauma-informed and person-centered approach that takes into account important individual factors like culture, recognizing the substance intoxication and withdrawal symptoms that overlap with PTSD symptoms, and attending to potential differential diagnoses. Several screening and assessment tools can assist a counselor in making a diagnosis, and often the biopsychosocial assessment is an effective approach alone. Treatment of co-occurring PTSD-SUD is complex, and counselors should either be skilled at both addiction and trauma treatment or be supervised by a skilled clinician in both of these areas. Treatment approaches include CBT-based exposure and nonexposure treatments, EMDR, and mindfulness-based approaches. In addition to scope or practice concerns, counselors need to be aware of issues related to duty to report, boundaries, privacy and confidentiality, and treating minors.

DISCUSSION QUESTIONS

1. Considering what you read, what could be changed to improve therapeutic outcomes for individuals with co-occurring PTSD and SUDs?

2. What role should counselors play in advocating for advancements in pharmacotherapeutic treatments for co-occurring PTSD and SUDs?
3. How does stigma toward addiction and mental health issues effect the development and use of evidence-based treatments?
4. What cultural and ethnic considerations need to be accounted for when assessing for and treating co-occurring PTSD and SUDs?

REFERENCES

American Psychiatric Association. (1980). *Diagnostic and statistical manual of mental disorders* (Third edition). American Psychiatric Association.

American Psychiatric Association. (2000). *Diagnostic and statistical manual of mental disorders: DSM-IV-TR.* (4th ed., text revision.). American Psychiatric Association.

American Psychiatric Association. (2013). *Diagnostic and statistical manual of mental disorders* (5th ed.). https://doi.org/10.1176/appi.books.9780890425596

Back, S. E., Foa, E. B., Killeen, T. K., Mills, K. L., Teesson, M., Cotton, B. D., Carroll, K. M., & Brady, K. T. (2014). *Concurrent treatment of PTSD and substance use disorders using prolonged exposure (COPE): Therapist Guide.* Oxford University Press, Incorporated.

Baer, R. A. (2003). Mindfulness training as a clinical intervention: A conceptual and empirical review. *Clinical Psychology: Science and Practice, 10*(2), 125–143. https://doi.org/10.1093/clipsy.bpg015

Bilevicius, E., Sommer, J. L., Asmundson, G. J. G., & El-Gabalawy, R. (2018). Posttraumatic stress disorder and chronic pain are associated with opioid use disorder: Results from a 2012-2013 American nationally representative survey. *Drug and Alcohol Dependence, 188,* 119–125. https://doi.org/10.1016/j.drugalcdep.2018.04.005

Blanco, C., Xu, Y., Brady, K., Pérez-Fuentes, G., Okuda, M., & Wang, S. (2013). Comorbidity of posttraumatic stress disorder with alcohol dependence among US adults: Results from national epidemiological survey on alcohol and related conditions. *Drug and Alcohol Dependence, 132*(3), 630–638. https://doi.org/10.1016/j.drugalcdep.2013.04.016

Blevins, C. A., Weathers, F. W., Davis, M. T., Witte, T. K., & Domino, J. L. (2015). The posttraumatic stress disorder checklist for DSM-5 (PCL-5): Development and initial psychometric evaluation. *Journal of Traumatic Stress, 28*(6), 489–498. https://doi.org/10.1002/jts.22059

Bowen, S., Chawla, N., Grow, J., & Marlatt, G. A., (2021). *Mindfulness-based relapse prevention for addictive behaviors: A clinician's guide* (2nd ed.). The Guilford Press.

Bowen, S., De Boer, D., & Bergman, A. L. (2017). The role of mindfulness as approach-based coping in the PTSD-substance abuse cycle. *Addictive Behaviors, 64,* 212–216. https://doi.org/10.1016/j.addbeh.2016.08.043

Boyd, J. E., Lanius, R. A., & McKinnon, M. C. (2018). Mindfulness-based treatments for posttraumatic stress disorder: A review of the treatment literature and neurobiological evidence. *Journal of Psychiatry & Neuroscience, 43*(1), 7–25. https://doi.org/10.1503/jpn.170021

Briere, J. N., & Scott, C. (2015). *Principles of trauma therapy: A guide to symptoms, evaluation, and treatment, 2nd ed., DSM-5 update* (pp. ix, 428). Sage Publications, Inc.

Brown, S., Stowasser, J., & Shapiro, F. (2016). *EMDR Therapy and the Treatment of Substance Abuse and Addiction.* 69–100. https://doi.org/10.1007/978-3-319-43172-7_5

Carr, A., Duff, H., & Craddock, F. (2020). A systematic review of reviews of the outcome of noninstitutional child maltreatment. *Trauma, Violence & Abuse, 21*(4), 828–843. https://doi.org/10.1177/1524838018801334

Centers for Disease Control and Prevention. (2020). *6 guiding principles to a trauma-informed approach.* Infographic: 6 Guiding Principles to a Trauma-Informed Approach. https://www.cdc.gov/cpr/infographics/6_principles_trauma_info.htm

Chou, S. P., Goldstein, R. B., Smith, S. M., Huang, B., Ruan, W. J., Zhang, H., Jung, J., Saha, T. D., Pickering, R. P., & Grant, B. F. (2016). The epidemiology of *DSM-5* nicotine use disorder: Results from the national epidemiologic survey on alcohol and related conditions-III. *The Journal of Clinical Psychiatry, 77*(10), 1404–1412. https://doi.org/10.4088/JCP.15m10114

Danovitch, I. (2016). Post-traumatic stress disorder and opioid use disorder: A narrative review of conceptual models. *Journal of Addictive Diseases, 35*(3), 169–179. https://doi.org/10.1080/10550887.2016.1168212

Debell, F., Fear, N. T., Head, M., Batt-Rawden, S., Greenberg, N., Wessely, S., & Goodwin, L. (2014). A systematic review of the comorbidity between PTSD and alcohol misuse. *Social Psychiatry and Psychiatric Epidemiology, 49*(9), 1401–1425. https://doi.org/10.1007/s00127-014-0855-7

Dworkin, E. R., Bergman, H. E., Walton, T. O., Walker, D. D., & Kaysen, D. L. (2018). Co-occurring post-traumatic stress disorder and alcohol use disorder in U.S. military and veteran populations. *Alcohol Research, 39*(2), E1–E9. eLibrary; ProQuest Central.

Elman, I., & Borsook, D. (2019). The failing cascade: Comorbid post traumatic stress- and opioid use disorders. *Neuroscience & Biobehavioral Reviews, 103*, 374–383. https://doi.org/10.1016/j.neubiorev.2019.04.023

Fallot, R. D., & Harris, M. (2001). A trauma-informed approach to screening and assessment. *New Directions for Mental Health Services, 2001*(89), 23–31. https://doi.org/10.1002/yd.23320018904

Federation of State Medical Boards. (April, 2021). *Medical marijuana state-by-state overview*. https://www.fsmb.org/siteassets/advocacy/key-issues/medical-marijuana-requirements-by-state.pdf

Figley, C. R. (2012). *Encyclopedia of trauma an interdisciplinary guide*. SAGE.

Foa, E. B., Riggs, D. S., Dancu, C. V., & Rothbaum, B. O. (1993). Reliability and validity of a brief instrument for assessing post-traumatic stress disorder. *Journal of Traumatic Stress, 6*(4), 459–473. https://doi.org/10.1002/jts.2490060405

Ford, J. D., & Courtois, C. A. (2020). *Treating complex traumatic stress disorders in adults: Scientific foundations and therapeutic models* (2nd ed.). Guilford Press.

Gentes, E. L., Schry, A. R., Hicks, T. A., Clancy, C. P., Collie, C. F., Kirby, A. C., Dennis, M. F., Hertzberg, M. A., Beckham, J. C., & Calhoun, P. S. (2016). Prevalence and correlates of cannabis use in an outpatient VA posttraumatic stress disorder clinic. *Psychology of Addictive Behaviors, 30*(3), 415–421. https://doi.org/10.1037/adb0000154

Gilpin, N. W., & Weiner, J. L. (2017). Neurobiology of comorbid post-traumatic stress disorder and alcohol-use disorder: Neurobiology of comorbid PTSD and AUD. *Genes, Brain and Behavior, 16*(1), 15–43. https://doi.org/10.1111/gbb.12349

Goldstein, R. B., Smith, S. M., Chou, S. P., Saha, T. D., Jung, J., Zhang, H., Pickering, R. P., Ruan, W. J., Huang, B., & Grant, B. F. (2016). The epidemiology of *DSM-5* posttraumatic stress disorder in the United States: Results from the national epidemiologic survey on alcohol and related conditions-III. *Social Psychiatry and Psychiatric Epidemiology, 51*(8), 1137–1148. https://doi.org/10.1007/s00127-016-1208-5

Grant, B. F., Goldstein, R. B., Saha, T. D., Chou, S. P., Jung, J., Zhang, H., Pickering, R. P., Ruan, W. J., Smith, S. M., Huang, B., & Hasin, D. S. (2015). Epidemiology of *DSM-5* alcohol use disorder: Results from the national epidemiologic survey on alcohol and related conditions III. *JAMA Psychiatry, 72*(8), 757–766. https://doi.org/10.1001/jamapsychiatry.2015.0584

Gray, M. J., Elhai, J. D., Owen, J. R., & Monroe, R. (2009). Psychometric properties of the Trauma Assessment for Adults. *Depression and Anxiety, 26*(2), 190–195. https://doi.org/10.1002/da.20535

Hasin, D. S. (2018). US epidemiology of cannabis use and associated problems. *Neuropsychopharmacology: Official Publication of the American College of Neuropsychopharmacology, 43*(1), 195–212. PubMed. https://doi.org/10.1038/npp.2017.198

Hassan, A. N., Le Foll, B., Imtiaz, S., & Rehm, J. (2017). The effect of post-traumatic stress disorder on the risk of developing prescription opioid use disorder: Results from the national epidemiologic survey on alcohol and related conditions III. *Drug and Alcohol Dependence, 179*, 260–266. https://doi.org/10.1016/j.drugalcdep.2017.07.012

Hawn, S. E., Cusack, S. E., & Amstadter, A. B. (2020). A systematic review of the self-medication hypothesis in the context of posttraumatic stress disorder and comorbid problematic alcohol use. *Journal of Traumatic Stress, 33*(5), 699–708. https://doi.org/10.1002/jts.22521

Hayes, S. C., Strosahl, K. D., & Wilson, K. G. (2012). *Acceptance and commitment therapy: The process and practice of mindful change* (2nd ed). The Guilford Press.

Herman, J. L. (1992). Complex PTSD: A syndrome in survivors of prolonged and repeated trauma. *Journal of Traumatic Stress, 5*(3), 377–391. https://doi.org/10.1007/BF00977235

Hooper, L. M., Stockton, P., Krupnick, J. L., & Green, B. L. (2011). Development, use, and psychometric properties of the trauma history questionnaire. *Journal of Loss & Trauma, 16*(3), 258–283. https://doi.org/10.1080/15325024.2011.572035

Imperatori, C., Innamorati, M., Bersani, F. S., Imbimbo, F., Pompili, M., Contardi, A., & Farina, B. (2017). The association among childhood trauma, pathological dissociation and gambling severity in casino gamblers. *Clinical Psychology & Psychotherapy, 24*(1), 203–211. Academic Search Premier.

Kabat-Zinn, J. (2013). *Full catastrophe living: Using the wisdom of your body and mind to face stress, pain, and illness* (2nd ed.). Random House.

Kalman, D., Morissette, S. B., & George, T. P. (2005). Co-morbidity of smoking in patients with psychiatric and substance use disorders. *The American Journal on Addictions, 14*(2), 106–123. https://doi.org/10.1080/10550490590924728

Kessler, R. C., Hwang, I., LaBrie, R., Petukhova, M., Sampson, N. A., Winters, K. C., & Shaffer, H. J. (2008). DSM-IV pathological gambling in the national comorbidity survey replication. *Psychological Medicine, 38*(9), 1351–1360. Cambridge Core. https://doi.org/10.1017/S0033291708002900

Killeen, T. K., Back, S. E., & Brady, K. T. (2011). The use of exposure-based treatment among individuals with PTSD and co-occurring substance use disorders: Clinical considerations. *Journal of Dual Diagnosis, 7*(4), 194–206. PubMed. https://doi.org/10.1080/15504263.2011.620421

Kilpatrick, D. G., Resnick, H. S., Milanak, M. E., Miller, M. W., Keyes, K. M., & Friedman, M. J. (2013). National estimates of exposure to traumatic events and PTSD prevalence using *DSM-IV* and *DSM-5* criteria. *Journal of Traumatic Stress, 26*(5), 537–547. https://doi.org/10.1002/jts.21848

Kratzer, L., Heinz, P., Pfitzer, F., Padberg, F., Jobst, A., & Schennach, R. (2018). Mindfulness and pathological dissociation fully mediate the association of childhood abuse and PTSD symptomatology. *European Journal of Trauma & Dissociation, 2*(1), 5–10. https://doi.org/10.1016/j.ejtd.2017.06.004

Kullack, C., & Laugharne, J. (2016). Standard EMDR protocol for alcohol and substance dependence comorbid with posttraumatic stress disorder: Four cases with 12-month follow-up. *Journal of EMDR Practice and Research, 10*(1), 33–46. ProQuest Central. https://doi.org/10.1891/1933-3196.10.1.33

Lazowski, L. E., & Geary, B. B. (2019). Validation of the Adult Substance Abuse Subtle Screening Inventory-4 (SASSI-4). *European Journal of Psychological Assessment: Official Organ of the European Association of Psychological Assessment, 35*(1), 86–97. https://doi.org/10.1027/1015-5759/a000359

Ledgerwood, D. M., & Milosevic, A. (2015). Clinical and personality characteristics associated with post traumatic stress disorder in problem and pathological gamblers recruited from the community. *Journal of Gambling Studies, 31*(2), 501–512. https://doi.org/10.1007/s10899-013-9426-1

Linehan, M. (2015). *DBT skills training manual* (2nd ed.). The Guilford Press.

Loignon, A., Ouellet, M.-C., & Belleville, G. (2020). A systematic review and meta-analysis on PTSD following TBI among military/veteran and civilian populations. *The Journal of Head Trauma Rehabilitation, 35*(1), E21–E35. https://doi.org/10.1097/HTR.0000000000000514

López-Martínez, A. E., Reyes-Pérez, Á., Serrano-Ibáñez, E. R., Esteve, R., & Ramírez-Maestre, C. (2019). Chronic pain, posttraumatic stress disorder, and opioid intake: A systematic review. *World Journal of Clinical Cases, 7*(24), 4254–4269. PubMed. https://doi.org/10.12998/wjcc.v7.i24.4254

Madison, C. A., & Eitan, S. (2020). Buprenorphine: Prospective novel therapy for depression and PTSD. *Psychological Medicine, 50*(6), 881–893. Applied Social Sciences Index & Abstracts (ASSIA); ProQuest Central. https://doi.org/10.1017/S0033291720000525

Marijuana Policy Project. (May 27, 2021). PTSD and medical cannabis programs. https://www.mpp.org/issues/medical-marijuana/ptsd-medical-cannabis-programs/

McCauley, J. L., Killeen, T., Gros, D. F., Brady, K. T., & Back, S. E. (2012). Posttraumatic stress disorder and co-occurring substance use disorders: Advances in assessment and treatment. *Clinical Psychology: Science and Practice, 19*(3), 283–304. https://doi.org/10.1111/cpsp.12006

McLellan, A. T., Luborsky, L., O'Brien, C. P., & Woody, G. E. (1980). An improved diagnostic instrument for substance abuse patients: The Addiction Severity Index. *Journal of Nervous & Mental Diseases, 168*, 26–33.

Messman-Moore, T. L., & Bhuptani, P. H. (2017). A review of the long-term impact of child maltreatment on posttraumatic stress disorder and its comorbidities: An emotion dysregulation perspective. *Clinical Psychology: Science and Practice, 24*(2), 154–169. https://doi.org/10.1111/cpsp.12193

Mestre-Pintó, J. I., Domingo-Salvany, A., Martín-Santos, R., Torrens, M., & PsyCoBarcelona Group. (2014). Dual diagnosis screening interview to identify psychiatric comorbidity in substance users: Development and validation of a brief instrument. *European Addiction Research*, *20*(1), 41–48. https://doi.org/10.1159/000351519

Miller, G. A. (1985). *The Substance Abuse Subtle Screening Inventory (SASSI) manual*. The SASSI Institute.

Mills, K. L., Teesson, M., Back, S. E., Brady, K. T., Baker, A. L., Hopwood, S., Sannibale, C., Barrett, E. L., Merz, S., Rosenfeld, J., & Ewer, P. L. (2012). Integrated exposure-based therapy for co-occurring posttraumatic stress disorder and substance dependence: A randomized controlled trial. *JAMA*, *308*(7), 690–699. https://doi.org/10.1001/jama.2012.9071

Moore, L. H., & Grubbs, J. B. (2021). Gambling disorder and comorbid PTSD: A systematic review of empirical research. *Addictive Behaviors*, *114*, 106713. https://doi.org/10.1016/j.addbeh.2020.106713

Najavits, L. M. (2002). *Seeking Safety: A treatment manual for PTSD and substance abuse*. The Guilford Press.

Najavits, L. M., Meyer, T., Johnson, K. M., & Korn, D. (2011). Pathological gambling and posttraumatic stress disorder: A study of the co-morbidity versus each alone. *Journal of Gambling Studies*, *27*(4), 663–683. https://doi.org/10.1007/s10899-010-9230-0

Petrakis, I. L., & Simpson, T. L. (2017). Posttraumatic stress disorder and alcohol use disorder: A critical review of pharmacologic treatments. *Alcoholism: Clinical and Experimental Research*, *41*(2), 226–237. https://doi.org/10.1111/acer.13297

Pietrzak, R. H., Goldstein, R. B., Southwick, S. M., & Grant, B. F. (2011). Prevalence and axis I comorbidity of full and partial posttraumatic stress disorder in the United States: Results from wave 2 of the national epidemiologic survey on alcohol and related conditions. *Journal of Anxiety Disorders*, *25*(3), 456–465. https://doi.org/10.1016/j.janxdis.2010.11.010

Rawson, R. A., Huber, A., McCann, M., Shoptaw, S., Farabee, D., Reiber, C., & Ling, W. (2002). A comparison of contingency management and cognitive-behavioral approaches during methadone maintenance treatment for cocaine dependence. *Archives of General Psychiatry*, *59*(9), 817. https://doi.org/10.1001/archpsyc.59.9.817

Roberts, N. P., Kitchiner, N. J., Kenardy, J., Bisson, J. I., & Roberts, N. P. (2010). Early psychological interventions to treat acute traumatic stress symptoms. *Cochrane Library*, *2012*(1), CD007944–CD007944. https://doi.org/10.1002/14651858.CD007944.pub2

Rogier, G., Beomonte Zobel, S., Marini, A., Camponeschi, J., & Velotti, P. (2021). Gambling disorder and dissociative features: A systematic review and meta-analysis. *Psychology of Addictive Behaviors*, *35*(3), 247–262. https://doi.org/10.1037/adb0000693

Saunders, E. C., Lambert-Harris, C., McGovern, M. P., Meier, A., & Xie, H. (2015). The prevalence of posttraumatic stress disorder symptoms among addiction treatment patients with cocaine use disorders. *Journal of Psychoactive Drugs*, *47*(1), 42–50. Academic Search Premier.

Saunders, J. B., Aasland, O. G., Babor, T. F., de la Fuente, J. R., & Grant, M. (1993). Development of the Alcohol Use Disorders Identification Test (AUDIT): WHO collaborative project on early detection of persons with harmful alcohol consumption—II. *Addiction (Abingdon, England)*, *88*(6), 791–804. https://doi.org/10.1111/j.1360-0443.1993.tb02093.x

Segal, Z. V., Williams, J. M. G., & Teasdale, J. D. (2013). *Mindfulness-based cognitive therapy for depression* (2nd ed.). The Guildford Press.

Selzer, M. L. (1971). The Michigan alcoholism screening test: The quest for a new diagnostic instrument. *American Journal of Psychiatry*, *127*, 1653–1658.

Shapiro, F. (1989). Eye movement desensitization: A new treatment for post-traumatic stress disorder. *Journal of Behavior Therapy and Experimental Psychiatry*, *20*(3), 211–217. https://doi.org/10.1016/0005-7916(89)90025-6

Shorter, D., Hsieh, J., & Kosten, T. R. (2015). Pharmacologic management of comorbid post-traumatic stress disorder and addictions. *American Journal on Addictions*, *24*(8), 705–712. Academic Search Premier.

Simpson, T. L., Lehavot, K., & Petrakis, I. L. (2017). No wrong doors: Findings from a critical review of behavioral randomized clinical trials for individuals with co-occurring alcohol/drug problems and posttraumatic stress disorder. *Alcoholism: Clinical and Experimental Research*, *41*(4), 681–702. https://doi.org/10.1111/acer.13325

Skinner, H. A. (1982). The drug abuse screening test. *Addictive Behaviors*, *7*(4), 363–371. https://doi.org/10.1016/0306-4603(82)90005-3

Smedley, B. D., Stith, A. Y., & Nelson, A. R. (2003). *Unequal treatment: Confronting racial and ethnic disparities in health care*. National Academies Press.

Smith, N. D. L., & Cottler, L. B. (2018). The epidemiology of post-traumatic stress disorder and alcohol use disorder. *Alcohol Research: Current Reviews*, *39*(2), 113–120. PubMed.

Substance Abuse and Mental Health Services Administration (SAMHSA). (2014). *Trauma-informed care in behavioral health services. Treatment Improvement Protocol (TIP) Series 57*. https://store.samhsa.gov/product/TIP-57-Trauma-Informed-Care-in-Behavioral-Health-Services/SMA14-4816

Substance Abuse and Mental Health Services Administration (SAMHSA). (2020). *Substance use disorder treatment for people with co-occurring disorders. Treatment Improvement Protocol (TIP) series, No. 42. SAMHSA publication No. PEP20-02-01-004* (No. PEP20-02-01-004; Treatment Improvement Protocol (TIP)). Substance Abuse and Mental Health Services Administration. https://store.samhsa.gov/product/tip-42-substance-use-treatment-persons-co-occurring-disorders/PEP20-02-01-004

Verplaetse, T. L., McKee, S. A., & Petrakis, I. L. (2018). Pharmacotherapy for co-occurring alcohol use disorder and post-traumatic stress disorder: Targeting the opioidergic, noradrenergic, serotonergic, and GABAergic/glutamatergic systems. *Alcohol Research: Current Reviews*, *39*(2), e1–e13. CINAHL Complete.

WHO ASSIST Working Group. (2002). The Alcohol, Smoking and Substance Involvement Screening Test (ASSIST): Development, reliability and feasibility. *Addiction*, *97*(9), 1183–1194. https://doi.org/10.1046/j.1360-0443.2002.00185.x

World Health Organization. (2013). *Guidelines for the management of conditions specifically related to stress*. WHO. http://www.ncbi.nlm.nih.gov/books/NBK159725/

World Health Organization. (2018). *International classification of diseases for mortality and morbidity statistics* (11th Revision). World Health Organization.

CHAPTER 14

CO-OCCURRING PERSONALITY AND SUBSTANCE USE DISORDERS

LATASHA Y. HICKS BECTON, JILLIAN Q. VAN WAGENEN, AND JENNIFER C. BARROW

LEARNING OBJECTIVES

After reading this chapter, you will be able to:
- Describe the basic features of personality disorders.
- Compare and contrast symptoms of personality disorders and effects of substance use.
- Demonstrate an understanding of treatment modalities utilized for treatment of co-occurring substance use and personality disorders.
- Identify legal and ethical concerns that may be associated with treatment for people who are dually diagnosed with personality and substance use disorders.

INTRODUCTION

While there have been significant efforts to reduce stigma that individuals living with mental health disorders are exposed to, negative attitudes continue to be pervasive in our society. This stigma is notable for folks living with personality disorders (PDs), and healthcare workers themselves have been shown to have negative attitudes when working with this population (Sheehan et al., 2016). There is a significant need to explore how to reduce this stigma (Sheehan et al., 2016) and education has been shown to be a powerful tool to use in behavioral health (Sulzer et al., 2021). This chapter explores PDs and their propensity for co-occurrence with substance use disorders (SUDs), and thus provides an educational opportunity for future counselors to reflect on this category of disorders. The chapter continues with an overview of the symptoms of PDs, differentiating them one from another as well as from the effects of substance use. Suggestions for assessment are included in addition to a discussion of aspects of treatment that may be helpful. The chapter ends with a case study followed by a brief discussion of diagnosis and treatment related to that specific case.

PERSONALITY DISORDERS: *DSM-5* DIAGNOSTIC CRITERIA AND DESCRIPTION

OVERVIEW OF DIAGNOSTIC FEATURES

The *Diagnostic and Statistical Manual for Mental Disorders, Fifth Edition* (*DSM-5*) published by the American Psychiatric Association (APA; 2013) outlines the criteria for PDs, separating them into three distinct groups: (a) Cluster A, (b) Cluster B, and (c) Cluster C. Cluster A includes paranoid, schizoid, and schizotypal PDs, which are characterized by a pervasive pattern of odd or eccentric behavior. Cluster B includes antisocial, borderline, histrionic, and narcissistic PDs, which are characterized by patterns of behavior with a focus on getting one's own needs met and/or a disregard for the rights or needs of others. Cluster C includes avoidant, dependent, and obsessive-compulsive PDs, which are often characterized by patterns of fearfulness or anxiety. There may be co-occurrence of PDs among Clusters A, B, and C.

PDs may be challenging to diagnose. In order to justify a diagnosis of PD, there must be evidence of an enduring and inflexible pattern of internal experiences and external behaviors over time, usually traceable to early adolescence or emerging adulthood, and these patterns must represent a deviation from established cultural norms for communication, habits, or behaviors (APA, 2013). For example, it would be improper to diagnosis a person with historically marginalized identities who is guarded or suspicious at an initial interview with paranoid PD without further exploration and consideration of cultural factors, as they may be unfamiliar with the process and the interviewer leading to the identified behaviors. Typically, people with PDs will demonstrate patterns of impairment in cognition, or ways of thinking, affectivity or emotional intensity and expression, interpersonal functioning, and impulse control that lead to clinically significant problems in their lives. Notably, there may be cases when the personality characteristics or patterns appear problematic to the clinician or collateral informants, yet the individual being evaluated has no insight into how their behavior impacts others. Additionally, the symptoms must not be better accounted for by the physiologic effects of substance use or another mental or physical health problem (APA, 2013).

A full description of the developmental course of PDs is beyond the scope of this chapter, so readers are referred to the *DSM-5* to obtain a comprehensive review of the diagnostic features as well as differential diagnoses, potential co-occurrence of more than one personality disorder, and potential for co-occurrence with SUDs (APA, 2013). Despite reported relationships between co-occurrence of PDs and SUDs, the symptoms are distinctly different. Throughout the section on PDs, the *DSM-5* lists the differential diagnosis for each PD which contains a statement similar to "must be distinguished from symptoms that may develop in association with persistent substance use" (APA, 2013, p. 647) in all but once case: antisocial personality disorder (ASPD; APA, 2013). So, while it is important to differentiate, the *DSM-5* offers minimal guidance on how to do so.

In the case of ASPD, the *DSM-5* (APA, 2013) is clear that one must have substantial evidence that the signs of the personality disorder were present in childhood (and thus likely evident prior to the onset of substance use). In addition, these symptoms must persist into adulthood for the diagnosis to be made. If the circumstances are such that both the antisocial behavior and substance use began in childhood, then both the diagnosis of SUD and ASPD may be made even if the antisocial acts are related to the sale or use of substances. As a note, a diagnosis of ASPD also requires that there was evidence of conduct disorder in childhood. There is no related diagnostic feature for other PDs. Additionally, the diagnosis of conduct disorder does not specifically mention substance use, though it can be inferred that there may be a relationship between some items of conduct disorder criterion A and consequences of childhood onset substance use.

INTERPLAY WITH SUBSTANCE USE DISORDERS

In the previous section, diagnostic features of PDs were briefly discussed. Now the focus turns to how the diagnostic features of PDs may interact with intoxication and withdrawal symptoms associated with various classes of substances, including how certain symptoms may interact with one another. Brief attention is also given to other addictive disorders.

DIFFERENTIAL DIAGNOSIS

When considering a diagnosis for PDs in people who also consume potentially impairing substances, it is important to consider the differences between an enduring pattern of personality characteristics and either episodic or regular substance use. Several symptoms of substance intoxication or withdrawal mimic the symptoms of various PDs. Additionally, the pattern of behavior associated with long-term substance use may appear as a PD. It is important, therefore, to consider the developmental course of the SUD prior to making a PD diagnosis.

Substance Intoxication and Withdrawal Symptoms

Symptoms of cannabis withdrawal include irritability, anger, aggression, and depressed mood (APA, 2013). To the untrained clinician, this withdrawal syndrome may appear to be symptoms of a PD, so it is important to differentiate between the two. Phencyclidine (PCP) intoxication symptoms include impulsivity and belligerence (APA, 2013), which may be mistaken for symptoms of borderline PD. Other symptoms of PCP or PCP-like intoxication, such as dissociation or stupor, may mimic the odd or eccentric behavior characteristic of psychosis or Cluster A PDs. People experiencing sedative-hypnotic type substance intoxication may present with stupor, coma, or impaired cognitions about life circumstances (APA, 2013), which may seem like schizoid or schizotypal PDs. While this is not an exhaustive list of mimicking symptoms of intoxication or withdrawal syndromes and PDs, these examples highlight the complexity involved with differential diagnosis of PDs from SUDs. In addition, just as it is important to differentiate PDs from symptoms of SUDs, it is important to clearly differentiate PDs from symptoms of behavioral/process addictions.

Behavioral/Process Addictions Characteristics

Behavioral/process addictions may also be closely associated with PDs, making differentiation difficult. Specifically, for problem gambling, there may be a pattern of deceitfulness, relationship problems, and mood lability, which are often associated with borderline, antisocial, or even narcissistic PDs. Sex addiction (although yet to be classified as an official disorder in the *DSM*) is often associated with impulsivity, deceitfulness, and relationship problems (APA, 2013). Relatedly, symptoms may be misinterpreted as histrionic, borderline, or antisocial PDs (Faridhosseini et al., 2019). Additionally, due to the repetitive patterns in substance and nonsubstance addictive behaviors, they may quite easily be mistaken for obsessive-compulsive personality disorder. It is important, therefore, to fully assess symptoms prior to rendering a diagnosis.

Legal Problem Criterion

In the transition from the *Diagnostic and Statistical Manual for Mental Disorders, Fourth Edition, Text Revision*, (*DSM-IV-TR*; APA, 2000) to the Fifth Edition (*DSM-5*), the criterion for legal problems related to substance use was removed. Of note, however, there remains a criterion (A.6.) in alcohol use disorder (AUD) for social problems associated with substance use; these social problems often include consequences of engaging in illegal activities. There are also criteria for continued use in dangerous situations (A.8 and A.9 for AUD) or with known negative consequences (APA, 2013, p. 491). These criteria cover many of the legal consequences that were directly addressed in the *DSM-IV-TR* (APA, 2000).

Antisocial PD and borderline personality disorder are both characterized by degrees of impulsivity. There may be a relationship between impulsivity and likelihood of legal involvement. When combined with the fact that simple possession of some substances is illegal at the federal level, it is likely that there may be significant legal involvement for people with either SUDs, PDs, or both.

PREVALENCE, STATISTICS, AND DEMOGRAPHICS

PDs are relatively rare in the U.S. population. Prevalence estimates in the general population range from .2% to 7.9% according to the *DSM-5* (APA, 2013). It is noted, however, that that the prevalence rates of PDs significantly increases if there is a comorbid SUD. Individuals with PDs are three times more likely to have a comorbid SUD than the general population (Karterud et al., 2009). Relatedly, Parmar and Kaloiya (2018) note the percentage of comorbid PDs and SUDs range from 38.8% to 73%. The authors assert that if someone has a diagnosable PD, their chance of developing an AUD increases five-fold, while the chance of developing some type of SUD increases 12-fold. Similarly, Straussner and Nemenzik (2007) state that 14.8% of adults meet the criteria for one PD, but that this percentage rises to 28% for those with an AUD, and to 47.7% for those with a SUD. Even more specifically, Trull et al. (2010) found the rate of Cluster B PDs, specifically borderline and antisocial, have been shown to have the highest rates of co-occurrence with SUDs. Relatedly, a 2018 study by Trull et al. (as cited in Substance Abuse Mental Health Services Administration [SAMHSA] 2020) notes the prevalence of borderline personality disorder in SUD treatment settings is as high as 53% in some cases. Additionally, Grant et al. (2016) found increased odds of being diagnosed with borderline personality disorder when there is a current or lifetime presence of a drug use disorder. Even among adolescents, there is a significant association between symptoms of PDs and co-occurrence with SUDs (Korsgaard et al., 2016).

There is evidence that the presence of a SUD greatly increases a person's chance of also having a PD (and vice versa). The reason for this high co-occurrence is still under investigation with researchers hypothesizing common factors or common causal pathways including genetics, trauma and abuse, and the common diagnosis criteria among disorders (Høye et al., 2021). Parmar and Kaloiya (2018) asserted that the high percentage of co-occurrence suggests the disorders are causally linked. The exact link is difficult to determine because of the complex nature of PDs coupled with the high prevalence of multiple diagnoses for these clients. Future research will be examining the theories of a primary SUD, primary PD, or a common factor that underlies both, like course of treatment, frequency of hospitalization, and gender (Høye et al., 2021).

ASSESSMENT AND DIAGNOSTIC CONSIDERATIONS

Aligned with what has been addressed thus far in this chapter, it is clearly seen how symptoms and manifestations of PDs may overlap with other mental health conditions, particularly PDs. As mentioned, diagnosing PDs is often difficult. Parmar and Kaloiya (2018) state that the difficulty in assessment leads to a blurry understanding of the epidemiology of PDs versus other mental illnesses as well. Exclusion criteria are useful for determining if the symptoms are present solely during an episode of another mental illness, such as differentiating between Cluster A disorders (i.e., characterized by odd or eccentric behavior) and a psychotic or manic episode. Also, a PD should not be diagnosed unless the defining characteristics are present before early adulthood, are a piece of the individual's long-term functioning, and are considered part of a pervasive pattern (APA, 2013). This information is typically received from subjective reports of the clients, yet confirmation with a family member is helpful, perhaps even necessary, to increase objectivity. Considering the frequency of co-occurrence and overlapping symptoms of PDs and SUDs as well as other mental health conditions, it is important to thoroughly and objectively assess symptoms.

When the individual being assessed has a PD as well as a co-occurring SUD, it is necessary to distinguish between the symptoms of the PD and the consequences of intoxication, withdrawal, or an associated issue. It is best if the person's body systems can be clear of impairing substances before a diagnosis of a PD is assigned, yet it is not always possible to delay assessment (Verheul & Van Den Brink, 2005). In order to properly differentiate, it is important to identify when the symptoms of the personality disorder began. More specifically, since PDs are reflective of patterns that may have begun in youth or adolescence and have continued into adult life, it is necessary to assess a person's behavior in childhood and early adulthood. For clients who began substance use in childhood or adolescence, however, this assessment may be quite difficult.

An example of the complexity when use begins in childhood or adolescence involves the relationship between an individual's use of substances and the presence of substance use in peer groups. When children, adolescents, or emerging adults are involved in "deviant" peer or social groups, there is a sharing of norms within the group, and in some cases, these norms are antisocial and may include substance use. There is a potential for substances to alter the behavior of the individual by changing their brain chemistry (Verheul & Van Den Brink, 2005) as well as potentially changing the behavior or character of the peer group. In some cases, consistent substance use may result in drug-related identity change (Anderson & Mott, 1998). These identity changes may appear as a persistent and pervasive pattern of personality characteristics, potentially reflecting symptoms of PDs. When personality symptoms are initiated close to the time substance use commences, it may be reasonable to rule out a PD. Specific training in assessment and diagnosis is helpful. Also, it may be helpful to utilize highly discriminative tests and diagnostic interviews (Vélez-Moreno et al., 2017). Failure to thoroughly assess and diagnose these co-occurring disorders (CODs) may result in development of a poor treatment plan. Importantly, an accurate and thorough assessment including collateral information may be necessary to ensure a proper diagnosis and is integral for proper treatment. Collateral information may come from the following sources: medical records, family members or others who live in the home, educational records if appropriate, and other professionals.

There is a poor prognosis for individuals with a comorbid SUD and PD. Those with PDs often have a difficult time connecting to others, and this limits the therapeutic relationship as well as the potential support network. One recent study identified poor patient/therapist relationships, higher dropout rates, nonadherence issues, poor motivation to change, earlier age of onset, frequent relapse, shorter periods of abstinence, increased psychological burden, poor social functioning, and an increased risk of suicide as factors that impact the treatment process (Parmar & Kaloiya, 2018). To ensure the best possible treatment outcomes, Vélez-Moreno et al. (2017) insist on a comprehensive evaluation and that the individual be treated holistically. As part of that comprehensive evaluation (often including biopsychosocial and spiritual assessment), it is important to fully assess the whole person by including topics such as cultural and gender differences. Although there are certainly many aspects to a person, these two sets of identity characteristics are addressed directly here.

CULTURAL CONSIDERATIONS

Culture should always be considered when assessing any client. Given the expectation that there be a pervasive and enduring pattern of behavior over time, it is possible that culture-specific behaviors may be misinterpreted as diagnostic information or symptoms to the untrained clinician. In order to meet the criteria for a PD, the client's personality traits must be maladaptive, inflexible, persistent, cause clinically significant distress, and be beyond acceptable patterns of behavior in their culture of origin. Failing to consider culture may result in misinterpretation of symptoms, thus conflating a person's cultural experiences, customs, or practices with symptoms of a diagnoseable mental health condition. Diagnosis and diagnostic features of mental health conditions were determined by people in positions of power and in a predominately White Western culture, and thus not providing specific criteria for assessing clients outside of industrialized nations that value independence over community.

For example, according to the text of the *DSM-5* (APA, 2013), rates of ASPD are higher in people who experience adverse socioeconomic and sociocultural situations (APA, 2013). Because participation in *illegal* or *countercultural* activities without remorse is a criterion, people who are disproportionately exposed to the legal system due to systemic injustice may be misdiagnosed (Høye et al., 2021). Additionally, there is a lack of consideration for how a person's economic situation may be related to their participation in behaviors that may be consistent with local cultural norms. This lack of diagnostic consideration may be reflective of bias and limited worldview on the part of *DSM-5* authors. Relatedly, when considering a diagnosis of ASPD, it is imperative to differentiate among true symptoms of PD symptoms and behaviors necessary for survival in adverse circumstances, such as having limited access to financial resources or basic needs or living in neighborhoods where there are cultural expectations of activity that may otherwise be considered countercultural or illegal. Counselors must also be aware of their own biases and values and how these might play into an inaccurate diagnosis of someone with a different worldview and cultural traditions.

GENDER DIFFERENCES

Differences between the manifestation of SUDs and PDs have been recorded between men and women, and there is a growing body of literature about trans and nonbinary people's experiences. Compared to men, women have a higher level of medical, psychological, and physical impairment that may be explained by differences in societal pressures, biological response, and medical consequences (Chen et al., 2019). Sher and colleagues (2015) reported gender differences in antisocial PDs and childhood trauma with 56.5% of men and 64.79% of women reporting childhood trauma. When assessing specifically for emotional, physical, and sexual abuse, women were more likely to have experienced sexual and emotional abuse than men. Though higher percentages of women experienced physical abuse than men, the difference was not clinically significant. Additionally, women tend to have a higher likelihood of borderline and histrionic PDs diagnosis in Cluster B, yet men are more likely to be diagnosed with narcissistic personality disorder (Sher et al., 2015).

Expanding the definition of gender to include transgender and gender diverse (T/GD) clients, Newcomb et al., (2020) found higher rates of substance use among T/GD clients when compared to cisgender populations. T/GD individuals' higher rates of substance use and CODs resulted from environmental factors, including abuse, trauma, negative psychosocial interactions, and loss of support systems. Disparities in health outcomes, access to healthcare, and CODs demonstrate a need for counselors to familiarize themselves with the unique cultural and health needs of T/GD clients. This may include accounting for social environment, stressors related to gender and/or sexual orientation, existing substance use, previous trauma, and economic/employment background (Day et al., 2017; Newcomb et al., 2020; Whitton et al., 2019).

Differences in gender is another reason why a thorough assessment is needed. Men with CODs and PDs are more likely to seek treatment for substance use, while women with the same comorbidity are more likely to seek treatment for problems related to PDs (Karterud et al., 2009). Among men and women with ASPD, men were more likely to exhibit antisocial behavior (Sher et al., 2015) and are more likely to be involved with violent and illegal actions versus the nonviolent antisocial behaviors (e.g., truancy, cancel social plans) of their female counterparts (Alegria et al., 2013). Furthermore, the nonviolent nature of ASPD in women may lead to the under-recognition of ASPD in women (Alegria et al., 2013). Relatedly, it is important that regardless of where a counselor encounters a client (e.g., hospital, community clinic, private practice), there should be a thorough assessment of personality, phenomenological, including gender, differences of symptom manifestation, in substance use treatment as well as assessment of substance use patterns in primary mental health treatment settings (Karterud et al., 2009). In addition to attending to differences in symptom presentation and experience by people who identify as men and women, it is also important to attend to cultural or community experiences for people who are nonbinary or have identities elsewhere on the gender continuum.

SCREENING AND ASSESSMENT TOOLS

Several considerations for assessment and diagnosis were considered in the previous section. There are several screening and assessment tools available for the assessment of both PDs and substance use. Since a primary factor in proper treatment planning is thorough assessment, an overview of tools and approaches is offered in this section. Although it is not feasible to offer a detailed overview of every available instrument or tool, a description of some of the key screening and assessment tools is provided. It is important to point out that while standardized screening and assessment tools are certainly useful, there is no substitute for a thorough clinical interview and ongoing assessment.

To properly treat co-occurring PDs and SUDs, an accurate diagnosis is essential. This means an extensive knowledge and use of screening and assessment tools is going to be an asset to each individual client's case. Screening for other mental disorders is needed to make sure the diagnosis of a PD is warranted. In addition to fully understanding the characteristics of personality, it is important to thoroughly assess the severity of clinical impact on the person and the temporal relationship between symptom development and onset of substance use. The severity of substance use also needs to be accurately assessed with appropriate screening tools and clinical assessment. Any assessment, questionnaire, or screening tool must align with the current standards of professional practice and properly assess symptoms represented in the most current versions of the *DSM* and the *International Statistical Classification of Diseases and Related Health Problems* (ICD). Further, it is a best practice to administer assessments in a client's first or primary language.

It is important to assess dangerousness with any clinical population and specifically with co-occurring PDs and SUDs. There is a high risk of suicidal behaviors, self-harm, and impulsivity with this population (Parmar & Kaloiya, 2018). These clinical issues, particularly the most severe and life-threatening symptoms (i.e., active suicidal and homicidal ideation with plan and/or intent) will need to be stabilized before other treatment can begin (Atkins, 2021).

STANDARDIZED INSTRUMENTS

Personality Disorders

Borderline and antisocial PDs are the most common PDs to co-occur with SUDs (Karterud et al., 2009; Parmar & Kaloiya, 2018; Straussner & Nemenzik, 2007). Relatedly, clients are more frequently and specifically screened for these two PDs in the context of SUD treatment. In their study on borderline features in substance use patients, Vest and Tragesser (2019) used the Personality Assessment Inventory for Borderlines (PAI-BOR; Morey, 1991) and asserted that the scale has demonstrated strong validation among both clinical and nonclinical samples. This scale looks at the specific features of borderline personality disorder as it relates to substance use (i.e., affective instability, identity disturbances, negative relationships, and self-harm/impulsivity). The Revised Diagnostic Interview for Borderlines (DIB-R; Zanarini et al., 1989) is also popular for this group and has excellent inter-rater and test/retest reliability, but results should still be confirmed with clinical assessment of symptoms as identified in the most current *DSM* (APA, 2013) or *ICD* manual (Heath et al., 2018). Since impulsiveness and emotional dysregulation are major contributors to borderline personality disorder, the Barratt Impulsiveness Scale (BIS-11; Patton et al., 1995) can be helpful for measuring a client's impulsivity. There is evidence of internal consistency and test/retest reliability for the BIS-11 (Heath et al., 2018).

For a measure that is not focused specifically on people with borderline personality disorder, the Structured Interview for *DSM-IV* Personality (SIDP-IV; Pfohl et al., 1997) is a good start; however, it will need to be modified as necessary to be consistent with the diagnostic criteria for the most current edition of the *DSM*. The International Personality Disorder Examination Screening Questionnaire (IPDE-SQ) has also been used in some clinical studies (e.g., Korsgaard et al., 2016; Loranger et al., 1994; Magallón-Neri et al., 2013). The IPDE-SQ follows the *ICD-10* criteria rather than the *DSM-5* and is selected because it is easy to administer and has adequate psychometric properties. As a matter of emphasis, it is often useful to use clinical questionnaires or standardized screening instruments to assist in the diagnostic process; yet, it is still the counselor's clinical responsibility to assess how symptoms align with diagnostic criteria as set forth in the *DSM* or *ICD* manual.

Substance Use Disorders

The Addictions Severity Index (ASI; McLellan et al., 1980, 1992) is commonly used to measure SUDs. Not only does this measure substance use, but it explores lifetime and past month issues in medical, educational, employment, legal, family/social, and psychiatric domains. Therefore, it may be a good supplement to the clinical interview. The ASI has excellent psychometric properties and a quantitative severity index, based on number, duration, frequency, and intensity of symptoms is produced within each domain (Heath et al., 2018). There is also a European Version of the ASI (Fureman et al., 1990; Vélez-Moreno et al., 2017).

It is also helpful to assess alcohol and other drug use in the recent past. Approaches to assessment used in treatment settings include assessment in quantity/frequency of use and modified timeline-follow back as well as other approaches. There are also major alcohol and other drug-related studies that assess for recent substance use. The National Survey on Drug Use and Health (NSDUH) published by SAMHSA measures substance use (including tobacco) in the past 90 days (Miller & Del Boca, 1994). Owens et al. (2018) used items from the NSUDH to assess the alcohol and drug use of clients receiving dialectical behavioral therapy (DBT; Linehan, 1993) in the 90 days prior to treatment as well as lifetime use to get a picture of where they are starting. The NSDUH items have strong internal consistency and can be modified to look at specific substance use by pulling items relating to the substance in question (Vest & Tragesser, 2019).

In addition to standardized assessments traditionally administered in SUD treatment, such as the Alcohol Use Disorders Identification Test (AUDIT; Babor et al., 2001), Drug Abuse Screening Test (DAST; Skinner, 1982), or other items mentioned previously, it may also be helpful to assess for various forms of impulsivity. Given the relationship between impulsivity and substance use, as well as the impulsive characteristics of people with PDs, assessing impulsivity may be an important step in determining the most appropriate care. In fact, Hershberger et al. (2017) suggested assessing for the impulsivity factor negative urgency, stating "there is a need to assess negative urgency and a lack of premeditation in SUD psychotherapy, particularly prior to treatment planning" (p. 413). Assessing these sorts of traits may prove challenging with standardized instruments, so the clinical interview is likely a helpful addition or follow-up to any assessment process.

Self-Harm

The Self-Harm Behavior Questionnaire (SHBQ; Gutierrez et al., 2001) is used to measure a client's current suicidal behaviors or ideations as well as self-damaging tendencies. The questionnaire has good test/retest reliability, internal consistency, and convergent validity with other valid measures of suicidality and self-harm (Heath et al., 2018). The SHBQ explores the client's preferred method of harm, the age of onset, frequency, and the need for medical treatment. This should be administered before treatment in case a more intensive route is needed. Along with this measure, the Profile of Mood States (POMS; McNair et al., 1971) is another self-report questionnaire that is helpful at this stage as it measures fluctuating mood states, anger/hostility, tension/anxiety, depression/dejection, vigor/activity, fatigue/inertia, and confusion/bewilderment (McNair et al., 1971) and has excellent internal consistency and test/retest reliability (Heath et al., 2018).

Clinical Interview

The clinical interview is a useful tool for understanding nuance in client reports and presents an opportunity to identify collateral informants. Sometimes people who exhibit symptoms of PDs and/or SUDs lack insight to the presence or prevalence of their symptoms, so it is helpful to collect collateral information. In addition to being an opportunity to build rapport with the client, the clinical interview is also useful for building the foundations and expectations for the treatment process. The stability of the relationship and a solid foundation and orientation to treatment is helpful for people diagnosed with PDs and SUDs alike.

Although standardized paper/pencil or electronic assessments and the clinical interview are based on the client's self-report, the clinical interview offers an opportunity for information exchange and interaction resulting in a more indepth assessment. The clinical interview may also be used to administer interviewer versions of some instruments (such as the AUDIT) and can specifically assess patterns of personality characteristics over time. Clinical interviews may also be used to assess change over time, particularly evaluating improvements (or deterioration) in quality of life and participation in maladaptive behaviors not addressed in standardized instruments.

TREATMENT MODALITIES

PDs are known to be difficult to treat. This is likely given the long duration of symptoms and the challenge of fully assessing them. Thus, a primary factor for treatment success is length of engagement in the treatment process. However, this may be a challenge as diagnostic features associated with borderline personality (for example) include impulsivity, emotional lability, and anger, which all may play a role in contributing to treatment dropout (Wnuk et al., 2013). This is also true for SUDs. Thus, treatment modalities designed to treat co-occurring substance use or other addictive disorders and borderline personality are best designed to address these potential barriers to treatment retention and subsequent efficacy. The treatments that have had the best results with this co-occurring personality and SUDs are cognitive behavioral therapy (CBT), particularly DBT, and 12-Step mutual support groups (Giannelli et al., 2019; Parmar & Kaloiya, 2018; Straussner & Nemenzik, 2007). Other interventions, such as motivational interviewing (MI; Miller & Rollnick, 2002, 2013), comprehensive validation therapy (CVT; Linehan et al., 1996), and assertive community treatment have also been shown to be beneficial when combined with the acceptance and validation aspects of DBT (Bornovalova & Daughters, 2007; Straussner & Nemenzik, 2007). Additionally, MI is a useful approach to implementing each of the previously mentioned treatment modalities as it has been linked to increasing a client's motivation to change as well as increasing a client's commitment to treatment (Bornovalova & Daughters, 2007).

Regardless of treatment modality, it is also important to assess and treat impulsivity. Impulsivity is associated with a reduction in outcomes (Hershberger et al., 2017). SUD treatment needs to address characteristics of impulsivity including negative urgency and sensation-seeking to improve treatment outcomes. Treatment interventions that target impulsive traits may be helpful for reducing symptoms of SUDs and a variety of mental health conditions (Hershberger et al., 2017).

COGNITIVE BEHAVIORAL THERAPIES

Cognitive behavioral therapies (CBTs) are a treatment of choice for primary mental health disorders and SUDs. These therapies are designed to identify problematic behaviors and challenge unhelpful thoughts and identify different behavioral options. There are many types of cognitive behavioral-informed therapies, including DBT, acceptance and commitment therapy (ACT; Hayes et al., 2012), and rational emotive behavior therapy (REBT; Ellis, 1996). Primary attention is given to DBT here because it is a treatment of choice for PDs and is also useful as an enhancement to traditional CBT for relapse prevention (Bornovalova & Daughters, 2007; Parmar & Kaloiya, 2018; Straussner & Nemenzik, 2007).

Dialectical Behavior Therapy

DBT (Linehan, 1993; Linehan et al., 1999) is a manualized modality for therapy grounded in a combination of CBT, mindfulness, and dialectics, which is the recognition that there can be multiple, seemingly conflicting truths. The core of DBT is radical acceptance while, at the same time, aiding the client in changing maladaptive and harmful behaviors and thoughts. DBT integrates individual therapy, group skills training, case management, psychoeducation, frequent contact measures such as telephone consultation, mutual self-help groups, and sometimes, collaboration with a prescribing physician. DBT is the standard intervention for borderline personality disorder specifically, and is a promising treatment for co-occurring PDs and SUDs (Bornovalova & Daughters, 2007; Linehan, 1993; Linehan et al., 1999; Owens et al., 2018; Parmar & Kaloiya, 2018). DBT may also be indicated for other addictive disorders; however, the scholarly literature is relatively silent on nonsubstance addictions.

Premature treatment dropout is a concern with clients with PDs, so increasing treatment retention is a necessary means of improving positive outcomes. Treatment outcomes for SUDs are highly related to time spent in treatment (Moggi et al., 2010). DBT is suggested as a useful addendum to the treatment process and may decrease attrition (Bornovalova & Daughters, 2007). Components of DBT that are speculated to reduce premature dropout are mindfulness training, validation and acceptance techniques, role induction, and perceived utility of the treatment. Bornovalova and Daughters (2007) reported perceived utility of treatment as one of the strongest predictors of treatment retention, but that evidence leans more toward generating hope and role induction for reducing dropout rates. Validation regarding therapeutic alliance is emphasized in DBT but there is little evidence to support its role in reducing dropout (Bornovalova & Daughters, 2007).

Comprehensive validation therapy (CVT; Linehan et al., 1996) utilizes the acceptance-based strategies from DBT, such as therapeutic warmth, responsiveness, and empathy, but does not include the formal problem solving or skills training. It has shown, however, higher treatment retention than DBT (Bornovalova & Daughters, 2007; Straussner & Nemenzik, 2007). The high retention seen in DBT can be attributed to the positive effects of the validation and acceptance components versus behavior change training (Bornovalova & Daughters, 2007; Straussner & Nemenzik, 2007).

Reducing self-damaging behavior and emotional dysregulation is another positive outcome common to DBT. Other encouraging results show that DBT is an effective modality for decreasing suicidal and nonsuicidal self-injurious behavior (NSSI) and in decreasing hospitalization and improving quality of life, and has been effective in treating those with co-occurring SUDs (Atkins, 2021). Decreasing self-mutilation and parasuicidal behavior is another positive aspect of DBT (Karterud et al., 2009). By learning techniques for managing volatile emotions, clients can avoid the emotional crises that often lead to substance use and other self-destructive behaviors (Straussner & Nemenzik, 2007). Since symptom presentations with comorbidity between SUDs and PDs have been shown to have more severe PD symptoms, removing substance use from the equation is highly important.

It may be helpful to offer additional treatment options, including contingency management. Mathias (1996; as cited by Straussner & Nemenzik, 2007) discussed contingency management type modifications for treatment. When the client has co-occurring ASPD and SUDs, offering quick and progressively greater rewards may increase treatment engagement (Mathias, 1996; Straussner & Nemenzik, 2007); however, doing so may conflict with the need to teach delayed gratification as part of relapse prevention skills in substance use treatment. Furthermore, when working with individuals with co-occurring borderline personality disorder and substance use, it is possible that the client's overriding desire to be safe can be used for their benefit by educating about how substance use can get in the way of their goal (Straussner & Nemenzik, 2007). Both PDs can increase the likelihood of the client not being completely honest about their substance use, so requiring collateral contacts to verify their information is helpful.

General Format of Dialectical Behavioral Therapy

Whereas there is a manualized protocol for DBT in treatment settings (Linehan, 2015), treatment may result in better outcomes when tailored to the client's individual needs. Atkins (2014, 2021) provides an example of a typical DBT treatment format for people with CODs based on Linehan's seminal and subsequent work (Linehan, 1993; Linehan et al., 1993, 1999). Since this population has a high occurrence of suicidality, step one of this model necessitates a thorough assessment. Suicidality/homicidality, medical concerns, and serious withdrawal or intoxication need to be stabilized before moving on to the skills-based treatment protocol (Atkins, 2014, 2021). Assessment should include evaluation of safety concerns and level of care determination as well as readiness for change, and other components of a full biopsychosocial assessment.

Based on the assessment in step one, step two consists of constructing a problems/need list that is categorized as substance use, mental health, or medical. Atkins (2014; 2021) explained that by following this three-item list, it will incorporate most issues and help the counselor focus on what is emergent, urgent, and what will be focused on in long-term treatment. This list will also inform the types of techniques needed, goals, and help the counselor to personalize the treatment for the client.

Step three of Atkins's (2014) format establishes the initial short-term and long-term goals for treatment. The previous steps listed are used as a guide with the most urgent or life-threatening issues addressed first (Linehan et al., 1993). It is important to have clear, measurable goals that are collaboratively created and are perceived by the client as possible. Longer episodes of care consistently show better outcomes for co-occurring SUD and PD clients (Moggi et al., 2010). Typically, programs include meetings with the client two times per week for 1 year: once a week for individual therapy and once a week for group skills training. As the treatment progresses, modifications to goals, techniques used, and skills taught can be made for each client.

SUGGESTED ADJUNCT INTERVENTIONS

Bornovalova and Daughters (2007) emphasized the benefit of relapse prevention models, contingency management, MI, frequent contact, strong therapeutic alliance, acceptance-based strategies, assertive community treatment, mindfulness, and 12-step group affiliation. Additionally, psychoeducation is an often-necessary tool in the beginning of treatment and periodically throughout. Straussner and Nemenzik (2007) advocated for the importance of treatment emphasizing education, more adaptive coping skills, normalizing interpersonal relationships, and family involvement. Medication for specific symptom control is used, but otherwise there are no specific FDA-approved medications for this combination of CODs. In a case study using DBT with a man diagnosed with comorbid borderline personality disorder and SUD, Owens et al. (2018) identified the following tools as effective:

- Mindfulness,
- Hierarchical behavior targets,

- Opposite emotion action,
- Contact between sessions,
- Safety planning,
- Daily diary of substance use,
- Behavior chains,
- Interpersonal effectiveness skills,
- Communication skills,
- Problem-solving skills,
- Pros/cons lists, and
- Acronyms such as DEAR MAN (a skill of DBT), which aids the client with effectively communicating their needs. According to Owens et al. (2018) the D is for describing the situation, E is for expressing one's feelings using "I" statements, A is to assert oneself, R is for reinforcing their reasons why what they want is important, M is to be mindful and not get off topic, A is for appearing confident, and N is to negotiate or compromise.

Twelve-Step Facilitation

In addition to traditional involvement in 12-step community groups, 12-step facilitation is also sometimes used in clinic-based care for substance use and co-occurring mental disorders. Utilizing a group counseling format, 12-step groups are designed to share experiences and build a community of support, while addressing triggers and responses through peer support and accountability (i.e., chips and tokens for anniversaries). While many clients are quite successful using these methods, results are difficult to duplicate in research studies. In the scholarly literature, there are mixed results about the relationship between 12-step facilitation and treatment outcomes. Without examining confounding variables such as genetic history, duration of use, previous counseling/treatment, and drug history, it may be difficult to account for the positive outcomes of 12-step facilitation as the sole treatment modality for successful recovery. Despite differences in efficacy, Bogenschutz et al. (2014) suggested that providers should not abandon 12-step facilitation as an approach to treatment of people who experience severe mental illness along with an AUD. It may, however, be useful for researchers to consider strategies to maximize exposure to 12-step facilitation, thus maximizing the effects of the treatment approach.

Regardless of mixed results in the scholarly literature, there are numerous benefits for 12-step facilitation as an addition to treatment. People with co-occurring substance use and PDs often have strained familial relationships, which lead to smaller support networks (Straussner & Nemenzik, 2007). Involvement in a 12-step group can make a positive impact on their support system. Increasing family and social functioning is just one aspect of the suggested integrated treatment (Vélez-Moreno et al., 2017). Moggi et al. (2010) found that increased patient involvement, a flexible/personalized program, and an emphasis on the importance of 12-step group membership was indicative of longer periods of abstinence when following up with patients 1 year post treatment. Longer episodes of care have been shown to be effective as well and 12-step groups are often attended for life (Moggi et al., 2010).

Another reason 12-step groups are promoted within this population is the importance of maintaining abstinence. The connection between substance use and higher severity of PD symptoms is demonstrated in a study of outpatient borderline personality and SUD patients (Heath et al., 2018).

Twelve-step groups directly work with abstinence from all substances, plus they are free, available at numerous times and locations, and, as previously noted, offer a large support network. This allows for flexibility and some control over their own treatment. In addition to traditional 12-step programs, other free recovery-focused support groups such as SMART Recovery, Recovery Dharma, LifeRing Secular Recovery, and other peer-based support groups serve a parallel purpose.

Relatedly, Straussner and Nemenzik (2007) suggested some modifications to the traditional 12-step program for clients with co-occurring PDs and SUDs. Examples of possible alterations to the program are having concrete goals instead of (or perhaps in addition to) the abstract goal of spiritual awakening. Straussner and Nemenzik (2007) explained that individuals with borderline personality disorder, for example, greatly fear being out of control, so it may be helpful to modify the language being used or clarify concepts regarding the 12 steps, such as the idea of integrating a higher power into one's life. Membership with these types of mutual support groups is increasingly popular and can help clients learn how to build a better, more manageable life and to take problems as they come.

Dialectical Behavior Therapy and 12-Step Facilitation

Although there is evidence of treatment efficacy for PDs treated with DBT (Panos et al., 2013), there is question about whether DBT is additive to the effects of 12-step facilitation and vice versa. In their meta-analysis of DBT and 12-step facilitation for SUDs, Giannelli et al. (2019) found no differential impacts on substance use for each of the treatment modalities regardless of whether substance use was measured by self-report, urinalysis, or treatment retention/attrition. They concluded that both DBT and 12-step facilitation are beneficial treatments for SUDs, yet one is no more effective than the other.

LEGAL AND ETHICAL CONSIDERATIONS
CONFIDENTIALITY

The privacy of individuals in substance use disorder treatment is legally protected under federal regulations (i.e., 42 U.S.C. 290dd-2), which is commonly referred to as 42 CFR Part 2, or simply, *Part 2*. These regulations specifically restrict the disclosure of client records related to SUD treatment. Though a full review of 42 CFR Part 2 is beyond the scope of this chapter, counselors are urged to consider the implications of current and historical legal involvement on SUD treatment and how legal involvement can impact treatment goals or outcomes. For example, mandated treatment as a part of release programs may improve client outcomes. Utilizing work release, halfway house placement, bonding out for treatment as a condition of release, or mandated treatment as a condition of probation all provide structure through placement, supervision, and with a built-in accountability, and clients may benefit from community of formal and informal supports.

Counselors also need to be aware that this population of co-occurring clients may be involved with various parts of the legal system. There is specific focus on ASPD given the likelihood of co-occurrence with SUDs, and the likelihood of legal involvement explored in the diagnostic section. There is also a need to consider how legal involvement may impact a person's ability to participate in treatment. For example, house arrest may impede the radius of accessible care and ability to access reliable transportation services (e.g., public transportation). Developing a network of referral sources near a client's home may improve attendance and participation in treatment programs by addressing the home's proximity to services.

MANDATED TREATMENT

Clients with ASPD may have frequent involvement with the legal system. Relatedly, it is possible they may be mandated to treatment as part of a probation, parole, or diversion program agreement. Collaborating with legal system professionals may be key to the client's success in treatment. Anecdotally, these collaborations often involve an agreement for the client to remain in treatment, follow the treatment recommendations, and regular drug screens within the legal system, as well as at the treatment site. Counselors sometimes have difficulty reconciling their own beliefs and values about treatment and the need to collaborate with the legal system as a stakeholder in the client's care. It is important for the counselors to challenge their own biases and refocus on the needs of the client, which may be to meet the requirements set forth by the legal system.

It seems important here to direct attention to counselor tasks associated with working with mandated clients. When initiating the therapeutic relationship, it is necessary to collect the appropriate written agreements to release information for the collaboration and communication process to occur between the treatment entity and referring organizations. Clients must be made aware of treatment expectations and facility guidelines, as failure to abide by them may not only impact services at the treatment site, but also may have legal or other consequences. For people who are mandated to treatment, it is important to help them understand the relationship between their treatment engagement, ability to abide by guidelines, and potential legal impacts as part of the informed consent process. Clients should be made aware of what information will be shared with the referring entity and how their decision to share (or not share) information may also impact their legal outcomes. Counselors also need to be clear about what information they are required to disclose, and then ensure they remain within those limits.

SUICIDE RISK ASSESSMENT

Clients with borderline personality disorder, specifically, may have a high propensity for suicidal ideation and may frequently require referral for hospitalization (Oldham, 2006). Care should be taken to describe symptoms behaviorally and provide the minimum necessary information to medical staff for the patient to get appropriate care. It may be helpful to have pre-existing plans in place, including written agreements for release of confidential information involving substance use history that may impact the assessment and treatment process in a hospital setting.

Assessing suicide in clients with co-occurring SUDs may be more complicated than assessing those who do not use substances. What may appear to the untrained person as a drug overdose or natural event in a person's pattern of drug use may indeed be a suicide attempt. For counselors working in hospital settings, it is important to thoroughly assess a person's motives for substance use and develop an understanding of their patterns of use over time. Repeated overdose in a short period may be reminiscent of other ritualistic parasuicidal or suicidal behaviors, which are often present in people who are diagnosed with borderline personality disorder.

CLINICAL CASE ILLUSTRATION AND DISCUSSION

CASE OF KENDALL

Kendall Blevins is a 27-year-old White male in opioid maintenance treatment for heroin use. Kendall was previously assigned to a counselor who has since left the agency, so he was recently transferred to a new counselor, Trinh. During a review of Kendall's treatment record, Trinh learns Kendall has been in the treatment program for about 2 years and is on a stable daily dose of 117 milligrams of methadone. The counselor also learns that Kendall has a legal history of petty theft as well as a history of harming animals as a child, stating he would catch squirrels or chipmunks, squeeze their necks and "watch them squirm until they stopped moving." Despite being in treatment for 2 years, Kendall has not been fully engaged as evidenced by irregularly attending group and individual counseling sessions as well as not following other regulations and guidelines of the opioid maintenance treatment program—some of which are designed to meet federal regulations for opioid maintenance treatment.

In the first meeting with Kendall, the counselor spends time getting to know him, doing a brief assessment, and updating his treatment plan. Kendall is quite pleasant, cooperative, and charming. He has requested information to be shared with his probation officer and signed the appropriate document for release of confidential information. As the discussion continues, Trinh asks about Kendall's history of mental health symptoms and suicidality. Kendall explained he has cut his wrists in the past and has some scarring as a result. When asked to see Kendall's scars, the counselor noted they are indeed quite fresh, deep, yet healing lacerations, so Kendall does not seem to require immediate wound care. When asked about the lacerations, Kendall explains that he got into an argument with his parents while he was visiting them over the weekend several weeks ago. Kendall's parents refused to give him any money, and he was angry at them, so he cut himself while they were watching. There was blood was all over the living room of his parent's home. Kendall left when his parents tried to call emergency services. Currently, Kendall denies wanting to die, but wanted to teach his parents a lesson. The counselor observes that while he was speaking, there is a relatively flat affect as well as a sense of emptiness in Kendall's eyes. When the counselor begins to talk with Kendall about potential for hospitalization, he becomes tearful and says he is worried that he will not be able to return to see Trinh for counseling. Additionally, Kendall stated that Trinh is "the best person [I] ever worked with," despite it being their first meeting.

After Kendall signed appropriate releases for contact, Trinh consulted with Kendall's father who provides financial support for Kendall's care. Kendall's father, Derek, retells the story of Kendall cutting his wrists while his mother watched screaming in horror, and how this has happened multiple times over. Derek also disclosed that Kendall regularly visits on the weekends and is initially charming, telling the parents how much he adores them and how they are "the best parents ever" but eventually asks for money. When his parents refuse, he becomes both physically and verbally assaultive, stating they are terrible people who do not deserve to live. These encounters often end with Kendall making a threat to harm himself by cutting his wrists or with an intentional overdose.

Derek becomes tearful and states the family is getting to be in financial trouble because they have simply started giving Kendall the money to prevent him from harming himself. Additionally, his parents pay for Kendall's apartment because they do not feel safe with him in their home. Kendall was previously employed and had a roommate to cover part of the bills; however, the roommate moved out because Kendall would get angry, punch holes in the walls, and physically fight his roommate on some occasions. Additionally, Kendall lost his job due to an angry outburst at work.

The next week, Trinh receives a phone call from the local police department stating Kendall is a suspect in multiple crimes: sale of counterfeit controlled substance to an undercover police officer (purported to be methadone but was actually pink liquid fabric softener) and armed robbery of a convenience store near the treatment center. Kendall was already on probation for a previous charge of possession with intent to sell and deliver a counterfeit controlled substance.

CASE DISCUSSION

Kendall demonstrates a pattern of disregard for and violation of the rights of others around him since he was a young child. He has failed to conform to social norms by participating in unlawful behavior and conning others. He demonstrates a pattern of impulsivity, irritability, and aggressiveness. There is no apparent remorse for his behavior; in fact, there is rationalization of it. Kendall seems to have a real fear of abandonment as evidenced by his behavior with the counselor in the first meeting, as well as affective instability and mood reactivity. The transitions from being charming to aggressive as reported by his parents and his relationship with the old roommate are evidence of inappropriate expressions of anger as well as instability in interpersonal relationships. There is also a pattern of substance use resulting in admission to opioid maintenance treatment. Based upon all of the gathered information, the counselor believes the appropriate diagnoses to be:

1. Opioid use disorder, severe, in sustained remission, on agonist therapy;
2. Antisocial personality disorder; and
3. Borderline personality disorder.

The counselor working with Kendall believes that primary treatments that are most appropriate for his plan of care include ongoing opioid maintenance therapy and outpatient treatment using DBT with weekly check-in appointments. There is a clear understanding between Kendall and his counselor that when Kendall threatens suicide, the next step is a referral to the local hospital emergency department, potentially with involuntary commitment. Kendall is asked to complete a treatment contract stating what he will participate in and what the consequences are for nonparticipation. Kendall is expected to have individual check-in sessions once a week and to attend group counseling twice per week to maintain access to opioid maintenance medication. He is also expected to attend at least two 12-step meetings in his community per week while he is in treatment. Goals for his care include improving the relationship with his parents as well as working toward employment and financial stability. Relatedly, Kendall is to follow the parameters set forth by his probation office to minimize future legal problems.

CHAPTER SUMMARY

PDs and SUDs often co-occur. In order to diagnose a PD, there must be evidence of a pervasive pattern of symptoms over time. Several symptoms of PDs and SUDs overlap, so it is important to understand which symptoms are a result of the substance use and which symptoms are characteristics of the person's personality structure regardless of whether a substance is in their body. A primary factor in determining diagnoses is doing a thorough assessment that includes a discussion of early life factors to establish a timeline for symptom development.

Assessment should not only evaluate for the presence of symptoms, but it should also review the impact that the symptoms have on the client's level of functioning. In identifying the clinical impact or significance, counselors can properly determine the appropriate level of care as well as design an effective treatment plan. CBTs in general, and DBT specifically, are useful treatment modalities for both SUDs and PDs. Establishment of a support group is particularly helpful for both classes of disorders, and involvement in the 12-step fellowship or other recovery-focused support group outside of treatment may be a good way to increase the size of a support network very quickly. Additionally, it may be helpful for the clinician to also utilize 12-step facilitation in the treatment setting.

DISCUSSION QUESTIONS

1. Given the relationship between suicidal ideation and borderline personality disorder, what are important factors for suicide assessment when there are co-occurring SUDs?
2. How do you differentiate between the pattern of behavior/personality characteristics associated with substance use and the presence of a true personality disorder?
3. Considering your specialty treatment setting, which screening or assessment instruments might best meet the needs of your current or future clients?
4. How can DBT and 12-step facilitation work together to enhance the quality and efficacy of client care for co-occurring SUDs and PDs?
5. What do you still need to learn more about when it comes to the intersection of PDs and addictive disorders?

REFERENCES

Alegria, A. A., Blanco, C., Petry, N. M., Skodol, A. E., Liu, S.-M., Grant, B., & Hasin, D. (2013). Sex differences in antisocial personality disorder: Results from the national epidemiological survey on alcohol and related conditions. *Personality Disorders*, *4*(3), 214–222. https://doi.org/10.1037/a0031681

American Psychiatric Association. (2013). *Diagnostic and statistical manual of mental disorders: DSM-5* (5th ed.). American Psychiatric Association.

American Psychiatric Association. & American Psychiatric Association. (2000). *Diagnostic and statistical manual of mental disorders: DSM-IV-TR.* (4th ed., text revision.). American Psychiatric Association.

Anderson, T. L., & Mott, J. A. (1998). Drug-related identity change: Theoretical development and empirical assessment. *Journal of Drug Issues*, *28*(2), 299–328. a9h.

Atkins, C. (2014). *Co-occurring disorders: Integrated assessment and treatment of substance use and mental disorders* (1st ed.). Premier Publishing and Media.

Atkins, C. (2021). *Co-occurring disorders: A whole-person approach to the assessment and treatment of substance use and mental disorders* (2nd ed.). PESI.

Babor, T. F., Higgins-Biddle, J. C., Saunders, J. B., & Monteiro, M. G. (2001). *The alcohol use disorders identification test. Guidelines for use in primary health care.* (Vol. 2). World Health Organization.

Bogenschutz, M. P., Rice, S. L., Tonigan, J. S., Vogel, H. S., Nowinski, J., Hume, D., & Arenella, P. B. (2014). 12-step facilitation for the dually diagnosed: A randomized clinical trial. *Journal of Substance Abuse Treatment*, *46*(4), 403–411.

Bornovalova, M. A., & Daughters, S. B. (2007). How does dialectical behavior therapy facilitate treatment retention among individuals with comorbid borderline personality disorder and substance use disorders? *Clinical Psychology Review*, *27*(8), 923–943.

Chen, F., Yang, H., Bulut, O., Cui, Y., & Xin, T. (2019). Examining the relation of personality factors to substance use disorder by explanatory item response modeling of *DSM-5* symptoms. *PLoS ONE*, *14*(6), 1–17.

Day, J. K., Fish, J. N., Perez-Brumer, A., Hatzenbuehler, M. L., & Russell, S. T. (2017). Transgender youth substance use disparities: Results from a population-based sample. *The Journal of Adolescent Health:*

Official Publication of the Society for Adolescent Medicine, 61(6), 729–735. https://doi.org/10.1016/j.jadohealth.2017.06.024

Ellis, A. 1913–2007. (1996). *Better, deeper, and more enduring brief therapy: The rational emotive behavior therapy approach*. Brunner/Mazel Publishers.

Faridhosseini, F., Saghebi, A., & Mirzadeh, M. (2019). Personality disorders and substance use disorders: A narrative review. *Electronic Physician, 11*(2), 7558–7563.

Fureman, B., Parikh, G., Braga, A., & McLellan, A. T. (1990). *Addiction Severity Index: A guide to training and supervising ASI interviews based on the past ten years* (5th ed.). The University of Pennsylvania/Veterans Administration, Center for Studios of Addiction.

Giannelli, E., Gold, C., Bieleninik, L., Ghetti, C., & Gelo, O. C. G. (2019). Dialectical behaviour therapy and 12-step programmes for substance use disorder: A systematic review and meta-analysis. *Counselling & Psychotherapy Research, 19*(3), 274–285. Academic Search Complete.

Grant, B. F., Saha, T. D., Ruan, W. J., Goldstein, R. B., Chou, S. P., Jung, J., Zhang, H., Smith, S. M., Pickering, R. P., Huang, B., & Hasin, D. S. (2016). Epidemiology of *DSM-5* drug use disorder: Results from the national epidemiologic survey on alcohol and related conditions-III. *JAMA Psychiatry, 73*(1), 39–47. https://doi.org/10.1001/jamapsychiatry.2015.2132

Gutierrez, P. M., Osman, A., Barrios, F. X., & Kopper, B. A. (2001). Development and initial validation of the self-harm behavior questionnaire. *Journal of Personality Assessment, 77*(3), 475–490. https://doi.org/10.1207/S15327752JPA7703_08

Hayes, S. C., Strosahl, K., Wilson, K. G., Strosahl, K., & Wilson, K. G. (2012). *Acceptance and commitment therapy: The process and practice of mindful change* (2nd ed.). Guilford Press.

Heath, L. M., Laporte, L., Paris, J., Hamdullahpur, K., & Gill, K. J. (2018). Substance misuse is associated with increased psychiatric severity among treatment-seeking individuals with borderline personality disorder. *Journal of Personality Disorders, 32*(5), 694–708.

Hershberger, A. R., Um, M., & Cyders, M. A. (2017). The relationship between the UPPS-P impulsive personality traits and substance use psychotherapy outcomes: A meta-analysis. *Drug & Alcohol Dependence, 178*, 408–416.

Høye, A., Jacobsen, B. K., Bramness, J. G., Nesvåg, R., Reichborn-Kjennerud, T., & Heiberg, I. (2021). Total and cause-specific mortality in patients with personality disorders: The association between comorbid severe mental illness and substance use disorders. *Social Psychiatry and Psychiatric Epidemiology, 56*(10), 1809–1819. https://doi.org/10.1007/s00127-021-02055-3

Karterud, S., Arefjord, N., Andresen, N. E., & Pedersen, G. (2009). Substance use disorders among personality disordered patients admitted for day hospital treatment. Implications for service developments. *Nordic Journal of Psychiatry, 63*(1), 57–63.

Korsgaard, H. O., Torgersen, S., Wentzel-Larsen, T., & Ulberg, R. (2016). Substance abuse and personality disorder comorbidity in adolescent outpatients: Are girls more severely ill than boys? *Child & Adolescent Psychiatry & Mental Health, 10*, 1–9.

Linehan, M. M. (1993). *Cognitive-behavioral treatment of borderline personality disorder*. The Guilford Press.

Linehan, M. M. (2015). *DBT skills training manual* (2nd ed.). The Guilford Press.

Linehan, M. M., Heard, H. L., & Armstrong, H. E. (1993). Naturalistic follow-up of a behavioral treatment for chronically parasuicidal borderline patients. *Archives of General Psychiatry, 50*(12), 971–974. https://doi.org/10.1001/archpsyc.1993.01820240055007

Linehan, M. M., Schmidt, H., Dimeff, L. A., Craft, J. C., Kanter, J., Comtois, K. A., (1999). Dialectical behavior therapy for patients with borderline personality disorder and drug-dependence. *American Journal on Addictions, 8*(4), 279–292.

Linehan, M. M., Tutek, D. A., & Dimeff, L. A. (1996). *Comprehensive validation therapy for substance abusers*. University of Washington.

Loranger, A. W., Sartorius, N., Andreoli, A., Berger, P., Buchheim, P., Channabasavanna, S. M., Coid, B., Dahl, A., Diekstra, R. F. W., Ferguson, B., Jacobsberg, L. B., Mombour, W., Pull, C., Ono, Y., & Regier, D. A. (1994). The international personality disorder examination: The World Health Organization/alcohol, drug abuse, and mental health administration international pilot study of personality disorders. *Archives of General Psychiatry, 51*(3), 215–224. https://doi.org/10.1001/archpsyc.1994.03950030051005

Magallón-Neri, E. M., Forns, M., Canalda, G., De La Fuente, J. E., García, R., González, E., Lara, A., & Castro-Fornieles, J. (2013). Usefulness of the International Personality Disorder Examination screening questionnaire for borderline and impulsive personality pathology in adolescents. *Comprehensive Psychiatry, 54*, 301–308. 10.1016/j.comppsych.2013.07.064

Mathias, R. (1996). Specialized approach shows promise for treating antisocial drug abuse patients. *NIDA Notes, 11*(4), 3–5.

McLellan, A. T., Kushner, H., Metzger, D., Peters, R., Smith, I., Grissom, G., Pettinati, H., & Argeriou, M. (1992). The fifth edition of the addiction severity index. *Journal of Substance Abuse Treatment, 9*(3), 199–213. https://doi.org/10.1016/0740-5472(92)90062-S

McLellan, A. T., Luborsky, L., Woody, G. E., & O'Brien, C. P. (1980). An improved diagnostic evaluation instrument for substance abuse patients: The addiction severity index. *The Journal of Nervous and Mental Disease, 168*(1). https://journals.lww.com/jonmd/Fulltext/1980/01000/An_Improved_Diagnostic_Evaluation_Instrument_for.6.aspx

McNair, D. M., Lorr, M., & Droppleman, L. F. (1971). *Profile of Mood States (POMS)*. Educational and Industrial Testing Service.

Miller, W. R., & Del Boca, F. K. (1994). Measurement of drinking behavior using the form 90 family of instruments. *Journal of Studies on Alcohol, Supplement, s12*, 112–118. https://doi.org/10.15288/jsas.1994.s12.112

Miller, W. R., & Rollnick, S. (2002). *Motivational interviewing: Preparing people for change* (2nd ed.). Guilford Press.

Miller, W. R., & Rollnick, S. (2013). *Motivational interviewing: Helping people change* (3rd ed.). Guilford Press.

Moggi, F., Giovanoli, A., Buri, C., Moos, B. S., & Moos, R. H. (2010). Patients with substance use and personality disorders: A comparison of patient characteristics, treatment process, and outcomes in Swiss and U.S. substance use disorder programs. *American Journal of Drug & Alcohol Abuse, 36*(1), 66–72.

Morey, L. C. (1991). *The Personality Assessment Inventory Professional Manual*. Psychological Assessment Resources.

Newcomb, M. E., Hill, R., Buehler, K., Ryan, D. T., Whitton, S. W., & Mustanski, B. (2020). High burden of mental health problems, substance use, violence, and related psychosocial factors in transgender, non-binary, and gender diverse youth and young adults. *Archives of Sexual Behavior, 49*(2), 645–659. https://doi.org/10.1007/s10508-019-01533-9

Oldham, J. M. (2006). Borderline personality disorder and suicidality. *American Journal of Psychiatry, 163*(1), 20–26. https://doi.org/10.1176/appi.ajp.163.1.20

Owens, M. D., Nason, E., & Yeater, E. (2018). Dialectical behavior therapy for multiple treatment targets: A case study of a male with comorbid personality and substance use disorders. *International Journal of Mental Health & Addiction, 16*(2), 436–450.

Panos, P. T., Jackson, J. W., Hasan, O., & Panos, A. (2013). Meta-analyses and systematic review assessing the efficacy of dialectical behavior therapy (DBT). *Research on Social Work Practice, 24*(2), 213–223. https://doi.org/10.1177/1049731513503047

Parmar, A., & Kaloiya, G. (2018). Comorbidity of personality disorder among substance use disorder patients: A narrative review. *Indian Journal of Psychological Medicine, 40*(6), 517–527.

Patton, J. H., Stanford, M. S., & Barratt, E. S. (1995). Factor structure of the Barratt Impulsiveness Scale. *Journal of Clinical Psychology, 51*(6), 768–774.

Pfohl, B., Blum, N., & Zimmerman, M. (1997). *The Structured Interview for DSM-IV Personality (SIDP-IV)*. American Psychiatric Press.

Sheehan, L., Nieweglowski, K., & Corrigan, P. (2016). The stigma of personality disorders. *Current Psychiatry Reports, 18*(11). https://doi.org/10.1007/s11920-015-0654-1

Sher, L., Siever, L. J., Goodman, M., McNamara, M., Hazlett, E. A., Koenigsberg, H. W., & New, A. S. (2015). Gender differences in the clinical characteristics and psychiatric comorbidity in patients with antisocial personality disorder. *Psychiatry Research, 229*(3), 685–689.

Skinner, H. A. (1982). The drug abuse screening test. *Addictive Behaviors, 7*(4), 363–371. https://doi.org/10.1016/0306-4603(82)90005-3

Straussner, S. L. A., & Nemenzik, J. M. (2007). Co-occurring substance use and personality disorders: Current thinking on etiology, diagnosis, and treatment. *Journal of Social Work Practice in the Addictions, 7*(1-2), 5–23. https://doi.org/10.1300/J160v07n01_02

Substance Abuse and Mental Health Services Administration. (2020). *TIP 42: Substance use treatment for persons with co-occurring disorders.* https://store.samhsa.gov/product/tip-42-substance-use-treatment-persons-co-occurring-disorders/PEP20-02-01-004

Sulzer, S. H., Prevedel, S., Barrett, T., Voss, M. W., Manning, C., & Madden, E. F. (2021). Professional education to reduce provider stigma toward harm reduction and pharmacotherapy. *Drugs: Education, Prevention and Policy.* https://doi.org/10.1080/09687637.2021.1936457

Trull, T. J., Jahng, S., Tomko, R. L., Wood, P. K., & Sher, K. J. (2010). Revised NESARC personality disorder diagnoses: Gender, prevalence, and comorbidity with substance dependence disorders. *Journal of Personality Disorders, 24*(4), 412–426. https://doi.org/10.1521/pedi.2010.24.4.412

Vélez-Moreno, A., Rojas, A., Rivera, F., Fernández-Calderón, F., Torrico-Linares, E., Ramírez-López, J., González-Saiz, F., & Lozano, Ó. (2017). The impact of personality disorders and severity of dependence in psychosocial problems. *International Journal of Mental Health & Addiction, 15*(5), 1008–1022.

Verheul, R., & Van Den Brink, W. (2005). Causal pathways between substance use disorders and personality pathology. *Australian Psychologist, 40*(2), 127–136.

Vest, N., & Tragesser, S. (2019). Borderline features and prescription opioid misuse in a substance use disorder treatment sample. *Substance Use & Misuse, 54*(1), 166–175.

Whitton, S. W., Dyar, C., Mustanski, B., & Newcomb, M. E. (2019). Intimate partner violence experiences of sexual and gender minority adolescents and young adults assigned female at birth. *Psychology of Women Quarterly, 43*(2), 232–249. https://doi.org/10.1177/0361684319838972

Wnuk, S., McMain, S., Links, P. S., Habinski, L., Murray, J., & Guimond, T. (2013). Factors related to dropout from treatment in two outpatient treatments for borderline personality disorder. *Journal of Personality Disorders, 27*(6), 716–726. https://doi.org/10.1521/pedi_2013_27_106

Zanarini, M. C., Gunderson, J. G., Frankenburg, F. R., & Chauncey, D. L. (1989). The revised diagnostic interview for borderlines: discriminating BPD from other Axis II disorders. *Journal of Personality Disorders, 3*(1), 10–18. https://doi.org/10.1521/pedi.1989.3.1.10

SECTION IV

SPECIAL POPULATIONS

CHAPTER 15

LIFESPAN DEVELOPMENT AND CO-OCCURRING DISORDERS

ANDREA JUNE, CAROLYN R. FALLAHI, AND CARISSA D. DAIGLE

LEARNING OBJECTIVES

After reading this chapter, you will be able to:
- Recognize age-specific risk factors in the development of a substance use disorder (SUD).
- Explain relevant diagnostic considerations for co-occurring disorders (CODs) among children, adolescents, and older adults.
- Identify empirically informed adaptations to therapeutic interventions to maximize successful outcomes across the lifespan.
- Describe the importance of the intersectionality of age with other multicultural considerations when working from a lifespan perspective.
- Recognize and address common ethical and legal considerations when working with children, adolescents, and older adults.

INTRODUCTION

Age is an important contextual variable within multicultural competence; its influence is present in the complex intersectionality that overlays co-occurring disorders (CODs) present in clients. The purpose of this chapter is to provide a general foundation for the impact of developmental age on the presentation and treatment of CODs. Given the more sizeable foundation of knowledge about CODs in adulthood, this chapter highlights current understanding of how those of the younger and older lifespans compare. Admittedly, there are limitations to providing overall group guidelines by chronological age rather than functional ability or other biopsychosocial markers; therefore, counselors are encouraged to be mindful of the heterogeneity within any group. Developmental considerations on the scope of CODs are addressed first, followed by treatment, multicultural, and then legal and ethical considerations. A case example and discussion conclude the chapter.

PREVALENCE, STATISTICS, AND DEMOGRAPHICS

TABLE 15.1 Prevalence Statistics Reported: 2019 Percentages

	ALCOHOL USE	MARIJUANA USE	Rx PAIN RELIEVER MISUSE	ILLICIT DRUG USE[a]	SUD[b]	MENTAL ILLNESS DISORDER	CO-OC-CURRING DISORDERS
AGE GROUP (YEARS)							
Adolescents (12–17)	9.4	13.2	2.3	7.5	4.5	15.7	1.7
Young adults (18–25)	54.3	35.4	5.2	17.2	14.1	29.4	7.6
Middle adults (26–49)	61.6	21.7	4.7	10.9	6.7[c]	25.0	5.2
Middle adults (50+)	49.2	9.5	2.3	4.3	-	14.1	1.5[d]
Older adults (65+)	43.9	5.1	1.7	2.7	-	11.8	-
RACE (18+ YEARS)							
White	74.0	55.1	3.8	9.2	2.9	22.2	1.5
Black	61.1	46.1	3.3	6.7	3.3	17.3	1.2
American Indian or Alaska Native	53.4	52.2	5.3	10.5	4.5	18.7	1.5
Native Hawaiian or Pacific Islander	55.1	42.7	2.3	5.9	2.9	16.6	1.3
Asian	54.3	21.5	1.8	5.2	1.7	14.4	0.9
Hispanic or Latino	64.1	37.0	3.8	8.6	2.9	18.0	1.2
Two or more races	72.3	66.7	5.5	13.8	5.9	31.7	3.1

Note: All results are reported as percentages from the 2019 National Survey on Drug Use and Health (Center for Behavioral Health Statistics and Quality, 2020).
[a] Illicit drug use excludes marijuana.
[b] SUD (substance use disorder) includes illicit drugs or alcohol.
[c] Reported only for 26+ age group.
[d] Reported only for 50+ age group.

SUBSTANCE USE AMONG ADOLESCENTS

Significant decreases in alcohol use in adolescence has been reported across all grade levels from 8th grade through 12th grade. The Monitoring the Future Survey (MTF) is a nationwide survey that is administered annually to 8th-, 10th-, and 12th-grade students since 1975 (National Institute on Drug Abuse [NIDA], 2020). The MTF examines alcohol and substance use and abuse as well as attitudes among adolescent students. Heavy episodic or binge drinking for adolescents born in the 1990s is lower than those during earlier periods of time. While vaping of nicotine and cannabis among 10th and 12th graders was increasing rapidly over the last few years, it seems to have leveled off in 2020. Marijuana is the most commonly used illicit substance by adolescents. Survey data administered before the COVID-19 pandemic revealed increases in amphetamine use, inhalant use, and over-the-counter cough medicines. Adolescents using other illicit drugs remains low for 12th graders.

Kuhn (2015) reviewed research on adolescent prevalence rates for substance use and found that adolescent males and females start using substances at similar rates, but once they start using, males' rates of substance use increase faster. NIDA (2003) reported on the work of Dr. William Latimer and colleagues who found that male teenagers who abused substances were more likely to be diagnosed with disruptive disorders (e.g., attention deficit/hyperactivity disorder [ADHD] or conduct disorder [CD]) and female abusers with depressive disorders. Large numbers of their samples were diagnosed with alcohol use disorders (AUDs), substance use disorders (SUDs), and polysubstance disorders. Girls were more likely to be diagnosed with abuse or dependence on one drug, while boys showed abuse or dependence on more than one drug. In a study examining racial and ethnic differences in 7th and 8th graders in California, 29.2% of 8th graders reported lifetime alcohol use, similar to the rates of other national studies (Shih et al., 2010).

SUBSTANCE USE INITIATION AND COURSE CONSIDERATIONS

Adolescence Into Adulthood

In a study based on substance abuse treatment admissions in 2011 (Substance Abuse and Mental Health Services Administration [SAMHSA], 2014), 74% of those in treatment initiated their use of substances at the age of 11 or younger while only 30.4% started using substances at 25 or older. Adolescents who start using alcohol or substances before the age of 18 is one of the significant risk factors in developing an AUD or SUD in adulthood as compared to those who exhibit delayed initiation (Dawson et al., 2008; King & Chassin, 2007). Later alcohol and substance use is more normative, possibly serving as a protective factor against developing an addiction in adulthood.

Experimentation with alcohol often begins during early adolescence (Brown et al., 2008). The age group that represents the greatest risk of developing an AUD involves those individuals in late adolescence who are aged 18 to 20. The increase in drinking often parallels the increased time away from home and time away from parental oversight and influence, older sibling influences, and peer influences (Brown et al., 2008). During the transition from high school to college, more experiences with binge drinking are seen. Brown et al. (2008) also reported that those in later adolescence who work 20 or more hours per week, get married, or become a parent are at increased risk for developing an AUD.

Research has demonstrated that serious substance users in adulthood follow a progression from high school to adulthood (Mackesy-Amiti et al., 1997; Stenbacka, 2003). Serious users may follow a typical pattern with the use of alcohol and cannabis followed by illicit drug use, or follow an atypical pattern that is often associated with earlier initiation of illicit drugs other than cannabis and a pattern in adolescence of increasing use of illicit substances through adulthood to more lifelong drug involvement. The trajectory of use may also influence adulthood patterns of substance use with the timing of the onset (earlier is more problematic) and changing the trajectory of the pattern of use (increasing the amounts used more quickly) can lead to more problematic use in adulthood (Nelson et al., 2015). Normative trends for alcohol and cannabis have supported the idea that the level of substance use at age 18 is an important predictor of use in adulthood (Patrick et al., 2011).

Other risk factors may include: (a) familial substance abuse, increasing the risk 10 to 50 times if there is a parent who abuses substances (Jennison & Johnson, 2001); (b) a history of adverse childhood experiences (ACES) or abuse (Khoury et al., 2010); (c) a history of divorce or partner substance use (Agrawal et al., 2005); and (d) being a member of a sexual minority (Brecht et al., 2004).

Middle Adulthood

For the majority of adults who fall in the middle adulthood range, substance use decreases during this age period (M. R. Lee et al., 2010). This is referred to as the aging out pattern (Sarabia & Martin, 2013). However, the proportion of adults still using and abusing alcohol and illicit substances at the age of 35 is still relatively high for both males and females (Merline et al., 2004).

The reduction in substance use varies by both sex and race. Vogt Yuan (2011) found that Blacks have lower rates of substance use in adolescence and early adulthood as compared to Whites, but by middle adulthood, those rates are similar, possibly explained by a lifetime of disadvantages. M. R. Lee et al. (2010) found no differences in the aging out process for alcohol use among Black and White women. Cannabis use decreased 8% every 10 years for Black women and 4% for White women, while Black women decreased their illicit drug use by 8% every 10 years and White women maintained their same level of use.

Schulenberg et al. (2016) found that in early midlife at the age of 35, binge drinking and cannabis use at 18 were the strongest predictors of alcohol and cannabis use disorders. Other predictors included overall health, satisfaction with a spouse or partner, and cognitive difficulties which included trouble remembering or learning new things, and/or difficulties in thinking or concentration.

For middle-aged adults, increases in cannabis use and prescription opioid misuse (and for some, subsequent heroin use) are on the rise (NIDA, 2019). This trend may be explained by the increases in prescriptions for pain relief as well as past experiences with recreational drug use. Furthermore, as mental health disorders go untreated, it is not uncommon for individuals to turn to substances for relief of their symptoms.

Etiological explanations for substance use (specifically nicotine, alcohol, and cannabis) find that environmental influences are strongest in adolescence, with familial environmental influences more strongly influencing cannabis use as compared to alcohol use (Kendler et al., 2008). As these participants got older, by middle adulthood, genetic influences have a stronger influence on substance use. Further, victimization during childhood increases the risk for substance use in middle adulthood (Spatz Widom et al., 2006).

DIAGNOSTIC CONSIDERATIONS: ADOLESCENTS AND YOUNG ADULTS

SUBSTANCE USE DISORDER CRITERIA CLASSIFICATION ISSUES

Several classification issues exist when utilizing the *Diagnostic and Statistical Manual of Mental Disorders, Fifth Edition* (*DSM-5*; American Psychiatric Association [APA], 2013) to diagnose a SUD in adolescents. Much of the research on the SUD classification in the *DSM-5* involved adults, not adolescents (SAMHSA, 2016). Furthermore, no studies were conducted on children. The merging of the abuse and dependence categories and the elimination of the legal criterion in the *DSM-5* seems to have improved the validity of the SUD for adolescents. Some criteria, such as tolerance, are overidentified in adolescents when compared to adults (C. T. Lee et al., 2011). Tolerance takes years to potentially develop in adults but is more rapidly acquired in adolescence. In addition, adolescents are more likely to over-endorse time spent on acquiring a drug than adults. Finally, maturation may play a role in adolescents over-endorsing some criteria (e.g., hazardous use). Adolescents are more impulsive and less likely to think about the long-term consequences of their behavior as compared to adults.

CO-OCCURRING MENTAL AND SUBSTANCE USE DISORDERS

Kaminer et al. (2007) noted that psychiatric comorbidity with SUDs (or dual-diagnosis) is "the rule rather than the exception" (p. 32).

MOOD DISORDERS

By late adolescence, approximately 10% to 20% of adolescents will experience a major depressive episode (MDE) and 25% subthreshold symptoms of depression. Approximately 358,000 adolescents, or 1.5%, had a co-occurring SUD and MDE in the past year (SAMHSA, 2019). Gottfredson and Hussong (2011) found that adolescents with negative affect endorsed symptoms of sadness, worry, anger, and stress, and were more at risk for daily drinking when they lacked parental involvement once they started high school. Early-onset bipolar disorder (BD), or pediatric BD, occurs in childhood or adolescence in approximately 50% of individuals and is associated with a poorer prognosis in adulthood (Miklowitz, 2012). Adolescents with BD are five times more likely to develop a co-occurring SUD. Notably, adolescents may develop a SUD before or after a diagnosis of BD. A meta-analytic review of the literature also shows significant differences between subthreshold BD in children and adolescents when compared to non-BD controls, including higher rates of comorbid disruptive behavior, mood, and SUDs (Vaudreuil et al., 2019).

ANXIETY DISORDERS

Like mood disorders, the prevalence of co-occurring anxiety disorders and SUDs is high. Between 21.9% and 24.1% report the use of alcohol and/or illicit drugs as a method for dealing with their symptoms according to a narrative review performed across all age groups (Turner et al., 2018). Wu et al. (2010), however, found that increases in SUDs depended upon the specific type of anxiety disorder. These authors report that social phobia (now considered as social anxiety disorder in the *DSM-5*) was more prevalent in boys and associated with tobacco use, where social phobia was negatively associated for girls. Other anxiety disorders, including agoraphobia, generalized anxiety disorder, obsessive-compulsive disorder, and separation anxiety disorders, were associated with an increase in SUDs for girls, including smoking, drinking, and illicit substance use (Wu et al., 2010). In contrast, other studies have found that anxiety may protect adolescents from SUDs by avoiding experimentation or other risky behaviors (Nelemans et al., 2014; Siebenbruner, et al., 2006).

ATTENTION DEFICIT/HYPERACTIVITY DISORDER AND CONDUCT DISORDER

The prevalence of ADHD is 6% to 9%, with children and adolescents showing more relationship problems and more academic underachievement compared to their non-ADHD peers (Merikangas et al., 2010). In addition to comorbidities with substance use, those diagnosed with ADHD are frequently diagnosed with learning disabilities and other psychological problems across the lifespan, including oppositional defiant disorder, CD, and mood and anxiety disorders (Biederman et al., 2006; Wilens & Spencer, 2010). Those adolescents diagnosed with ADHD are at an increased risk to abuse marijuana and alcohol, or a combination of the two. If also diagnosed with CD, those rates rise significantly, up to four times the prevalence. They often have a history of cigarette smoking as well as exhibit early signs of having a SUD that runs a chronic course over time. The risk for early onset and atypical heavy substance use in adolescence and adulthood increases with a diagnosis of ADHD and/or oppositional defiant disorder (ODD)/CD (Howard et al., 2020).

Adolescent males who show symptoms of CD often increase their use of substances, especially alcohol and marijuana (Cerdá et al., 2016). Interestingly, these researchers found that when alcohol use increased, so too did their risk for anxiety disorders. This co-occurrence is possibly due to an increase in social or economic problems (e.g., arrests, crime, unemployment) or neurochemical changes that possibly increase the risk for vulnerability to an anxiety disorder. Increased drinking was found in early to mid adolescence, where an increase in marijuana was found in later adolescence.

Posttraumatic Stress Disorder

Early ACEs, such as maltreatment, victimization, neglect, and exposure to parent stress and substance use, place adolescents at risk for SUDs (McCrory & Mayes, 2015). These experiences might set the stage for problems with emotional regulation or impulsivity (Chambers et al., 2003), therefore adding to their vulnerabilities. Childhood and adolescents with histories of traumatic experiences had an increased rate of SUDs, specifically, 39% alcohol, 34.1% cocaine, 6.2% heroin or opiates, and 44.8% cannabis (Khoury et al., 2010). Conversely, adolescents who experienced early substance use initiation placed them at increased risk for further traumatic experiences (including sexual assault and further victimization) often because early substance use was related to greater risk taking and delinquent peer relationships (Kingston & Raghavan, 2009). Furthermore, the prevalence of posttraumatic stress disorder (PTSD) and trauma are significantly high in those diagnosed with SUDs (Gielen et al., 2012).

Psychotic Disorders

Substance misuse was twice that of the general population in a group of young people with first-episode psychosis (Barnett et al., 2007). Increased rates for young males were reported with an increased chance of being diagnosed with a SUD over time (Cantwell et al., 1999). In a study examining first-episode psychosis, 62% of patients in an early psychosis prevention program were diagnosed with SUDs (Lambert et al., 2005). The most prevalent combination of illicit drugs used included cannabis, alcohol, and amphetamines. It is not known why certain people can stop using substances and their symptoms will abate, and yet others will go on to have unrelenting symptoms. There is widespread acceptance that heavy and long-term cannabis use can increase the risk of psychosis, with psychotic symptoms worsening if substances are used over a long-term basis (Barkus & Murray, 2010).

DIAGNOSTIC CONSIDERATIONS: OLDER ADULTS
A GLOBAL TREND OF AGING

Gerontologists define older adulthood beginning at 65 years and further delineate our growing longevity into the young old (65–74 years), the old-old (75–84 years), and the oldest-old (85+

years) to acknowledge the varied biopsychosocial needs. Worldwide, due to increases in education, technology, and medicine, people are living longer. The population of individuals in the United States age 65 and older numbered 52.4 million in 2018, which represents an increase of 35% since 2008 (Administration for Community Living [ACL], 2020). And it is expected that this trend will only continue. By 2040, it is estimated there will be about 80.8 million older adults, more than twice as many as in 2000 (ACL, 2020). Consistently, older women outnumber older men (29.1 million to 23.3 million in 2018), and nearly one in 10 older adults live below the poverty level (ACL, 2020). Society must take the mental health and substance use needs of this growing demographic seriously.

SUBSTANCE USE PREVALENCE

Historically, older adults have had lower levels of reported substance abuse. Many argue, however, that substance abuse among older adults has been under identified, ignored, or misdiagnosed for decades (Benshoff et al., 2003; Carew & Comiskey, 2018; Kuerbis et al., 2014). Several often overlapping factors may account for this assertion of a hidden problem. Healthcare professionals, out of misinformation or bias, may inadequately assess for substance use among older adults. Differential diagnosis is complicated by shared symptoms common in SUDs as well as in cognitive disorders and other age-related problems (e.g., falls, poor memory, slurred speech, poor personal hygiene), and, therefore, may be overlooked. Even when carefully assessed, the *DSM-5* diagnostic criteria's emphasis on the impact of use on social and occupational responsibilities may contribute to subclinical findings because these may be less apparent among older adults whose lives may be less public than younger adults. Family members may wrongly use age to explain away problematic drinking behavior (e.g., "*At his age Grandpa can drink whatever he wants*") or be ashamed of it. Because of these potential variables, substance abuse among older adults may not be brought to a healthcare professional's attention. Additionally, older adults themselves may not fully understand or recognize the symptoms as a disorder and appreciate the negative health impact (Segal et al., 2018).

Acknowledging the limitations to our current understanding of the full scope of the problem, the mental health literature emphasizes that the need for services among this population is growing (Carew & Comiskey, 2018). With the combined surge in older adults and the higher reported use rates among the "Baby Boomer" cohort (i.e., people born between 1946 and 1964), researchers are predicting higher rates of unhealthy use (Choi et al., 2015; Han & Moore, 2018). Distinct from previous generations, the Baby Boomer generation came of age during a period of changing attitudes toward drug and alcohol use, with the prevalence rates of SUD remaining high among this group as they age (Moore et al., 2009; SAMHSA, 2013).

ALCOHOL

Among adults and older adults alike, alcohol is the most commonly used and abused substance (Moore et al., 2009; Segal et al., 2018). Most of the available information on substance use among older adults focuses on alcohol abuse. While lower than that of younger adults, prevalence rates for at-risk and problem drinking among older adults range between 1% and 16%, with higher levels among men (Barry & Blow, 2016; Kuerbis et al., 2014; Lehmann & Fingerhood, 2018). Estimates vary based on the definitions of "older adult," "at-risk," or "problem" drinking, as well as on the year and methodology of collecting the estimates. The National Institute on Alcohol Abuse and Alcoholism (NIAAA), a commonly referenced source of drinking definitions, recommends that adults aged 60 years or older consume no more than two drinks on a given day for men and no more than one drink on a given day for women (U.S. Department of Agriculture & U.S. Department of Health and Human Services, 2020). Recommendations for alcohol intake are often lower for older adults compared to younger adults due to normative age-related changes in the body's response to chemical substances. These changes in absorption and metabolism make older adults more susceptible to the adverse effects of alcohol.

OVER-THE-COUNTER AND PRESCRIPTION DRUGS

Where information is available on drug use, it has mainly highlighted over-the-counter (OTC) and prescription drugs because these tend to be more commonly used among older adults compared to younger adults. As one study found, 87% of older adults used at least one of these substances while 36% used five or more (Qato et al., 2016). Medical exposure to prescription drugs with abuse potential has been identified as a strong risk factor associated with abuse (Simoni-Wastila & Yang, 2006). And, while OTC substances are available without a prescription, use in sufficient quantities without the oversight of a prescriber can lead to adverse health outcomes. Older adults are among the most likely to receive a prescription for benzodiazepines and opioids—substances with high abuse potential (Lehmann & Fingerhood, 2018). In addition to using benzodiazepines for the treatment of anxiety, these substances are often prescribed for sleep disturbance and pain (conditions that disproportionately impact older adults) and older adults are more likely to experience chronic health conditions and visit their primary medical provider (Centers for Disease Control and Prevention [CDC], 2013; Patel et al., 2013). Moreover, out of misinformation or bias, providers may be more likely with an older adult than a younger adult to prescribe a solution rather than advise an environmental or behavioral intervention (e.g., akin to the belief that old dogs cannot learn new tricks) when effective therapeutic intervention exists for older adults (American Psychological Association, 2014).

Polypharmacy, prescriptions written by multiple different providers without collaboration, is also more common among older adults and is associated with increased risk for abuse and adverse health outcomes such as delirium, falls or other accidents, and even mortality (Maree et al., 2016). It is worth mentioning again that older adults are more susceptible than younger adults to adverse drug reactions, drug interactions, and drug toxicity due to changes in the way the aging body responds to chemical substances. For example, older adults prescribed benzodiazepines are more sensitive to its side effects (e.g., dizziness, fall risk). Additionally, this class of drugs can lead to delirium and more lasting impacts on cognitive functioning (Salmon & Forester, 2012).

ONSET OF CHRONIC SUBSTANCE USE

Harmful substance use among older adults is often categorized into two groups: (a) those with chronic use across the lifespan and (b) those with later-life onset. These two distinct patterns of use have been most clearly evidenced among older abusers of alcohol; however, this trend has also been found with other substances as well (Edgell et al., 2000; Gfroerer et al., 2003; Lehmann & Fingerhood, 2018). Later-life onset is more commonly associated with stressful life events such as loss of loved ones, change in living situation, retirement, a new impairment affecting daily functioning, or social isolation. Chronic users began before the age of 60 and are more likely to have higher co-occurring psychiatric and medical disorders, more serious financial and legal trouble, previous treatment history, and a less solid social support system (Salmon & Forester, 2012; Segal et al., 2018). With regard to alcohol specifically, about two thirds of older alcohol abusers are chronic users; however, women represent a higher proportion of the later-life group compared to the chronic-user group (Lehmann & Fingerhood, 2018).

MENTAL, PHYSICAL, AND SUBSTANCE USE DISORDER COMORBIDITY

Mental Disorders

Most older adults live functional and emotionally stable lives. Despite many persisting societal myths, the presence of a mental health disorder is not more "expected" or "natural" during older age. Consistent with the general population, however, mood and anxiety disorders are the most prevalent mental disorders to appear among older adults and do co-occur frequently (Segal et al., 2018; Yochim & Woodhead, 2018). Extensive research also links higher rates of anxiety and depression (and associated behaviors) among older adults with serious medical problems, as both a precipitating and exacerbating factor (Zarit & Zarit, 2007). This may help explain the higher prevalence rates of mental health disorders within long-term care and rehabilitation settings. Moreover, since mental health conditions and medical problems are known to be associated independently with SUDs, it can be especially problematic when found together. For example, one study found that among people aged 57 to 85 years, those with multiple chronic conditions and depression were nearly five times as likely to experience problem drinking as older adults with multiple chronic conditions and no depression (Mowbray et al., 2017).

Data from the 2019 National Survey on Drug Use and Health show rates of co-occurring mental health and SUDs are lower in older age but still impact millions of people (SAMHSA, 2020). Reported as adults aged 50 or older, 1.5% (or 1.7 million people) had both any mental illness and a SUD in the past year. A study by Choi et al. (2015) examined persons aged 50 to 64 years with older adults over the age of 65. They found any illicit drug or tobacco use was associated with higher odds of having a past-year mental health problem in both groups. Binge drinking was also associated with increased odds among those aged 65 years and older. Indeed, depression and AUD combined is one of the frequently noted CODs in older adults in the research literature. Older adults with co-occurring mental health disorders have higher healthcare utilization, increased complexity of the course and prognosis of mental and physical illnesses, increased disability and impairment, increased caregiver stress, heightened mortality, and higher risk of suicide (Bartels et al., 2006).

Chronic Health Conditions

While the overall health status for older Americans has improved for the past several decades, it is estimated that two thirds of older Americans experience multiple chronic conditions (CDC, 2013). The presence of multiple chronic conditions, in and of itself, is associated with adverse health outcomes. The addition of substance misuse further amplifies the risk of developing additional chronic health conditions, increasing disability associated with chronic health conditions, producing negative medication interactions, and undermining effective management of chronic diseases (Mowbray et al., 2017; Wu et al., 2018).

Chronic conditions have become the primary reason that many older adults seek medical care and more chronic conditions mean more visits. Medicare beneficiaries data show that while 4% of those with no or one chronic conditions had 13 or more doctor visits per year; the statistic jumps to 92% for those with six or more chronic conditions (Centers for Medicare and Medicaid Services [CMS], 2012). Polypharmacy and its associated risks, thus, are higher. Compared to younger adults, older adults account for a disproportionately higher rate of emergency medical services (37 vs. 60 visits per 100 persons) and are more likely to have overnight hospitalizations (139.8 vs. 259.4 visits per 100 persons; Institute of Medicine [IOM], 2008).

In one study examining a large sample of electronic medical records, SUDs were identified to be more prevalent among adults with hepatitis, chronic obstructive pulmonary disease (COPD), ischemic heart disease, and chronic kidney disease—conditions more likely to impact older adults—and were associated with a significantly higher risk of hospitalization (Wu et al., 2018). Consistent with nonmedical samples, Wu et al. (2018) found that alcohol and tobacco use disorders were higher among older adults while drug use disorders were higher among younger adults. Multiple comorbidities of SUDs and chronic health conditions among older adults warrant attention in our healthcare system.

PHYSICAL PAIN

According to data collected by the U.S. Census Bureau in 2018, 34% of adults aged 65 and older reported having some type of disability (Administration for Community Living, 2020). Pain has been identified as one of the most widely cited symptoms underlying disability among older adults. According to data from the 2011 National Health and Aging Trends Study, 52.9% of those over 65 years of age reported bothersome pain in the last month (Patel et al., 2013). In a review of persistent pain by Molton and Terrill (2014), the authors acknowledged the significant role pain can have in developing depression, decreased physical activity and weight gain, and the negative health sequela of sleep problems. The types of pain most reported by older adults—osteoarthritic back pain, peripheral neuropathic pain, chronic joint pain—add yet another layer to the already complex SUD comorbidity picture due to their association with chronic conditions such as arthritis and diabetes. Most reviews note that the among the current cohorts of older adults, a SUD may begin with using prescribed pain medications (e.g., oxycodone) to address genuinely experienced pain. Many older adults may initially be cautious and fearful about addiction, but as mentioned previously, this may change with the aging Baby Boomers. Once misuse has begun, "doctor shopping" for pain medications among multiple providers may be as common among older adults as younger adults (Maree et al., 2016).

TREATMENT CONSIDERATIONS
ADOLESCENTS AND YOUNG ADULTS

Although abstinence is still presented to adolescents as the best way to deal with substance use problems, the need to be abstinent is not seen as important or realistic for many adolescents (Kelly et al., 2008). Moreover, abstinence-based programs do not take adolescents diagnosed with mental health disorders into account, even though these adolescents typically start using at an earlier age than those without a mental health disorder (Henderson et al., 2017). For many clinicians, pushing abstinence results in what Phillips and Labrow (2000) referred to as the "you'll never see them again" method (p. 283). For adolescents who have co-occurring mental disorders and SUDs, it is especially important to understand how harm reduction methods can be beneficial. Philips and Labrow explained that adolescents with SUDs may be using drugs to self-medicate. Although clinicians do not condone drug use, a harm reduction model may be beneficial for some adolescents with co-occurring mental and SUDs.

MOTIVATIONAL ENHANCEMENT AND COGNITIVE-BEHAVIORAL THERAPIES

There is evidence that abstinence-based programs can help some adolescents stop using alcohol and marijuana when used in combination with motivational enhancement therapy/

cognitive-behavioral therapy (MET/CBT) and parent-training curricula (Stanger et al., 2017). However, MET/CBT has been shown effective independent of abstinence-based incentives as well. MET is designed to work on motivating the adolescent to not want to participate in drugs through empathic stances focusing on reflective listening and self-efficacy for change (Cornelius et al., 2011). CBT, typically paired with MET, emphasizes learning triggers and consequences of drug use by assessing high-risk situations and how to cope with them as well as cravings (Cornelius et al., 2011).

Other Psychotherapeutic Treatment Modalities

Other successful treatment modalities with adolescents and young adults with co-occurring mental disorders and SUDs include functional family therapy (FFT), dialectical behavioral therapy (DBT), and multidimensional family therapy (MDFT).

Functional Family Therapy

FFT addresses the CODs of mental health and substance use together with the environmental factors of family and community for a well-rounded treatment method (Hartnett et al., 2017). It is an evidence-based model comprised of three steps: (a) engagement and motivation, (b) behavior change, and (c) generalization to future challenges. FFT is in the top 5% of programs used in over 300 countries around the world for addressing CODs involving behavior and substance use (Hartnet et al., 2017).

Dialectical Behavioral Therapy

Henderson et al. (2017) demonstrated the effectiveness of DBT, focusing on teaching coping strategies for emotional and behavioral control to families and adolescents. The idea behind DBT is to use strategies to better control emotions, leading to better control of behaviors, and help with eliminating the dependency on substance use as a coping technique.

Multidimensional Family Therapy

MDFT, similarly to FFT, uses a three-stage method for treatment: (a) developing alliances and motivation, (b) promoting change in thinking and behaviors, and (c) reinforcing changes (Liddle et al., 2018). MDFT differs from FFT by focusing on (a) the adolescent individually and as part of the family, (b) the parents separately and as part of the family, (c) the entire family entity, and (d) the community involvement in the adolescent's life. Adolescents with more severe mental health issues, or those participating in dangerous or violent behaviors, would still need inpatient therapy over MDFT.

Harm Reduction Practices

Notably, none of these aforementioned treatment methods eliminated substance use for all participants, which may highlight the added value of harm reduction methods. Any method used that does not directly encourage the elimination of drug use altogether is a part of harm reduction practices (Kleinig, 2004). Harm reduction is a way to control drug use and limit it to manageable levels under the supervision of a clinician. Examples of these programs for opioid use may include needle exchanges, methadone clinics, or safe injection sites where drugs can be taken while under medical supervision. The goal of the harm reduction model for intravenous drug use is to decrease the chance of contracting a medical disease or prevent death by accidental overdose.

Other forms of harm reduction may involve psychoeducational programs designed to inform adolescents and young adults of the consequences of their choices when using any substances ranging from alcohol to opioids. Psychoeducational approaches, such as providing informative materials, have shown some effectiveness in lowering risky drinking behaviors (Quinn et al., 2019) and improving depression scores (Conejo-Cerón et al., 2020). Research suggests that adolescents whose parents push abstinence may feel more resentment which limits treatment success, while parents who implement harm reduction strategies with evidence-based guidance are able to help their adolescents both limit substance use and participate in safer substance use practices (Slemon et al., 2019).

Medical/Behavioral Care Coordination

Adolescents and young adults also need access to coordinated services that will competently address co-occurring mental disorders and substance use disorders. Most adolescents and their families rely on their primary medical provider to link the adolescent with additional services for both substance use and mental health care (Stiffman et al., 2004). However, mental health treatment and substance use treatment are siloed, and many professionals do not have sufficient education to confidently cross the divide when treating CODs. Unfortunately, lack of cross-training combined with the barriers created by a division between mental health and substance use specialties make identifying and treating substance use among adolescents, who are already engaged in mental health services, extremely difficult (Anthony et al., 2011). The "no wrong door" approach (Henderson et al., 2017, p. 111), having all resources equally available no matter what type of provider is seen first, would help families of adolescents with CODs find treatment faster and with less stress as all services would be connected. If there existed true collaboration and coordination among fields that provide mental health, medical, and substance use services, then adolescents could access the best treatment for their circumstance no matter what "door" they enter.

OLDER ADULTS

Unfortunately, many inaccurate stereotypes persist about older adults that can negatively affect assessment and treatment. Research has shown that providers are less likely to screen older adults for mental health and substance use, may lower expectations for treatment, assume older adults are too old to change, or are less likely to benefit from therapy (American Psychological Association, 2014). Counselors must be mindful to recognize any false belief about the value of treatment for older adults and then work to reduce internalized bias, in both themselves and their clients, to avoid impeding therapeutic progress. Actively querying about substance use among older adults and knowing that treatment can be effective for this demographic is essential.

Screening and Assessment

It is recommended that counselors ask about substance use in a similar way to other health behaviors and chronic diseases, with the discussion focused on improved functioning and high quality of life. Broad, open-ended questions are recommended, and any stigmatizing or judgmental language should be avoided. Older adults who lived through the "War on Drugs" may be particularly sensitive to the tone of the inquiry and may be less forthcoming (Han & Moore, 2018). Counselors should be mindful that an older adult's report of a history of falls, accidents, disorientation, poor nutrition, or self-neglect may be indicative of a SUD and, therefore, should be assessed accordingly (Segal et al., 2018). Screening tools specifically designed for and validated with older adults are available for alcohol. Among these, the Michigan Alcohol Screening Test-Geriatric Version (MAST-G; Willenbring et al., 1987), the Alcohol Use Disorders Identification Test (AUDIT; Saunders et al., 1993), and the Comorbidity-Alcohol Risk Evaluation Tool (CARET; Fink et al., 2002) are recommended. A validated approach to screening for SUDs among older adults is currently lacking; however, the Alcohol, Smoking and Substance Involvement Screening Test (ASSIST; WHO ASSIST Working Group, 2002) is widely used in clinical practice and research (Han & Moore, 2018; Lehmann & Fingerhood, 2018).

THERAPEUTIC INTERVENTIONS, EVIDENCE-BASED PRACTICES, AND CARE COORDINATION SERVICES

Research indicates older adults can benefit from therapeutic interventions for SUDs as much as younger adults (American Psychological Association, 2014). However, the presentation of CODs among older adults carries added complexity because of normal age-related changes as well as disease processes that are more common with increased age. Interventions may need to be modified to accommodate for cognitive or sensory changes (e.g., reducing extraneous noise, slower pace); include more psychoeducation about normal aging processes and typical reactions to common older-age experiences than is usually the case with younger adults (e.g., older bodies process alcohol differently); or adapt to varied clinical settings (e.g., shared home, long-term care community; American Psychological Association, 2014).

As with other age groups, counselors are encouraged to use evidence-based practices with older adults. Motivational interviewing (MI; Miller & Rollnick, 2013) is a common treatment approach to examining current health behaviors and adopting a committed attitude to change. Reasons for changing substance use behaviors among older adults may be more focused on preserving functional independence and maintaining cognitive abilities compared to younger adults (Lehmann & Fingerhood, 2018). For most older adults who misuse alcohol, research has demonstrated that brief interventions delivered in health and social settings are effective and specialized substance use treatment is not required (Barry & Blow, 2016). However, once committed to a treatment program, older adults appear to stay in treatment longer and demonstrate more sobriety for alcohol and opioid use disorders when compared to younger adults (Carew & Comiskey, 2018; Kuerbis et al., 2014). Not surprisingly, those with a later onset of substance use have better treatment outcomes. Cognitive-behavioral interventions are also recommended as they are effective for mental health and SUDs among older adults (American Psychological Association, 2014; Kuerbis et al., 2014; Segal et al., 2018). Despite these indications, there remain significant gaps in the treatment literature for older adults. Smaller sample sizes of older adults admitted to treatment facilities continue to limit research, and larger scale longitudinal research tracking treatment and health outcomes for SUDs needs to include more older adults.

Han (2018) made a compelling argument about the need for a coordinated care approach—integrating chronic medical care with addiction treatment rooted in harm reduction principles of geriatric medicine. Although not the first to advocate for more integrated and multidisciplinary support for individuals with SUDs, Han clearly articulated the natural connection between the common goals for treatment for SUDs, for chronic medical diseases (of which SUDs could be considered), and for older adults. The greatest benefit to older adult clients may come from more collaboration between the addiction treatment models and the geriatric care models for chronic disease management, with a patient-centered (rather than disease-centered) focus on maximizing functional status, maintaining independence, symptom management, and the anticipation and management of transitions of care and advance care planning.

MULTICULTURAL CONSIDERATIONS

ADOLESCENTS AND YOUNG ADULTS

Counseling diverse adolescents and young adults may require some modifications in both the initial assessment and treatment regimen in order to provide effective counseling and retain youth who might drop out of treatment because the interventions are not sensitive to their background or culture (Tubman et al., 2002). When treatment is adapted to reflect their unique experiences and cultural characteristics, better outcomes are often seen when compared to more generic treatments (Santisteban et al., 2013). Liu and Clay (2002) offered a five-step framework to guide counselors working with diverse child clients:

1. Evaluate which cultural aspects are relevant.
2. Determine the level of skills and information necessary for competent treatment and possible referral.
3. Determine how much, when, and how to incorporate cultural issues.
4. Examine the potential treatments and the cultural assumptions of each.
5. Implement the treatment using the cultural strengths.

Common developmental experiences, expectations, and pressures will be interwoven with other important sociodemographic influences on the issues clients bring to therapy (Baruth & Manning, 2000; Liu & Clay, 2002). Conceptualization of abstract constructs of race and culture are still developing among children and adolescents. Moral judgments—our sense of right and wrong—are also evolving at this age. Evaluation and acceptance by peer groups garners greater attention during this phase of the lifespan and must be reconciled with pre-existing family values and goals. Counselors should also be mindful of academic experiences and how exceptional or remedial placements may be relevant to CODs (Tummala-Narra & Yang, 2019). Another salient cultural dimension being defined during this age of development is gender, influenced by the biological marker of puberty.

In addition to these developmental considerations, minority adolescents and young adults may also have culture-specific beliefs and experiences that impact expression of CODs and engagement with treatment. For example, many Asian American adolescents may be reluctant to share their psychological distress with parents and family members out of fear of burdening them or concern that their parents will not understand (Tummala-Narra & Yang, 2019). Counselors should also be mindful of minority adolescent and young adult experiences with immigration, forced separation from parents, adoption, language barriers, acculturative stress, as well as any ideological, emotional, or physical conflict within the family. Equally important to understand is an individual's history of prejudice and discrimination. The negative impact of stereotyping and discrimination on identity and well-being can be profound. As Liu and Clay (2002) emphasized, it is important for counselors to understand if, when, and how these various considerations may be most helpful to helping their clients. Concepts of resilience should also be culturally embedded, with counselors utilizing cultural narratives and symbols that are meaningful and empowering (Tummala-Narra & Yang, 2019).

OLDER ADULTS

Existing multicultural frameworks for counseling can be applied to working with minority older adults, especially when age is included as a critical component of diversity (Committee on Aging,

2009). Health and treatment behaviors are influenced by a wide variety of sociodemographic variables—race, ethnicity, gender, sexual orientation, socioeconomic status—and age is interwoven in that intersectional complexity. Clinical presentation of mental health and SUDs and treatment-seeking behaviors among older adults will reflect the interactions of these factors (American Psychological Association, 2014). Moreover, generational cohorts will have different formative beliefs and values. Older cohorts who value self-reliance may be less likely to admit to needing help, whereas younger cohorts of older adults (like the Baby Boomer generation) may be more accepting of mental health support. Even so, they will still carry more internalized mental health stigma than younger adults.

The growing diversity of the older adult population is notable. While 80% of older adults aged 65 years and older in 2010 were non-Hispanic White, the number is projected to drop to 58% by 2050 (Administration for Community Living, 2017; CDC, 2013). Conversely, the proportion of older Latino/a Americans will almost triple (7% to 20%), the proportion of older Asian Americans will more than double (3.3% to 8.5%), and both the African American and American Indian and Alaskan Native older adult population will also see an increase (3% and 1%, respectively) (Administration for Community Living, 2017; CDC, 2013). And, while the U.S. Census has never included LGBT persons in its measure, estimates suggest that LGBT adults over the age of 50 will steadily grow from 3 million to 7 million by 2030 (SAGE, 2020).

Counselors should be mindful that many older minority adults faced bias, prejudice, and discrimination in the pursuit of education, careers, housing, and healthcare. Limiting or denying resources over decades means that economic insecurity is more common among minority older adults and that excessive death, morbidity, and disability are prevalent among minority elders (Administration for Community Living, 2020; Office of Ethnic Minority Affairs, 2009). Unfortunately, biases in the criminal justice system also contribute to higher lifetime prevalence rates of incarceration among older minorities with SUDs. Racial, ethnic, and sexual minority older adults may also express distrust in or delay engagement with physical and mental health care due to the historically disparate or unethical treatment (e.g., conversion therapy, Tuskegee study, lobotomies). Counselors working with diverse older adults must be mindful that the adverse impact of social, financial, legal, and health inequities are compounded over the life course.

At the same time, it behooves counselors to acknowledge the strengths of their minority older adult clients. Afterall, these older adults are the survivors. Counselors are encouraged to build upon the strengths and skills older adults have developed over a lifetime of experience. Compared to younger clients, older adults have more experience in coping with life's stressors and building support networks and have developed notable resilience. As some of this resilience may be rooted in specific cultural values and beliefs, counselors should approach their work from the perspective of supplementing existing coping strategies and support networks rather than replacing them with mainstream approaches to care (Committee on Aging, 2009).

LEGAL AND ETHICAL CONSIDERATIONS
ADOLESCENTS AND YOUNG ADULTS

Recognizing the need for substance use and mental health treatment to be accessible for minors under the age of 18 even without parental consent, a federal law—The Health Insurance Portability and Accountability Act of 1996 (HIPAA)—has been cited protecting the confidentiality of minors in some cases (Weddle & Kokotailo, 2005). This federal law defers to states on how to handle disclosures. If a state requires a disclosure to parents, HIPAA allows the program to do that. If the state does not require a disclosure, then it is up to the treatment program and/or the treating clinician. This understanding of a need for privacy for the minor seeking treatment has led to a debate regarding if the minor fully understands all the risks associated with treatment and has the cognitive capacity to truly consent for that treatment (Kerwin et al., 2015). This is not the case for most minors, however, as they do not frequently self-refer for treatment. More often, they are sent for treatment by the criminal justice system. The United States Department of Health and Human Services, SAMHSA, and the Center for Behavioral Health Statistics and Quality (2012) reported that 45.6% of all referrals for minors come from the legal system. While many state laws favor consent of a minor as sufficient for inpatient and outpatient substance use and mental health treatment, it does vary state by state (Kerwin et al., 2015). Nonetheless, it is important that mental health professionals explain the limitations to confidentiality to all concerned parties. For example, when there is a risk for harm to self or others, confidentiality will be broken, or when utilizing healthcare insurance, a breach to confidentiality can be the result. It is important to understand the laws in the state where the mental health professional is practicing.

In addition, harm reduction treatments are engulfed in ethical and legal concerns. The most obvious is that engaging in substance use is often an illegal activity. The risk of legal consequences needs to be fully addressed and consented to. Carter and Hall (2008) found that opioid users can consent to treatment so long as they are not in a state of withdrawal or intoxication. Methadone clinics are an example of how to eliminate the legality problem as it changes from an illegal substance to a prescribed one. Harm reduction opponents suggest that there are three main ethical concerns and debates regarding harm reduction practices. These opponents believe harm reduction encourages drug use, sends conflicting and mixed messages, and does not stop drug use (Christie et al., 2008). However, in contrast to the views of the opponents, outcomes of scientific research show harm reduction encourages safety as well as avoidance of overdosing (CDC, 2019). Harm reduction does not encourage or advocate for substance use, and, in fact, substance use does not usually increase with harm reduction methods. Rather, more referrals are made to abstinence-based incentives and other recovery programs from harm reduction facilities (Christie et al., 2008). With the concern for mixed signals, programs such as needle exchanges have shown no increase in drug use but rather a decrease in the spread of infections such as HIV (CDC, 2019). Furthermore, parents who participate in harm reduction practices help their adolescents and young adults access treatment when ready and engage in substance use more safely in the meantime (Slemon et al., 2019). It is true that harm reduction is not an immediate removal of substance use, but research suggests it helps prevent overdose and other negative consequences associated with addictive behavior (CDC, 2019; Slemon et al., 2019).

OLDER ADULTS

Working with older adults demands balancing the desire to guard the adult's safety with recognizing the individual's right to make their own decisions (American Psychological Association, 2014). With this in mind, three issues counselors need to consider when working with older adults with CODs are highlighted: (a) capacity, (b) confidentiality, and (c) mandatory reporting. Older adults should be assumed to retain capacity to make independent decisions (i.e., participation in care, refusal of services, discharge plans). Unfortunately, delirium, mild cognitive impairment, and neurocognitive disorders (formerly labeled dementia) commonly co-occur in older adults with SUDs, which forces the question of capacity to the forefront of treatment planning (Salmon & Forester, 2012). Neuropsychological testing and capacity assessments may be necessary to ascertain the degree of impairment and likelihood of regaining capacity to participate in the varied health and living situation decisions (Moye et al., 2013). For example, capacity may be regained after benzodiazepine intoxication and toxicity are resolved but long-term alcohol abuse may have destroyed so much brain tissue that the impairment is now permanent. In the latter case, care will involve a healthcare power of attorney or, in the absence of a support system, a court-appointed guardian. As with younger adults with capacity, older adults share the protection of confidentiality. Counselors may have more interactions with concerned family members or caregivers when working with older adults compared to younger adults and must be mindful not to violate this ethical foundation (American Psychological Association, 2014). However, as with other potentially vulnerable populations, confidentiality must be broken in the case of elder mistreatment.

CLINICAL CASE ILLUSTRATION AND DISCUSSION

CASE OF MRS. JOHNSON

Mrs. Johnson is a 75-year-old retired, widowed, African American woman who lives alone in her home of 50 years. Her husband died 6 months ago. Her daughter lives nearby and her grandson occasionally visits to "check-in on her" and "help around the house." One evening when her grandson came to visit, he found Mrs. Johnson on the floor. She needed help standing up, could not focus on him, and was slurring her words. She was taken to the hospital where she reluctantly admitted that she fell and had some trouble getting up. Nothing was broken, but her examination revealed multiple bruise sites on her arms and legs in various stages of healing. Mrs. Johnson has a medical history of inconsistently managed type II diabetes, high cholesterol, and new complaints of frequent dizziness. When the medical provider asked Mrs. Johnson if she is drinking enough water, she quipped with a smile, "Does the afternoon retirement cocktail count?" The provider laughed and moved on, believing he had his answer. Her A1C blood sugar levels were elevated but the review of her current medications on file showed no adverse interactions. The provider referred her to the nutritionist who addressed the importance of staying hydrated to decrease dizziness associated with orthostatic hypotension and reviewed healthy eating habits for diabetes self-management. Mrs. Johnson returned home but was admitted to the hospital again 3 months later after another fall. This time it was evident that she hit her head.

Despite earlier reservations about speaking with his grandmother's providers, the grandson now felt compelled to share his observations about the significant increase in his grandmother's drinking since her husband died. Since the previous hospital visit, he reported that she has been more forgetful, found sleeping in her bathrobe on the couch at all hours during the day (a behavior previously uncommon), eating significantly less, and been infrequently adherent to her medication schedule. Initially angry with her grandson for "speaking out of turn" she finally admitted that life has been more difficult since her husband died but insisted that she was "not losing my mind," was safe to return to her home to live independently despite the falling, and did not have any problems with alcohol. While still skeptical, she finally agreed to speak with a counselor about the loss of her husband at the encouragement of her grandson. She also told her grandson that she would reach out to her pastor whom she has not spoken with since her husband's funeral; her attendance at church has also been sporadic.

CASE DISCUSSION

As in Mrs. Johnson's case, many older adults with SUDs first present in a medical setting. However, initial presentations are complicated by medical conditions. In this example, the medical providers focused primarily on her uncontrolled chronic medical conditions as the primary cause for her fall (and associated slurring and bruises) and failed to accurately assess for the influence of substance use. Perhaps out of discomfort with the topic of substance use or internalized bias about older adults, the provider accepted her joking deflection about drinking and moved on. This was a missed opportunity to assess the potential contribution of the sugar in alcohol exacerbating her diabetes and to provide education to Mrs. Johnson, which can be an effective intervention with older adults. Additionally, while medications on file were reviewed, older adults are more likely to take over-the-counter medications and these can also contribute to medication interactions. A second hospitalization due to a more dangerous fall may have been avoided with a more comprehensive, while still nonjudgmental, and aging-informed assessment of Mrs. Johnson when she first presented.

Her counselor will need to work to establish trust with Mrs. Johnson, understanding her current beliefs about the need for and effectiveness of therapy. The role of religion and her pastor in supporting community members during times of difficulty may also be important cultural considerations to explore. While discussing the loss of her husband, careful assessment will elucidate the most appropriate mental health diagnosis, without over-pathologizing her grief, and determine the possible role of her increased alcohol intake as a maladaptive coping mechanism. Given the fall where she hit her head and the potentially excess alcohol intake recently, Mrs. Johnson's cognitive status should be monitored, and a capacity evaluation should be completed if there are safety concerns about her decision-making abilities. Although not readily apparent, elder abuse should also be monitored. Her bruising is most likely associated with her frequency of falls, but like many younger victims of abuse, Mrs. Johnson may feel ashamed and embarrassed and thus reluctant to admit to any mistreatment. Finally, Mrs. Johnson's love for her grandson is an important character strength and motivator that may be helpful in reducing or eliminating her drinking and increasing other positive health behaviors.

CHAPTER SUMMARY

The purpose of this chapter was to provide a general foundation for the impact of developmental age on the presentation and treatment of co-occurring mental and SUDs. Age is an important contextual variable within multicultural competence; CODs impact individuals of all ages and the counselors who can adapt to the unique biopsychosocial contexts across the lifespan will be in a better position to create meaningful change in partnership with their clients. Examining mental health and substance use by age reveals different patterns of use and different risk factors for initial and chronic use. While therapeutic approaches are similarly effective, different access points to treatment are noted and modalities may be tailored according to a client's age. Commonly, across the lifespan, the best therapeutic outcomes result from coordinated and integrated mental health, physical health, and substance use care.

DISCUSSION QUESTIONS

1. Summarize the most common CODs across the lifespan, noting similarities and differences across the various age groups.
2. Multicultural competence begins with self-reflection. What bias might you have internalized about the younger or older lifespan that would be important to monitor in your work?
3. Do you believe harm reduction practices are more effective than abstinence-based models? Please explain your answer.
4. How would the implementation of true collaboration between mental health and medical health fields be helpful across the lifespan? Explain for adolescents, young adults, middle adults, and older adults.
5. Research the mandatory reporting laws in your state related to age. What are the requirements for minors as well as for older adults?

REFERENCES

Administration for Community Living. (2017). *Profile of American Indians and Alaska Natives age 65 and over.* U.S. Department of Health and Human Services. https://acl.gov/sites/default/files/Aging%20and%20Disability%20in%20America/2017OAProfileAIAN508.pdf

Administration for Community Living. (2020). *2019 profile of older Americans.* U.S. Department of Health and Human Services. https://acl.gov/sites/default/files/Aging and Disability in America/2019ProfileOlderAmericans508.pdf

Agrawal, A., Gardner, C. O., Prescott, C. A., & Kendler, K. S. (2005). The differential impact of risk factors on illicit drug involvement in females. *Social Psychiatry and Psychiatric Epidemiology, 40*(6), 454–466. https://doi.org/10.1007/s00127-005-0907-0

American Psychiatric Association. (2013). *Diagnostic and statistical manual of mental disorders* (5th ed.). https://doi.org/10.1176/appi.books.9780890425596

American Psychological Association (2014). Guidelines for psychological practice with older adults. *The American Psychologist, 69*(1), 34–65. https://doi.org/10.1037/a0035063

Anthony, E. K., Taylor, S. A., & Raffo, Z. (2011). Early intervention for substance abuse among youth and young adults with mental health conditions: An exploration of community mental health practices. *Administration and Policy in Mental Health and Mental Health Services Research, 38*(3), 131–141. https://doi.org/10.1007/s10488-010-0308-x

Barkus, E., & Murray, R. M. (2010). Substance use in adolescence and psychosis: Clarifying the relationship. *Annual Review of Clinical Psychology, 6*, 365–389. https://doi.org/10.1146/annurev.clinpsy.121208.131220

Barnett, J. H., Werners, U., Secher, S. M., Hill, K. E., Brazil, R., Masson, K., Pernet, D. E., Kirkbride, J. B., Murray, G. K., Bullmore, E. T., & Jones, P. B. (2007). Substance use in a population-based clinic sample of people with first-episode psychosis. *British Journal of Psychiatry, 190*(6), 515–520. https://doi.org/10.1192/bjp.bp.106.024448

Barry, K. L., & Blow, F. C. (2016). Drinking over the lifespan: Focus on older adults. *Alcohol Research: Current Reviews, 38*(1), 115–120. https://www.researchgate.net/publication/302592549_Drinking_Over_the_Lifespan_Focus_on_Older_Adults

Bartels, S., Blow, F., Van Critters, A., & Brockmann, L. (2006). Dual diagnosis among older adults: Co-occurring substance abuse and psychiatric illness. *Journal of Dual Diagnosis, 2*(3), 9–30. https://doi.org/10.1300/J374v02n03_03

Baruth, L. G., & Manning, M. L. (2000). A call for multicultural counseling in middle schools. *The Clearing House, 73*(4), 243–246. https://doi.org/10.1080/00098650009600962

Benshoff, J. J., Harrawood, L. K., & Koch, D. S. (2003). Substance abuse and the elderly: Unique issues and concerns. *Journal of Rehabilitation, 69*(2), 43–48. http://www.kvccdocs.com/KVCC/2016-MHT/MHT216/lessons/L-12/SubstanceElderly.pdf

Biederman, J., Monuteaux, M. C., Mick, E., Spencer, T., Wilens, T. E., Silva, J. M., Snyder, L. E., & Faraone, S. V. (2006). Young adult outcome of attention deficit hyperactivity disorder: A controlled 10-year follow-up study. *Psychological Medicine, 36*(2), 167–179. https://doi.org/10.1017/S0033291705006410

Brecht, M.-L., O'Brien, A., von Mayrhauser, C., & Anglin, M. D. (2004). Methamphetamine use behaviors and gender differences. *Addictive Behaviors, 29*(1), 89–106. https://doi.org/10.1016/S0306-4603(03)00082-0

Brown, S. A., McGue, M., Maggs, J., Schulenberg, J., Hingson, R., Swartzwelder, S., Martin, C., Chung, T., Tapert, S. F., Sher, K., Winters, K. C., Lowman, C., & Murphy, S. (2008). A developmental perspective on alcohol and youths 16 to 20 years of age. *Pediatrics, 121*(Suppl. 4), S290–S310. https://doi.org/10.1542/peds.2007-2243D

Cantwell, R., Brewin, J., Glazebrook, C., Dalkin, T., Fox, R., Medley, I., & Harrison, G. (1999). Prevalence of substance misuse in first-episode psychosis. *British Journal of Psychiatry, 174*(2), 150–153. https://doi.org/10.1192/bjp.174.2.150

Carew, A. M., & Comiskey, C. (2018). Treatment for opioid use and outcomes in older adults: A systematic literature review. *Drug and Alcohol Dependence, 182*, 48–57. https://doi.org/10.1016/j.drugalcdep.2017.10.007

Carter, A., & Hall, W. (2008). Informed consent to opioid agonist maintenance treatment: Recommended ethical guidelines. *International Journal of Drug Policy, 19*(1), 79–89. https://doi.org/10.1016/j.drugpo.2007.09.007

Center for Behavioral Health Statistics and Quality. (2020). *Results from the 2019 national survey on drug use and health: Detailed tables.* Substance Abuse and Mental Health Services Administration. https://www.samhsa.gov/data/

Centers for Disease Control and Prevention. (2013). *The state of aging and health in America.* U.S. Department of Health and Human Services. https://www.cdc.gov/aging/pdf/State-Aging-Health-in-America-2013.pdf

Centers for Disease Control and Prevention. (2019). *Summary of information on the safety and effectiveness of syringe services programs (SSPs).* U.S. Department of Health and Human Services. https://www.cdc.gov/ssp/syringe-services-programs-summary.html

Centers for Medicare and Medicaid Services (2012). *Chronic Conditions among Medicare Beneficiaries.* U.S. Department of Health and Human Services. https://www.cms.gov/Research-Statistics-Data-and-Systems/Statistics-Trends-and-Reports/Chronic-Conditions/Downloads/2012Chartbook.pdf

Cerdá, M., Prins, S. J., Galea, S., Howe, C. J., & Pardini, D. (2016). When psychopathology matters most: Identifying sensitive periods when within-person changes in conduct, affective and anxiety problems are associated with male adolescent substance use. *Addiction, 111*(5), 924–935. https://doi.org/10.1111/add.13304

Chambers, R. A., Taylor, J. R., & Potenza, M. N. (2003). Developmental neurocircuitry of motivation in adolescence: A critical period of addiction vulnerability. *American Journal of Psychiatry, 160*(6), 1041–1052. https://doi.org/10.1176/appi.ajp.160.6.1041

Choi, N. G., DiNitto, D. M., & Marti, C. N. (2015). Alcohol and other substance use, mental health treatment use, and perceived unmet treatment need: Comparison between baby boomers and older adults. *American Journal on Addictions, 24*(4), 299–307. https://doi.org/10.1111/ajad.12225

Christie, T., Groarke, L., & Sweet, W. (2008). Virtue ethics as an alternative to deontological and consequential reasoning in the harm reduction debate. *International Journal of Drug Policy, 19*(1), 52–58. https://doi.org/10.1016/j.drugpo.2007.11.020

Committee on Aging. (2009). *Multicultural competency in Geropsychology.* American Psychological Association. https://www.apa.org/pi/aging/programs/pipeline/multicultural-competency.pdf

Conejo-Cerón, S., Bellón, J. Á., Motrico, E., Campos-Paíno, H., Martín-Gómez, C., Ebert, D. D., Buntrock, C., Gili, M., & Moreno-Peral, P. (2020). Moderators of psychological and psychoeducational interventions for the prevention of depression: A systematic review. *Clinical Psychology Review, 79*, Article 101859. https://doi.org/10.1016/j.cpr.2020.101859

Cornelius, J. R., Douaihy, A., Bukstein, O. G., Daley, D. C., Wood, S. D., Kelly, T. M., & Salloum, I. M. (2011). Evaluation of cognitive behavioral therapy/motivational enhancement therapy (CBT/MET)

in a treatment trial of comorbid MDD/AUD adolescents. *Addictive Behaviors, 36*(8), 843–848. https://doi.org/10.1016/j.addbeh.2011.03.016

Dawson, D. A., Goldstein, R. B., Chou, S. P., Ruan, W. J., & Grant, B. F. (2008). Age at first drink and the first incidence of adult-onset DSM-IV alcohol use disorders. *Alcoholism: Clinical and Experimental Research, 32*(12), 2149–2160. https://doi.org/10.1111/j.1530-0277.2008.00806.x

Edgell, R. C., Kunik, M. E., Molinari, V. A., Hale, D., & Orengo, C. A. (2000). Nonalcohol-related use disorders in geropsychiatric patients. *Journal of Geriatric Psychiatry and Neurology, 13*(1), 33–37. https://doi.org/10.1177/089198870001300105

Fink, A., Morton, S. C., Beck, J. C., Hays, R. D., Spritzer, K., Oishi, S., Moore, A. A. (2002). The alcohol-related problems survey: Identifying hazardous and harmful drinking in older primary care patients. *Journal of the American Geriatrics Society, 50*(10),1717–1722. https://doi.org/10.1046/j.1532-5415.2002.50467.x

Gfroerer, J., Penne, M., Pemberton, M., & Folsom, R. (2003). Substance abuse treatment need among older adults in 2020: The impact of the aging baby-boom cohort. *Drug and Alcohol Dependence, 69*(2), 127–135. https://doi.org/10.1016/s0376-8716(02)00307-1

Gielen, N., Havermans, R. C., Tekelenburg, M., & Jansen, A. (2012). Prevalence of post-traumatic stress disorder among patients with substance use disorder: It is higher than clinicians think it is. *European Journal of Psychotraumatology, 3*(1), Article 17734. https://doi.org/10.3402/ejpt.v3i0.17734

Gottfredson, N. C., & Hussong, A. M. (2011). Parental involvement protects against self-medication behaviors during the high school transition. *Addictive Behaviors, 36*(12), 1246–1252. https://doi.org/10.1016/j.addbeh.2011.07.035

Han, B. H. (2018). Aging, multimorbidity, and substance use disorders: The growing case for integrating the principles of geriatric care and harm reduction. *International Journal of Drug Policy, 58*, 135–136. https://doi.org/10.1016/j.drugpo.2018.06.005

Han, B. H., & Moore, A. A. (2018). Prevention and screening of unhealthy substance use by older adults. *Clinics in Geriatric Medicine, 34*(1), 117–129. https://doi.org/10.1016/j.cger.2017.08.005

Hartnett, D., Carr, A., Hamilton, E., & O'Reilly, G. (2017). The effectiveness of functional family therapy for adolescent behavioral and substance misuse problems: A meta-analysis. *Family Process, 56*(3), 607–619. https://doi.org/10.1111/famp.12256

Henderson, J. L., Brownlie, E. B., McMain, S., Chaim, G., Wolfe, D. A., Rush, B., Boritz, T., & Beitchman, J. H. (2017). Enhancing prevention and intervention for youth concurrent mental health and substance use disorders: The research and action for teens study. *Early Intervention in Psychiatry, 13*(1), 110–119. https://doi.org/10.1111/eip.12458

Howard, A. L., Kennedy, T. M., Mitchell, J. T., Sibley, M. H., Hinshaw, S. P., Arnold, L. E., Roy, A., Stehli, A., Swanson, J. M., & Molina, B. S. G. (2020). Early substance use in the pathway from childhood attention-deficit/hyperactivity disorder (ADHD) to young adult substance use: Evidence of statistical mediation and substance specificity. *Psychology of Addictive Behaviors, 34*(2, Suppl.). https://doi.org/10.1037/adb0000542.supp

Institute of Medicine (US) Committee on the Future Health Care Workforce for Older Americans. (2008). *Retooling for an aging America: Building the health care workforce.* National Academies Press. https://www.ncbi.nlm.nih.gov/books/NBK215400/

Jennison, K. M., & Johnson, K. A. (2001). Parental alcoholism as a risk factor for DSM-IV-defined alcohol abuse and dependence in American women: The protective benefits of dyadic cohesion in marital communication. *The American Journal of Drug and Alcohol Abuse, 27*(2). 349–374. https://doi.org/10.1081/ADA-100103714

Kaminer, Y., Connor, D. F., & Curry, J. F. (2007). Comorbid adolescent substance use and major depressive disorders: a review. *Psychiatry (Edgmont), 4*(12), 32–43. https://www.ncbi.nlm.nih.gov/pmc/articles/PMC2861513/

Kelly, J. F., Myers, M. G., & Rodolico, J. (2008). What do adolescents exposed to Alcoholic Anonymous think about 12-step groups? *Substance Abuse, 29*(2), 53–62. https://doi.org/10.1080/08897070802093122

Kendler, K. S., Schmitt, E., Aggen, S. H., & Prescott, C. A. (2008). Genetic and environmental influences on alcohol, caffeine, cannabis, and nicotine use from early adolescence to middle adulthood. *Archives of General Psychiatry, 65*(6), 674–682. https://doi.org/10.1001/archpsyc.65.6.674

Kerwin, M. E., Kirby, K. C., Speziali, D., Duggan, M., Mellitz, C., Versek, B., & McNamara, A. (2015). What can parents do? A review of state laws regarding decision making for adolescent drug abuse and mental health treatment. *Journal of Child & Adolescent Substance Abuse, 24*(3), 166–176. https://doi.org/10.1080/1067828X.2013.777380

Khoury, L., Tang, Y. L., Bradley, B., Cubells, J. F., & Ressler, K. J. (2010). Substance use, childhood traumatic experience, and posttraumatic stress disorder in an urban civilian population. *Depression and Anxiety, 27*(12), 1077–1086. https://doi.org/10.1002/da.20751

King, K. M., & Chassin, L. (2007). A prospective study of the effects of age of initiation of alcohol and drug use on young adult substance dependence. *Journal of Studies on Alcohol and Drugs, 68*(2), 256–265. https://doi.org/10.15288/jsad.2007.68.256

Kingston, S., & Raghavan, C. (2009). The relationship of sexual abuse, early initiation of substance use, and adolescent trauma to PTSD. *Journal of Traumatic Stress, 22*(1), 65–68. https://doi.org/10.1002/jts.20381

Kleinig, J. (2004). Ethical issues in substance use intervention. *Substance Use & Misuse, 39*(3), 369–398. https://doi.org/10.1081/JA-120029983

Kuerbis, A., Sacco, P., Blazer, D. G., & Moore, A. A. (2014). Substance abuse among older adults. *Clinics in Geriatric Medicine, 30*(3), 629–654. https://doi.org/10.1016/j.cger.2014.04.008

Kuhn, C. (2015). Emergence of sex differences in the development of substance use and abuse during adolescence. *Pharmacology & Therapeutics, 153,* 55–78. https://doi.org/10.1016/j.pharmthera.2015.06.003

Lambert, M., Conus, P., Lubman, D. I., Wade, D., Yuen, H., Moritz, S., Naber, D., McGorry, P. D., & Schimmelmann, B. G. (2005). The impact of substance use disorders on clinical outcome in 643 patients with first-episode psychosis. *Acta Psychiatrica Scandinavica, 112*(2), 141–148. https://doi.org/10.1111/j.1600-0447.2005.00554.x

Lee, C. T., Rose, J. S., Engel-Rebitzer, E., Selya, A., & Dierker, L. (2011). Alcohol dependence symptoms among recent onset adolescent drinkers. *Addictive Behaviors, 36*(12), 1160–1167. https://doi.org/10.1016/j.addbeh.2011.07.014

Lee, M. R., Chassin, L., & MacKinnon, D. (2010). The effect of marriage on young adult heavy drinking and its mediators: Results from two methods of adjusting for selection into marriage. *Psychology of Addictive Behaviors, 24*(4), 712–718. https://doi.org/10.1037/a0020983

Lehmann, S. W., & Fingerhood, M. (2018). Substance-use disorders in later life. *New England Journal of Medicine, 379,* 2351–2360. https://doi.org/10.1056/NEJMra1805981

Liddle, H. A., Dakof, G. A., Rowe, C. L., Henderson, C., Greenbaum, P., Wang, W., & Alberga, L. (2018). Multidimensional family therapy as a community-based alternative to residential treatment for adolescents with substance use and co-occurring mental health disorders. *Journal of Substance Abuse Treatment, 90,* 47–56. https://doi.org/10.1016/j.jsat.2018.04.011

Liu, W. M., & Clay, D. L. (2002). Multicultural counseling competencies: Guidelines in working with children and adolescents. *Journal of Mental Health Counseling, 24*(2), 177–187. https://psycnet.apa.org/record/2002-13525-008

Mackesy-Amiti, M. E., Fendrich, M., & Goldstein, P. J. (1997). Sequence of drug use among serious drug users: Typical vs atypical progression. *Drug and Alcohol Dependence, 45*(3), 185–196. https://doi.org/10.1016/S0376-8716(97)00032-X

Maree, R. D., Marcum, Z. A., Saghafi, E., Weiner, D. K., & Karp, J. F. (2016). A systematic review of opioid and benzodiazepine misuse in older adults. *The American Journal of Geriatric Psychiatry, 24*(11), 949–963. https://doi.org/10.1016/j.jagp.2016.06.003

McCrory, E. J., & Mayes, L. (2015). Understanding addiction as a developmental disorder: An argument for a developmentally informed multilevel approach. *Current Addiction Reports, 2*(4), 326–330. https://doi.org/10.1007/s40429-015-0079-2

Merikangas, K. R., He, J., Burstein, M., Swanson, S. A., Avenevoli, S., Cui, L., Benjet, C., Georgiades, K., & Swendsen, J. (2010). Lifetime prevalence of mental disorders in U.S. adolescents: Results from the national comorbidity survey replication--Adolescent supplement (NCS-A). *Journal of the American Academy of Child and Adolescent Psychiatry, 49*(10), 980–989. https://doi.org/10.1016/j.jaac.2010.05.017

Merline, A. C., O'Malley, P. M., Schulenberg, J. E., Bachman, J. G., & Johnston, L. D. (2004). Substance use among adults 35 years of age: Prevalence, adulthood predictors, and impact of adolescent substance use. *American Journal of Public Health, 94*(1), 96–102. https://doi.org/10.2105/ajph.94.1.96

Miklowitz, D. J. (2012). Family treatment for bipolar disorder and substance abuse in late adolescence. *Journal of Clinical Psychology, 68*(5), 502–513. https://doi.org/10.1002/jclp.21855

Miller, W. R., & Rollnick, S. (2013). *Motivational interviewing: Helping people change* (3rd ed.). Guilford.

Molton, I. R., & Terrill, A. L. (2014). Overview of persistent pain in older adults. *American Psychologist, 69*(2), 197–207. http://doi.org/10.1037/a0035794

Moore, A. A., Karno, M. P., Grella, C. E., Lin, J. C., Warda, U., Liao, D. H., & Hu, P. (2009). Alcohol, tobacco, and nonmedical drug use in older U.S. adults: Data from the 2001/02 national epidemiologic survey of alcohol and related conditions. *Journal of the American Geriatrics Society, 57*(12), 2275–2281. https://doi.org/10.1111/j.1532-5415.2009.02554.x

Mowbray, O., Washington, T., Purser, G., & O'Shields, J. (2017). Problem drinking and depression in older adults with multiple chronic health conditions. *Journal of the American Geriatrics Society, 65*(1), 146–152. https://doi.org/10.1111/jgs.14479

Moye, J., Marson, D. C., & Edelstein, B. (2013). Assessment of capacity in an aging society. *American Psychologist, 68*(3), 158–171. https://doi.org/10.1037/a0032159

National Institute on Drug Abuse. (2003, June 1). *Substance-abusing adolescents show ethnic and gender differences in psychiatric disorders.* Retrieved January 12, 2021, from https://archives.drugabuse.gov/news-events/nida-notes/2003/06/substance-abusing-adolescents-show-ethnic-gender-differences-in-psychiatric-disorders

National Institute on Drug Abuse. (2019, July 10). *Drug use and its consequences increase among middle-aged and older adults.* Retrieved August 3, 2021, from https://www.drugabuse.gov/news-events/nida-notes/2019/07/drug-use-its-consequences-increase-among-middle-aged-older-adults

National Institute on Drug Abuse. (2020). *Monitoring the future.* https://www.drugabuse.gov/drug-topics/trends-statistics/monitoring-future

Nelemans, S. A., Hale, W. W., III., Branje, S. J. T., Raaijmakers, Q. A. W., Frijns, T., van Lier, P. A. C., & & Meeus, W. H. J. (2014). Heterogeneity in development of adolescent anxiety disorder symptoms in an 8-year longitudinal community study. *Development and Psychopathology, 26*(1), 181–202. https://doi.org/10.1017/S0954579413000503

Nelson, S. E., van Ryzin, M. J., & Dishion, T. J. (2015). Alcohol, marijuana, and tobacco use trajectories from age 12 to 24 years: Demographic correlates and young adult substance use problems. *Development and Psychopathology, 27*(1), 253–277. https://doi.org/10.1017/S0954579414000650

Office of Ethnic Minority Affairs. (2009). *Psychological and behavioral perspectives on health disparities.* American Psychological Association.

Patel, K. V., Guralnik, J. M., Dansie, E. J., & Turk, D. C. (2013). Prevalence and impact of pain among older adults in the United States: Findings from the 2011 National Health and Aging Trends Study. *Journal of the International Association for the Study of Pain, 154*(12), 2649–2657. https://doi.org/10.1016/j.pain.2013.07.029

Patrick, M. E., Schulenberg, J. E., O'Malley, P. M., Maggs, J. L., Kloska, D. D., Johnston, L. D., & Bachman, J. G. (2011). Age-related changes in reasons for using alcohol and marijuana from ages 18 to 30 in a national sample. *Psychology of Addictive Behaviors, 25*(2, Suppl.). https://doi.org/10.1037/a0022445.supp

Phillips, P., & Labrow, J. (2000). Dual diagnosis—does harm reduction have a role? *International Journal of Drug Policy, 11*(4), 279–283. https://doi.org/10.1016/S0955-3959(00)00058-X

Qato, D. M., Wilder, J., Schumm, L. P., Gillet, V., & Alexander, G. C. (2016). Changes in prescription and over-the-counter medication and dietary supplement use among older adults in the United States, 2005 vs 2011. *JAMA Internal Medicine, 176*(4), 473–482. https://doi.org/10.1001/jamainternmed.2015.8581

Quinn, C. A., Hides, L., de Andrade, D., Pocuca, N., Wilson, M., & Kavanagh, D. J. (2019). Impact of a brief psychoeducational intervention for reducing alcohol use and related harm in school leavers. *Drug and Alcohol Review, 38*(4), 339–348. https://doi.org/10.1111/dar.12920

SAGE: Advocacy & Service for LGBT Elders (2020). *LGBT aging.* https://www.sageusa.org/resource-category/lgbt-aging/

Salmon, J. M., & Forester, B. (2012). Substance abuse and co-occurring psychiatric disorders in older adults: A clinical case and review of the relevant literature. *Journal of Dual Diagnosis, 8*(1), 74–84. https://doi.org/10.1080/15504263.2012.648439

Santisteban, D. A., Mena, M. P., & Abalo, C. (2013). Bridging diversity and family systems: Culturally informed and flexible family-based treatment for Hispanic adolescents. *Couple and Family Psychology: Research and Practice, 2*(4), 246–263. https://doi.org/10.1037/cfp0000013

Sarabia, S., & Martin, J. (2013). Aging effects on substance use among midlife women: The moderating influence of race and substance. *Journal of Social Work Practice in the Addictions, 13*(4), 417–435. https://doi.org/10.1080/1533256X.2013.842799

Saunders, J. B., Aasland, O. G., Babor, T. F., De La Fuente, J. R., & Grant, M. (1993). Development of the alcohol use disorders identification test (Audit): WHO collaborative project on early detection of persons with harmful alcohol consumption-II. *Addiction, 88*(6), 791–804. https://doi.org/10.1111/j.1360-0443.1993.tb02093.x

Schulenberg, J. E., Patrick, M. E., Kloska, D. D., Maslowsky, J., Maggs, J. L., & O'Malley, P. M. (2016). Substance use disorder in early midlife: A national prospective study on health and well-being correlates and long-term predictors. *Substance Abuse: Research and Treatment, 9*(Suppl. 1), S41–S57. https://doi.org/10.4137/SART.S31437

Segal, D. L., Qualls, S. H., & Smyer, M. A. (2018). *Aging and mental health* (3rd ed.). John Wiley & Sons, Inc. https://doi.org/10.1002/9781119133186

Shih, R. A., Miles, J. N. V., Tucker, J. S., Zhou, A. J., & D'Amico, E. J. (2010). Racial/ethnic differences in adolescent substance use: Mediation by individual, family, and school factors. *Journal of Studies on Alcohol and Drugs, 71*(5), 640–651. https://doi.org/10.15288/jsad.2010.71.640

Siebenbruner, J., Englund, M. M., Egeland, B., & Hudson, K. (2006). Developmental antecedents of late adolescence substance use patterns. *Development and Psychopathology, 18*(2), 551–571. https://doi.org/10.1017/S0954579406060287

Simoni-Wastila, L., & Yang, H. K. (2006). Psychoactive drug abuse in older adults. *The American Journal of Geriatric Pharmacotherapy, 4*(4), 380–394. https://doi.org/10.1016/j.amjopharm.2006.10.002

Slemon, A., Jenkins, E. K., Haines-Saah, R. J., Daly, Z., & Jiao, S. (2019). 'You can't chain a dog to a porch': A multisite qualitative analysis of youth narratives of parental approaches to substance use. *Harm Reduction Journal, 16*(26), Article 26. https://doi.org/10.1186/s12954-019-0297-3

Spatz Widom, C., Marmorstein, N. R., & Raskin White, H. (2006). Childhood victimization and illicit drug use in middle adulthood. *Psychology of Addictive Behaviors, 20*(4), 394–403. https://doi.org/10.1037/0893-164X.20.4.394

Stanger, C., Scherer, E. A., Babbin, S. F., Ryan, S. R., & Budney, A. J. (2017). Abstinence based incentives plus parent training for adolescent alcohol and other substance misuse. *Psychology of Addictive Behaviors, 31*(4), 385–392. https://doi.org/10.1037/adb0000279

Stenbacka, M. (2003). Problematic alcohol and cannabis use in adolescence—risk of serious adult substance abuse? *Drug and Alcohol Review, 22*(3), 277–286. https://doi.org/10.1080/0959523031000154418

Stiffman, A. R., Pescosolido, B., & Cabassa, L. J. (2004). Building a model to understand youth service access: The gateway provider model. *Mental Health Services Research, 6*(4), 189–198. https://doi.org/10.1023/B:MHSR.0000044745.09952.33

Substance Abuse and Mental Health Services Administration. (2013). *Results from the 2012 national survey on drug use and health: Summary of national findings* (NSDUH Series H-46, HHS Publication No. (SMA) 13-4795). https://www.samhsa.gov/data/sites/default/files/NSDUHresults2012/NSDUHresults2012.pdf

Substance Abuse and Mental Health Services Administration. (2016). *Impact of the DSM-IV to DSM-5 changes on the national survey on drug use and health [internet]*. https://www.ncbi.nlm.nih.gov/books/NBK519702/

Substance Abuse and Mental Health Services Administration. (2019). *Key substance use and mental health indicators in the United States: Results from the 2018 national survey on drug use and health* (HHS Publication No. PEP19-5068, NSDUH Series H-54). Center for Behavioral Health Statistics and Quality. https://www.samhsa.gov/data/sites/default/files/cbhsq-reports/NSDUHNationalFindingsReport2018/NSDUHNationalFindingsReport2018.pdf

Substance Abuse and Mental Health Services Administration. (2020). *Key substance use and mental health indicators in the United States: Results from the 2019 National Survey on Drug Use and Health* (HHS Publication No. PEP20-07-01-001, NSDUH Series H-55). Center for Behavioral Health Statistics and Quality. https://www.samhsa.gov/data/sites/default/files/reports/rpt29393/2019NSDUHFFRPDFWHTML/2019NSDUHFFR1PDFW090120.pdf

Substance Abuse and Mental Health Services Administration, Center for Behavioral Health Statistics and Quality. (2014, July 14). *The TEDS report: Age of substance use initiation among treatment admissions aged 18 to 30*. https://www.samhsa.gov/data/sites/default/files/WebFiles_TEDS_SR142_AgeatInit_07-10-14/TEDS-SR142-AgeatInit-2014.htm

Tubman, J. G., Wagner, E. F., Gil, A. G., & Pate, K. N. (2002). Brief motivational intervention for substance-abusing delinquent adolescents: Guided self-change as a social work practice innovation. *Health & Social Work, 27*(3), 208–212. https://doi.org/10.1093/hsw/27.3.208

Tummala-Narra, P., & Yang, E. J. (2019). Asian American adolescent girls: Navigating stress across multiple contexts. In T. Bryant-Davis (Ed.), *Multicultural feminist therapy: Helping adolescent girls of color to thrive* (pp. 113–153). American Psychological Association. https://doi.org/10.1037/0000140-005

Turner, S., Mota, N., Bolton, J., & Sareen, J. (2018). Self-medication with alcohol or drugs for mood and anxiety disorders: A narrative review of the epidemiological literature. *Depression and Anxiety, 35*(9), 851–860. https://doi.org/10.1002/da.22771

United States Department of Health and Human Services, Substance Abuse and Mental Health Services Administration, & Center for Behavioral Health Statistics and Quality. (2012). *Treatment episode data set -- Admissions (TEDS-A)* (ICPSR 35037) [Data set]. Substance Abuse and Mental Health Data Archive. https://doi.org/10.3886/ICPSR35037.v1

U.S. Department of Agriculture & U.S. Department of Health and Human Services. (December 2020). *Dietary Guidelines for Americans, 2020–2025* (9th ed.). https://www.dietaryguidelines.gov/sites/default/files/2020-12/Dietary_Guidelines_for_Americans_2020-2025.pdf

Vaudreuil, C. A. H., Faraone, S. V., Di Salvo, M., Wozniak, J. R., Wolenski, R. A., Carrellas, N. W., & Biederman, J. (2019). The morbidity of subthreshold pediatric bipolar disorder: A systematic literature review and meta-analysis. *Bipolar Disorders, 21*(1), 16–27. https://doi.org/10.1111/bdi.12734

Vogt Yuan, A. S. (2011). Black-white differences in aging out of substance use and abuse. *Sociological Spectrum, 31*(1), 3–31. https://doi.org/10.1080/02732173.2011.525694

Weddle, M., & Kokotailo, P. K. (2005). Confidentiality and consent in adolescent substance abuse: An update. *Virtual Mentor, 7*(3), 239–243. **Error! Hyperlink reference not valid.**https://doi.org/10.1001/virtualmentor.2005.7.3.pfor1-0503

WHO ASSIST Working Group. (2002). The alcohol, smoking and substance involvement screening test (ASSIST): Development, reliability and feasibility. *Addiction, 97*(9), 1183–1194. https://doi.org/10.1046/j.1360-0443.2002.00185.x

Wilens, T. E., & Spencer, T. J. (2010). Understanding attention-deficit/hyperactivity disorder from childhood to adulthood. *Postgraduate Medicine, 122*(5), 97–109. https://doi.org/10.3810/pgm.2010.09.2206

Willenbring, M. L., Christensen, K. J., Spring, W. D., Jr., & Rasmussen, R. (1987). Alcoholism screening in the elderly. *Journal of the American Geriatrics Society, 35*(9), 864–869. https://doi.org/10.1111/j.1532-5415.1987.tb02339.x

Wu, L.-T., Zhu, H., & Ghitza, U. E. (2018). Multicomorbidity of chronic diseases and substance use disorders and their association with hospitalization: Results from electronic health records data. *Drug and Alcohol Dependence, 192*, 316–323. https://doi.org/10.1016/j.drugalcdep.2018.08.013

Wu, P., Goodwin, R. D., Fuller, C., Liu, X., Comer, J. S., Cohen, P., & Hoven, C. W. (2010). The relationship between anxiety disorders and substance use among adolescents in the community: Specificity and gender differences. *Journal of Youth and Adolescence, 39*(2), 177–188. https://doi.org/10.1007/s10964-008-9385-5

Yochim, B., & Woodhead, E. (2018). *Psychology of aging: A biopsychosocial perspective.* Springer Publishing Company, LLC.

Zarit, S. H. & Zarit, J. M. (2007). *Mental disorders in older adults: Fundamentals of assessment and treatment* (2nd ed.). Guilford Press.

CHAPTER 16

GENDER AND CO-OCCURRING DISORDERS

GENEVA M. GRAY, ASHA DICKERSON, AND VERONICA M. WANZER

LEARNING OBJECTIVES

After reading this chapter, you will be able to:
- Analyze the statistical gender differences present in relation to co-occurring disorders (CODs) and treatment options.
- Identify unique treatment issues experienced by individuals who identify as cisgender.
- Evaluate treatment considerations when working with individuals who are transgender.
- Recognize various gender differences that are present according to the research that is available.

INTRODUCTION

The term *co-occurring disorders* (CODs) denotes that not only does an individual have a substance use diagnosis, but that there are other diagnosed mental disorders concurrently present as well. Many theories attempt to explain why some people have CODs. These range from a person's need to self-medicate or manage existing mental health symptoms to informing that the symptoms of mental illness are a consequence of using substances. Although substance use and CODs do not discriminate, especially concerning gender, there are some clear demographic differences counselors need to be aware of that are present based on the research that is available.

According to Bockting et al. (2013), minority stress theory states that many health conditions, both physical and mental, are caused by the stress associated with mistreatment and discrimination that is experienced by members of underrepresented groups. This theory proposes that these stressors are unique and not experienced by majority/privileged populations. The theory also states that said stressors are institutional and chronic.

Treatment needs of women are complex as are the definitions of femininity and masculinity. When gender was defined decades ago, only two strict categories were largely recognized and given consideration by our social systems. This is known as the *binary gender system* because only two gender categories were considered to exist: male and female. In contemporary times, many have come to understand that the concept of gender can be far more complex and fluid. People who identify outside of the binary gender system (e.g., transgender, non-binary, gender non-conforming) have unique experiences and multicultural issues. Therefore, gender must always be considered with all clients. The discussion surrounding diversity of gender is still fairly new, and research concerning CODs and genders other than cisgender male or cisgender female are scarce.

PREVALENCE, STATISTICS, AND DEMOGRAPHICS

The Substance Abuse and Mental Health Services Administration (SAMHSA) administers the National Survey on Drug Use and Health (NSDUH) yearly. According to SAMHSA's 2019 NSDUH, two in five women surveyed reported struggling with illicit drug abuse while three in four of those same women reported struggling with alcohol use. This total for women using illicit drugs was approximately 7.2 million, representing 5.6% of the female population. These numbers were the exact same numbers reported in 2018 (SAMHSA, 2018). In 2019, 24.5% of women reported having a mental illness. The total: 31.7 million women reported having a substance disorder or other mental illness while 4.6 million had both simultaneously (SAMHSA, 2019).

GENDER DIVERSE

When considering gender, it is important not to negate the importance of sexual orientation and gender identity. People who identify as lesbian, gay, bisexual, transgender, or questioning (LGBTQ) often experience depression and other mental health issues as a result of the stigma associated with their sexual orientation and/or gender identity. Sexual and gender minorities, as a whole, have an increased risk of mental health issues, including substance use disorders (SUDs). Whereas the general rate for substance abuse is 9%, the rate for substance use within the LGBTQ+ population has greatly increased by at least three times that rate (SAMHSA, 2018).

Seeking treatment for SUDs or CODs is just the first step. Unfortunately, transgender individuals face obstacles even before treatment can begin. One issue with treatment options for individuals who are transgender is placement within residential treatment. Treatment centers that receive certain funding are often bound by government rules for client placement (i.e., a transgender female who has not undergone gender confirmation surgery may only have the option of living in the same area as cisgender males). This can be a very uncomfortable position for a woman, cisgender or transgender, to be in. Surveys continue to show that many of the facilities that assist people with CODs, are not equipped with staff who understand transgender identities and the associated attitudes, laws, and other factors. In addition, facilities are not prepared to meet the unique needs of people who are transgender (Finnegan & McNally, 2002).

TRANSGENDER MEN

The majority of research analyzes people who are transgender as one group but more recent research has begun to look at the differences within the populations (Ruppert et al., 2021). A study completed in 2016 found that 42.2% of transmen reported heavy episodic drinking (HED) usage of alcohol in comparison to 22.7% of the transwomen who were surveyed (Scheim et al., 2016). It is important to note that there is no statistical difference in the reports of HED in transmen and cisgender men. Transgender men who received gender-affirming medical interventions reported less depression following the interventions but reported higher prevalence rates of alcohol abuse (Ruppert et al., 2021).

Transgender Women

Transgender individuals, especially transgender children and adolescents, are highly susceptible to depression and eating disorders with self-harm and suicidal behaviors, particularly before receiving gender-affirming medical treatment (Connolly et al., 2016). Further research also notes the increased prevalence reported by transgender women (Hughes & Ellison, 2002). Although there is still limited research on substance use among people who are transgender, there is sufficient research concerning other mental health diagnoses within the population. Even though the overall rates of usage are hard to know exactly, there is research available that suggests that people who are transgender tend to seek treatment for SUDs more than those who are not transgender (Keuroghlian et al., 2015).

Gender Non-Conforming

Azagba et al.'s (2019) study found that gender non-conforming individuals had the highest rate of binge drinking when compared to other gender minorities. Some research has explored the experiences of gender non-conforming individuals by their gender assigned at birth. This research highlights that those who were assigned male at birth had 80% higher alcohol usage than transgender men and over twice as high as transgender women and people who were gender non-conforming assigned female (Newcomb et al., 2020). There is very little research on gender non-conformity and illicit drug use. This is an area needing further research. According to Newcomb et al. (2020) gender non-conforming individuals do not have heightened illicit drug usage when compared to transmen or transwomen.

TREATMENT CONSIDERATIONS

Many of the symptoms associated with CODs are "persistent, severe, and resistant to treatment" (Ruiz, 2017, p.10). In general, the treatment needs of all people with co-occurring mental disorders and SUDs are complex and require support that is integrated because individuals will be less likely to seek and participate in treatment if it is fragmented (Miquel et al., 2013). Treatment for CODs should include care for both the mental illness as well as the SUDs (Watkins et al., 1999). Therefore, treatment for people with CODs requires collaborative care by multidisciplinary teams (Manuel et al., 2018). According to researchers, an integrated approach is preferred, rather than parallel (simultaneous treatment for SUD and mental health without collaboration among providers) or sequential care (Drake et al., 2008). Sequential care is an approach that involves resolving one disorder before being able to move on to treat the other disorder. Moore (2009) suggested that treatment providers develop integrated and collaborative care that includes the use of existing community resources like medication management, family counseling, individual counseling, and group counseling in order to support long-term recovery efforts. It is assumed that all of the aforementioned efforts are key factors to continuity of care for people with CODs (Moore, 2009).

GENDER-BASED RATES OF TREATMENT USAGE

Despite the high rates of individuals diagnosed with CODs, few people receive treatment for both SUDs as well as mental health disorders. Manuel et al. (2018) indicate that low rates of treatment usage among people with CODs may be related to societal stigma and negative attitudes about mental illness and substance abuse. Also, it is likely that many people with CODs experience structural barriers (fragmented services) and financial barriers (e.g., lack of insurance, inability to pay) to treatment access (Manuel et al., 2018).

In addition, because of the complexities associated with CODs for women, treatment requires longer periods of time and increased staff involvement than that of non-COD-based treatment (SAMHSA, 2020). Therefore, long-term inpatient programs are more likely to include treatment for CODrs (Chen et al., 2011). Involvement in long-term inpatient treatment presents a major barrier for women with CODs, due to inability to pay for treatment, lack of access to inpatient treatment programs, and existing parenting responsibilities (Chen et al., 2011; SAMHSA, 2020).

GENDER-BASED TREATMENT NEEDS

Individuals diagnosed with CODs have specific gender-based treatment needs (Manuel et al., 2018). Regardless of the particular co-occurring diagnosis, both men and women report unmet needs associated with treatment for CODs (Manuel et al., 2018). In fact, within the past 6 years, women received more treatment for both substance abuse and mental health than men only when combining the two numbers. Men seek substance use treatment more and women seek mental health treatment more. This may be due to women's individual perceptions of the underlying problem (SAMHSA, 2020). In addition, it is likely that this occurs because mental health treatment (in comparison to SUD treatment) is more accessible, people perceive that mental health treatment is more important than treatment for SUDs, and/or there is a lack of knowledge on whether substance use is a mental illness (Manuel et al., 2018). Even though women use mental health treatment more often, they reported higher unmet treatment needs of mental health disorders than SUDs. The gap in services may be related to a lack of recognition for men that distress is possibly a mental health need (Manuel et al., 2018).

Among cisgender people with CODs, men are more likely to engage in drug use at age 18 whereas women initiate drug use at age 22 (Manuel et al., 2018) and women are more likely than men to be diagnosed with a COD (Miquel et al., 2013). Men are more likely than women to be diagnosed with a psychotic disorder co-occurring with SUDs (Miquel et al, 2013). Also, men with CODs are more likely to use stimulants and cannabis (Manuel et al., 2018). While women are more likely to be diagnosed with a COD than men, they also have higher rates of mood and anxiety disorders (Manuel et al., 2018). In addition, Chen et al. (2011) and Ruiz (2017) reported that women have higher rates of diagnosed major depressive disorder, anxiety, and posttraumatic stress disorder (PTSD). Women with a diagnosis of alcohol use disorder have higher rates of diagnosed CODs than men (Holzhauer & Gamble, 2017). Also, women with a history of cocaine dependence are three times more likely than men to exhibit psychotic symptoms (Miquel et al., 2013). The documented gender-based differences associated with CODs warrants treatment with a greater emphasis on alcohol use disorder and drug problems. The greater emphasis may include the use of community-based prevention programs to assist with addressing the higher vulnerability to mood disorders and depressant abuse/dependence (Manuel, et al., 2018).

FAMILY AND SOCIAL RELATIONSHIPS

There are gender-based differences in family relationships, marital status, cohabitation, and parenting for people with CODs that should be considered during treatment. Women appear

TABLE 16.1 Gender-Based Statistics for CODs With Individuals 18 to 65 Years Old

NON-BINARY, GENDER DIVERSE AND/OR GENDER FLUID IDENTIFYING	TRANSGENDER WOMEN	TRANSGENDER MEN	WOMEN	MEN
Gender diverse individuals experience significantly higher prevalence of nicotine, cannabis, cocaine, and opioid use disorder than cisgender counterparts and the overall U.S. population (Hughto et al., 2021)	Gender minority stressors are more consistent predictors of substance use (Gonzalez et al., 2017)	Report significantly higher frequency of cannabis and illicit drug use, as compared to gender-diverse counterparts (Gonzalez et al., 2017)	Higher rates of diagnosis of major depressive disorder, anxiety disorders, and PTSD (Chen, 2011; Manuel et al., 2018; Ruiz, 2017)	More likely to use stimulants and cannabis (Manuel et al., 2018)
Gender diverse individuals frequently use substances to cope with discrimination (Hughto et al., 2021)	Sexual orientation and gender incongruence are predictors of excessive alcohol, cannabis, and illicit drug use (Gonzalez et al., 2017)	Sexual orientation and gender incongruence are predictors of excessive cannabis use (Gonzalez et al., 2017)	Most likely to be diagnosed with CODs (Manuel et al., 2018)	Higher rates of SUDs than women (SAMHSA, 2020)
Geographic location differences among gender-diverse populations is a significant predictor of substance choice and rate of use (Hughto et al., 2021)	Internalized stigma associated with cannabis use among transgender women (Gonzalez et al., 2017)	Internalized stigma associated with excessive alcohol use among transgender men (Gonzalez et al., 2017)	When diagnosed with alcohol use disorder, higher rates of co-occurring diagnosis than men (Holzhauer & Gamble, 2017)	Less diagnosed with MH disorders (SAMHSA, 2020)
Substance use and COD research with gender-diverse populations is scarce (Gonzalez et al., 2017; Hughto et al., 2021)	Young adults (18–25) in both groups experience the most significant rates of mental health disorders and SUDs relative to older gender-diverse individuals and the overall population of cisgender people (Hughto et al., 2021)		Three times more likely to exhibit psychotic symptoms with a history of cocaine dependence (Miquel et al., 2013)	More likely than women to be diagnosed with a psychotic disorder co-occurring with substance use disorders (Miquel et al., 2013)

COD, co-occurring disorder; SUD, substance use disorder.

to have closer familial and social relationships than men; however, often due to consequences associated with substance use, those relationships may be strained (Katz-Saltsman et al., 2008). Also, women identified more concerns with family and social problems. They are more willing than men to address family problems in treatment yet not in a co-ed treatment environment (DiNitto et al., 2002). Whereas more men may be just as impacted by strained relationships with family and others, they are possibly unable/unwilling to recognize the conflict (DiNitto et al., 2002). Internalized stereotypical concepts of masculinity or being "manly" may contribute to denial or minimizing of the problem.

Women are more likely to be primary caregivers for children than men regardless of the diagnosis and were often pregnant or actively parenting when treatment was needed (Manuel et al., 2018). However, parenting responsibilities often present as a primary barrier to entering treatment and/or treatment completion (Agterberg et al., 2020; Jeong et al., 2015). With this in mind, the effective treatment should be both collaborative and comprehensive in nature (Baird, 2008). Collaborative treatment involves the inclusion of several social service entities like child protective services, medical professionals, legal systems, community case workers, psychiatrists, and counselors. Women who are pregnant or parenting need comprehensive care that includes treatment programs with childcare, healthcare, prenatal care, psychiatric care and vocational training (Baird, 2008).

Although men with CODs are less likely than women to be involved in parenting, Stover et al. (2018) suggested that men would benefit from the inclusion of parenting support during treatment. Researchers included a fatherhood-based parenting program in men's treatment. The program included skills training, cognitive restructuring, and reflective functioning. Results indicated that men experienced greater interest in active parenting as well as co-parenting with the mother of their children. In addition, men reported an increased understanding of the value of fatherhood (Stover et al., 2018).

Prior to treatment entry/engagement women are more likely than men to live with family, partners, and spouses who are addicted or use substances (DiNitto et al., 2002). Therefore, it is likely that upon treatment completion, women are likely to return to the same environment. With this in mind, women in treatment for CODs need education on the risks of returning to the environment (DiNitto et al., 2002). Women also need realistic and practical support on breaking previous associations with individuals who are addicted or use substances. Support should include details on alternative living arrangements, financial/money management, employment skills, and overall life skills. Also, there is a need for the inclusion of partners, spouses, and other family members in treatment (Agterberg et al., 2020; Katz-Saltzman et al., 2008; Mueser et al., 2009).

HISTORY OF TRAUMA AND ABUSE

Men and women with CODs report a strong relationship to violent victimization, sexual abuse, and psychological or emotional distress (de Waal et al., 2018; Lowenthal et al., 2018). People with CODs who have a history of trauma and victimization, if left untreated, can lead to an exacerbation of symptoms associated with co-occurring disorders (de Waal et al., 2018). Sullivan et al. (2016) highlighted a strong association between substance use and increases in PTSD symptoms for people with a history of intimate partner violence. Also, women who have a history of sexual abuse and victimization require mental health treatment (Lowenthal et al., 2018). Further, McKee and Hilton (2017) indicated that helping professionals can expect to interact with women who have CODs that consist of substance use, PTSD, and intimate partner violence. Sullivan et al. (2016) noted that women with a recent history of intimate partner violence were 15 times more likely to engage in alcohol and drug use. Kail (2010) suggested that treatment providers facilitate trauma-focused substance use treatment that includes motivational interviewing. Warshaw et al. (2013) suggested that treatment providers utilize "modified cognitive behavioral therapy protocols" to consider psychoeducation, trauma history, safety needs, and risk of further victimization (p. 17). Because many women with CODs have a history of violent victimization, they exhibit fear of being harmed while in treatment, therefore co-occurring treatment should include a safe and nonthreatening environment (McKee & Hilton, 2017).

According to de Waal et al. (2018) men are less likely than women to disclose a history of violent trauma. These researchers indicated that young men with CODs have a "self-sacrificing" (p. 74) and accommodating personality style that may be connected to childhood physical abuse. The men would benefit from treatment that addresses developing and maintaining appropriate boundaries with others. Overall, men and women require gender specific prevention efforts and treatment groups should address victimization, trauma, and sexual abuse (McKee & Hilton, 2017).

SOCIOECONOMIC FACTORS

In comparison to individuals with a sole diagnosis, individuals with CODs have higher rates of unemployment and are prone to struggles in daily life (Pérez-López et al., 2018). Both men and women with CODs who initiate treatment have a history of unemployment, homelessness, and poverty (SAMHSA, 2020). However, women are more likely than men to be unemployed. Therefore, DiNitto et al. (2002) suggest that treatment for CODs should also address identifying and engaging activities that are meaningful and productive. Treatment efforts should include courses or training related to basic living skills and money management. Robertson et al. (2020) found that extremely low employment rates at baseline were partially related to direct admission from prison or jail into a treatment facility. Six months after transition from incarceration to treatment, most of the participants in the study were still unemployed and had not completed vocational training. Administrators of the treatment facility hired a vocational trainer to assist with employment and education upon discharge from the program. The addition of vocational training corresponded with increased rates of employment and decreased rates of homelessness and poverty among people with CODs.

LEGAL AND ETHICAL CONSIDERATIONS

DiNitto et al. (2002) denoted gender-based differences in history of illegal activity among people with CODs. Young men are more likely to have a history of property offenses like theft or breaking and entering (de Waal et al., 2018). Men have a history of arrests and charges for more serious crimes and experience longer periods of jail time than women, while women have a history of sexual solicitation and drug possession offenses (DiNitto et al., 2002).

Regardless of the offense, it is possible that both men and women exhibit fear of legal consequences and thus engage in either substance abuse or mental health treatment to avoid incarceration. Men are also motivated to continue with treatment as a result of fear of committing violent acts (Watkins et al., 1999). Overall, people with CODs benefit from support in avoiding behaviors that might lead to incarceration because involvement in the legal system may contribute to the exacerbation of symptoms associated with the COD (de Waal et al., 2018).

The connection between CODs warrants that treatment providers include anger management training, social skills training, and offense-related prevention efforts. Watkins et al. (1999) also suggest the inclusion of motivational interviewing techniques that encourage the risks and benefits for continued engagement in illegal acts. Women are likely to benefit from co-occurring-based treatment to address guilt, shame, and feelings of worthlessness associated with their criminal charges. Offenses like prostitution and other sex work activities are heavily stigmatized in our society and can result in internalized oppressive beliefs.

SCREENING AND ASSESSMENT TOOLS

SAMHSA stresses the importance of screening and assessment with populations experiencing CODs. Screening is described as "a process for evaluating the possible presence of a particular problem" (SAMHSA, 2013, p. 58). Screening outcomes are used to determine whether an evaluation is necessary. Should a screening tool indicate the need for an evaluation, assessment tools are used to define, diagnose, and treat the problem (SAMHSA, 2013). When screening and assessing CODs with SUDs, it is important to consider population demographics and identities, including gender, race, and other cultural considerations. Common screening and evaluation tools used to identify the prevalence of CODs and SUDs with gender-based cultural considerations are included in Table 16.2.

MULTICULTURAL CONSIDERATIONS

Culturally diverse populations are at higher risk for experiencing the co-occurrence of mental health challenges and substance use/abuse issues (Gainsbury, 2017). According to Gainsbury (2017), positive outcomes and retention among culturally diverse clients is dependent on the provision of culturally competent treatment and equitable practices. Additionally, the integration of treatment for clients with diverse identities reduces overall costs related to care and treatment (Gainsbury, 2017). The benefits of cultural competence with individuals experiencing co-occurring mental health and substance use issues outweigh the risks associated with omitting, avoiding, or diminishing the necessity of such practices. Thus, clinicians are encouraged to acquire a working knowledge and understanding of the complex intersection of culture and CODs in the lives of the diverse clients served (Hickling, 2012).

Historically in the field of counseling, multicultural considerations and competence were not a critical aspect of clinical practice. In fact, foundational psychotherapeutic perspectives, theories, and treatment were based on the interactions and innovations derived from Anglo-European/White psychologists and their client counterparts (Raja, 2016). The expansion of and greater access to mental health services made apparent the need for the acquisition of multicultural competence to support a growing diverse client population, mitigating the increasing risk for client harm based on their multilayered cultural identities (Raja, 2016). Early ideas to address this disconnect in the field included demographic matching within the therapist/client relationship; however, studies contraindicated both the benefits and risks for doing so. For example, gender matching among therapists and clients is considered most significant only when other factors are included (i.e., age, client diagnosis) rather than considering gender alone (Raja, 2016). Additionally, Raja (2016) suggests clinicians take a client-centered stance, allowing the client's needs, preferences, and cultural identities to be the guiding light toward ensuring multicultural competence. Hickling (2012) indicated that providing opportunities for exploring ethnicity with a client opens the door to learning about the client's ever-evolving culture.

To obtain this client-centered information, Hickling (2012) offered *psychohistoriography* as a means of uncovering the intricate complexities of a client's rich diverse identity and experiences.

TABLE 16.2 **Common Screening and Assessment Tools**

SCREENING/ASSESSMENT	DESCRIPTION	RESOURCE URL/WEBSITE
SAMHSA TIP 42: Screening and Assessment of Co-Occurring Disorders	Complete Screening and Assessment Process, pages 31–68	https://store.samhsa.gov/sites/default/files/SAMHSA_Digital_Download/PEP20-02-01-004_Final_508.pdf
DSM-5 Level 2 Cross-Cutting Symptoms Measure–Substance Abuse–Adult	The 15-item measure is used to assess the pure domain of prescription medicine, and illicit substance use in adults age 18 and older	https://www.psychiatry.org/psychiatrists/practice/dsm/educational-resources/assessment-measures
AUDIT	A simple and effective method of screening for unhealthy alcohol use defined as risky or hazardous consumption or any alcohol use disorder	https://auditscreen.org/
CAGE	Identifies alcohol problems over the lifetime. Two positive responses are considered a positive test and indicate further assessment is warranted	CAGE Screening Tool
TWEAK	A five-item scale developed originally to screen for risk drinking during pregnancy (however, the items are not gender specific and the scale can be used with either women or men)	https://adai.uw.edu/instruments/pdf/TWEAK_252.pdf
Mental Health Screening Form-III (MHSF-III)	A 17-item instrument designed as a mental health screening tool for clients seeking admission to substance abuse treatment programs. Preliminary examination of the instrument has shown it to be reliable and valid	The Mental Health Screening Form-III
PTSD Screening and Assessment	Proper assessment of trauma exposure and PTSD is best accomplished with validated measures. Using the link, information and online courses about assessment tools and best practices are found	https://www.ptsd.va.gov/professional/assessment/overview/index.asp
Suicide Screening and Assessment Tools	Ask Suicide-Screening Questions (ASQ) tool is a set of four brief suicide screening questions that takes 20 seconds to administer	Adult ASQ Toolkit

Specifically, "psychohistoriography is an analytic tool used to create *insight* and to *incite* change in individuals or collectives by examining their psychopathology within the historical context of that person or group" (Hickling, 2012, p. 213). Doing so helps bridge the gap between the client's experience and the helper's understanding of the client experience by focusing on the client's cultural background and experiences.

The overlapping and intersecting identities of gender, CODs, and culture are rarely researched, yet is a critically important aspect of clinical treatment and intervention for these clients. For example, Davis and colleagues (2015) were the first researchers to empirically determine that "the intersection of African American woman substance abusers' ethnic, gender, and clinical identities foster distinctive life experiences that dictate special treatment needs" (p. 132). Clinicians who affirmatively respond to the identities and experiences of diverse clients with CODs will experience positive treatment outcomes and a strong therapeutic alliance with these clients (Davis et al., 2015). Data from the study showed that the ability to establish a working alliance with African American women substance abusers is "significantly increased when therapists are multiculturally competent, egalitarian, and empowering, in addition to demonstrating empathy, unconditional positive regard, and genuineness" (Davis et al., 2015, p. 132).

Similarly in their research, Oberheim and colleagues (2017) explored the unique needs related to the gender identity of transgender individuals entering treatment for SUDs. Both the incidences of mental health and substance use issues remain extremely high for transgender individuals, with SUDs affecting over 25% of this population (Oberheim et al., 2017). Mental health challenges and substance use plague the transgender community due to their experience of "stigma, discrimination, bullying, family conflict, and abuse" (Oberheim et al., 2017, p. 33). Ill-equipped clinicians who are unaware of the unique needs of transgender individuals with CODs will potentially do harm by jeopardizing the client's ability to successfully complete treatment (Oberheim et al., 2017). Hence the need for "trans-competent" clinicians who are able to effectively and affirmatively treat CODs and meet the unique needs of this group (Oberheim et al., 2017, p. 38).

Oberheim and colleagues (2017) engaged in breakthrough original research highlighting the need to educate and train trans-competent counselors and design facilities, with these clients in mind, that effectively treat CODs. Achieving this goal requires professional helpers to look to the literature and research to inform our practices for working with transgender clients (Oberheim et al., 2017). Overall, clinicians must be prepared to understand the needs of the transgender population seeking treatment for CODs through the acquisition of knowledge, taking a nonjudgmental therapeutic stance, and examining one's personal beliefs and biases on gender (Oberheim et al., 2017).

Gainsbury (2016) revealed that clinicians are "one of the primary sources of racial/ethnic disparities in mental health treatment outcomes" (p. 990). A nonjudgmental approach with clients requires the clinician to remain humble, curious, "non-assuming, open and respectful of one's cultural identities" (Gainsbury, 2016, p. 990). During sessions, clinicians must inquire about and actively work to include the client's cultural identities in practice, specifically treatment planning, as well as discussing culture-specific behaviors to avoid pathologizing the client/family (Gainsbury, 2016). Learning information about the client and client's family, especially family of origin, is critically important for enhancing cultural sensitivity in treatment for CODs (Gainsbury, 2016). Salom et al.'s (2015) novel research examined the familial factors associated with the development of CODs. The researchers discovered that "maternal smoking and low mother-child warmth appear to be involved with the development of comorbidity in young adults" and "adolescent behavior and drinking are early markers of this comorbidity" (Salom et al., 2015, pp. 254–255).

Uncovering the client's familial dynamics can help support clinicians in learning about the client/family's help-seeking behaviors, family involvement in developing and maintaining CODs; working with the family simultaneously may mitigate these challenges, that is, diminish enabling behaviors (Gainsbury, 2016). Clinicians failing to address and process cultural identities and differences with their clients out of concern that doing so would cause more challenges are providing less than efficacious services (Gainsbury, 2016). Instead, "openly acknowledging, querying and addressing cultural issues" can help resolve and reduce any barriers to effective treatment (Gainsbury, 2016, p. 990). Maintaining an open dialogue around culture with clients experiencing CODss is critically important, especially toward the conclusion of treatment. These discussions include processing cultural factors that represent stressors and strengths to support the client in maintaining positive treatment outcomes (Gainsbury, 2016).

CLINICAL CASE ILLUSTRATION AND DISCUSSION

CASE OF CHRISTINE

Christine is a 27-year-old White, cisgender female from a rural county in Alabama. During her childhood, her father was in recovery from methamphetamine use and her mother was prescribed alprazolam for severe anxiety. Christine recalled on special occasions both her mother and father would take extra alprazolam for fun. At age 14, her parents relinquished custody of her due to behavioral issues and also because she formed an intimate relationship with an African American male from her school. While in foster care, she began experimenting with marijuana with her foster brother. One day when they were home alone, he sexually assaulted her. After the assault, Christine became withdrawn from her foster family and peers. She experienced depressed moods and self-blame for assault. Christine also experienced frequent flashbacks of the assault. She felt afraid, alone, and ashamed. During a routine home visit, Christine's foster care case worker noticed changes in Christine's behavior and mood. After an extended period of probing and questions, Christine disclosed the assault to her case worker. Upon reporting the assault, she was removed from the home and placed in a group home.

At age 15, while in the group home, she began to use various pills including ecstasy, oxycodone hydrochloride, and hydromorphone hydrochloride provided by other residents. At age 17, she became pregnant and later gave birth to a son. After the child was born, Christine moved in with the child's biological father, Ben, who was a drug dealer and convicted felon. Ben, 10 years Christine's senior, was from a neighborhood near the group home where Christine lived. Christine began engaging in prostitution in order to support her and Ben's crack cocaine addiction. When the child was 7 months old, Ben physically abused Christine to the point of requiring hospitalization. Child protective services were contacted, and they removed the child from the home. Christine's parents would not accept custody of the baby because the child was biracial and the child was placed in foster care. Before Christine would be eligible to regain custody, she was ordered to complete a 15-week parenting class, complete a residential treatment program, remain drug free for at least 6 months, secure legal income, and secure clean and safe housing.

The child's foster parents are interested in adoption and if Christine does not reach all of her goals within the next 12 months, Christine's parental rights may be terminated and her child will be eligible for adoption.

CASE DISCUSSION

Situations such as those experienced by Christine are a reality for many women with children who are also addicted to drugs. Traumatic situations lead to psychiatric symptoms and development of CODs. Those who do not have access to mental health care, or are untrusting of mental health professionals, will often self-medicate in an attempt to numb the negative feeling associated with traumatic events or current struggles. Women have also noted that a fear of losing their children or lack of childcare are reasons that they avoid going to treatment.

CHAPTER SUMMARY

There are several theories as to why individuals experience co-occurring mental and substance use disorders. Chronic societal stressors, stigma, and discrimination are among the many reasons individual continue to experience CODs. In considering this experience, counselors must include the impact of gender, specifically the ever-expanding gender experiences of the clinical populations served. These considerations are critical regarding the treatment needs of cisgender and transgender women and LGBTQ+-identifying individuals who experience CODs at alarmingly higher rates than cisgender males. Additionally, the likelihood of gender-diverse clients receiving a COD diagnosis is exponentially higher than that of the remaining population. Accurately diagnosing CODs with this population is one step toward meeting their treatment needs. Further considerations for gender-diverse clients include facility placement.

Meeting the treatment needs of all clients with CODs must include care for both substance use and mental illness through the use of a multidisciplinary team of professionals who collaborate in care for the client. Otherwise, many of the clients' needs will go unmet. Variances among men and women who seek treatment for CODs are significant and must be understood to provide the most effective treatment plan, emphasizing a focus on either more substance or mental health support. Other supports needed are also influenced by the client's gender experience (e.g., family dynamics, trauma history, employment and housing statuses).

Ethical and legal considerations for clients with CODs include understanding the relationship between gender and illegal activity, as well as gender related to avoidance of legal consequences. These engagements in the legal system could be the catalyst for many individuals to seek, maintain, and complete treatment, regardless of gender. Treatment support connected to the client's legal history must include attention to the offense and weighing of the risks and benefits of engaging in illegal activity.

The high-risk needs of individuals experiencing CODs requires clinicians to do their best to address the holistic needs of these clients through cultural exploration and understanding. This exploration strengthens the therapeutic relationship and allows for shared collaboration regarding culture-specific themes related to treatment. To include, maintain, and enhance multicultural competence with this group, it is imperative that clinicians remain curious, nonjudgmental, educated/trained, and open to all of the client's unique needs. After all, it is these unique needs that embody the client's personality, being, and personal culture.

TABLE 16.3 **Mental Health and Substance Use Disorder Support Resources**

NAME	DESCRIPTION	WEBSITE
Drug and alcohol support groups	Links to resources and various alcohol and drug support groups	https://www.therecoveryvillage.com/treatment-program/aftercare/related/support-groups/
12-step programs	Links to listing for 12-step programs, designed to support people struggling with addiction	https://www.therecoveryvillage.com/treatment-program/aftercare/related/types-12-step-programs/
Support groups for families	Links to support for family members of people with substance use disorders	https://www.therecoveryvillage.com/family-friend-portal/support-groups-for-families/
Al-Anon	Support for family and friends of people with alcohol use disorders	https://al-anon.org/
Nar-Anon	Support for family and friends of people with substance use disorders and addiction	https://www.nar-anon.org/naranon/
The Trevor Project	The Trevor Project is the world's largest suicide prevention and crisis intervention organization for LGBTQ (lesbian, gay, bisexual, transgender, queer, and questioning) young people	https://www.thetrevorproject.org/get-help/
National Suicide Prevention Hotline	The Lifeline provides 24/7, free and confidential support for people in distress, prevention and crisis resources for individuals and their loved ones, and best practices for professionals in the United States	https://suicidepreventionlifeline.org
Trans Lifeline	Trans Lifeline provides trans peer support for our community that's been divested from police since day one. It's run by and for trans people	https://translifeline.org/

DISCUSSION QUESTIONS

1. What are some specific treatment considerations among transgender individuals with CODs? How might counselors effectively support transgender individuals in treatment?
2. What approaches can counselors utilize to help women with CODs to prepare for returning to an environment where family members, partners, or spouses are engaging in substance use post-treatment?

3. Identify some of the major treatment concerns for men with CODs. What type of treatment environment would you develop to support men toward treatment completion?
4. What are some of the key factors to consider when including family members, partners, and/or spouses in counseling for people with CODs?
5. When considering the case of Christine, how can she benefit from collaborative and comprehensive treatment?
6. When considering Christine's situation, is placing a woman's children in foster care used as a punishment?

REFERENCES

Agterberg, S., Schubert, N., Overington, L., & Corace, K., (2020). Treatment barriers among individuals with co-occurring substance use and mental health problems: Examining gender differences. *Journal of Substance Abuse Treatment, 112*, 29–35. https://doi.org/10.1016/j.jsat.2020.01.005

Azagba S., Latham K., Shan L. (2019). Cigarette, smokeless tobacco, and alcohol use among transgender adults in the United States. *International Journal of Drug Policy, 73*, 163–169. https://doi.org/10.1016/j.drugpo.2019.07.024

Baird, C. (2008). Improving outcomes for women with co-morbid conditions: Look to the evidence. *Journal of Addictions Nursing, 19*(2), 45–47. https://doi.org/10.1080/10884600802173358

Bockting, W. O., Miner, M. H., Romine, R. E. S., Hamilton, A., & Coleman, E. (2013). Stigma, mental health, and resilience in an online sample of the US transgender population. *American Journal of Public Health, 103*(5), 943–951. https://doi.org/10.2105/AJPH.2013.301241

Chen, K. W., Banducci, A. N., Guller, L., Macatee, R. J., Lavelle, A., Daughters, S. B., & Lejuez, C. W. (2011). An examination of psychiatric comorbidities as a function of gender and substance type within an inpatient substance use treatment program. *Drug and Alcohol Dependence, 118*(2-3), 92–99.

Connolly, M. D., Zervos, M. J., Barone, C. J., Johnson, C. C., & Joseph, C. L. M. (2016) The mental health of transgender youth: advances in understanding. *Journal of Adolescent Health, 59*(5), 489–495. https://doi.org/10.1016/j.jadohealth.2016.06.012.

Davis, T. A., Ancis, J. R., & Ashby, J. S. (2015). Therapist effects, working alliance, and African American women substance users. *Cultural Diversity and Ethnic Minority Psychology, 21*(1), 126–135.

DiNitto, D. M., Webb, D. K., & Rubin, A. (2002). Gender differences in dually-diagnosed clients receiving chemical dependency treatment. *Journal of Psychoactive Drugs, 34*(1), 105–17.

Drake, R. E., O'Neal, E. L., & Wallach, M. A. (2008). A systematic review of psychological research on psychosocial interventions for people with co-occurring severe mental and substance use disorders. *Journal of Substance Abuse Treatment, 34*(1), 123–138. https://doi.org/10.1016/j.jsat.2007.01.011

Finnegan, D. G., McNally, E. B. (2002). *Counseling lesbian, gay, bisexual and transgender substance abusers*. New York, NY: Haworth Press.

Gainsbury, S. M. (2016). Cultural competence in the treatment of addictions: Theory, practice, and evidence. *Clinical Psychology and Psychotherapy, 24*, 987–1001. https://doi.org/10.1002/cpp.2062

Gainsbury, S. M. (2017). Cultural competence in the treatment of addictions: Theory, practice and evidence. *Clinical Psychology & Psychotherapy, 24*(4), 987–1001.

Gonzalez, C. A., Gallego, J. D., & Bockting, W. O. (2017). An examination of demographic characteristics, components of sexuality and gender, and minority stress as predictors of excessive alcohol, cannabis, and illicit (noncannabis) drug use among a large sample of transgender people in the United States. *Journal of Primary Prevention, 38*(4). https://doi.org/10.1007/s10935-017-0469-4

Hickling, F. W. (2012). Understanding patients in multicultural settings: A personal reflection on ethnicity and culture in clinical practice. *Ethnicity & Health, 17*(1-2), 203–216.

Holzhauer, C. G., & Gamble, S. A. (2017). Depressive symptoms mediate the relationship between changes in emotion regulation during treatment and abstinence among women with alcohol use disorders. *Psychology of Addictive Behaviors, 31*(3), 284–295. https://doi.org/10.1037/adb0000274

Hughes, T. L., Elinson, M. (2002). Substance use and abuse in lesbian, gay, bisexual, and transgender populations. *Journal of Primary Prevention, 22*, 263–298.

Hughto, J. M. W., Quinn, E. K., Dunbar, M. S., Rose, A. J., Shireman, T. I., & Jasuja, G. K. (2021). Prevalence and co-occurrence of alcohol, nicotine, and other substance use disorder diagnoses among US transgender and cisgender adults. *JAMA Network Open, 4*(2). https://doi.org/10.1001/jamanetworkopen.2020.36512

Jeong, J. J., Pepler, D. J., Motz, M., DeMarchi, G., & Espinet, S. (2015). Readiness for treatment: Does it matter for women with substance use problems who are parenting? *Journal of Social Work Practice in the Addictions, 15*(4), 394–417. https://doi.org/10.1080/1533256X.2015.1091002

Kail, B. L. (2010). Motivating women with substance abuse and intimate partner violence. *Journal of Social Work Practice in the Addictions, 10*(1), 25–43. https://doi.org/10.1080/15332560903526002

Katz-Saltsman, S., Biegel, D., & Townsend, A. (2008). The impact of caregiver-care recipient relationship quality on family caregivers of women with substance-use disorders or co-occurring substance and mental disorders. *Journal of Family Social Work, 11*(2), 141–165. https://doi.org/10.1080/10522150802169012

Keuroghlian, A. S., Reisner, S. L., White, J. M., & Weiss, R. D. (2015). Substance use and treatment of substance use disorders in a community sample of transgender adults. *Drug and Alcohol Dependance, 152*, 139–146. https://doi.org/10.1016/j.drugalcdep.2015.04.008

Lowenthal, M., Surratt, H. L., Buttram, M. E., & Kurtz, S. P. (2018). Serious mental illness among young adult women who use drugs in the club scene: Co-occurring biopsychosocial factors. *Psychology, Health & Medicine, 23*(1), 82–88. https://doi.org/10.1080/13548506.2017.1330545

Mangrum, L. F., Spence, R. T., & Lopez, M. (2006). Integrated versus parallel treatment of co-occurring psychiatric and substance use disorders. *Journal of Substance Abuse Treatment, 30*(1), 79–84. https://doi.org/10.1016/j.jsat.2005.10.004

Manuel, J. I., Stebbins, M. B., & Wu, E. (2018). Gender differences in perceived unmet treatment needs among persons with and without co-occurring disorders. *The Journal of Behavioral Health Services & Research, 45*(1), 1–12. https://doi.org/10.1007/s11414-016-9530-y

McKee, S. A., & Hilton, N. Z. (2017). Co-occurring substance use, PTSD, and IPV victimization: Implications for female offender services. *Trauma, Violence, & Abuse, 20*(3), 303–314.

Miquel, L., Roncero, C., García-García, G., Barral, C., Daigre, C., Grau-López, L., Bachiller, D., & Casas, M. (2013). Gender differences in dually diagnosed outpatients. *Substance Abuse, 34*(1), 78–80. https://doi.org/10.1080/08897077.2012.709223

Moore, K. A., Young, M. S., Barrett, B., & Ochshorn, E. (2009). A 12-month follow-up evaluation of integrated treatment for homeless individuals with co-occurring disorders. *Journal of Social Service Research, 35*(4), 322–335.

Mueser, K. T., Glynn, S. M., Cather, C., Zarate, R., Fox, L., Feldman, J., Wolfe, R., & Clark, R. E. (2009). Family intervention for co-occurring substance use and severe psychiatric disorders: Participant characteristics and correlates of initial engagement and more extended exposure in a randomized controlled trial. *Addictive Behaviors, 34*(10), 867–877. https://doi.org/10.1016/j.addbeh.2009.03.025

Newcomb M. E., Hill R., Buehler K., Ryan D. T., Whitton S. W., & Mustanski B. (2020). High burden of mental health problems, substance use, violence, and related psychosocial factors in transgender, non-binary, and gender diverse youth and young adults. *Archives of Sexual Behavior, 49*, 645–659. https://doi.org/10.1007/s10508-019-01533-9

Oberheim, S. T., DePue, M. K., & Hagedorn, W. B. (2017). Substance use disorders (SUDs) in transgender communities: The need for trans-competent SUD counselors and facilities. *Journal of Addictions & Offender Counseling, 38*(1), 33–47.

Pérez-López, A., Marín-Navarrete, R., Villalobos-Gallegos, L., Sánchez-Domínguez, R., Toledo-Fernández, A., & Ambriz-Figueroa, A. K. (2018). Effects of co-occurring disorders on the perception of family functioning. *Journal of Substance Use, 23*(5), 528–534. https://doi.org/10.1080/14659891.2017.1405092

Raja, A. (2016). Ethical considerations for therapists working with demographically similar clients. *Ethics & Behavior, 26*(8), 678–687. https://doi.org/10.1080/10508422.2015.1113133

Robertson, A. J., Easter, M. M., Hsiu-Ju, L., Khoury, D., Pierce, J., Swanson, J., & Swartz, M. (2020). Gender specific participation and outcomes among jail diversion clients with co-occurring substance abuse and mental health disorders. *Journal of Substance Abuse Treatment, 115*, 1–7. https://doi.org/10.1016/j.jsat.2020.108035

Ruiz, P. (2017). Addressing co-occurring disorders. *Focus, 15*, 9–10. https://doi.org/10.1176/appi.focus.154S11

Ruppert, R., Kattari, S. K., & Sussman, S. (2021). Review: Prevalence of addiction among transgender and gender diverse subgroups. *International Journal of Environmental Research and Public Health, 18*(16). https://doi.org/10.3390/ijerph18168843

Salom, C. L., Williams, G. M., Najman, J. M., & Alati, R. (2015). Familial factors associated with development of alcohol and mental health comorbidity. *Addiction, 110*(2), 248–257. https://doi.org/10.1111/add.12722

Scheim, A. I., Bauer, G. R., & Shokoohi, M. (2016). Heavy episodic drinking among transgender persons: Disparities and predictors. *Drug and Alcohol Dependence, 167*, 156–162. https://doi.org/10.1016/j.drugalcdep.2016.08.011

Stover, C. S., Carlson, M. Patel, S., & Manalich, R. (2018). Where's dad? The importance of integrating fatherhood and parenting programming into substance use treatment for men. *Child Abuse Review, 27*(4), 280–300. https://doi.org/10.1002/car.2528

Substance Abuse and Mental Health Services Administration. (2013). *Substance abuse treatment: Addressing the specific needs of women. Treatment Improvement Protocol (TIP) series* Rockville, MD: Substance Abuse and Mental Health Services Administration, Center for Substance Abuse Treatment. DHHS Publication SMA13-4426.

Substance Abuse and Mental Health Services Administration. (2018). *National Survey on Drug Use and Health.* Rockville, MD: Substance Abuse and Mental Health Services Administration, Center for Substance Abuse Treatment. https://www.samhsa.gov/data/release/2018-national-survey-drug-use-and-health-nsduh-releases.

Substance Abuse and Mental Health Services Administration. (2019). *National Survey on Drug Use and Health.* Rockville, MD: Substance Abuse and Mental Health Services Administration, Center for Substance Abuse Treatment. https://www.samhsa.gov/data/release/2019-national-survey-drug-use-and-health-nsduh-releases.

Substance Abuse and Mental Health Services Administration. (2020). *TIP 42: Substance use treatment for persons with co-occurring disorders. Treatment Improvement Protocol [TIP] Series*, HHS Publication No. (SMA) PEP20-02-01-004). U. S. Department of Health and Human Services. https://store.samhsa.gov/product/tip-42-substance-use-treatment-persons-co-occurring-disorders/PEP20-02-01-004

Sullivan, T. P., Weiss, N. H., Flanagan, J. C., Willie, T. C., Armeli, S., & Tennen, H. (2016). PTSD and daily co-occurrence of drug and alcohol use among women experiencing intimate partner violence. *Journal of Dual Diagnosis, 12*(1), 36–42. https://doi.org/10.1080/15504263.2016.1146516

de Waal, M. M., Christ, C., Dekker, J. J. M., Kikkert, M. J., Lommerse, N. M., van den Brink, W., & Goudriaan, A. E. (2018). Factors associated with victimization in dual diagnosis patients. *Journal of Substance Abuse Treatment, 84*, 68–77.

Warshaw, C., Sullivan, C. M., & Rivera, E. A. (2013). *A systematic review of trauma-focused interventions for domestic violence survivors.* Retrieved from http://www.nationalcenterdvtraumamh.org/wp-content/uploads/2013/03/NCDVTMH_EBPLitReview2013.pdf

Watkins, K. E., Shaner, A., & Sullivan, G. (1999). Addictions services: The role of gender in engaging the dually diagnosed in treatment. *Community Mental Health Journal, 35*(2), 115–26.

CHAPTER 17

MILITARY POPULATION AND CO-OCCURRING DISORDERS

BENJAMIN V. NOAH

LEARNING OBJECTIVES

After reading this chapter, you will be able to:
- Distinguish facts concerning military populations from fiction.
- Choose appropriate therapy for posttraumatic stress disorder (PTSD) and moral injury.
- Describe alcohol use disorders place as a co-occurring factor when counseling military populations.
- Describe suicide indication in treatment beyond PTSD.

AUTHOR'S PERSONAL STATEMENT

I have a passion and a mission to provide counseling to military service members and veterans. I served 25 years active duty in the U.S. Air Force—I enlisted the day after I graduated from high school and spent 15 years in the enlisted ranks and my last 10 years were as a commissioned officer (for an explanation of the rank system, please see Department of Defense, n.d.; Prosek et al., 2018). During my career, I earned three college degrees (including a master's degree in counseling), served three combat tours, and was involved in five humanitarian missions. I started providing counseling in the Air Force as a volunteer. After my retirement from the Air Force in 1992, I became a professor of counseling and still teach as an adjunct faculty member. I am the founding editor of the *Journal of Military and Government Counseling,* and the majority of my research involves the military and veterans. I struggled with alcoholism and posttraumatic stress disorder (PTSD) like so many others within this population, thus I rely on my first-person experience as well as available research while writing this very important chapter.

—Benjamin V. Noah, PhD

INTRODUCTION

The United States has a long and proud history rooted in military culture. There is, however, also a history of the country neglecting veterans soon after the guns go silent, a concern amplified following the Vietnam War (Burkett & Whitley, 1998; Childers, 2009). The question is: Will today's veterans find themselves facing the same disregard as their counterparts reported after Vietnam? — "In time our battles were forgotten, our sacrifices were discounted, and both our sanity and our suitability for life in polite American society were publicly questioned" (Moore & Galloway, 1992, p. xix). This is a particularly important question with the recent collapse of Kabul, Afghanistan on August 15, 2021, and with it the end of U.S. military action that began in the shadow of September 11, 2001.

The National Center for Veterans Analysis and Statistics estimated that there are 19 million veterans in the United States (U.S. Department of Veteran Affairs, 2021c). The Defense Manpower Data Center (DMDC; 2022) provides current statistics for active-duty military, reserve, and national guard personnel. However, the released information is only representative of folks with unclassified status leaving the numbers incomplete as those serving on classified missions or in classified locations are not included. As of December 31, 2021, there were approximately 1,359,194 service members on active-duty and 793,522 in the reserves and national guard. The Army is the largest branch (470,519), the Navy is second (344,778), the Air Force/Space Force third (333,269), the Marine Corps is fourth (176,259), and the Coast Guard is the smallest (41,261; DMDC, 2022). As of this writing the Space Force is still being organized. Using a current U.S. population estimate of 332 million (Census Bureau, 2021), almost 6% of the U.S. population is currently serving or are veterans.

It is fair to assume that many people (including counselors) get their impressions of the military and veterans from Hollywood, mass media, and social media. Alcohol and drug use in the military are themes in many movies. Examples include *The Sands of Iwo Jima* (1949), *The Outsider* (1961), *Platoon* (1986), and *The Hurt Locker* (2008). Recent research by Delphi Behavioral Health Group (DBHG; 2022) found the military to be the profession with members who reportedly consume the most alcohol in the country. Ergo, when counseling with service members and veterans, alcohol use disorder (AUD) will be a focus area for treatment. The therapy approaches used with veterans and service members are, in most cases, the same as for others seeking treatment—the difference comes in the uniqueness of the military culture.

A common belief among veterans is that those who have not served simply have no respect for the military (Springer, 2021). Therefore, it is essential for counselors to understand the basics of the culture first and foremost, and hopefully this will allow the appropriate treatment to be successful. A foundational knowledge to understanding military culture begins with understanding the vocabulary. The vocabulary can seem like learning a new language. A short list of terms is available in Prosek et al. (2018). For a more complete list, look to the Department of Defense's *DOD Dictionary of Military and Associated Terms* (2021). When in a counseling session and a term comes up that is not known, ask the client. This may result in a look of frustration from the client but most will take time to educate a civilian (i.e., anyone who is not in the military or a veteran).

Military service can be hard, and trauma may be found, not just in combat but in the many humanitarian missions (e.g., responding to natural disasters, helping war refugees), normal training missions, and in sexual and personal violence encounters. "There is a myth that veterans are broken … that what we do somehow rips apart our humanity and damages us beyond repair…" (Fannin, 2018, para 2). The majority of service members return to civilian life and proudly wear their veteran label while becoming successful. Many service members return to their families and feel themselves to be "outsiders." This outsider status may result in increased drinking and the development of depression while harming the family relationship. The family, especially the children, of service members and veterans also feel the impact of service, develop their own mental health issues, and may also need to seek counseling (Matsakis, 2007; Petty, 2009).

PREVALENCE, STATISTICS, AND DEMOGRAPHICS

The mental health professional seeking prevalence information about co-occurring disorders (CODs) among the military population, such as specific incidents or numbers of service members or veterans with behavioral health (BH) issues or numbers of those currently in treatment, will run into a series of walls. For example, not all service members seek treatment within the military and not all veterans are in the Department of Veterans Affairs (VA) health system (Gade & Huang, 2021; Springer, 2021). Additional reasons include that some veterans may not have VA health services within commuting distance or there is a long wait time for treatment, which has been an ongoing issue within the VA system (Gade & Huang, 2021). The warrior culture does not want to be seen as "weak"; thus, shame and stigma may cause this population to seek treatment "off post" with civilian professionals (Prosek et al., 2018; Springer, 2021). Members of the National Guard and Reservist are not always eligible for the BH services that are available to active-duty service members, which places them with civilian providers (TRICARE, n.d.). Stoicism—the ability to suffer in silence—also keeps this population from seeking services. This stoicism is shown in the "suck it up" or "embrace the suck" attitude that keeps many from seeking help (Springer, 2021; Stebnicki, 2021).

DIAGNOSTIC INFORMATION

The Department of Defense (DOD) provides BH data in its annual *Health of the Force* report for the active component (AC; used interchangeably with active-duty) service members. According to the DOD report (2020b):

> A Servicemember was identified as having a BH disorder if they had at least two inpatient, outpatient, or in-theater encounters for a BH condition of any type within 365 days with at least one of the diagnoses occurring during 2019. (p. 9)

BH estimates are provided, in order of prevalence, for adjustment disorders, depressive disorders, anxiety disorders, PTSD, alcohol-related disorders, bipolar disorders, substance-related disorders, and psychoses (DOD, 2020b). Women had a higher prevalence for all disorders except alcohol-related disorders and substance-related disorders where the men prevailed. For all AC service members in 2019, 8.4% of were diagnosed with a BH disorder. The occurrence of BH disorders has been relatively stable for the last 4 years (DOD, 2020b). When looking at prevalence of disorders for AC service members, it is important to remember that those who are not mission capable/deployable are often discharged. This helps to explain the low percentage for the AC when compared to those counted in the VA.

The DOD and the VA do not report data using the same conventions. The VA does not provide a single report on the mental health of veterans; therefore, this requires the curious to look at research outside of the VA or to cherry-pick data from the articles written within the VA Office of Research and Development. This is frustrating to any researcher, and even those within the VA system must mine the data from multiple sources (VA researcher requested anonymity, personal communication, date redacted). A significant contributing factor in the lack of veteran mental health data is a general lack of trust in the VA system among veterans. My (the chapter author's) father and his six brothers all served in World War II; they would refer to the VA as "the place to go to die." I have heard this same sentiment among veterans of my generation (i.e., Vietnam). It can still be heard today and is reflected in an approximate 62% use rate among veterans since 2003 (VA, 2017). There is a hesitancy among veterans and their families to report military service to mental health professionals; thus, screening for military service is needed during all intake appointments (Inoue et al., 2021).

The Substance Abuse and Mental Health Services Administration (SAMHSA) conducts yearly surveys on drug use among veterans; even though it is based on a sample, it does provide an indication of the extent of mental health and substance use issues among veterans. The 2019 SAMHSA survey found that 3.9 million veterans had a substance use disorder (SUD) and/or a mental illness. The number of veterans with a mental illness was 833,000 (26.6%); while 1,000,000 (80.8%) battled alcohol use; 343,000 (26.9%) reported illicit drug use; and 98,000 (7.7%) used both alcohol and illicit drugs. Just over 2% reported a COD (SAMHSA, 2020), but this number is suspected to be higher than acknowledged by those surveyed.

Adjustment Disorders

Approximately 8.1% of women and 3.8% of the men AC service members were diagnosed and treated for adjustment disorders in 2019 (DOD, 2020b). No comparable data could be found reported by the VA. The *Diagnostic and Statistical Manual of Mental Disorders, Fifth Edition-Text Revision (DSM-5-TR*; American Psychiatric Association [APA], 2022) reports a prevalence of 5% to 20% among the general population. If it is assumed that the veteran population is representative of the rest of the country, then AC service members may have a lower occurrence of adjustment disorders.

Depressive Disorders

Among AC service members, 5.1% women and 2.4% men were seen for major depressive disorder in 2019 (DOD, 2020b). In 2008, however, it was estimated that one in eight to 10 veterans visiting VA primary care clinics had major depression (VA, 2021a). The *DSM-5-TR* reports a 7% to 21% prevalence depending on age (APA, 2022). Blore et al. (2015) found that depression and dysthymia among Gulf War veterans were reported at twice the rate of the civilian population. After deployment, 15% of service members were seen for depression (Inoue et al., 2021). "Separation from loved ones and support systems, stressors of combat, and seeing oneself and others in harm's way are all elements that increase the risk of depression in active duty and veteran populations" (Inoue et al., 2021, Introduction). Prior to the *DSM-III*, combat-related stress was often diagnosed as an anxiety disorder or depression with anxiety features (the diagnosis was given to this chapter's author by the VA in 1979).

Anxiety Disorders

Anxiety disorders were reported for 5.1% of female AC service members and 2.2% of male AC service members (DOD, 2020b). Again, no comparable data could be found from the VA. The *DSM-5-TR* lists anxiety disorders by type; however, the prevalence rates are typically under 5% (APA, 2022). It is important to consider that an anxiety disorder may be comorbid with PTSD (APA, 2022).

Posttraumatic Stress Disorder

Of the AC service members who were diagnosed with PTSD in 2019, 2.6% were women and 1.2% were men (DOD, 2020b). Perhaps this number is low in comparison to veterans, as service members who are not deemed fit for deployment are typically medically discharged from service. Additionally, the diagnosis may be with delayed expression and does not express itself until the service member leaves the structured environment of active duty. Among veterans of all ages with PTSD, 10% to 20% is the typical range reported (Inoue et al., 2021; National Center for PTSD, 2022a; Springer, 2021). This statistic, however, may not include those service members who have yet to exhibit active symptoms of PTSD until the next traumatic event occurs.

The VA's National Center for PTSD (NCPTSD, 2022b) recommends three well-researched trauma-focused therapies for treating PTSD: (a) prolonged exposure (PE), (b) cognitive processing therapy (CPT), and (c) eye movement desensitization and reprocessing (EMDR). Regardless of the therapy approach used, counselors should allow the veteran to lead the speed and direction of treatment. For example, some veterans may hold on to grief and nightmares as these symptoms can represent maintaining a connection to fallen comrades (Springer, 2021). Additionally, the veteran may not be able to remember important experiences connected to the trauma, otherwise known as dissociative amnesia (APA, 2022), or the events may never rise to the surface. Although these gaps in memory will slow the therapeutic progress, it is important for counselors to accept an "I do not know" response and not assume the veteran is engaged in avoidance or resistance.

When considering a diagnosis, counselor should look beyond combat as a source of PTSD. To illustrate, deployment on humanitarian missions provides many incidents that can lead to PTSD. Military or National Guard units are typically the first large resources deployed to a national disaster. Additionally, military sexual trauma (MST) has been a focus of recent media coverage and is a cause of PTSD for both female and male service members. The most recent DOD survey in 2018 reported that 6.2% of active-duty women and 0.7% of active-duty men experienced sexual assault, and 24.2% of active-duty women and 6.3% of active-duty men experienced sexual harassment (as cited in Street et al., 2022). The VA's universal screening program found about one in three women and one in 50 men experienced MST at some point during their military service (as cited in Street et al., 2022). Finally, the day-to-day operations of the military provide any number of ways to witness death: aircraft accidents, training accidents, and a standard off-base car accident. To put this in perspective, between 2006 and 2021, 5,419 active-duty service personnel died in accidents compared to 2,723 killed in combat (Congressional Research Service [CRS], 2021). Counselors are encouraged to ask the client about exposures and proceed where the answers take the session.

ALCOHOL-RELATED DISORDERS

Alcohol use is an ingrained piece of the military culture. Reporting for duty with a hangover or still under the influence is not uncommon. Incidents off-installation or being "drunk on-duty" are dealt with in the military justice system and may result in a fine, loss of rank, or being mandated to counseling. The stated alcohol use disorder data included in the *Department of Defense Health of the Force* report (DOD, 2020b) involve those service members who were hospitalized: 1.1% of women and 1.5% of men. Repeated alcohol-related incidents typically result in discharge from service. Veterans' use of alcohol is found in over 50% of the population with approximately 25% heavy drinkers; the use rises for those with combat exposure (Teeters et al., 2017). Counselors should always inquire about alcohol use, both past and present, during intake and assessment sessions with service members and veterans. For those who are currently abstaining from alcohol, ask about current thoughts of drinking as this could indicate craving, which is a significant factor in relapse (APA, 2022). Lastly but very importantly, alcohol use is an important contributing factor in suicide risk and completed suicides among veterans (VA, 2020a); therefore, counselors should conduct a thorough screening at intake and an ongoing assessment throughout counseling for those at risk.

Bipolar Disorders, Substance-Related Disorders, and Psychoses

Bipolar disorder, nonalcohol substance-related disorders, and psychoses are combined into a single topic because the occurrence among AC service members is less than 0.3% for both women and men combined (DOD, 2020b). Once diagnosed, these disorders result in discharge from service. Use of illicit drugs is handled within the military justice system and results in prison or discharge. Such drug use will typically be found during routine random drug testing. Veterans use illicit drugs at a similar rate to civilians (Teeters et al., 2017). Teeters et al. found a 24% increase in opioid prescriptions by the VA between 2001 and 2009 with a high percentage being given for PTSD and other mental health disorders.

Traumatic Brain Injury

While it is not a mental disorder, the prevalence of traumatic brain injury (TBI) among service members and veterans must be a treatment consideration. The rate of TBI in the AC is not reported in the Department of Defense's annual *Health of the Force* report. "Traumatic brain injury has become known as a 'signature wound' of Operation Enduring Freedom (OEF) and Operation Iraqi Freedom (OIF), because the incidence of TBI is higher in these conflicts than it has been in previous conflicts" (CRS, 2013, p. 1). TBI is often comorbid with anxiety, depression, substance use, and/or PTSD (CRS, 2013; Summerall, 2017). An estimated 22% of all combat casualties during OEF/OIF were TBI, and up to 80% of military personnel who reported blast injuries may have TBI (Summerall, 2017).

Moral Injury

The concept of moral injury is relatively new to the mental health literature, yet the struggle between actions in war and the warrior's moral code is as old as combat. The guilt and shame over actions taken or witnessed are found in Homer (Shay, 1994) and the Old Testament (e.g., Psalms 7 and 51). The term itself, however, is evolving (Springer, 2021). Litz et al. (2009) proposed an early definition: "… moral injury involves an act of transgression that creates dissonance and conflict because it violates assumptions and beliefs about right and wrong and personal goodness" (p. 698). A moral injury may occur by acts of omission or commission or "… in response to acting or witnessing behaviors that go against an individual's values and moral beliefs" (Norman & Maguen, n.d., para. 1). Witnessing the death of civilians (especially children) or encountering the dead after the fact creates moral conflict for many veterans. There is overlap between moral injury and PTSD and could be considered as co-occurring in certain incidents (Norman & Maguen, n.d.; Springer, 2021). A combination of moral injury, PTSD, and depression may be lethal (Norman & Maguen, n.d.), so it is vital that counselors assess for these variables and treat accordingly to mitigate risk and harm. Springer (2021) quotes one veteran's letter: "my God has forgiven me, and what I need now is to forgive myself" (p. 83). This citation suggests a need to explore the religious and spiritual beliefs of veterans as they work toward their own self-forgiveness. Should the veteran or the counselor be uncomfortable with the spiritual aspects, a contemplative approach such as Frankl's logotherapy (1959/2006) or Marinoff's philosophical counseling (1999) could be used. PE therapy, CPT, and acceptance and commitment therapy adapted for moral injury are recommended treatment approaches (Norman & Maguen, n.d.).

Suicide

Military and veteran suicide has been a concern in the media and a focus of VA research since 2001. The growing number of those serving, and the increased operational tempo during the War on Terror, are often listed as creating a rise in veteran suicide. Even though counselors should not assume that military clients who disclose suicidal ideation were deployed and/or have PTSD, they should always inquire (Sloan & Noah, 2018). The decrease in operational tempo starting in 2017 has seen a reduction in the suicide rate. Any suicide is a loss and a tragedy, and the yearly average of suicides has been above 6,000 (VA, 2021b). This means that since 2003 more service members and veterans have been lost to suicide than to combat. Much of the media focus has been on PTSD and suicide; however, there is more to consider. For example, there were 902 suicide deaths in 2016 among National Guard and Reserve members who were never federally active; thus, never deployed (VA, 2018). Several studies identified depression co-occurring with PTSD to be particularly fatal (Bryan & Anestis, 2011; Bryan et al., 2013; Finley et al., 2015). In 2019, the highest rate of suicide (38.6%) was among veterans over 55 years of age (VA, 2021b). Meichenbaum (2014) highlights the clinical challenge counselors face:

> *There are no treatments to take away the emotional pain and the interpersonal aftermath, but the clinical challenge is how psychotherapists can help such clients continue their life's journey and help them transform their losses and pain into a life still worth living. (p. 330)*

SCREENING AND ASSESSMENT TOOLS

There are numerous diagnostic interviews, self-report scales, and assessment tools available for various mental and SUDs; however, since PTSD and trauma exposure are primary occurrences among service members and veterans, an abbreviated list for these clinical issues is offered here.

Counselors are encouraged to visit the website of the National Center for PTSD (NCPTSD, 2022e) where a comprehensive catalogue of measures for PTSD and trauma exposure is listed, described, and marked if available for direct download, by request, or via other authors and organizations.

TABLE 17.1 **Select PTSD and Trauma Exposure Diagnostic Interviews, Self-Report Scales, and Assessment Tools**

TYPE	NAME	ABBREVIATION
Adult Interviews	Clinician-Administered PTSD Scale for *DSM-5*	CAPS-5
	PTSD Symptom Scale-Interview for *DSM-5*	PSS-I-5
	Structured Clinical Interview for the *DSM-IV* Axis I Disorders	SCID PTSD Module
	Structured Interview for PTSD	SI-PTSD
Adult Self-Report	Davidson Trauma Scale	DTS
	Impact of Event Scale-Revised	IES-R
	Posttraumatic Diagnostic Scale for *DSM-5*	PDS-5
	Trauma Symptom Checklist-40	TSC-40
	Trauma Symptom Inventory	TSI
	Well-Being Inventory	WBI
Deployment Measures	Deployment Risk and Resilience Inventory-2	DRRI-2

(continued)

TABLE 17.1 **Select PTSD and Trauma Exposure Diagnostic Interviews, Self-Report Scales, and Assessment Tools (*Continued*)**

TYPE	NAME	ABBREVIATION
DSM-5 Measures	Life Events Checklist for *DSM-5*	LEC-5
	Primary Care PTSD Screen for *DSM-5*	PC-PTSD-5
PTSD Screens	Trauma Screening Questionnaire	TSQ
	Startle, Physically Upset by Reminders, Anger, and Numbness (SPAN) Self-Report Screen	SPAN
	Short Post-Traumatic Stress Disorder Rating Interview	SPRINT
Trauma Exposure Measures	Brief Trauma Questionnaire	BTQ
	Combat Exposure Scale	CES
	Trauma History Questionnaire	THQ
	Trauma History Screen	THS

TREATMENT CONSIDERATIONS

Service members may have a *duty profile* (i.e., a physical or mental condition that places them on limited duty or non-deployable status) while veterans may need a *disability assessment*. Both types provide the opportunity for the counselor to examine an array of mental and physical issues involving the use of *ICD-10* codes. These assessments are often based on one visit with medical personnel; however, time should be taken to explore the thoughts of clients as well as add supplemental assessments when clinically indicated. It is important to point out that many service members and veterans may have little interest (as well as patience) for approaches that focus on feelings. Instead, some may prefer a more direct "get the job done" approach. Counselors should, nevertheless, be flexible as there will be times in the therapy session when the processing of emotions must occur.

TREATMENT MODALITIES

Three preferred treatment modalities recommended by the NCPTSD were mentioned earlier in this chapter: (a) CPT, (b) PE therapy, and (c) EMDR. A concise overview of each is provided here as well as a brief mention of various ancillary approaches that may be integrated into counseling services when working with the military population.

Cognitive Processing Therapy

CPT assumes that posttraumatic cognitions contribute to and maintain PTSD. CPT, developed by Resick and Schnicke (1993), is formatted as a 12-session, three-phased approach involving individual, group, or a combination of both depending on each client's need (Resick et al., 2008). Multiple clinical trials and other research attest to CPT's efficacy (VA, 2020b). The first phase of CPT involves building rapport and providing education on PTSD. Counselors may present PTSD as a "normal reaction to an abnormal situation" in order to soften the "clinical" focus while humanizing the client's experience during the discussion. The second phase moves to where the client is asked to write a detailed story of their worst trauma experience (which may be very difficult for many clients). The story is then processed using Socratic questioning. The third phase builds on the second in that it helps the client modify beliefs about the trauma (Resick et al., 2008). The National Center for PTSD within the U.S. Department of Veteran Affairs offers a foundational continuing education course on CPT as a first-line treatment for military and veteran clients as well as those with co-occurring mental and substance use conditions (NCPTSD, 2022c).

Prolonged Exposure Therapy

PE therapy is another cognitive-behavioral approach with extensive empirical support (Foa et al., 2019). Like CPT, it has a manual for clinicians with the addition of a workbook for the client. Ninety-minute sessions allow the client to work through emotional processing (Foa et al., 2019). The client tells the story of the nightmare but pulls out sites, people, or events connected to the event. These people, places, and events that can trigger the client are subsequently placed into a hierarchy for in vivo exposure (Foa et al., 2019). In vivo exposure then has the client repeatedly confront the trigger (Foa et al., 2019). PE therapy is especially effective in treating female veterans with PTSD who exhibit avoidance and numbing (Schnurr & Lunney, 2015). The National Center for PTSD within the U.S. Department of Veteran Affairs offers a foundational continuing education course on PE for PTSD, so interested counselors are directed to obtain more information through their *Treatment Essentials* webpage (NCPTSD, 2022d).

Eye Movement Desensitization and Reprocessing

EMDR was developed by Francine Shapiro in the 1980s to treat PTSD. EMDR moves the client through an eight-phase process. During the process phase, the client visualizes the nightmare while engaged in bilateral stimulation such as tapping the side of the body or side-to-side eye movement (Shapiro, 2001). Studies on EMDR use with veterans supports a 3-month treatment period (Beauvais et al., n.d.). Additional information on EMDR is made available by the National Center for PTSD (2022d), which is accessible on the U.S. Department of Veteran Affairs website.

Other Treatment Approaches

Service members and veterans are resilient due to training that emphasizes never giving up and going the extra mile (Springer, 2021; Stebnicki, 2021). In the past 20 years, the military services have introduced resiliency and wellness programs to strengthen earlier training (Stebnicki, 2021). Some service members and veterans who have not been successful with standard counseling approaches have been helped by mindfulness-based stress reduction, yoga, meditation, and/or religion/spirituality (Stebnicki, 2021). In addition to these ancillary approaches, there are internet resources available to counselors that provide information and training on a number of preferred treatment modalities for working with service members, veterans, and their families; however, three are highlighted here:

1. U.S. Department of Veterans Affairs (VA; 2021d) *Mental Health* webpage

2. National Center for PTSD (2022f), which includes a specific section dedicated to providers where an abundance of information on trauma, PTSD, and treatment is offered

3. Substance Abuse and Mental Health Services Administration (SAMHSA; 2022) Service Members, Veterans, and their Families Technical Assistance Center

MULTICULTURAL CONSIDERATIONS

On July 26, 1948, President Harry S. Truman signed Executive Order 9981 desegregating the United States Armed Forces (Truman Library Institute, 2022). "Despite the issuing of the order, there was considerable resistance from the military. The full effects would not be felt until the end of the Korean War. The Army's last segregated units were finally disbanded in 1954" (Feng, 2021, para. 6). John Allen (2020), President of the Brookings Institute, wrote that the military has made significant progress in addressing racism in the ranks. When one considers that the military is an all-volunteer force, the racial/minority makeup is strikingly similar between the military and the country that it serves.

TABLE 17.2 **Race/Ethnicity of the Military Compared to the U.S. Population**

POPULATION TYPE	RACE/ETHNICITY			
	HISPANIC OR LATINO	BLACK OR AFRICAN AMERICAN	RACIAL MINORITIES GROUPS[a]	WHITE
Total Military Force[b] (Department of Defense, 2020a)	16.1%	16.8%	13%	54.1%
U.S. Population (Jensen et al., 2021)	18.7%	12.1%	11.4%	57.8%

[a] Racial minority includes Asian, American Indian or Alaska Native, Native Hawaiian or Other Pacific Islander, Multiracial, and Other/Unknown.
[b] Total military force consist of active-duty and reserve not including state guard members.

The author of this chapter served in the Air Force during a period when lesbian, gay, and bisexual (LGB) service members were routinely discharged. Of the LGB individuals who continued to serve, they only did so by not disclosing their sexual orientation. "Homosexuality" was deemed to be "incompatible" to military service—over 17,000 LGB personnel were discharged through the 1980s (Pruitt, 2019). Although this was changed during the Clinton administration with the passage of the *Policy Concerning Homosexuality in the Armed Forces* (1993)—colloquially known as "Don't Ask, Don't Tell"—LGB service members were still, nonetheless, discharged because of their sexual orientation. With the repeal of this policy in 2010, President Barrack Obama allowed full military service regardless of a person's sexual orientation (Obama, 2010). The Council on Foreign Relations (2020) indicated that the DOD does not report the number of LGBTQ+ service members; this is confirmed by the lack of such data in the DOD 2020 demographics report (DOD, 2020a). It is estimated, however, that 74,000 LGBTQ+ service members have served since 2010 (McNamara et al., 2020). McNamara et al. (2020, 2021) emphasized the marginalization of LGBTQ+ within the larger culture of the military "… policy change alone, without assurances that being LGBT will not be held against them, may not be enough to fully integrate LGBT service members into the fighting force" (McNamara et al., 2021, p. 524). If the history of other minority service is any guide, it may be several more years before the LGBTQ+ service members are fully viewed as part of the team.

It is important to keep in mind that the military is more than its demographic makeup—it is a distinct culture unto itself with each branch comprising distinct subcultures (Fenell, 2008; Prosek et al., 2018). These branches include the Army, Navy, Marine Corps, Air Force, Space Force, and Coast Guard. According to Fasoli (2020), "culture is a shared and historical system of ideas, values, and practices of a community" (p. 299). The American Counseling Association (ACA) expands on the definition of culture: "membership in a socially constructed way of living, which incorporates collective values, beliefs, norms, boundaries, and lifestyles that are cocreated with others who share similar worldviews comprising biological, psychosocial, historical, psychological, and other factors" (ACA, 2014, p. 20). The shared experience can create limited understanding of the cultural dynamics for civilian counselors and even counselors with military service in their background may find themselves limited in their cultural understanding of the other services (Springer, 2021). The author of this chapter served 25 years on active duty with the last combat tour (Desert Storm) occurring before many of today's veterans were born. So, when conducting the first counseling session with a new veteran, it will be emphasized that their war experiences are not comparable to older veterans; however, he will diligently work to travel with them as they share their lived military experiences. Nevertheless, whether a counselor does or does not have personal experience or direct military involvement, Meichenbaum (2014) offers this advice: "When treating returning service members, there is a need to understand and appreciate military culture. There is a need for the therapist to 'stand close' to the suffering of the client without being overwhelmed" (p. 332).

Service members and veterans are always concerned that counselors will not respect or understand their "warrior" culture. Springer (2021) describes being a warrior:

A "warrior" is someone who lives by a code—a set of values that helps them make decisions between what is right and wrong. A warrior is someone who endures challenges and makes personal sacrifice in the service of these values. (p. 209)

An excellent, and short, expression of the warrior values is General Douglas MacArthur's "*Duty, Honor, Country*" speech at West Point in 1962 (West Point Association of Graduates, 2013).

A primary value among the military is that the mission comes first. Each service has a specific mission set forth in Title 10, Section 8062 of the U.S. Code, and each branch has a shortened version of its mission that its members learn in initial training. For example, "The mission of the United States Air Force is to fly, fight, and win" (U.S. Air Force, n.d.). The men and women of the Air Force are held to this mission 24 hours a day, 365 days a year. Mission is an inclusive term as each deployment, each exercise, and each flight of an aircraft has an assigned mission—that is an objective or goal. A deployment or mission may also be classified and be referenced to vaguely by the service member or veteran. This is further reinforced by the enlistment oath taken by all who enter the military:

I, _____, do solemnly swear (or affirm) that I will support and defend the Constitution of the United States against all enemies, foreign and domestic; that I will bear true faith and allegiance to the same; and that I will obey the orders of the President of the United States and the orders of the officers appointed over me, according to regulations and the Uniform Code of Military Justice. So help me God. (Enlistment Oath-Who May Administer, 1956)

Many, if not most, veterans carry this oath as a sacred value through their lives—it does not have a statute of limitations. It, too, is part of the warrior ethos: "A warrior is someone who endures challenges and makes personal sacrifice in the service of these values" (Springer, 2021, p. 209).

It is necessary for the civilian provider to understand that this is not an "individualist" culture. Initial military training is designed to take individuals and turn them into members of a cohesive team. This team identification applies to each service member's "battle buddies," the unit, and the unit's mission (Lutrell, 2006; Moore & Galloway, 1992; Springer, 2021). Service members place the group above the individual, and they carry this group ethos into civilian life (Springer, 2021). This intense focus on the unit and mission often means that families are in a subordinate position (Matsakis, 2007; Petty, 2009). Physical pain may also be repressed to stay with the unit. As one Marine said, "embrace the suck … lean into the pain and you will get through it" (Springer, 2021, p. 187).

There is also an attitude among this population that civilians (counselors included) will denigrate their service and sacrifice. "Today's Veterans tell me that they feel no better understood by society than our Vietnam Veterans did" (Springer, 2021, p. xxv). Something as simple as how to address or what name to use can easily trip the unaware counselor as first name, last name, rank, specialty, or call sign are all options (Stebnicki, 2021). Another tripping point is the use of acronyms and abbreviations as a normal part of the language. A veteran may use a string of acronyms when talking to a counselor to determine if the counselor will be a "good fit." It is better for the counselor to admit not knowing what is being "thrown" at them than to try to bluff through the conversation. Counselors should not be shy about asking what an acronym, or anything else said, may mean.

Fenell (2008) expressed a need for counselors to receive culturally appropriate training to work with the military/veteran population. This need is still being identified in current research of counselor training programs (Arcuri-Sanders & Forziat-Pytel, 2022a; Carter & Watson, 2018) and of other mental health professionals training (Arcuri-Sanders & Forziat-Pytel, 2022b). The lack of appreciation of military culture may be part of the reason service members are reluctant to talk to mental health providers in time of stress (Springer, 2021).

LEGAL AND ETHICAL CONSIDERATIONS

Counselors should be aware that military members will be, and veterans may be, under the Uniformed Code of Military Justice (UCMJ; 1951). The UCMJ applies to all active-duty members of the uniformed services, students at the military academies, members of the reserves and National Guard (at specified times), and retired members of the uniformed services who receive pay (for a complete list see UCMJ, 1951, §802. Art. 2.). A counselor with a military-related client may be asked for certain information by military authorities should the client be under investigation or subject to charges. This may also place the counselor in tension with the *2014 ACA Code of Ethics* (see §B.1.c.). Should such a request be made, seeking legal advice is the preferred course of action. Military commanders may mandate a service member to mental health services and would, naturally, want to know when the service member was fit for duty. This reinforces "the common thread in the military is that mental health providers serve in evaluative roles" (Springer, 2021, p. 23).

A commander or the service member may want a counselor's input before implementation of nonjudicial punishment (UCMJ, 1951, §815. Art. 15.). More information may be sought should the service member be facing a general court-martial (UCMJ, 1951, §832. Art. 32., §834. Art. 34., §835. Art. 35.). The request for a support letter could come from the service member seeking a defense for lack of mental responsibility (UCMJ, 1951, §850a. Art. 50a.). Again, the primary concern of military authorities will simply be whether the service member is fit for duty. Members of state guards will be under a similar state legal code. For example, the members of the Texas Military Department are subject to the Texas Code of Military Justice (TCMJ) when not in federal service (TCMJ, 1987, §432.002). There may be a conflict between military regulations and state regulations; therefore, a review of each counselor's state licensure board rules and regulations is recommended. And, when in doubt, counselors should seek legal counsel.

Counselors need to be aware of ethical considerations regardless of working with the military and/or civilian population, hence, the ACA *Code of Ethics* (2014) is the primary resource for this information. The ACA ethics code reminds counselors to include cultural considerations in areas of confidentiality (§B.1.a.), values conflicts (§I.1.c.), imposition of personal values (§A.4.b.), multicultural differences (§A.2.c., §C.5.), counselor impairment (§C.2.g.), competence boundaries (§C.2.a.), and treatment modalities (§C.7.a.). When working with a client's trauma, counselor impairment is a critical concern. When working with service members or veterans, vicarious trauma can build on a counselor quickly. Consequently, proactive self-care becomes a life necessity.

CLINICAL CASE ILLUSTRATION AND DISCUSSION

These case illustrations are composites of several veterans. In each case, the experiences of two or three veterans have been consolidated into one person. The typical period of therapy was 12 to 14 sessions.

CASE OF KEN

Ken is a 30-year-old active-duty Air Force recruiter referred to counseling for reporting suicidal ideation. Ken saw combat as security police and was previously treated for PTSD (F43.10) and alcohol use disorder (F10.20). The symptoms of PTSD had abated, and he had been abstinent for 14 months and attended Alcoholics Anonymous weekly. He came home from work and was "blindsided" by an empty house—his wife and daughter were gone. His wife later called and told him she was leaving and had filed for divorce. Ken went into a "hole." Two weeks later he reported to his commander that he had spent the night with a loaded pistol in his lap but did not use it because of his dog laying its head on the pistol.

CASE OF MARY

Mary is a 26-year-old Army veteran. She was in Iraq as a military policewoman and guarded convoys in and out of Baghdad. An improvised explosive device (IED) landed her in hospitals for a year and ended her Army career. Because Mary suffered a TBI (S06.2X0 diffuse TBI without loss of consciousness) and loss of both legs (S88.919 complete traumatic bilateral amputation of lower leg, level unspecified), her counselor had to become familiar with the *ICD-10* S-category codes used for physical injuries. While in the hospital, Mary was diagnosed with PTSD (F43.10) with dissociation (derealization) and developed opioid use disorder (F11.20) from the hydrocodone she used for pain. She stated that she learned how to work the system to keep herself "well supplied" from the VA.

CASE OF KENNETTA

Kennetta is a 29-year-old former Army nurse who spent 3 years assigned to a hospital in Germany where casualties from both Iraq and Afghanistan were sent for stabilization before moving to hospitals in the states. She reported that the continuous strain of long shifts, little sleep, and working with the "wreckage of war" caused her to develop negative emotions. Listening to the patients tell how they were wounded and the emotions they expressed created feelings of guilt and horror. Early in her time in Germany, she had started drinking to "relax" so that she could sleep. However, the longer her time in Germany, the more she drank. She was diagnosed with vicarious PTSD (F43.10) and moderate alcohol use disorder (F10.20).

CASE OF ROBERT

Robert was a Marine rifle platoon commander in Desert Storm. At the urging of his wife, he came to counseling expressing disgust with himself for the return of symptoms of PTSD and that he started drinking after 20 years of sobriety. He said after the birth of his first grandchild he noticed feelings of shame when he was around the child. When a second grandchild arrived, the feelings of shame increased as did his drinking.

CASE DISCUSSIONS

Ken

He reported to the counselor that his nightmares had returned but he managed to stay sober. Ken expressed that he could "get the nightmares back in the box" if the feelings of failure and worthlessness from losing his daughter and wife were "fixed." A diagnosis of major depressive disorder (F32.1) was given and was the focus for treatment. A combination of cognitive therapy and reality therapy were used for 12-weeks to help Ken re-establish his sense of being in control of his life and his career. He set new life goals for moving forward as a single. He said his biggest plus from the therapy was staying sober through the process.

Mary

She reported that she needed to find a new "mission" in life. Since she was having issues with use of her pain medication, she did not want medication for the PTSD so PE therapy (Foa et al., 2019) was used to help resolve the PTSD. At first, she was resistant to the breath exercises and the workbook. He counselor asked her to try for a few weeks. After this, she was on-board for the therapy. Mary knew she needed some pain medication but wanted a way to control her intake. Person-centered therapy was used to develop boundaries in her use. She transferred her pain management to a local doctor who accepted her TRICARE health insurance plan. They established a protocol that allowed Mary one hydrocodone before bed. If she still could not sleep, a second pill could be taken but she would email her doctor of the additional pill use—this gave her accountability for her use. Existential therapy was used to explore an appropriate new "mission." Mary settled on going back to school to become a middle school social studies teacher.

Kennetta

After discussing the alcohol use, it was decided to use CPT (Resick et al., 2008) to treat the PTSD and determine if the alcohol use decreased to a non-clinical level. At the end of 12 sessions, Kennetta reported the emotions of the PTSD had subsided as well as her use of alcohol. During one of her counseling sessions, Kennetta decided to change her specialization from being a trauma nurse to an area that was less emotional, so she began working in the neonatal work at a local hospital.

Robert

When asked to describe some of the events that led to the PTSD diagnosis, Robert related a series of events during the fighting into Iraq when his platoon had come across some dead civilians, including children. He was fairly sure the casualties were not by his platoon, but it still "haunted" him because of the children. His commander at the time told him to "Forget it, it is war." Robert was describing a moral injury. A combination of person-centered therapy and logotherapy was used to help Robert reframe the experience and decrease the feelings of shame. Robert discussed his religious history with his counselor, which had been strong when he was a child. He decided to try going back to church, and once he did, Robert surprisingly felt like he "had returned home." As the shame lessened, so did his drinking, and he was then able to be the type of grandfather he wanted to be for his grandchildren.

CHAPTER SUMMARY

"Veterans are capable of tolerating a *massive* amount of pain and suffering" (Springer, 2021, 168). This stoic position is a factor in many veterans not seeking help until it is too late or nearly so. The high rate of alcohol use is another factor that keeps veterans away from counseling. When working with service members or veterans, counselors need to be conscious of any personal bias toward this population. Veterans have seen their service denigrated by society in the past and thus will be cautious in developing a relationship with the civilian provider. Military personnel are proud of their unique culture and this pride carries into their entry of veteran status.

Co-occurring disorders are common for the military and veteran population due to the common and high use of alcohol. Multiple disorders are not uncommon as a service member recently returned from deployment may have alcohol issues, a TBI, and PTSD from combat then develops anxiety and depression when trying to reconnect to family members. When developing a treatment plan with such a veteran, it may be helpful for counselors to ask, "What do you think is the easiest obstacle to overcome?" The movement forward will depend on the answer. Counselors should also utilize evidence-based treatments such as CPT, PE, or EMDR for PTSD. With other disorders, a wellness model, reality therapy, person-centered, and existential approaches are useful. The military are trained to be flexible and to move when encountering an obstacle. Counselors should also be flexible and change approaches as needed.

It is common practice among Memorial Day speakers to compress lines from two of Associate Justice Oliver Windell Holmes's Memorial Day speeches into one paragraph. Holmes' speeches were given some 20 and 30 years after his service in the Civil War. Like many Memorial Day speakers, this chapter's author has spoken these words on Memorial Day but also at the funerals of veterans as they best sum up the experience of war for the veteran:

> But the truth is that war is the business of youth and early middle age (p. 91)...We have shared the incommunicable experience of war; we have felt, we still feel, the passion of life to its top (p. 93)...Through our great good fortune, in our youth our hearts were touched with fire. (Holmes, 1992, p. 86)

DISCUSSION QUESTIONS

1. Summarize the issues with statistics provided by the Department of Veteran Affairs.
2. Describe the deployment cycle.

3. Summarize the major ethical and legal issues when working with service members and veterans.

4. Describe the warrior ethos.

5. Describe when contemplative therapy approaches may be useful for a veteran.

REFERENCES

Allen, J. R. (2020). *The U.S. military has made progress in ending racial discrimination. The rest of our country must as well.* https://www.brookings.edu/blog/up-front/2020/02/06/the-us-military-has-made-progress-in-ending-racial-discrimination-the-rest-of-our-country-must-as-well/

American Counseling Association. (2014). *The 2014 code of ethics.* Author.

American Psychiatric Association. (2022). *Diagnostic and statistical manual of mental disorders* (5th ed., text rev.). https://doi.org/10.1176/appi.pn.2022.03.3.28

Arcuri-Sanders, N. M., & Forziat-Pytel, K. (2022a). Effectively counseling the military population: Training needs for counselors. *Journal of Multicultural Counseling and Development*, 1–12. https://doi.org/10.1002/jmcd.12236

Arcuri-Sanders, N. M., & Forziat-Pytel, K. (2022b). Mental health professionals serving the Military: Who has access? *Journal of Counseling Research and Practice*, 7(2), p. 108–132. https://egrove.olemiss.edu/jcrp/vol7/iss2/6

Blore, J. D., Sim, M. R., Forbes, A. B., Creamer, M. C., & Kelsall, H. L. (2015). Depression in Gulf War veterans: A systematic review and meta-analysis. *Psychol Med*, 45(8), 1565–1580. https://doi.org/10.1017/S0033291714001913

Bryan, C., & Anestis, M. (2011). Reexperiencing symptoms and the interpersonal-psychological theory of suicidal behavior among deployed service members evaluated for traumatic brain injury. *Journal of Clinical Psychology*, 67(9), 856–865. https://doi.org/10.1002/jclp.20808

Bryan, C. J., Hernandez, A. M., Allison, S., & Clemans, T. (2013). Combat exposure and suicide risk in two samples of military personnel. *Journal of Clinical Psychology*, 69(1), 64–77. https://doi.org/10.1002/jclp.21932

Burkett, B. G., & Whitley, G. (1998). *Stolen valor: How the Vietnam generation was robbed of its heroes and its history.* Verity Press.

Carter, T. T., & Watson, T. I. (2018). Infusing military culture into counselor education. *Journal of Military and Government Counseling*, 6(3), 155–170. https://mgcaonline.org/wp-content/uploads/2018/10/JMGC-Vol-6-Is-3.pdf

Census Bureau. (2021). *U.S. and world population clock.* https://www.census.gov/popclock/

Childers, T. (2009). *Soldier from the war returning: The greatest generation's troubled homecoming from World War II.* Houghton Mifflin Harcourt.

Congressional Research Service. (2013). *Traumatic brain injury among veterans.* http://www.ncsl.org/documents/statefed/health/TBI_Vets2013.pdf

Congressional Research Service. (2021). *Trends in active-duty military deaths since 2006.* https://crsreports.congress.gov/product/pdf/IF/IF10899

Council on Foreign Relations. (2020). *Demographics of the U.S. military.* https://www.cfr.org/backgrounder/demographics-us-military

Defense Manpower Data Center. (2022). *DoD personnel, workforce reports & publications* (December, 2021). https://dwp.dmdc.osd.mil/dwp/app/dod-data-reports/workforce-reports

Delphi Behavioral Health Group. (2022). *Drinking habits by industry.* https://delphihealthgroup.com/drinking-habits-by-industry/

Department of Defense. (n.d.). *U.S. military rank insignia.* https://www.defense.gov/Resources/Insignia/

Department of Defense. (2020a). *2020 demographics profile of the military community.* https://download.militaryonesource.mil/12038/MOS/Reports/2020-demographics-report.pdf

Department of Defense. (2020b). *Health of the Force.* https://health.mil/Reference-Center/Reports/2020/11/24/DoD-Health-of-the-Force-2019

Department of Defense. (2021, November). *DOD dictionary of military and associated terms.* https://irp.fas.org/doddir/dod/dictionary.pdf

Dunlap, S. L., Holloway, I. W., Pickering, C. E., Tzen, M., Goldbach, J. T., Castro, C. A. (2021). Support for transgender military service from active duty United States military personnel. *Sexuality Research and Social Policy 18*, 137–143. https://doi.org/10.1007/s13178-020-00437-x

Enlistment Oath: Who May Administer, Title 10 U.S.C. §502 (1956). https://www.govregs.com/uscode/expand/title10_subtitleA_partII_chapter31_section520#uscode_1

Fannin, J. (2018, Feb 4). Veterans are not broken. *Military Times.* https://www.militarytimes.com/opinion/commentary/2018/02/04/veterans-are-not-broken/

Fasoli, A. D. (2020). Interpretive approaches to culture: Understanding and investigating children's psychological development. *Applied Developmental Science, 24*(4), 299–309. https://doi.org/10.1080/10888691.2020.1789357

Fenell, D. (2008, June 14). A distinct culture. *Counseling Today.* https://ct.counseling.org/2008/06/a-distinct-culture/

Feng, P. (2021). *Executive order 9981: Integration of the armed forces.* https://armyhistory.org/executive-order-9981-integration-of-the-armed-forces/

Finley, E. P., Bollinger, M., Noel, P. H., Amuan, M. E., Copeland, L. A., Pugh, J. A., Dassori, A., Palmer, R., Bryan, C., Pugh, M. J. V. (2015). A national cohort study of the association between the polytrauma clinical triad and suicide-related behavior among US Veterans who served in Iraq and Afghanistan. *American Journal of Public Health, 105*(2), 380–387. https://doi.org/10.2105/AJPH.2014.301957

Foa, E., Hembree, E. A., Rothbaum, B. O., & Rauch, S. (2019). *Prolonged exposure therapy for ptsd: Emotional processing of traumatic experiences - therapist guide* (2nd ed.). Oxford University Press USA - OSO. https://doi.org/10.1093/med-psych/9780190926939.001.0001

Frankl, V. E. (2006). *Man's search for meaning.* Beacon Press. (Original work published 1959)

Gade, D., & Huang, D. (2021). *Wounding warriors: How bad policy is making Veterans sicker and poorer.* Ballast Books.

Holmes, O. W., Jr. (1992). *The essential Holmes: Selections from the letters, speeches, judicial opinions, and other writings of Oliver Wendell Holmes, Jr.* (R, A. Posner, Ed.). University of Chicago Press.

Inoue, C., Shawler, E., Jordan, C. H., & Jackson, C. A. (2021, May 24). *Veteran and military health issues.* StatPearls. https://www.ncbi.nlm.nih.gov/books/NBK572092/

Jensen, E., Jones, N., Rabe, M., Pratt, B., Medina, L., Orozco, K., & Spell, L. (2021). *The chance that two people chosen at random are of different race or ethnicity groups has increased since 2010.* https://www.census.gov/library/stories/2021/08/2020-united-states-population-more-racially-ethnically-diverse-than-2010.html

Litz, B. T., Stein, N., Delaney, E., Lebowitz, L., Nash, W. P., Silva, C., & Maguen, S. (2009). Moral injury and moral repair in war veterans: A preliminary model and intervention strategy. *Clinical Psychology Review, 29*, 695–706. https://doi.org/10.1016/j.cpr.2009.07.003

Lutrell, M. (2006). *Lone survivor.* Little, Brown, and Company.

Marinoff, L. (1999). *Plato, not Prozac!* HarperCollins.

Matsakis, A. (2007). *Back from the front: combat trauma, love, and the family.* Sidran Institute Press.

McNamara, K. A., Lucas, C. L., Goldbach, J. T., Castro, C. A., & Holloway, I. W. (2021). "Even if the policy changes, the culture remains the same": A mixed methods analysis of LGBT service members' outness patterns. *Armed Forces & Society, 47*(3), 505–529. https://doi.org/10.1177/0095327X20952136

McNamara, K. A., Lucas, C. L., Goldbach, J. T., Holloway, I. W., & Castro, C. A. (2020). "You don't want to be a candidate for punishment": A qualitative analysis of LGBT service member "outness." *Sexuality Research and Social Policy, 18*, 144–159. https://doi.org/10.1007/s13178-020-00445-x

Meichenbaum, D. (2014). Ways to bolster resilience in traumatized clients: Implications for psychotherapists. *Journal of Constructivist Psychology, 27*(4), 329–336. https://doi.org/10.1080/10720537.2013.833064

Moore, H. G., & Galloway, J. L. (1992). *We were soldiers once…and young.* Random House.

National Center for PTSD. (2022a, March, 23). *How Common is PTSD in Veterans?* https://www.ptsd.va.gov/understand/common/common_veterans.asp

National Center for PTSD. (2022b, March, 23). *PTSD treatment basics.* https://www.ptsd.va.gov/understand_tx/tx_basics.asp

National Center for PTSD. (2022c, April 6). *Cognitive processing therapy for PTSD.* https://www.ptsd.va.gov/professional/treat/txessentials/cpt_for_ptsd_pro.asp

National Center for PTSD. (2022d, April 25). *Treatment essentials.* https://www.ptsd.va.gov/professional/treat/txessentials/index.asp

National Center for PTSD. (2022e, May 23). *PTSD screening instruments.* https://www.ptsd.va.gov/professional/assessment/list_measures.asp

National Center for PTSD. (2022f, June 30). *PTSD: National Center for PTSD.* https://www.ptsd.va.gov/index.asp

Norman, S. B., & Maguen, S. (n.d.) *Moral injury.* https://www.ptsd.va.gov/professional/treat/cooccurring/moral_injury.asp

Obama, B. (2010, December). *Remarks by the President and Vice President at signing of the Don't Ask, Don't Tell Repeal Act of 2010.* https://obamawhitehouse.archives.gov/the-press-office/2010/12/22/remarks-president-and-vice-president-signing-dont-ask-dont-tell-repeal-a

Petty, K. (2009). *Deployment: Strategies for working with kids in military families.* Redleaf Press.

Policy Concerning Homosexuality in the Armed Forces, 10 U.S.C. § 654 (1993). https://www.govinfo.gov/content/pkg/USCODE-2010-title10/pdf/USCODE-2010-title10-subtitleA-partII-chap37-sec654.pdf

Prosek, E. A., Burgin, E. E., Atkins, K. M., Wehrman, J. D., Fenell, D. L., Carter, C., & Green, L. (2018). Competencies for counseling military populations. *Journal of Military and Government Counseling,* 6(2), 87–99. https://mgcaonline.org/wp-content/uploads/2018/07/JMGC-Vol-6-Is-2.pdf

Pruitt, S. (2019). *Once banned, then silenced: How Clinton's Don't Ask Don't Tell policy affected LGBT military.* Retrieved from https://www.history.com/news/dont-ask-dont-tell-repeal-compromise

Resick, P. A., & Schnicke, M. K. (1993). *Cognitive processing therapy for rape victims: A treatment manual.* Sage Publications.

Resick, P. A., Monson, C. M., & Chard, K. M. (2008). *Cognitive processing therapy: Veteran/military version.* Department of Veterans' Affairs.

Schnurr, P. P., & Lunney, C. A. (2015). Differential effects of prolonged exposure on posttraumatic stress disorder symptoms in female veterans. *Journal of Consulting and Clinical Psychology,* 83(6),1154–1160. https://doi.org/10.1037/ccp0000031

Shapiro, F (2001). *Eye movement desensitization and reprocessing: Basic principles, protocols, and procedures.* Guildford Press.

Shay, J. (1994). *Achilles in Vietnam: Combat trauma and the undoing of character.* Scribner.

Sloan, A., & Noah, B. V. (2018). Suicide in the military – more than PTSD. *Journal of Military and Government Counseling,* 6(4), 270–280. https://mgcaonline.org/wp-content/uploads/2019/10/JMGC-Vol-6-Is-4.pdf

Springer, S. (2021). *Warrior: How to support those who protect us* (2nd ed.). Hidden Ivy.

Stebnicki, M. A. (2021). *Clinical military counseling: Guidelines for practice.* American Counseling Association.

Street, A., Skidmore, C., Gyuro, L., & Bell, M. (2022). *Military sexual trauma.* https://www.ptsd.va.gov/professional/treat/type/sexual_trauma_military.asp#four

Substance Abuse and Mental Health Services Administration. (2020). *2019 National survey on drug use and health: veterans.* https://www.samhsa.gov/data/report/2019-nsduh-veterans

Substance Abuse and Mental Health Services Administration. (2022, June 16). *SAMHSA Service Members, Veterans, and their Families Technical Assistance (SMVF TA) Center.* https://www.samhsa.gov/smvf-ta-center

Summerall, E. L. (2017). *Traumatic brain injury and PTSD: Focus on veterans.* Retrieved from https://www.ptsd.va.gov/professional/co-occurring/traumatic-brain-injury-ptsd.asp

Teeters, J. B., Lancaster, C. L., Brown, D. G., & Back, S. E. (2017). Substance use disorders in military veterans: Prevalence and treatment challenges. *Substance abuse and rehabilitation,* 8, 69–77. https://doi.org/10.2147/SAR.S116720

Texas Code of Military Justice, Chapter 432 (1987). https://statutes.capitol.texas.gov/Docs/GV/htm/GV.432.htm

TRICARE. (n.d.) *National guard or reserve members.* https://www.tricare.mil/Plans/New/NewNGRM

Truman Library Institute. (2022). *Executive order 9981: Desegregation of the armed forces, July 26, 1948.* https://www.trumanlibrary.gov/library/research-files/executive-order-9981-desegregation-armed-forces?documentid=NA&pagenumber=1

Uniform Code of Military Justice, 10 USC Ch. 47 (1951). https://uscode.house.gov/view.xhtml?path=/prelim@title10/subtitleA/part2/chapter47&edition=prelim

U.S. Air Force (n.d.). *We do the impossible everyday: Find your path*. U.S. Air Force. Retrieved July 8, 2022, from https://www.airforce.com/mission

U.S. Department of Veterans Affairs. (2017). Analysis of VA health care utilization among Operation Enduring Freedom (OEF), Operation Iraqi Freedom (OIF), and Operation New Dawn (OND) veterans. https://www.publichealth.va.gov/docs/epidemiology/healthcare-utilization-report-fy2015-qtr3.pdf

U.S. Department of Veterans Affairs. (2018). *VA national suicide data report 2005–2016*. https://www.mentalhealth.va.gov/docs/datasheets/OMHSP_National_Suicide_Data_Report_2005-2016_508-compliant.pdf

U.S. Department of Veterans Affairs. (2020a). *Alcohol use disorder and suicide among veterans*. https://www.mentalhealth.va.gov/suicide_prevention/docs/FSTP-Alcohol-Use.pdf

U.S. Department of Veterans Affairs. (2020b). *Clinical trials database: PTSD-repository*. https://www.ptsd.va.gov/ptsdrepository/index.asp

U.S. Department of Veterans Affairs. (2021a, January). *Depression*. https://www.research.va.gov/topics/depression.cfm

U.S. Department of Veterans Affairs. (2021b, September). *National veteran suicide prevention annual report*. https://www.mentalhealth.va.gov/docs/data-sheets/2021/2021-National-Veteran-Suicide-Prevention-Annual-Report-FINAL-9-8-21.pdf

U.S. Department of Veterans Affairs. (2021c, April). *Veteran population*. https://www.va.gov/vetdata/Veteran_Population.asp

U.S. Department of Veterans Affairs. (2021d, July 1). *Mental health*. https://www.mentalhealth.va.gov/index.asp

West Point Association of Graduates. (2013). *Remarks by General Douglas MacArthur upon receiving the Sylvanus Thayer Award West Point – 1962*. https://www.westpointaog.org/sslpage.aspx?pid=2229

CHAPTER 18

LGBTQ+ COMMUNITIES AND CO-OCCURRING DISORDERS

TIFFANY SOMERVILLE, BREON ROSE, RATTANAKORN RATANASHEVORN, DEB CRAWFORD, AND SUSAN KASHUBECK-WEST

LEARNING OBJECTIVES

After reading this chapter, you will be able to:
- Describe the role that holding an LGBTQ+ identity may have on the prevalence, etiology, and treatment of co-occurring disorders (CODs).
- Explain relevant statistics around the prevalence of CODs in the LGBTQ+ community.
- Apply relevant multicultural and ethical treatment strategies to working with LGBTQ+ individuals with CODs.
- Evaluate one's understanding using the case example of an LGBTQ+ individual with CODs.

INTRODUCTION

Sexual identity and gender identity are two important characteristics to consider when working with individuals with co-occurring mental and substance use disorders (SUDs); therefore, the goal of this chapter is to highlight some of the important aspects of working with LGBTQ+ individuals with co-occurring disorders (CODs). Many different identities fall within the LGBTQ+ spectrum, each with different lived experiences and different disparities in mental health outcomes. This chapter covers relevant statistics around prevalence of both mental disorders and SUDs, important multicultural and conceptualization factors, ethical concerns, and specific treatment considerations for working with this population. Where possible, the differentiation between sexual and gender minorities is addressed; however, the research base for gender minorities is considerably smaller than that for sexual minorities. To provide context for this chapter, *sexual minorities* and *gender minorities* are first briefly discussed.

PREVALENCE, STATISTICS, AND DEMOGRAPHICS
SEXUAL MINORITIES

Sexual minorities can be defined as individuals who typically identify as follows:

- **Lesbian:** a woman-identified individual who is attracted to women,
- **Gay:** a man-identified individual attracted to men,
- **Bisexual:** an individual attracted to men or women,
- **Pansexual:** an individual attracted to any gender, and
- **Queer:** an individual who identifies on the sexual minority spectrum that may not ascribe to one of the previously mentioned labels; an individual who is romantically, physically, or sexually attracted to individuals of their same gender identity, or to multiple gender identities.

Sexual minorities have been shown to experience greater mental health concerns than their heterosexual counterparts (Mays & Cochran, 2001; Williams & Mann, 2017). Going further, sexual minorities experience higher rates of anxiety, depression, and substance use than heterosexual individuals (Mays & Cochran, 2001; Williams & Mann, 2017), and this is often linked to discrimination. It is important to note that although many studies compare mental health outcomes of LGBTQ+ people with cisgender, heterosexual individuals, sometimes comparing the stigmatized minority to the dominant majority can make the minority appear sick, deficient, or damaged. These disparities should not be understood as a characteristic of these populations, but rather, a result of the stigma and societal oppression this group experiences. For example, sexual minority individuals who experienced lifetime or daily discrimination were one to two times more likely to report the presence of a psychiatric disorder than heterosexuals (Mays & Cochran, 2001). Large scale studies have also shown that sexual minority individuals are more likely to get treatment for anxiety disorders, depressive disorders, mood disorders, and SUDs than individuals who identify as heterosexual (Bränström, 2017).

Although much of the literature on sexual and gender minority mental health discusses the prevalence of both substance use and mental health-related outcomes, research on these CODs is more limited. Sexual minorities have been shown to be two to three times more likely to have co-occurring psychological distress and SUDs than heterosexual individuals (Bränström & Pachankis, 2018). Kerridge et al. (2017) found that in a nationally representative sample of individuals, sexual minority individuals displayed elevated rates of 12-month and lifetime alcohol use disorder and major depressive disorder, persistent depressive disorder, panic disorder, agoraphobia, social phobia, generalized anxiety disorder, posttraumatic stress disorder, borderline personality disorder, and schizotypal personality disorder, as compared to their heterosexual counterparts. More specifically, sexual minority men with alcohol use disorder were more likely than heterosexual men with alcohol use disorder to have a mood disorder, anxiety disorder, and lifetime drug use disorder (Lee et al., 2015). Sexual minority men have also been shown to have two to four times higher odds of experiencing co-occurring depressive symptoms and SUDs than heterosexuals (Felner et al., 2021). Similarly, sexual minority women with alcohol use disorder displayed a higher prevalence of mood disorder, dysthymic disorder, or panic disorder than heterosexual women with alcohol use disorder (Mereish et al., 2015). Additionally, sexual minority women were also shown to be three to nine times more likely to experience co-occurring substance use and depressive symptoms than heterosexual women (Felner et al., 2021).

GENDER MINORITIES

Gender minorities can be defined as individuals who typically identify as follows:

- **Transgender:** an individual who does not identify with their sex assigned at birth,
- **Nonbinary:** an individual who does not identify with the gender binary of male or female, and
- **Gender non-conforming:** an individual who presents their gender identity in a way that is inconsistent with gender norms; an individual who either does not identify with their sex assigned at birth or has a gender identity that falls outside of the gender binary.

Gender minorities also experience mental health outcomes that differ from their cisgender counterparts. An integrative review of gender minority mental health by Valentine and Shipherd (2018) found that in samples of transgender/gender nonconforming individuals, roughly 50 studies reported depressive symptoms in participants, 26 studies reported suicidality, 20 reported anxiety, 15 reported posttraumatic stress symptoms, and 26 reported general psychological distress. Additionally, over 31 studies identified alcohol or substance use in this population. Research has also shown that transgender adolescents show greater risk for substance use outcomes than cisgender adolescents (Watson et al., 2020).

Although some studies are beginning to focus on the disparate mental health outcomes for gender minority individuals, very little research has focused specifically on prevalence of co-occurring substance use and other mental health problems in this population. Felner et al. (2021) found that gender minority individuals who were assigned male at birth were roughly three times more likely to experience co-occurring depressive symptoms and SUDs than their cisgender counterparts. Even this finding was a secondary analysis of the study, which primarily focused on sexual minority CODs. Overall, much more research needs to be done to better understand the prevalence of co-occurring substance use and other mental health disorders in gender minority populations.

MULTICULTURAL CONSIDERATIONS
THEORETICAL FRAMEWORKS
INTERSECTIONALITY

Intersectionality is the framework introduced by Kimberlé Crenshaw in 1989 to encourage a focus on multiple aspects and layers of a person rather than focusing on a single identity such as race, sexuality, or gender expression (Cho et al., 2013). Focusing on one aspect of a client may lead to an incomplete or stereotypical view of the client and their problems. Using an intersectional lens means focusing on the multiple sources of oppression and privilege that a person experiences. This lens, therefore, allows for a more holistic understanding of people and the ways their identities create a unique experience. An intersectional lens also addresses issues of power, social justice, and structural oppression. For example, what kinds of structural oppression are faced by LGBTQ+ people with CODs, and how do these impact their well-being and mental health? What type of supports are available for LGBTQ+ individuals with CODs? What are the structural barriers (e.g., access to resources, poverty, systemic racism) and systemic stressors (e.g., pathologizing in the mental health field, invisibility, lack of legal rights) for LGBTQ+ individuals with CODs?

Minority Stress Theory

A second useful model for understanding the lived experience of LGBTQ+ individuals is minority stress theory, which was introduced by Meyer (2003). The theory posits that the psychological issues that minority individuals in society experience are the result of the stigma, discrimination, and prejudice they face as a minority person. These negative experiences may trigger expectations of rejection, identity concealment, and internalized oppression in the sexual minority individual, and these may eventually lead to adverse mental health outcomes. Similar to intersectionality theory, minority stress theory expands the focus beyond the individual to an examination of external and structural causes of psychological difficulties. Therefore, it avoids perpetuating a "blaming the victim" narrative.

Minority stress theory has been used to illustrate how CODs might be caused by minority stress. Empirical evidence supports that internalized heterosexism (the internalization of negative messages about homosexuality by LGBTQ+ people; Szymanski et al., 2008) is associated with negative psychological consequences such as maladaptive coping, more alcohol use, psychopathology, and psychological disorders (Kuerbis et al., 2017). More specifically, Livingston et al. (2017) reported that experiences of discrimination and mistreatment were associated with greater odds of substance and nicotine use in sexual and gender minority individuals. Similarly, being exposed to stigma and heterosexism was correlated with negative mood and more craving for alcohol in lesbian, gay, and bisexual (LGB) youth (Mereish & Miranda, 2019).

Integrating Intersectionality and Minority Stress Theories

As previously noted, LGBTQ+ people have a higher risk of being diagnosed with CODs. Minority stress theory suggests that these disorders are a result of the stigma and discrimination faced by LGBTQ+ people. However, keeping in mind the importance of an intersectional lens, minority stress may affect the substance use and mental health of LGBTQ+ individuals differently depending on their cultural identities. For example, a recent study by Felt et al. (2020) looked at drug use in high school students in the United States across 12 years from 2005 to 2017. The researchers found that drug use decreased among all students over time but it decreased less among lesbian and gay participants than among bisexual and heterosexual participants. The results of this study highlight the importance of paying attention to intersectionality when working with LGBTQ+ individuals with CODs.

Gender

Thinking more specifically about potential subgroups within the larger LGBTQ+ population, such as those based on gender, one factor commonly focused on in men who have sex with men (MSM) is their risk for HIV infection (Balan et al., 2018; Klein et al., 2014). The link between substance use and sexual behavior is one that has been repeatedly examined because drug use may decrease the practice of safer sex behaviors. The term *chemsex,* primarily associated with queer culture and MSM, has been used to refer to the use of drugs such as methamphetamines, GHB ("date rape drug"), and amyl nitrate (poppers) to enhance sexual pleasure (Giorgetti et al., 2017). In addition, drug use may be a response to internalized oppression in MSM. For example, a study by Moody et al. (2018) found that more internalized heterosexism was associated with greater depression, which in turn was correlated with more drug use.

Sexual minority women are thought to be at higher risk for alcohol use disorders; indeed, the relationship between alcohol use and minority stress factors has been frequently studied in samples of sexual minority women. Hughes et al. (2014) found that sexual minority women with both childhood and adult experiences of being targets of oppression had the highest risk of having both depression and hazardous drinking. More specifically, bisexual women in this study reported the most depression. In addition, relationships among variables may be more nuanced than a simple positive correlation between stigma and CODs. For example, Dyar et al. (2020) studied a sample of sexual and gender minority individuals assigned female at birth over a period of 2 years. The results showed that when individuals reported more victimization and microaggressions than usual, their use of alcohol and cannabis was higher and more problematic. In addition, when they reported more minority stress than usual, they reported more anxiety and depression. The findings suggest that working with sexual minority women with co-occurring mental disorders and SUDs might require more sensitive and subtle detection as well as long-term observation to notice the adverse impact of oppression. In addition, different types of minority stress might have different impacts on mental health and substance use.

People of Color

Another area of intersecting identities that has been examined is the experience of LGBTQ+ people of color (POC). For example, Drazdowski et al. (2016) found that racism and LGBTQ+ discrimination experiences predicted more internalized oppression, and subsequently more illicit drug use. Results from a recent qualitative study (Noyola et al., 2020) showed that Latinx LGBTQ+ individuals experienced rejection and ambivalence from family based on their sexual and gender identities and they experienced marginalization from LGBTQ+ communities based on their race and ethnicity. In other words, LGBTQ+ POC have to deal with both racism and LGBTQ+ discrimination; therefore, problematic substance use may be an unhelpful coping strategy that leads to the development of co-occurring mental disorders and SUDs.

Understanding how race and ethnicity intersect with LGBTQ+ identities in POC with CODs is complicated because of the multiple disadvantaged identities (Demant et al., 2018). For example, Mereish and Bradford (2014) reported that sexual minority POC women have a higher substance abuse risk than heterosexual POC women and sexual minority women. Sexual minority POC men had similar risk levels to heterosexual POC men and lower levels of substance abuse risk compared to White sexual minority men (Mereish & Bradford, 2014). Looking more closely, even though Black individuals generally showed lower rates of common psychiatric disorders and SUDs in comparison to White individuals, Black sexual minority individuals have higher rates of these disorders than Black heterosexual individuals (Rodriguez-Seijas et al., 2019). These findings suggest that the minority stress associated with multiple marginalized identities takes a toll. As shown, the rates of CODs among subgroups of the LGBTQ+ community can be very different.

Another illustration of the importance of an intersectional lens was demonstrated in a study by Drabble et al. (2018), who examined spirituality, religiosity, mental health, and substance use across different racial and ethnic groups of LGBTQ+ individuals. Among the many findings was that highly religious Black sexual minority women reported more hazardous drinking than highly religious White sexual minority women, and highly spiritual Latina sexual minority women reported more drug use than White sexual minority women. The results of this study highlight the importance of examining whether religious and spiritual communities are sources of support or marginalization for different racial and ethnic LGBTQ+ individuals. Relationship status also mattered, as single sexual minority POC women reported more drinking than their cohabitating counterparts. Thus, there are multiple identity factors that may play a role in understanding risk for CODs. Importantly, much of the sparse research in this area of racial and ethnic differences has focused on Black and Latinx groups; more research with Asian, indigenous people, and other racial and ethnic minority groups is sorely needed.

In general, the majority of research on SUDs in the LGBTQ+ community has been with well-educated White participants and these findings may not generalize to LGBTQ+ POC. As demonstrated earlier, there are unique intersectional experiences and issues among LGBTQ+ people with CODs. The large number of cultural identities combined with an array of potential SUDs and mental health diagnoses makes it challenging to study risk and resilience factors among members of this diverse group. Nevertheless, findings based on one cultural group (such as White, well-educated, cisgender sexual minority men and women) cannot be expected to generalize to all of the many groups that fit under the LGBTQ+ umbrella. It is imperative that research be conducted with a variety of diverse samples to more fully understand LGBTQ+ clients with CODs. As with all clients, it is important to have cultural humility in working with this population. Failing to attend to diversity within a population with multiple marginalized identities may obscure important mental health distinctions (Rodriguez-Seijas et al., 2019).

LEGAL AND ETHICAL CONSIDERATIONS

Ethical considerations for counselors who serve LGBTQ+ persons with co-occurring mental disorders and SUDs are covered in this section. Unfortunately, there is a lack of specific research and training for working with sexual and gender minorities with dual diagnoses. This section integrates what is known about working with clients who have substance use and mental health disorders with what is currently known about working with LGBTQ+ populations. The focus is on fundamental principles of support, counselor competence, counselor self-awareness, and social advocacy as ethical obligations while serving LGBTQ+ communities with CODs.

FUNDAMENTALS OF SUPPORT

The fundamental principles of professional ethical behavior that guide counseling professionals are integral to providing sound care and support for sexual and gender minorities with CODs; therefore, *autonomy, non-maleficence, beneficence, justice, fidelity,* and *veracity* (American Counseling Association, 2014, p. 3) should be at the forefront of any clinical process, especially when working with this population. Although the core counseling principles have been noted as mandatory guidelines, they are especially important while working with those who are affected by substance misuse (Geppert & Roberts, 2008). For example, counselors should consider how to support gender minority clients and their autonomy at the same time that they might hold gatekeeping power for access to gender-affirming medical treatments, such as hormones or surgery. Counselors are reminded that respecting others, promoting well-being, and doing no harm are ethical principles that should be upheld when working with all clients, including those who have been stigmatized based on their sexual, gender, racial, ethnic, and other identities. Providers should be aware of client concerns related to fidelity, justice, and confidentiality, especially while working in facilities where sexual and gender minorities might be marginalized.

Stigma related to the abuse of substances should also be considered, as it has been found to be very common among persons who have CODs (Corrigan et al., 2009; Geppert & Roberts, 2008). Importantly, Luoma et al. (2007) found that experiences of internal and external acts of stigmatization posed additional challenges for the retention of participants in residential and outpatient substance treatment centers. In addition, Can and Tanriverdi (2015) found a negative correlation between internalized stigma and social functioning in patients diagnosed with a SUD.

Research has also highlighted the importance of addressing stigma at an organizational level. Antistigma and antidiscrimination programs have been found to improve staff attitudes and knowledge while working with patients who are affected by substance use (Khenti et al., 2019). This underscores the importance of not only recognizing the vast impact of stigma on sexual and gender minorities but also intentionally striving to dismantle it. Thus, counselors must be trained to be culturally sensitive to engage with LGBTQ+ people with CODs on an individual, organizational, and societal level.

COUNSELOR COMPETENCY

Recently, the movement within the counseling profession to provide effective therapy to minority clients has made numerous strides. In its 2016 standards, the Council for Accreditation of Counseling and Related Educational Programs (CACREP; 2015) included understanding the *sociocultural context* of clients in its tenets. The Society for Sexual, Affectional, Intersex, and Gender Expansive Identities (formerly known as the Association for Lesbian, Gay, Bisexual, and Transgender Issues in Counseling, 2013) developed counseling competencies for serving sexual and gender minorities. The Substance Abuse and Mental Health Services Administration (SAMHSA, 2020) updated its guiding principles for mental health professionals assisting clients who hold substance use and/or mental health diagnoses during recovery. These recovery principles urge addiction professionals to understand community, culture, respect, the impact of trauma, and strength-focused care as part of standard practice. Additionally, the American Counseling Association (ACA, 2014) requires counselors to support the lived experiences of clients while being ethically bound to *non-maleficence* (i.e., do no harm). Creating a safe environment, using empowerment-based interventions, and having awareness of how oppressive systems within the social environment intersect to negatively affect the wellbeing of sexual and gender minorities who use substances are essential for sound care.

Although there have been efforts to develop extensive multicultural competence in the counseling profession, there remains numerous barriers to training competent counselors. Troutman and Packer-Williams (2014) argued that the CACREP standards were vague concerning working with the LGBTQ+ population, which could lead to counselor training programs diminishing the value of preparing students to develop competencies for serving individuals in these communities. Relatedly, Chaney (2019) analyzed journal articles from the inception of the *Journal of Addictions & Offender Counseling* in 1980 through 2018 and found only five articles that specifically centered on the needs of LGBTQ+ persons with dual diagnoses, suggesting a notable lack of attention to this subject. Finally, much of the counseling and psychological literature has primarily focused on the deficits and risk behaviors that sexual and gender minorities contend with, rather than their resilience in navigating oppressive environments (Luke & Goodrich, 2015). The lack of training in counseling programs coupled with sparse research on LGBTQ+ individuals with CODs may mean clients are working with counselors who lack competence, increasing the likelihood of harm, which is antithetical to the principle of *beneficence.*

COUNSELOR SELF-AWARENESS

A major feature of competence is counselor self-awareness. Specifically, counselors are encouraged to engage in an ongoing process to educate themselves and to address their own personal bias while working with diverse populations (Ratts et al., 2016). Numerous studies have highlighted the importance of self-awareness and reflection to minimize heterosexist and cisnormative (i.e., the common assumption that people are cisgender) beliefs while working with LGBTQ+ communities. Salpietro et al. (2019) examined the experiences of cisgender counselors who provide care to transgender individuals. Participants reported numerous challenges posed by personal, societal, familial, and healthcare systems while working with trans persons. Notable examples from this study included: (a) witnessing gender minority clients being misgendered by staff; (b) transgender clients being ostracized from their families for not dressing according to their limited views of what constitutes gender-appropriate clothing choices; and (c) cisgender bias influencing the therapeutic alliance. Additionally, professional counselors from this study reported a lack of preparation and focus on sexual and gender competence development within their counseling training programs.

Several research studies have found that a lack of training predicts poorer outcomes for LGBTQ+ clients. For example, Mizock and Lundquist (2016) observed that a lack of competence and training on working with gender minorities was linked to poor therapy satisfaction for clients. In a qualitative study (Morris et al., 2020) examining microaggressions aimed at trans and gender-diverse persons, participants shared that the lack of competence in their providers exacerbated their distress and ultimately negatively affected their well-being.

Although there is a great deal of harm that can be caused by a lack of training, the benefits of provider awareness and competence has also been observed in several studies. Kattari et al. (2016) examined the impact of transgender inclusive providers who worked with gender-diverse persons. They found that gender minorities reported more favorable mental health outcomes when working with an inclusive, culturally sensitive provider. Anzani et al. (2019) observed that transgender participants reported feeling supported when counselors displayed their own understanding of identity disclosure and when therapists appeared to challenge cisnormative beliefs while normalizing acceptance and authentic gender expression in session. These findings corroborate the need for the counseling profession to be intentional about training providers to be culturally sensitive and competent.

ASSESSMENT CONSIDERATIONS

It is important to acknowledge that most assessment tools have been developed using a heteronormative and cisnormative framework (Oberheim et al., 2017). It is essential for counseling professionals to consider the numerous ways that heterosexist and cisnormative beliefs influence addiction screening, assessment, and diagnostic criteria while working with sexual and gender minorities (Chaney, 2019). Oberheim et al. (2017) also encouraged counselors to be mindful of the historical and modern inclination to over-pathologize minority individuals during assessments.

IMPORTANCE OF ADVOCACY

According to the American Civil Liberties Union (2021), there are numerous anti-LGBTQ+ laws in force, such as those that criminalize healthcare for gender minority youth, create barriers to receive affirming identification documents, or relegate sexual and gender minorities to use non-affirming facilities. The ACA describes advocacy as the "promotion of the well-being of individuals, groups, and the counseling profession within systems and organizations. Advocacy seeks to remove barriers and obstacles that inhibit access, growth, and development" (ACA, 2014, p. 20).

Alongside stigma that might derive from substance use, discriminatory laws pose a threat to the well-being of sexual and gender minorities. For example, Rostosoky et al. (2009) observed that state marriage amendments prohibiting same-sex marriage increased psychological and minority distress in LGB persons. Similarly, Hatzenbuehler et al. (2010) found that residing in areas with discriminatory policies and laws appeared to impact the well-being of LGB communities, increasing their vulnerability to the development of psychological and substance-related disorders. More recently, Grzanka et al. (2020) examined the impact of the *consciousness clause*, a discriminatory law passed in Tennessee that let therapists refuse service to LGBTQ+ clients. Participants in their study expressed perceptions that this clause was harmful and could be a catalyst for discrimination against other marginalized groups. Du Bois et al. (2018) found that trans persons experienced better health outcomes in alcohol consumption and mental wellness when residing in areas with trans-inclusive policies and state-wide protections. These findings underscore the importance of championing advocacy efforts to support sexual and gender minority communities.

Suggestions for individual advocacy might include counselors self-educating themselves on historic and contemporary sociocultural issues for LGBTQ+ persons. Rose (2020) noted that community and organizational advocacy could include joining initiatives that bolster the well-being of sexual and gender minorities or challenging anti-LGBTQ+ policies or rhetoric. State-wide advocacy might include letter-writing, political lobbying, or training other mental health professionals on sexual and gender minority-related concerns. Importantly, advocacy is a required component of the counseling process that promotes the well-being of sexual and gender minorities with CODs.

OVERALL IMPLICATIONS AND RECOMMENDATIONS

With a general lack of LGBTQ+-specific research and training within the counseling profession, it is imperative that professional counselors engage in opportunities to develop competencies while serving sexual and gender minorities. Counselors should be informed by the six fundamental principles of ethical behavior as outlined by the ACA (2014): *autonomy, non-maleficence, beneficence, justice, fidelity,* and *veracity* (p. 3). Additionally, in any professional setting the potential impact of stigma should be addressed. Sexual and gender minorities who use substances may be especially vulnerable to developing unhelpful coping strategies engendered by societal stigma and maltreatment in care. Providing affirmative, culturally sensitive care is not only best practice while working with these communities but also a professional obligation. Counselors are also encouraged to reflect on their own values and biases pertaining to substance use and LGBTQ+ communities. Furthermore, counselors should be aware of the historic and contemporary impact of oppression and how this influences screening, assessment, and diagnostic processes in counseling. Counselors need to remember the importance of an intersectional lens and to not see sexual and gender minorities as a monolithic community. Finally, counselors are reminded of their ethical obligation to advocate for the needs of sexual and gender minorities.

TREATMENT CONSIDERATIONS FOR LGBTQ+ INDIVIDUALS WITH CO-OCCURRING DISORDERS

As described earlier in the prevalence section of this chapter, it is clear that LGBTQ+ individuals are more likely to be diagnosed with co-occurring mental health and substance use conditions than their heterosexual and cisgender counterparts. Despite the documented need for appropriate interventions with this population due to the increased rates of diagnoses, there is a lack of research regarding culturally competent treatment options for LGBTQ+ individuals with co-occurring mental disorders and SUDs. LGBTQ+ individuals with co-occurring mental health disorders and SUDs have a myriad of unique treatment considerations that mental health providers should be aware of in order to most effectively meet the needs of this population. In this section, treatment considerations that apply broadly to LGBTQ+ individuals with CODs are described and then examples of more specialized treatment considerations for some sexual and gender minorities are provided.

IMPLICATIONS OF MINORITY STRESS

As previously noted, LGBTQ+ individuals are likely to struggle with the effects of minority stressors, including LGBTQ+- discrimination. This discrimination appears to be connected to mental health symptomology, including greater anxiety and worsened depressed mood (Livingston et al., 2020), as well as increased suicidal ideation (Carter et al., 2019). Hatzenbuehler et al. (2009) developed a framework to help mental health providers conceptualize the pervasive impacts of minority stress. Their framework explained that stigma from others results in minority stress which subsequently affects emotional regulation, social interactions, and thinking patterns. Treatment options that are informed in part by the implications of minority stress may be more impactful and helpful for LGBTQ+ individuals (Heck, 2015). Additionally, greater resilience and awareness of the impacts of structural stigma can help reduce psychological distress for LGBTQ+ individuals (Breslow et al., 2015), indicating that mental health providers can play an important role in helping clients develop these skills and understandings to partially mitigate the effects of minority stressors.

SUBSTANCE USE AS A COPING STRATEGY FOR TRAUMATIC EXPERIENCES

Substance use can be conceptualized as a means of coping with past traumatic experiences. Drawing from a large, nationwide survey of both LGB and non-LGB individuals, Sweet and Welles (2012) found that sexual minorities had much higher odds of experiencing childhood sexual abuse than their heterosexual counterparts. Mental health providers should not assume a causal relationship between childhood sexual abuse and sexual minority status as this is a dangerous and harmful stereotype; rather, this connection between childhood sexual abuse and sexual minority behavior is likely attributable to the subtle behaviors of these children that in some way indicated their sexual minority status, thereby making them more vulnerable to abuse from adult perpetrators (Sweet & Welles, 2012). Additionally, Banerjee et al. (2018) found that sexual minority men who had experienced childhood sexual abuse were more likely to engage in alcohol abuse, indicating the use of substances as a means of coping with past trauma.

LGBTQ+ individuals are also vulnerable to other types of trauma. Lifetime prevalence rates of sexual violence are often higher for sexual minority men and women as compared to their heterosexual counterparts (Walters et al., 2013). For example, the lifetime prevalence of violence by an intimate partner (rape, physical violence, and/or stalking) was 44% for lesbians, 61% for bisexual women, 35% for heterosexual women, 26% for gay men, 37% for bisexual men, and 29% for heterosexual men (Walters et al., 2013). These are only some of the examples of the traumatic experiences that can happen to LGBTQ+ individuals, so it is essential for mental health providers to utilize trauma-informed practices with all LGBTQ+ clients (Scheer & Poteat, 2018).

SUICIDALITY AND NONSUICIDAL SELF-INJURY

Counseling professionals should also keep in mind that substance use may serve as a maladaptive coping strategy in the wake of significant LGBTQ+-based discrimination. Mereish et al. (2014) found that substance use mediated the effects of gender and sexual minority stress on suicidal ideation, indicating that participants in this study used substances in part to cope with the challenges of minority stress. Remembering this perspective is helpful in more deeply empathizing with the experiences of clients and understanding patterns of behavior. Perhaps more importantly, this perspective also helps to destigmatize and depathologize SUDs in the LGBTQ+ population.

Counseling professionals should also be aware of the relatively higher occurrence of lifetime suicide attempts in the LGBTQ+ population as compared to heterosexual and cisgender individuals (King et al., 2008). Some of the stressors unique to LGBTQ+ individuals, including uncertainty around disclosing sexual or gender identity and experiences of discrimination, appear to partially explain their overall increased risk of suicide (Mustanski & Liu, 2013; Rivers et al., 2018). Additionally, a lack of positive family support after coming out appears to increase the risk of suicide (Scourfield et al., 2008).

In a meta-analysis of 86 studies on suicidal ideation, Liu et al. (2020) found that individuals with CODs and sexual minority status indicated a higher risk of suicidal ideation. LGBTQ+ individuals with CODs are at particular risk of developing suicidal ideation and attempting suicide; therefore, specialized assessment, monitoring, and interventions related to LGBTQ+ suicidality are particularly needed. For example, Goldbach et al. (2019) surveyed youth who received services from an LGBTQ+-specific crisis line, most of whom called the crisis line to discuss thoughts of suicide. Almost half (42%) of participants reported that they selected this crisis line because of the available counselors who provided services from an LGBTQ+-affirming perspective.

In addition to suicidal ideation and attempts, counseling professionals should also assess for nonsuicidal self-injury (NSSI), defined as physical harm to one's body without the intent to die by suicide (O'Brien et al., 2018). In a meta-analysis of 51 studies on NSSI in the LGBTQ+ population, Liu et al. (2019) found that lifetime prevalence rates of NSSI in sexual minority individuals (29.68%) were over twice that of heterosexual individuals (14.57%); gender minority individuals had the highest rates of lifetime NSSI (46.65%). Due to the significantly increased risk of NSSI, counselors working with LGBTQ+ individuals should ensure they can utilize appropriate assessment and intervention strategies for clients who engage in NSSI.

SOCIAL SUPPORT

Social support is another important factor in every individual's mental health and overall psychological well-being. LGBTQ+ individuals often struggle to feel a sense of belonging with their community due to homophobia, transphobia, discrimination, and oppression (Pakula et al., 2016). Low social support is connected with worse mental health and substance use outcomes for LGBTQ+ individuals with CODs (Klein & Golub, 2016; McConnell et al., 2015). Sexual minority individuals are less likely to feel strongly connected to their general community, leading to a greater chance of worsened mental health outcomes (Pakula et al., 2016). Rejection from family members due to LGBTQ+ identity is also connected to worsened mental health and substance use (Klein & Golub, 2016). Conversely, supportive relationships and programs for LGBTQ+ individuals can lead to better mental health outcomes. Family acceptance of LGBTQ+ identity is associated with higher self-esteem and better overall physical health, as well as lower rates of depression, substance use, and suicidality (Ryan et al., 2010). Acceptance and connection to others in the LGBTQ+ community also appear to decrease the overall risk of suicidal behaviors (Carter et al., 2019; Kaniuka et al., 2019).

TREATMENT BARRIERS

Unfortunately, LGBTQ+ individuals with CODs face some barriers to treatment that prevent them from engaging with treatments that could be helpful in reducing both mental health and substance use symptoms. In a study of 2,778 sexual and gender minority individuals, Ferlatte et al. (2019) found that 62.3% of participants reported that they could not pay for mental health services, and 52.2% reported having inadequate insurance for required services. In addition to financial barriers, 46% of participants reported feeling uncomfortable discussing their mental health concerns and 43% felt a sense of shame about their mental health struggles (Ferlatte et al., 2019). Past biased reactions from health professionals related to LGBTQ+ status also discourage folks from seeking needed services (McNair et al., 2018).

Gender minority individuals in particular also face additional barriers that complicate their mental health and substance use treatment. Unfortunately, there is even less research regarding the treatment needs of gender minorities with CODs in comparison to that of sexual minorities. While all LGBTQ+ individuals are likely to face discrimination, transgender individuals report being particularly vulnerable to discrimination in comparison to their cisgender LGB counterparts (Su et al., 2016). Additionally, mental health providers may find it challenging to properly assess whether mental health symptoms can be attributed to gender dysphoria or a separate mental health diagnosis (Janssen et al., 2019).

AFFIRMATIVE TREATMENTS

Many of the treatments that are efficacious for LGBTQ+ individuals with CODs can be generally described as LGBTQ+-affirmative treatments. These affirmative treatments are structured to provide support and acceptance for all sexual and gender minority identities. Affirmative treatments are in sharp contrast to approaches such as conversion therapy that attempt to change an individual's sexual orientation and/or gender identity; conversion therapy is increasingly being banned across the United States due to the harmful effects on LGBTQ+ individuals (Drescher et al., 2016). Furthermore, affirmative treatments are likely to include paradigms related to the significant impacts of minority stress (Pachankis et al., 2015, 2020). Pachankis (2018) identified several guiding principles of LGBTQ+-affirmative treatments such as: (a) encouraging insight into the relationship between minority stress and mental health; (b) reducing feelings of shame and guilt related to LGBTQ+ status; (c) challenging maladaptive thinking patterns that lead to decreased self-esteem; and (d) increasing resilience and connection with community.

Providers using affirmative treatments are also more likely to work with LGBTQ+ clients from a strengths-based perspective instead of pathologizing aspects of their identities. Lytle et al. (2014) developed a model for using a strengths-based approach with LGBTQ+ clients that is grounded in positive psychology rather than a psychopathology approach. This model includes recommendations for helping clients to use their resilience, personal character strengths, coping skills, and positive relationships with others to more effectively cope with the ramifications of discrimination and minority stress. Overall, LGBTQ+ individuals with CODs are likely to benefit from a therapeutic environment where they feel safe to discuss and integrate their identity into their work (Penn et al., 2013).

Substance use treatments for sexual minority men in particular also often focus on reducing or eliminating substance use in order to decrease sexual activity that could increase susceptibility to HIV (Carrico et al., 2016; Jaffe et al., 2007; Mimiaga et al., 2012). Jaffe et al. (2007) compared four conditions of substance use treatment for sexual minority men: (a) contingency management; (b) cognitive-behavioral therapy; (c) combined contingency management and cognitive-behavioral therapy; and (d) a gay-specific version of cognitive-behavioral therapy. Jaffe et al. found that the participants who engaged in the LGBTQ+-specific type of cognitive-behavioral therapy intervention showed the greatest reduction in substance use and sexual behaviors that may make these men more susceptible to HIV. Mental health symptoms and substance use issues may interact in such a way to increase sexual activity, thereby increasing HIV vulnerability for MSM and reducing the efficacy of HIV-prevention programs (Parsons et al., 2012; Safren et al., 2011). Additionally, CODs may decrease adherence to crucial HIV medications that can reduce HIV viral load, subsequently reducing the likelihood of HIV transmission to sexual partners (White et al., 2014). Mental health providers working in substance use programs should be sure to provide LGBTQ+-specific treatment options rather than providing identical treatment to all clients regardless of sexual or gender identity. For example, with LGBTQ+-specific approaches, sexual minority men may reduce their susceptibility to contracting HIV, increase their medication compliance, and better cope with their HIV status.

UNMET TREATMENT NEEDS AND FUTURE DIRECTIONS

Overall, there are numerous unmet needs for LGBTQ+ individuals with CODs. Significant numbers of LGBTQ+ individuals are not able to access needed treatment (McNair et al., 2018). Furthermore, racial and ethnic minorities within the LGBTQ+ community are even less likely to be able to access treatment for CODs (Jeong et al., 2016). There is also a lack of research on the unique treatment considerations for gender minorities. Much of the current research area refers to LGBTQ+ individuals in generalized, monolithic terms. Mental health providers must remain cognizant of the wealth of diverse experiences of individuals who fall under the LGBTQ+ umbrella.

Even when LGBTQ+ individuals are able to enter treatment, they are unlikely to find LGBTQ+-specific programs to meet their needs. Williams and Fish (2020) found that out of 13,044 treatment facilities in the United States, only 12.6% of mental health facilities and 17.6% of substance abuse facilities offered LGBTQ+-specific programs. LGBTQ+ treatment centers are also more frequently located in urban areas, further isolating individuals who live in rural areas without access to culturally competent treatment (Martos et al., 2017). Williams and Fish (2020) also speculated that many of the facilities that reported having LGBTQ+-specific programming may have been referring to only LGB-specific treatment due to an overall lack of transgender-specific treatment nationwide. Despite the evidence that LGBTQ+ individuals need culturally competent, affirmative services, they are not readily accessible by all who need them.

CLINICAL CASE ILLUSTRATION AND DISCUSSION

CASE OF RYAN

Ryan (they/them) is a 25-year-old first-generation Asian American medical student. Ryan's parents moved to the United States from China 2 years before Ryan was born. Ryan currently lives at home with their parents and their only sibling, a sister who is 2 years younger. They have been to seven counseling sessions at the university's counseling center and have committed to continuing with weekly counseling sessions. Ryan came to counseling for help with stress.

Ryan's sex assigned at birth was male, and they have identified as a cisgender male until recently. Over the past 6 months, they have begun exploring their gender identity and using they/them pronouns. About 2 months ago, Ryan also came out to their friends and family as bisexual. According to Ryan, their parents immediately became upset when they came out as bisexual and gender nonconforming. Ryan's parents have insisted that Ryan is male and heterosexual; they have largely ignored Ryan and threatened to kick them out several times since they came out. Throughout Ryan's gender and sexual identity exploration, their sister has always been extremely supportive.

Ryan has also reported experiencing biased reactions from others in their life. While most of their friends have been supportive, two of Ryan's relatively close friends have seemed to distance themselves lately, which has been hurtful for Ryan. Furthermore, Ryan has requested that their professors begin using they/them pronouns, and two of Ryan's professors have continued to use he/him pronouns. Ryan has felt anxious about speaking up to their professors regarding their pronouns. While Ryan has been exploring their gender identity, they have started dressing differently, including wearing some jewelry, makeup, and more traditionally feminine clothing. According to Ryan, they have noticed staring and "dirty looks" from strangers when they are out shopping, studying on campus, and riding the bus.

According to Ryan, they have been struggling to sleep for several months, and they typically get about 4 hours of sleep per night. Ryan has been having issues with overeating and having a hard time getting out of bed every day. These symptoms have begun to negatively affect their medical school work. Ryan reported feeling very worried that they will fail out of medical school if they cannot keep up with their work. Ryan also feels a lot of pressure from their parents to become a successful doctor. After a few counseling sessions, Ryan's counselor determined that they are experiencing symptoms of depression and anxiety.

Since coming out, Ryan has been trying to make connections with more LGBTQ+ friends as most of their long-time friends are heterosexual and cisgender. Ryan has made some LGBTQ+ friends at school who like to drink alcohol together frequently, often four to five nights per week. Ryan also reports consuming at least three tall liquor-based cocktails per day over the past month, with more drinking occurring on particularly stressful days.

CASE DISCUSSION

Ryan reported that their goals for treatment are to further explore their gender identity, cope with recent stresses due to coming out, and to reduce feelings of depression and their use of alcohol. Their counselor conducted a full mental health assessment in their first session, including a thorough multicultural assessment. Additionally, the counselor asked about Ryan's pronouns in the first session, and she has affirmatively used Ryan's pronouns correctly throughout their sessions. Ryan's counselor has been using a person-centered approach with an emphasis on affirming Ryan's gender and sexual minority identities. Much of the time in session has been spent exploring Ryan's experiences of discrimination and oppression since coming out.

Ryan has also been discussing their alcohol use in session. With the counselor, Ryan has explored their use of alcohol as a maladaptive coping skill for stress. Ryan reported feeling less guilt and shame related to alcohol use after understanding the factors that have contributed to their drinking. The counselor has helped them to explore healthier coping mechanisms to reduce frequency of alcohol use, including exercise and meditation. Ryan has reported a reduction in their alcohol use over the past couple of weeks, though they still feel that they are drinking too much. Their counselor has also provided additional resources for LGBTQ-specific substance use treatment should Ryan feel that they need more services to decrease their alcohol use.

Ryan expressed interest in learning more about hormone replacement therapy. Ryan's counselor explained the diagnosis of gender dysphoria that is typically required for hormonal treatment. She also suggested additional resources and professionals that could be helpful, including the university health services clinic and a local transgender health clinic. Ryan has scheduled appointments for a physical health screening and an appointment with a doctor at the trans health clinic so that they can learn more about hormone replacement therapy. Furthermore, Ryan's counselor has provided resources for LGBTQ+ groups at the university and in the community so that Ryan can make connections within the LGBTQ+ community.

Though early in their treatment, Ryan has reported that they are already feeling a bit better. They stated that having a counselor who is accepting of their identity and open to discussing the effects of minority stress has been really helpful for them. Additionally, Ryan stated that they are excited to connect with additional resources that can aid in their treatment.

CHAPTER SUMMARY

Counseling professionals should be cognizant of the unique needs of LGBTQ+ individuals. Instead of providing uniform treatment to all clients, clinicians should work to provide treatment specific to the needs of this population. Treatment options will vary depending on factors such as theoretical orientation and method of delivery, but there are several broad themes that counselors should incorporate into their treatment while working with LGBTQ+ persons with substance use challenges.

First, counselors should demonstrate an awareness of and ongoing acknowledgment of the influence of stress on minority persons. Treatment providers can utilize strategies to help clients tap into their resilience in the face of numerous stressors. Second, counselors should remember that substance use may function as a coping strategy for other mental health concerns, experiences of trauma, and/or minority stress. Keeping this perspective in mind is useful in reducing stigma around the use of substances in the LGBTQ+ population. Third, counselors should ensure that their treatment strategies are affirmative of LGBTQ+ identities and integrative with other healthcare professionals and facilities. Finally, it is important to remember that the LGBTQ+ community is not a monolith—each person has their own unique experiences and needs for their mental health, and substance use treatment needs to incorporate an intersectional lens. Counseling professionals are encouraged to keep these overall themes in mind as part of their development of culturally competent treatment strategies while working with sexual and gender minorities diagnosed with CODs.

DISCUSSION QUESTIONS

1. How might minority stress and stigma affect the mental health of an LGBTQ+ client? Their readiness for counseling and willingness to stay in counseling? How might their multiple identities be important?
2. How could you communicate to your LGBTQ+ clients that you practice affirmative treatment approaches? What are some examples of a nonaffirmative approach?
3. Knowing that LGBTQ+ individuals with CODs face higher rates of both suicide attempts and nonsuicidal self-injury, what strategies could you use to help your LGBTQ+ clients remain safe?
4. As a counselor, what can you do to advocate for systemic changes that could benefit the lives of your LGBTQ+ clients?

REFERENCES

ALGBTIC LGBQQIA Competencies Taskforce, Harper, A., Finnerty, P., Martinez, M., Brace, A., Crethar, H. C., Loos, B., Harper, B., Graham, S., Singh, A., Kocet, M., Travis, L., Lambert, S., Burnes, T., Dickey, L. M., & Hammer, T. R. (2013). Association for lesbian, gay, bisexual, and transgender issues in counseling competencies for counseling with lesbian, gay, bisexual, queer, questioning, intersex, and ally individuals. *Journal of LGBT Issues in Counseling, 7*(1), 2–43. https://doi.org/10.1080/15538605.2013.755444

American Civil Liberties Union (2021). *Legislation affecting LGBT rights.* https://www.aclu.org/legislation-affecting-lgbt-rights-across-country

American Counseling Association. (2014). *ACA code of ethics.* https://www.counseling.org/docs/default-source/default-document-library/2014-code-of-ethics-finaladdress.pdf

Anzani, A., Morris, E. R., & Galupo, M. P. (2019). From absence of microaggressions to seeing authentic gender: Transgender clients' experiences with microaffirmations in therapy. *Journal of LGBT Issues in Counseling, 13*(4), 258–275. https://doi.org/10.1080/15538605.2019.1662359

Balán, I. C., Frasca, T., Pando, M. A., Marone, R. O., Barreda, V., Dolezal, C., Carballo-Diéguez, A., & Ávila, M. M. (2018). High substance use and HIV risk behavior among young Argentine men who have sex with men. *AIDS and Behavior, 22*(4), 1373–1382. https://doi.org/10.1007/s10461-017-1987-z

Banerjee, N., Ironson, G., Fitch, C., Boroughs, M. S., Safren, S. A., Powell, A., & O'Cleirigh, C. (2018). The indirect effect of posttraumatic stress disorder symptoms on current alcohol use through negative cognitions in sexual minority men. *Journal of Traumatic Stress, 31,* 602–612. https://doi.org/10.1002/jts.22304

Bränström, R. (2017). Minority stress factors as mediators of sexual orientation disparities in mental health treatment: A longitudinal population-based study. *Journal of Epidemiology and Community Health, 71*(5), 446–452. https://doi.org/10.1136/jech-2016-207943

Bränström, R., & Pachankis, J. E. (2018). Sexual orientation disparities in the co-occurrence of substance use and psychological distress: A national population-based study (2008–2015). *Social Psychiatry and Psychiatric Epidemiology, 53*(4), 403–412. https://doi.org/10.1007/s00127-018-1491-4

Breslow, A. S., Brewster, M. E., Velez, B. L., Wong, S., Geiger, E., & Soderstrom, B. (2015). Resilience and collective action: Exploring buffers against minority stress for transgender individuals. *Psychology of Sexual Orientation and Gender Diversity, 2*(3), 253–265. https://doi.org/10.1037/sgd0000117

Can, G., & Tanrıverdi, D. (2015). Social functioning and internalized stigma in individuals diagnosed with substance use disorder. *Archives of Psychiatric Nursing, 29*(6), 441–446. https://doi.org/10.1016/j.apnu.2015.07.008

Carrico, A. W., Zepf, R., Meanley, S., Batchelder, A., & Stall, R. (2016). Critical review: When the party is over: A systematic review of behavioral interventions for substance-using men who have sex with men. *Journal of Acquired Immune Deficiency Syndrome, 73*(3), 299–306. https://doi.org/10.1097/QAI.0000000000001102

Carter, S. P., Allred, K. M., Tucker, R. P., Simpson, T. L., Shipherd, J. C., & Lehavot, K. (2019). Discrimination and suicidal ideation among transgender veterans: The role of social support and connection. *LGBT Health, 6*(2), 1–8. https://doi.org/10.1089/lgbt.2018.0239

Chaney, M. P. (2019). LGBTQ+ addiction research: An analysis of the *Journal of Addictions & Offender Counseling. Journal of Addictions & Offender Counseling, 40*(1), 2–16. https://doi.org/10.1002/jaoc.12053

Cho, S., Crenshaw, K. W., & McCall L. (2013). Toward a field of intersectionality studies: Theory, applications, and praxis. *Journal of Women in Culture and Society, 38*(4), 785–810. https://doi.org/10.1086/669608

Corrigan, P. W., Kuwabara, S. A., & O'Shaughnessy, J. (2009). The public stigma of mental illness and drug addiction: Findings from a stratified random sample. *Journal of Social Work, 9*(2), 139–147. https://doi.org/10.1177/1468017308101818

Council for Accreditation of Counseling and Related Educational Programs. (2015). *2016 CACREP Standards*. http://www.cacrep.org/wp-content/uploads/2017/08/2016-Standards-with-citations.pdf

Demant, D., Oviedo-Trespalacios, O., Carroll, J. A., Ferris, J. A., Maier, L., Barratt, M. J., & Winstock, A. R. (2018). Do people with intersecting identities report more high-risk alcohol use and lifetime substance use? *International Journal of Public Health, 63*(5), 621–630. https://doi.org/10.1007/s00038-018-1095-5

Drabble, L., Veldhuis, C. B., Riley, B. B., Rostosky, S., & Hughes, T. L. (2018). Relationship of religiosity and spirituality to hazardous drinking, drug use, and depression among sexual minority women. *Journal of Homosexuality, 65*(13), 1734–57. https://doi.org/10.1080/00918369.2017.1383116

Drazdowski, T., Perrin, P., Trujillo, M., Sutter, M., Benotsch, E., & Snipes, D. (2016). Structural equation modeling of the effects of racism, LGBTQ discrimination, and internalized oppression on illicit drug use in LGBTQ people of color. *Drug and Alcohol Dependence, 159*, 255–262. https://doi.org/10.1016/j.drugalcdep.2015.12.029

Drescher, J., Schwartz, A., Casoy, F., McIntosh, C. A., Hurley, B., Ashley, K., Barber, M., Goldenberg, D., Herbert, S. E., Lothwell, L. E., Mattson, M. R., McAfee, S. G., Pula, J., Rosario, V., & Tompkins, D. A. (2016). The growing regulation of conversion therapy. *Journal of Medical Regulation, 102*(2), 7–12.

Du Bois, S. N., Yoder, W., Guy, A. A., Manser, K., & Ramos, S. (2018). Examining associations between state-level transgender policies and transgender health. *Transgender Health, 3*(1), 220–224. https://doi.org/10.1089/trgh.2018.0031

Dyar, C., Sarno, E., Newcomb, M., & Whitton, S. (2020). Longitudinal associations between minority stress, internalizing symptoms, and substance use among sexual and gender minority individuals assigned female at birth. *Journal of Consulting and Clinical Psychology, 88*(5), 389–401. https://doi.org/10.1037/ccp0000487

Felner, J. K., Haley, S. J., Jun, H.-J., Wisdom, J. P., Katuska, L., & Corliss, H. L. (2021). Sexual orientation and gender identity disparities in co-occurring depressive symptoms and probable substance use disorders in a national cohort of young adults. *Addictive Behaviors, 117*, 106817. https://doi.org/10.1016/j.addbeh.2021.106817

Felt, D., Wang, X., Ruprecht, M. M., Turner, B., Beach, L. B., Philbin, M. M., Birkett, M., & Philips II, G. (2020). Differential decline in illicit drug use by sexual identity among United States high school students, 2005–2017. *LGBT Health, 7*(8), 420–430. https://doi.org/10.1089/lgbt.2020.0163

Ferlatte, O., Salway, T., Rice, S., Oliffe, J. L., Rich, A. J., Knight, R., Morgan, J., & Ogrodniczuk, J. S. (2019). Perceived barriers to mental health services among Canadian sexual and gender minorities with depression and risk of suicide. *Community Mental Health Journal, 55*, 1313–1321. https://doi.org/10.1007/s10597-019-00445-1

Geppert, C. M. A., & Roberts, L. W. (2008). *The book of ethics: Expert guidance for professionals who treat addiction*. Hazelden.

Giorgetti, R., Tagliabracci, A., Schifano, F., Zaami, S., Marinelli, E., Busardò, F.P. (2017) When "Chems" meet sex: A rising phenomenon called "ChemSex." *Current Neuropharmacology, 15*(5), 762–770. https://doi.org/10.2174/1570159X15666161117151148

Goldbach, J. T., Rhoades, H., Green, D., Fulginiti, A., & Marshal, M. P. (2019). Is there a need for LGBT-specific suicide crisis services? *Crisis, 40*(3), 203–208. https://doi.org/10.1027/0227-5910/a000542

Grzanka, P. R., DeVore, E. N., Frantell, K. A., Miles, J. R., & Spengler, E. S. (2020). Conscience clauses and sexual and gender minority mental health care: A case study. *Journal of Counseling Psychology, 67*(5), 551–567. https://doi.org/10.1037/cou0000396

Hatzenbuehler, M. L. (2009). How does sexual minority stigma "get under the skin"? A psychological mediation framework. *Psychological Bulletin, 135*(5), 707–730. https://doi.org/10.1037/a0016441

Hatzenbuehler, M. L., McLaughlin, K. A., Keyes, K. M., & Hasin, D. S. (2010). The impact of institutional discrimination on psychiatric disorders in lesbian, gay, and bisexual populations: A prospective study. *American Journal of Public Health, 100*(3), 452–259. https://doi.org/10.2105/AJPH.2009.168815

Heck, N. C. (2015). The potential to promote resilience: Piloting a minority stress-informed, GSA-based, mental health promotion program for LGBTQ youth. *Psychology of Sexual Orientation and Gender Diversity, 2*(3), 225–231. https://doi.org/10.1037/sgd0000110

Hughes, T. L., Johnson, T. P., Steffen, A. D., Wilsnack, S. C., & Everett, B. G. (2014). Lifetime victimization, hazardous drinking, and depression among heterosexual and sexual minority women. *LGBT Health, 1*(3), 192–203. https://doi.org/10.1089/lgbt.2014.0014

Jaffe, A., Shoptaw, S., Stein, J. A., Reback, C. J., & Rotheram-Fuller, E. (2007). Depression ratings, reported sexual risk behavior, and methamphetamine use: Latent growth curve models of positive change among gay and bisexual men in an outpatient treatment program. *Experimental and Clinical Psychopharmacology, 15*(3), 301–307. https://doi.org/10.1037/1064-1297.15.3.301

Janssen, A., Busa, S., & Wernick, J. (2019). The complexities of treatment planning for transgender youth with co-occurring severe mental illness: A literature review and case study. *Archives of Sexual Behavior, 48*, 2003–2009. https://doi.org/10.1007/s10508-018-1382-5

Jeong, Y. M., Veldhuis, C. B., Aranda, F., & Hughes, T. L. (2016). Racial/ethnic differences in unmet needs for mental health and substance use treatment in a community-based sample of sexual minority women. *Journal of Clinical Nursing, 25*, 3557–3569. https://doi.org/10.1111/jocn.13477

Kaniuka, A., Pugh, K. C., Jordan, M., Brooks, B., Dodd, J., Mann, A. K., Williams, S. L., & Hirsch, J. K. (2019). Stigma and suicide risk among the LGBTQ population: Are anxiety and depression to blame and can connectedness to the LGBTQ community help? *Journal of Gay and Lesbian Mental Health, 23*(2), 205–22 0. https://doi.org/10.1080/19359705.2018.1560385

Kattari, S. K., Walls, N. E., Speer, S. R., & Kattari, L. (2016). Exploring the relationship between transgender-inclusive providers and mental health outcomes among transgender/gender variant people. *Social Work in Health Care, 55*(8), 635–650. https://doi.org/10.1080/00981389.2016.1193099

Kerridge, B. T., Pickering, R. P., Saha, T. D., Ruan, W. J., Chou, S. P., Zhang, H., Jung, J., & Hasin, D. S. (2017). Prevalence, sociodemographic correlates and DSM-5 substance use disorders and other psychiatric disorders among sexual minorities in the United States. *Drug and Alcohol Dependence, 170*, 82–92. https://doi.org/10.1016/j.drugalcdep.2016.10.038

Khenti, A., Bobbili, S. J., & Sapag, J. C. (2019). Evaluation of a pilot intervention to reduce mental health and addiction stigma in primary care settings. *Journal of Community Health, 44*(6), 1204–1213. https://doi.org/10.1007/s10900-019-00706-w

King, M., Semlyen, J., Tai, S. S., Killaspy, H., Osborn, D., Popelyuk, D., & Nazareth, I. (2008). A systematic review of mental disorder, suicide, and deliberate self harm in lesbian, gay and bisexual people. *BMC Psychiatry, 8*(70), 1–17. https://doi.org/10.1186/1471-244X-8-70

Klein, H. (2014). Depression and HIV Risk taking among men who have sex with other men (MSM) and who use the internet to find partners for unprotected sex. *Journal of Gay & Lesbian Mental Health, 18*(2), 164–189. https://doi.org/10.1080/19359705.2013.834858

Klein, A. & Golub, S. A. (2016). Family rejection as a predictor of suicide attempts and substance misuse among transgender and gender nonconforming adults. *LGBT Health, 3*(3), 193–199. https://doi.org/10.1089/lgbt.2015.0111

Kuerbis, A., Mereish, E. H., Hayes, M., Davis, C. M., Shao, S., & Morgenstern, J. (2017). Testing cross-sectional and prospective mediators of internalized heterosexism on heavy drinking, alcohol problems, and psychological distress among heavy drinking men who have sex with men. *Journal of Studies on Alcohol and Drugs, 78*, 113–123. https://doi.org/10.15288/jsad.2017.78.113

Lee, J. H., Gamarel, K. E., Kahler, C. W., Marshall, B. D. L., van den Berg, J. J., Bryant, K., Zaller, N. D., & Operario, D. (2015). Co-occurring psychiatric and drug use disorders among sexual minority men with lifetime alcohol use disorders. *Drug and Alcohol Dependence, 151,* 167–172. https://doi.org/10.1016/j.drugalcdep.2015.03.018

Liu, R. T., Bettis, A. H., & Burke, T. A. (2020). Characterizing the phenomenology of passive suicidal ideation: A systematic review and meta-analysis of its prevalence, psychiatric comorbidity, correlates, and comparisons with active suicidal ideation. *Psychological Medicine, 50,* 367–383. https://doi.org/10.1017/S003329171900391X

Liu, R. T., Sheehan, A. E., Walsh, R. F. L., Sanzari, C. M., Cheek, S. M., Hernandez, E. M. (2019). Prevalence and correlates of non-suicidal self-injury among lesbian, gay, bisexual, and transgender individuals: A systematic review and meta-analysis. *Clinical Psychology Review, 74,* 1–41. https://doi.org/10.1016/j.cpr.2019.101783

Livingston, N. A., Flentje, A., Brennan, J., Mereish, E. H., Reed, O., & Cochran, B. N. (2020). Real-time associations between discrimination and anxious and depressed mood among sexual and gender minorities: The moderating effects of lifetime victimization and identity concealment. *Psychology of Sexual Orientation and Gender Diversity, 7*(2), 132–141. https://doi.org/10.1037/sgd0000371

Livingston, N., Flentje, A., Heck, N. C., Szalda-Petree, A., & Cochran, B. N. (2017). Ecological momentary assessment of daily prejudice experiences and nicotine, alcohol, and drug use among sexual and gender minority individuals. *Journal of Consulting and Clinical Psychology, 85*(12), 1131–1143. https://doi.org/10.1037/ccp0000252

Luke, M., & Goodrich, K. M. (2015). Working with family, friends, and allies of LBGT youth. *Journal for Social Action in Counseling and Psychology, 7*(1), 63–83. https://doi.org/10.33043/JSACP.7.1.63-83

Luoma, J. B., Twohig, M. P., Waltz, T., Hayes, S. C., Roget, N., Padilla, M., & Fisher, G. (2007). An investigation of stigma in individuals receiving treatment for substance abuse. *Addictive Behaviors, 32*(7), 1331–1346. https://doi.org/10.1016/j.addbeh.2006.09.008

Lytle, M. C., Vaughan, M. D., Rodriguez, E. M., & Shmerler, D. L. (2014). Working with LGBT individuals: Incorporating positive psychology into training and practice. *Psychology of Sexual Orientation and Gender Diversity, 1*(4), 335–347. https://doi.org/10.1037/sgd0000064

Martos, A. J., Wilson, P. A., & Meyer, I. H. (2017). Lesbian, gay, bisexual, and transgender (LGBT) health services in the United States: Origins, evolution, and contemporary landscape. *PLoS ONE, 12*(7), 1–18. https://doi.org/10.1371/journal.pone.0180544

Mays, V. M., & Cochran, S. D. (2001). Mental health correlates of perceived discrimination among lesbian, gay, and bisexual adults in the United States. *American Journal of Public Health, 91*(11), 1869–1876. https://doi.org/10.2105/AJPH.91.11.1869

McConnell, E. A., Birkett, M. A., & Mustanski, B. (2015). Typologies of social support and association with mental health outcomes among LGBT youth. *LGBT Health, 2*(1), 55–61. https://doi.org/10.1089/lgbt.2014.0051

McNair, R., Pennay, A., Hughes, T. L., Love, S., Valpied, J., & Lubman, D. I. (2018). Health service use by same-sex attracted Australian women for alcohol and mental health issues: A cross-sectional study. *BJGP Open,* 1–11. https://doi.org/10.3399/bjgpopen18X101565

Mereish, E. H., & Bradford, J. B. (2014). Intersecting identities and substance use problems: Sexual orientation, gender, race, and lifetime substance use problems. *Journal of Studies on Alcohol and Drugs, 75*(1), 179–188. https://doi.org/10.15288/jsad.2014.75.179

Mereish, E. H., Lee, J. H., Gamarel, K. E., Zaller, N. D., & Operario, D. (2015). Sexual orientation disparities in psychiatric and drug use disorders among a nationally representative sample of women with alcohol use disorders. *Addictive Behaviors, 47,* 80. https://doi.org/10.1016/j.addbeh.2015.03.023

Mereish, E. H., & Miranda Jr., R. (2019). Exposure to stigma elicits negative affect and alcohol craving among young adult sexual minority heavy drinkers. *Alcoholism: Clinical and Experimental Research, 43*(6): 1263–1272. https://doi.org/10.1111/acer.14055

Mereish, E. H., O'Cleirigh, C., & Bradford, J. B. (2014). Interrelationships between LGBT-based victimization, suicide, and substance use problems in a diverse sample of sexual and gender minority men and women. *Psychology, Health, and Medicine, 19*(1), 1–13. https://doi.org/10.1080/13548506.2013.780129

Meyer, I. H. (2003). Prejudice, social stress, and mental health in lesbian, gay, and bisexual populations: Conceptual issues and research evidence. *Psychological Bulletin, 129*(5), 674–697. https://doi.org/10.1037/0033-2909.129.5.674

Mimiaga, M. J., Reisner, S. L., Pantalone, D. W., O'Cleirigh, C., Mayer, K. H., & Safren, S. A. (2012). A pilot trial of integrated behavioral activation and sexual risk reduction counseling for HIV-uninfected men who have sex with men abusing crystal methamphetamine. *AIDS Patient Care and STDs, 26*(11), 681–693. https://doi.org/10.1089/apc.2012.0216

Mizock, L., Lundquist, C. (2016). Missteps in psychotherapy with transgender clients: Promoting gender sensitivity in counseling and psychological practice. *Psychology of Sexual Orientation and Gender Diversity, 3*(2), 148–155. https://doi.org/10.1037/sgd0000177

Moody, R. L., Starks, T. J., Grov, C., & Parsons, J. T. (2018). Internalized homophobia and drug use in a national cohort of gay and bisexual men: Examining depression, sexual anxiety, and gay community attachment as mediating factors. *Archives of Sexual Behavior, 47*(4), 1133–1144. https://doi.org/10.1007/s10508-017-1009-2

Morris, E. R., Lindley, L., & Galupo, M. P. (2020). "Better issues to focus on": Transgender microaggressions as ethical violations in therapy. *The Counseling Psychologist, 48*(6), 883–915. https://doi.org/10.1177/0011000020924391

Mustanski, B. & Liu, R. T. (2013). A longitudinal study of predictors of suicide attempts among LGBT youth. *Archive of Sexual Behavior, 42*, 437–448. https://doi.org/10.1007/s10508-012-0013-9

Noyola, N., Sánchez, M., & Cardemil, E. V. (2020). Minority stress and coping among sexual diverse Latinxs. *Journal of Latinx Psychology, 8*(1), 58–82. https://doi.org/10.1037/lat0000143

Oberheim, S. T., Swank, J. M., & DePue, M. K. (2017). Building culturally sensitive assessments for transgender clients: Best practices for instrument development and the adaptation process. *Journal of LGBT Issues in Counseling, 11*(4), 259–270. https://doi.org/10.1080/15538605.2017.1380554

O'Brien, K. H. M., Liu, R. T., Putney, J. M., Burke, T. A., & Aguinaldo, L. D. (2018). Suicide and self-injury in gender and sexual minority populations. In K. B. Smalley, J. C. Warren, & K. N. Barefoot (Eds.), *LGBT health: Meeting the needs of gender and sexual minorities* (pp. 181–198). Springer Publishing Company.

Pachankis, J. E. (2018). The scientific pursuit of sexual and gender minority mental health treatments: Toward evidence-based affirmative practice. *American Psychologist, 73*(9), 1207–1219. https://doi.org/10.1037/amp0000357

Pachankis, J. E., Hatzenbuehler, M. L., Rendina, H. J., Safren, S. A., & Parsons, J. T. (2015). LGB-affirmative cognitive-behavioral therapy for young adult gay and bisexual men: A randomized controlled trial of a transdiagnostic minority stress approach. *Journal of Consulting and Clinical Psychology, 83*(5), 875–889. https://doi.org/10.1037/ccp0000037

Pachankis, J. E., McConocha, E. M., Clark, K. A., Wang, K., Behari, K., Fetzner, B. K., Brisbin, C. D., Scheer, J. R., & Lehavot, K. (2020). A transdiagnostic minority stress intervention for gender diverse sexual minority women's depression, anxiety, and unhealthy alcohol use: A randomized controlled trial. *Journal of Consulting and Clinical Psychology, 88*(7), 613–630. https://doi.org/10.1037/ccp0000508

Pakula, B., Carpiano, R. M., Ratner, P. A., & Shoveller, J. A. (2016). Life stress as a mediator and community belonging as a moderator of mood and anxiety disorders and co-occurring disorders with heavy drinking of gay, lesbian, bisexual, and heterosexual Canadians. *Social Psychiatry and Psychiatric Epidemiology, 51*, 1181–1192. https://doi.org/10.1007/s00127-016-1236-1

Parsons, J. T., Grov, C., & Golub, S. A. (2012). Sexual compulsivity, co-occurring psychosocial health problems, and HIV risk among gay and bisexual men: Further evidence of a syndemic. *American Journal of Public Health, 102*(1), 156–162. https://doi.org/10.2105/AJPH.2011.300284

Penn, P. E., Brooke, D., Mosher, C. M., Gallagher, S. Brooks, A. J., & Richey, R. (2013). LGBTQ persons with co-occurring conditions: Perspectives on treatment. *Alcoholism Treatment Quarterly, 31*(4), 466–483. https://doi.org/10.1080/07347324.2013.831637

Ratts, M. J., Singh, A. A., Nassar-McMillan, S., Butler, S. K., & McCullough, J. R. (2016). Multicultural and social justice counseling competencies: Guidelines for the counseling profession. *Journal of Multicultural Counseling & Development, 44*(1), 28–48. https://doi.org/10.1002/jmcd.12035

Rivers, I., Gonzalez, C., Nodin, N., Peel, E., & Tyler, A. (2018). LGBT people and suicidality in youth: A qualitative study of perceptions of risk and protective circumstances. *Social Science & Medicine, 212*, 1–8. https://doi.org/10.1016/j.socscimed.2018.06.040

Rodriguez-Seijas, C., Eaton, N. R., & Pachankis, J. E. (2019). Prevalence of psychiatric disorders at the intersection of race and sexual orientation: Results from the national epidemiologic survey of alcohol and related conditions-III. *Journal of Consulting and Clinical Psychology, 87*(4), 321–331. https://doi.org/10.1037/ccp0000377

Rose, J. S. (2020). Advocacy and social justice within and on behalf of the LGBTGEQIAP⊠+⊠Community. *Journal of LGBT Issues in Counseling*, *14*(4), 362–373. https://doi.org/10.1080/15538605.2020.1827477

Rostosky, S. S., Riggle, E. D., Horne, S. G., & Miller, A. D. (2009). Marriage amendments and psychological distress in lesbian, gay, and bisexual (LGB) adults. *Journal of Counseling Psychology*, *56*(1), 56–66. https://doi.org/10.1037/a0013609

Ryan, C., Russell, S. T., Huebner, D., Diaz, R., & Sanchez, J. (2010). Family acceptance in adolescence and the health of LGBT young adults. *Journal of Child and Adolescent Psychiatric Nursing*, *23*(4), 205–213. https://doi.org/10.1111/j.1744-6171.2010.00246.x

Safren, S. A., Blashill, A. J., & O'Cleirigh, C. M. (2011). Promoting the sexual health of MSM in the context of comorbid mental health problems. *AIDS Behavior*, *15*, 30–34. https://doi.org/10.1007/s10461-011-9898-x

Salpietro, L., Ausloos, C., & Clark, M. (2019). Cisgender professional counselors' experiences with trans clients. *Journal of LGBT Issues in Counseling*, *13*(3), 198–215. https://doi.org/10.1080/15538605.2019.1627975

Scheer, J. R. & Poteat, V. P. (2018). Trauma-informed care and health among LGBTQ intimate partner violence survivors. *Journal of Interpersonal Violence*, *36*(13–14), 6670–6692. https://doi.org/10.1177/0886260518820688

Scourfield, J., Roen, K., & McDermott, L. (2008). Lesbian, gay, bisexual, and transgender young people's experiences of distress: Resilience, ambivalence, and self-destructive behaviors. *Health and Social Care in the Community*, *16*(3), 329–336. https://doi.org/10.1111/j.1365-2524.2008.00769.x

Su, D., Irwin, J. A., Fisher, C., Ramos, A., Kelley, M., Mendoza, D. A. R., & Coleman, J. D. (2016). Mental health disparities within the LGBT population: A comparison between transgender and nontransgender individuals. *Transgender Health*, *1*(1), 12–24. https://doi.org/10.1089/trgh.2015.0001

Substance Abuse and Mental Health Services Administration (2020). *Substance Use Disorder Treatment for People with Co-Occurring Disorders*. Treatment Improvement Protocol (TIP) Series, No 42. https://store.samhsa.gov/product/tip-42-substance-use-treatment-persons-co-occurring-disorders/PEP20-02-01-004

Sweet, T., & Welles, S. L. (2012). Associations of sexual identity or same-sex behaviors with history of childhood sexual abuse and HIV/STI risk in the United States. *JAIDS Journal of Acquired Immune Deficiency Syndromes*, *59*(4), 400–408. https://doi.org/10.1097/QAI.0b013e3182400e75

Szymanski, D. M., Kashubeck-West, S., & Meyer, J. (2008). Internalized heterosexism: A historical and theoretical overview. *The Counseling Psychologist*, *36*(4), 510–524. https://doi.org/10.1177/0011000007309488

Troutman, O., & Packer-Williams, C. (2014). Moving beyond CACREP standards: Training counselors to work competently with LGBT clients. *The Journal of Counselor Preparation and Supervision*, *6*(1), 1–17. https://doi.org/10.7729/61.1088

Valentine, S. E., & Shipherd, J. C. (2018). A systematic review of social stress and mental health among transgender and gender non-conforming people in the United States. *Clinical Psychology Review*, *66*, 24–38. https://doi.org/10.1016/j.cpr.2018.03.003

Walters, M. L., Chen J., & Breiding, M. J. (2013). *The National Intimate Partner and Sexual Violence Survey (NISVS): 2010 findings on victimization by sexual orientation*. Centers for Disease Control and Prevention. https://www.cdc.gov/violenceprevention/pdf/nisvs_sofindings.pdf

Watson, R. J., Fish, J. N., McKay, T., Allen, S. H., Eaton, L., & Puhl, R. M. (2020). Substance use among a national sample of sexual and gender minority adolescents: Intersections of sex assigned at birth and gender identity. *LGBT Health*, *7*(1), 37–46. https://doi.org/10.1089/lgbt.2019.0066

White, J. M., Gordon, J. R., & Mimiaga, M. J. (2014). The role of substance use and mental health problems in medication adherence among HIV-infected MSM. *LGBT Health*, *1*(4), 319–322. https://doi.org/10.1089/lgbt.2014.0020

Williams, N. D. & Fish, J. N. (2020). The availability of LGBT-specific mental health and substance abuse treatment in the United States. *Health Services Research*, *55*(6), 932–943. https://doi.org/10.1111/1475-6773.13559

Williams, S. L., & Mann, A. K. (2017). Sexual and gender minority health disparities as a social issue: How stigma and intergroup relations can explain and reduce health disparities. *Journal of Social Issues*, *73*(3), 450–461. https://doi.org/10.1111/josi.12225

INDEX

ACA. *See* American Counseling Association (ACA)
ACA ethics code (ACA code of ethics), 31, 109, 153, 154, 176, 266, 268, 394, 395
administration routes
    absorption, 57
    common administration routes, 57
    inhalation is the fastest administration route, 57
    injection, 57
    mucous membrane absorption, 57
    and psychoactive effects timeline, 57
alcohol, 49–50, 100, 101, 103, 104, 112, 145
alcohol use disorder (AUD), 98, 103, 104, 172, 281
    acamprosate and, 36, 173, 174
    disulfiram and, 173
    naltrexone and, 173–174
American Counseling Association (ACA), 31, 32, 109, 393
American Society of Addiction Medicine (ASAM), 43, 44
    ASAM continuum of care, 128–130
    six dimensions of multidimensional assessment, 127–128
amphetamines, 45–46, 49, 136, 237, 283, 285
anticonvulsants, 170
antihistamines, 167, 169
anxiety disorders and symptoms
    antihistamines for, 169
    barbiturates for, 167–168
    benzodiazepines for, 168–169
ASAM. *See* American Society of Addiction Medicine (ASAM)
AUD. *See* Alcohol use disorder (AUD)

barbiturates, 167–168
behavioral addictions, 57
    gambling addiction, 57–58
    internet gaming addiction, 58
    sexual addiction, 58–59
benzodiazepines, 50, 167, 168–169
bipolar and related disorders
    anticonvulsants, 170
    lithium, 169–170
blood alcohol concentration (BAC), 49–50

blood alcohol level (BAL). *See* Blood alcohol concentration (BAC)
brief psychotic disorder, 278–279
Buddhism, 185
buprenorphine, 175

CALOCUS. *See* Child and Adolescent Level of Care Utilization System (CALOCUS)
cannabis, 11, 12, 48, 53–54
cannabis use disorder, 281–282
central nervous system depressants
    alcohol, 49–50
    benzodiazepines, 50
    fentanyl, 51
    heroin, 51
    opioids, 51
    prescription pain medication, 52
Child and Adolescent Level of Care Utilization System (CALOCUS)
    evaluation parameters, 130
    level of care definitions, 130
    level of care guidelines, 127–132
    scoring methodology, 130
cocaine, 47–48
comorbidity, 236–237, 244, 297, 299, 306, 323, 327, 345, 353
    mental, physical, and substance use disorder
        chronic health conditions, 349–350
        mental disorders, 349
        physical pain, 350
    and multimorbidity, 4
    in young adults and adolescent behavior, 376
contemplation stage of change, 144
co-occurring anxiety, obsessive compulsive disorder and substance use disorder
    addictive process, empty self theory, 263
    American Counseling Association Code of Ethics, 266–267
    anxiety of guilt and condemnation, 254–255
    anxiety of meaninglessness, 254
    boundaries and dual relationship, 268
    burnout, 268
    counselor competence, 267–268
    DSM-5, 266

co-occurring anxiety (*cont.*)
  generalized anxiety disorder (GAD), 255
  multiculturalism and values, 269–271
    self-awareness, 267
co-occurring bipolar and substance use disorders
  and anxiety disorders, 14–15
  assessment and diagnostic considerations, 215–216
  assessment process, 19–20
    basics of, 19–20
    and bipolar disorders, 8, 14
    formal assessment to determine type and severity, 19
    six dimensions of multidimensional assessment, 20
    twelve steps in assessment process, 20–21
  bipolar I disorder, 235
  bipolar II disorder, 236
co-occurring disorders, screening and assessment
  establishing therapeutic relationships, 24
  guidelines for counselors, 26–27
  matching treatment to levels of care, 24–25
  providing integrated care, 24
  screening and assessment, difference between, 17–18
  special populations, 27
co-occurring disorders treatment, 28–31
  depressive disorders, 7–8, 13
    ASAM's continuum of care, 30–31
    disruptive mood dysregulation disorder, 210
    major depressive disorder, 210
    other specified and unspecified depressive disorder, 212
    persistent depressive disorder, 210
    premenstrual dysphoric disorder, 210–211
    substance-/medication-induced depressive disorder, 211–212
  etiological paradigms and risk factors, 11
    cannabis disorders co-occurring with anxiety disorders, 12
    gene expression changes, 11
  impact of, 12
  legal and ethical considerations, 31, 223–224
    each disorder will intensify the other, 12
    use substances to manage psychiatric symptoms, 11–12
  medical comorbidities, 239–240
    bipolar disorders, 236
      alcohol, 237–238
      cannabis and other illicit substances, 238
      and personality disorders, 10, 16–17
      tobacco, 238
    pharmacotherapy, 33
  mental disorders, impact of, 12–13
  and personality disorders, adverse effects, 16–17
  and posttraumatic stress disorder, 10, 16
  and posttraumatic stress disorder, adverse effects, 16
  prevalence, statistics and demographics
    adolescents, 214
    adults, 213–214
  professional competence
    advanced competencies, 32–33
  and schizophrenia, 9, 15
  screening and assessment instruments, 33
  screening and assessment tools, 217–219, 241
    Alcohol Use Disorders Identification Test (AUDIT), 218
    CAGE-AID substance misuse screening tool, 217
    depression outcome scale, 217
    Hamilton Depression Rating scale, 217
    integrated group therapy, 242–243
    integrated motivational interviewing and cognitive behavior therapy, 243
    NIDA-Modified ASSIST, 218
    patient health questionnaire-9, 217
  substance-use disorders, 212–213
  training, specialized credentialing and resources, 32
  treatment modalities
    adjunct services, 222
    biopsychosocial approaches, 222
    brief interventions, 220–221
    harm reduction, crisis mitigation and stigma management, 222–223
    SSRIs, 221
    wellness-promoting strategies, 221
co-occurring disorders, comprehensive assessment
  aftercare, 108–109
  aftercare recovery initiatives
    treatment plan, 105–107
    twelve-step assessment process, 104–105
  American Psychiatric Association's Global Assessment Functioning (GAF), 108
  American Society for Addiction Medicine criteria, 107–108
  assessment, 100
    assessment considerations, 109–110
    biopsychosocial evaluation, 98–99
    cultural considerations, 95, 110
    diagnostic considerations, 110
    motivational interviewing, 96
    initial interview, 94–95
    therapeutic relationship, 95–96
  intoxication and withdrawal, 100–101
  screening, 99–100
    clinical case illustration and discussion, 111
    cultural considerations, 95, 110
    screening and assessment tools, 101–103
co-occurring personality and substance use disorders
  assessment and diagnostic considerations
    confidentiality, 330–331
    gender differences, 322–323
    mandated treatment, 331
    prognosis, 321
    suicide risk assessment, 331
  clinical interview, 325–326

dialectical behavior therapy, 327–328
    diagnostic features, overview, 318–319
        interplay with substance use disorders, 3
        withdrawal symptoms, 319
        self-harm, 325
        substance use disorders, 324–325
    personality disorders (PD), 318–319, 324
    prevalence, statistics and demographics, 320
co-occurring schizophrenia, other psychotic disorder and substance use disorders
    assessment and diagnostic considerations
        alcohol use disorders, 281
        cannabis use disorders, 281–282
        diagnostic decision-making, 284–285
        intoxication and withdrawal, 283–284
        nicotine use disorder, 282–283
        opioid use disorder, 282
        stimulant use disorder, 282
    DSM-5 disorders and ICD-10 coding, 279–280
    prevalence, statistics and demographics, 281
        brief delusional disorder, 278
        brief psychotic disorder, 278–279
        schizoaffective disorder, 278
        schizophrenia, 277–278
        schizophreniform disorders, 278
    screening and assessment tools
        cognitive behavior therapy, 286
        DSM-5 clinician-rated dimensions of psychosis severity, 285–286
        DSM-5 self-rated level-1 cross-cutting symptom measure, 284–285
        mindfulness-based interventions, 287–288
        pharmacotherapy, 286
        positive and negative syndrome scale, 286
        substance-induced psychotic disorder, 283
        substance-/medication-induced psychotic disorder, 279
co-occurring trauma- and stressor-related and substance use disorders
    assessment and diagnostic considerations, 300–302
    legal and ethical considerations, 308
    prevalence, statistics and demographics
        alcohol use disorders, 298
        cannabis use disorder, 298–299
        common factors model, 297
        gambling disorder, 299–300
        mutual maintenance model, 297
        nicotine use disorder, 299
        opioid use disorder, 299
        PTSD susceptibility model, 297
        self-medication model, 297
        trauma and stressor-related disorders, 295–296

delusional disorders, 176–178
Department of Veterans Affairs (VA) health system, 385

determination stage of change, 145
Diagnostic and Statistical Manual of Mental Disorders, 32, 53, 210, 237, 256, 275, 295, 301, 344, 386
drug categories
    central nervous system stimulants
        amphetamines, 45–46
        cocaine, 47–48
        methamphetamine, 46
        prescription stimulants, 46–47
        tobacco/nicotine, 48–49
    psychedelics
        cannabis, 53–54
        ketamine, 54
drugs of abuse and addiction
    addiction, defined, 43
    administration routes
        common administration routes, 57
        contact absorption, 57
        inhalation, 57
        mucous membrane absorption, 57
    central nervous system depressants
        alcohol, 49–50
        benzodiazepines, 50
        fentanyl, 51
        heroin, 51
        opioids, 51
        prescription pain medications, 52
    drug categories
        central nervous system stimulants, 45–49
            amphetamines, 45–46
            cocaine, 47–48
            methamphetamine, 46
            prescription stimulants, 46–47
            tobacco/nicotine, 48–49
        psychedelics
            cannabis, 53–54
            ketamine, 54
            LSD, 54–55
            MDMA/Ecstasy, 55
            psilocybin, 55–56
    six degrees of addiction, 43
    three-stage cycle, 43–44
DSM-5 disorders and ICD-10 coding, 279–280

face validity, 101
fentanyl, 51

gender and co-occurring disorders
    legal and ethical considerations, 373–374
        client-centered information offered psychohistoriography, 374–376
        common screening and assessment tools, 375
        nonjudgmental approach, 376
        unique needs of transgender individuals, 376

gender and co-occurring disorders (*cont.*)
    prevalence, statistics and demographics
        gender non-confirming, 369
        transgender men, 368
        transgender women, 369
    screening and assessment tools, 374
    treatment considerations, 370–373
        family and social relationships, 370–372
        gender-based rates of treatment, 369–370
        socioeconomic factors, 373
        trauma and abuse, 372–373
generalized anxiety disorder (GAD), 255
Global Assessment of Functioning (GAF), 108

hallucinations, 276
heroin, 51

illicit drug use, 281

ketamine, 54
    in depression, 54
    in mental disorders, 54
    psychosis-like effects, 54
    for treating health and substance use disorders, 54
    in treatment of mood disorders, 54

level of care criteria
    abstinence model, 125
    American Society of Addiction Medicine (ASAM) criteria, 127–130
    harm reduction model, 125
    InterQual Behavioral Health Criteria, 131
    least restrictive level of care, 126
    level of care determination, 126
    LOCUS/CALOCUS, 130–131
    MCG care guidelines, 131
    most appropriate care, 126
    restrictive level, 126
levels of care
    day treatment/partial hospitalization program (PHP), 124–125
    inpatient, 125
        intensive outpatient program (IOP), 124
        outpatient counseling/medication management/employee assistance program, 124
        peer support/community support groups, 124
        residential, 125
LGBTQ+ communities and co-occurring disorders
    affirmative treatments, 414–415
    assessment considerations, 410
    counselor self-awareness, 409–410
    fundamentals of support, 408–409
    gender minorities, 405
    importance of advocacy, 410–411
    intersectionality, 405
    minority stress, 412
    minority stress theory, 406
    overall implications and recommendations, 411
    sexual minorities, 404
    social support, 413–414
    substance use, 412–413
    suicidality and non-suicidal self-injury, 413
    treatment barriers, 414
lithium, 169–170
lysergic acid diethylamide (LSD)
    for alcohol use disorder, 54
    common side effects of, 55

maintenance stage of change, 145
managed care
    case management, 134
    comparing level of care guidelines, 131–132
    incentive-based payment, 133
    legal and ethical considerations, 132–133
    managed care and provider relationship, 133
        health insurance, 120
        insurance benefits, 123–124
        managed care, defined, 120
        person's health, insurance considerations, 119–120
        private insurance, 123
        public sector, 122–123
    managed care organizations (MCOs) and counselors, 119
    peer specialists and behavioral health coaches, 135
    population health programs, 135
    social determinants of health, 134–135
    technology and telehealth, 135–136
    whole-person care, 122
managed care organizations (MCOs), 119
master addiction counselor (MAC), 34
MDMA/Ecstasy, 55
methadone, 174–175
methamphetamine, 46
military population and co-occurring disorders
    adjustment disorders, 386
    alcohol-related disorders, 387
    anxiety disorders, 386
    bipolar disorders, substance-related disorders and psychoses, 388
    cognitive processing therapy, 390–391
    depressive disorders, 386
    eye movement desensitization and reprocessing (EMDR), 391
    "individualist" culture, 394
    injury, 388

legal and ethical considerations, 394–395
LGB members, 392
military service and trauma, 384
"mission comes first," 393
moral race/ethnicity demographics, 392
other treatment approaches, 391
posttraumatic stress disorders, 386–387
prolonged exposure therapy, 391
screening and assessment tools, 389–390
suicide, 388–389
traumatic brain injury, 388
treatment modalities, 220–223
mindfulness-based practices
  for anxiety and obsessive-compulsive
      disorders, 192
  dialectical behavior therapy, 187–188
  historical origins
    Buddhism, 185
  mindfulness-based therapies
    acceptance and commitment therapy, 188–189
    cognitive therapy, 189–190
  for mood disorders, 191–192
  provider resources, 196
  psychotherapy, 197
  for schizophrenia spectrum and other psychotic
      disorders, 193
  for substance-use disorders, 194
  for trauma and stressor-related disorders, 192–193
monoamine oxidase inhibitors (MAOIs), 165–166
motivational interviewing (MI), 146–149
multicultural considerations
  complexities of a client's rich diverse identity,
      374–377
  psychohistoriography, 374–376
  screening and assessment tools, 375
multimorbidity, 4

naloxone, 175
National Institute of Alcohol Abuse and Alcoholism
    (NIAAA), 49, 131
National Institute on Drug Abuse (NIDA), 11
neuroscience of mental and substance use disorders
  addiction and mental health disorders, 78, 79
  basic brain anatomy
    glial cells, 72
    neurons, 72–73
  brain and nervous system, 72
    adverse childhood experiences, 76
    childhood and adolescence, 75–76
    neuroplasticity, 77
  brain regions and structures
    central brain, 74
    lower brain, 73
    upper brain, 74
  brain regions and systems involved in addictions,
      79–80

connectome, 74–75
implications for treatment, 81–82
seven systems, 75
substance use and mental disorders, relationship
    between, 81
three networks, 75
three-stage cycle, 80–81
neurotransmitters, 163
  psychoactive drug use, 163
nicotine use disorder, 282–283

older adults
  alcohol, 347–348
  chronic health conditions, 349–350
  chronic substance use, 348
  dialectical behavioral therapy, 351
  evidence-based practices and care coordination
      services, 353
  global trend of aging, 346–347
  legal and ethical considerations, 356–357
  mental disorders, 349
  multicultural considerations, 354–355
  over-the-counter and prescription drugs, 348
  physical pain, 350
  screening and assessment, 352–353
  therapeutic interventions, 353
opioid use disorder, 282
  buprenorphine, 175
  methadone, 174–175
  naloxone, 175
opioids, 51

partial hospitalization program (PHP), 104
persistent depressive disorder (PDD), 210, 404
precontemplation stage of change, 144
preparation stage of change, 144
psilocybin, 53, 56, 175
  effects of, 56
  mushrooms, 56
  nausea and, 55
  potency of, 56
  in treatment of mental and substance use
      disorders, 56
psychedelics
  cannabis, 53–54
  ketamine, 54
  LSD, 54–55
  MDMA/Ecstasy, 55
  psilocybin, 53, 55–56, 175
  psychedelic renaissance, 175–176
psychopharmacological interventions
  anxiety disorders and symptoms, medications for
    barbiturates, 167–168
    benzodiazepines, 168–169
  bipolar and related disorders, medications for

psychopharmacological interventions (cont.)
   anticonvulsants, 170
   lithium, 169–170
   depressive disorders and symptoms, medications for
      monoamine oxidase inhibitors (MAOIs), 165–166
      selective serotonin reuptake inhibitors, 166
      third-generation antidepressants, 166–167
      tricyclic antidepressants, 166
   legal and ethical considerations
      competence, 176
      legal authority to prescribe, 176–178
      neurotransmitters, 163
   pharmacology alliance, 159–161
   schizophrenia spectrum and other psychotic disorders, medications for
      second-generation (atypical) antipsychotics, 172
      third-generation antipsychotics, 172
      traditional antipsychotics, 171–172
   substance use disorders, medication-assisted treatment
      for alcohol-use disorders, 173–174
      for opioid misuse
         buprenorphine, 175
         methadone, 174–175
         naloxone, 175

schizoaffective disorder, 278
   schizophrenia, 277–279
   medications for
      second-generation (atypical) antipsychotics, 172
      third-generation antipsychotics, 172
      traditional antipsychotics, 171–172
   schizophreniform disorders, 278
   screening process, 18–19
   defined, 18
   mental disorder screening, 18
   substance misuse screening, 18
selective serotonin reuptake inhibitors (SSRIs), 166
sexual and gender minorities, 368, 403, 408–412, 417

six degrees of separation, 43
stages of change, 96, 97, 103, 106, 107, 114, 145, 149, 155, 156, 226, 302
stimulant use disorder, 282
Substance Abuse and Mental Health Services Administration (SAMHSA), 44
substance-/medication-induced psychotic disorder, 279
substance use disorders
   and anxiety disorders, 14–15
   and bipolar disorders, 8, 14
   and co-occurring disorders, 12, 17–18
   and depressive disorders, 7–8, 13
   etiological paradigms and risk factors, 11
   medications for, 172–173
   and mental disorders, impact of, 12–13
   and personality disorders, 10, 16–17
   and posttraumatic stress disorder, 10, 16
   prevalence, statistics and demographics, 4–7
   and schizophrenia, 9, 15

third-generation antidepressants, 166–167
tobacco/nicotine, 48–49
transtheoretical model (TTM), 141, 142–146, 149
trauma and abuse, 372–373
treatment engagement, therapeutic strategies, and recovery models
   building successful relationships, 142
   recovery maintenance, 152–153
   relapse, 151
   stages of change, 143
      action stage, 145
      client statements by stage of change, 144
      commonalities among theories, 142
      contemplation stage, 144
      maintenance stage, 145
      mandated clients, 153–154
      motivational interviewing (MI), 146–149
      precontemplation stage, 144
      preparation stage, 144
      processes of change, 146
      termination stage, 145
      tricyclic antidepressants, 166
tricyclic antidepressants, 166

www.ingramcontent.com/pod-product-compliance
Ingram Content Group UK Ltd.
Pitfield, Milton Keynes, MK11 3LW, UK
UKHW051848210426
5322IPUK00024B/617